PRINCIPLES OF EXERCISE TESTING AND INTERPRETATION, 2nd Ed.

Principles of Exercise Testing and Interpretation

Second Edition

KARLMAN WASSERMAN, M.D., Ph.D.
Professor of Medicine, UCLA School of Medicine
Chief, Division of Respiratory and Critical Care Physiology and Medicine
Harbor-UCLA Medical Center
Torrance, California

JAMES E. HANSEN, M.D.
Professor of Medicine Emeritus, UCLA School of Medicine
Division of Respiratory and Critical Care Physiology and Medicine
Harbor-UCLA Medical Center
Torrance, California

DARRYL Y. SUE, M.D.
Professor of Medicine, UCLA School of Medicine
Medical Director, Department of Respiratory Therapy
Director, Medical Critical Care
Harbor-UCLA Medical Center
Torrance, California

BRIAN J. WHIPP, Ph.D., D.Sc.
Professor and Chairman, Department of Physiology
St. George's Hospital Medical School
London, England

RICHARD CASABURI, Ph.D., M.D.
Associate Professor of Medicine, UCLA School of Medicine
Director, Clinical Respiratory Physiology Laboratory
Associate Chief, Division of Respiratory and Critical Care Physiology and Medicine
Department of Medicine
Harbor-UCLA Medical Center
Torrance, California

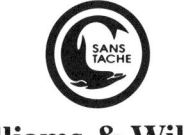

Williams & Wilkins

PHILADELPHIA · BALTIMORE · HONG KONG
LONDON · MUNICH · SYDNEY · TOKYO

A WAVERLY COMPANY

Williams & Wilkins
Rose Tree Corporate Center, Building II
1400 North Providence Road, Suite 5025
Media, PA 19063-2043 USA

Executive Editor—J. Matthew Harris
Development Editor—Lisa Stead
Project Editor—Dorothy DiRienzi
Production Manager—Michael De Nardo

Library of Congress Cataloging-in-Publication Data

Principles of exercise testing and interpretation / Karlman Wasserman
    ... [et al.]. — 2nd ed.
        p.   cm.
    Includes bibliographical references and index.
    ISBN 0-8121-1634-8
    1. Exercise tests.   2. Heart function tests.   3. Pulmonary
function tests.   4. Exercise—Physiological aspects.   I. Wasserman,
Karlman.
    [DNLM: 1. Exercise Test.   2. Exertion.   WG 141.5.F9 P957 1994]
RC71.8.P75   1994
616.07′5—dc20
DNLM/DLC
for Library of Congress   93-36939
                                                                CIP

ISBN 0-8121-1634-8

First Edition, 1987
Second Edition, 1994

NOTE: Although the author(s) and the publisher have taken reasonable steps to ensure the accuracy of the drug information included in this text before publication, drug information may change without notice and readers are advised to consult the manufacturer's packaging inserts before prescribing medications.

Print number: 5   4   3   2

Dedicated to our families

Preface

Whether individuals are unable to perform a physical task that they expect to accomplish without undue feelings of fatigue, shortness of breath, or pain, they usually complain of exercise intolerance. These symptoms are not restricted to specific diseases but may be found in patients with primary heart disease (coronary artery, valvular, congenital, and cardiomyopathic), disorders of the pulmonary or peripheral circulations, lung disease, obesity syndrome, and metabolic and neuromuscular disorders. The major objective of clinical exercise testing is to isolate the cause or causes of these symptoms of exercise intolerance. This book describes how to evaluate the patient with exercise intolerance using the physiology and pathophysiology of gas exchange as frames of reference.

Cellular respiration is a fundamental component of the bioenergetics of muscle contraction. Because the circulation couples cellular respiration with ventilation at the lung, diseases affecting cellular metabolism, the heart, peripheral or pulmonary circulations, or the lungs can affect gas exchange measured at the mouth. This concept was appreciated at least 65 years ago by physiologists, but utilization of gas exchange measurements for routine evaluation of patients was time consuming and therefore clinically impractical. Advances in instrumentation and computer technology, particularly over the past 15 years, have changed this situation. Now, rapid, precise, and continuous measurements of gas exchange during exercise are routinely made, with calculations and final data reports generated within minutes of testing. Thus, exercise testing can be used to assess rapidly and accurately the physiologic state of the metabolic, cardiovascular, and respiratory systems. Uniquely abnormal gas exchange patterns are now recognized in different diseases, allowing exercise testing to be used to identify the major pathophysiologic features accounting for a patient's symptoms.

The absence of detailed electrocardiographic displays in this book should not be interpreted to mean that we do not regard the electrocardiogram as an essential component of exercise tests. On the contrary, we record and analyze a 12-lead electrocardiogram at least every 2 minutes during exercise. Because many other sources are available for interpreting the exercise electrocardiogram, we provide only an interpretation of the records, rather than the records themselves.

Because an increasing number of cardiology and pulmonary diagnostic laboratories use gas exchange measurements to evaluate their patients' pathophysiologic features, we decided that several chapters were needed to describe the gas exchange responses to exercise in health and in different disease states. In later chapters, we provide our current knowledge of normal values and the options for exercise test protocols, with critiques of each. This allows the reader to have a basis for selecting the set of normal values and the exercise protocol best suited to their needs. One chapter describes a scheme by which the massive amount of generated data from short-duration exercise tests may be systematically reviewed. We find that conclusions on pathophysiology may be logically reached from this scheme.

The final chapter consists of 79 case presentations. Each case, illustrating common and not so common disorders, was selected to make a teaching point in pathophysiology. In this respect, this chapter serves as an atlas of disorders that result in exercise limitation.

Detailed practical information is provided in the Appendices to assist the reader in setting up a laboratory, in testing the subject, and in making necessary calculations. Although this is of special importance to anyone wishing to establish a labo-ratory, it also enhances the interpreter's understanding of the technical aspects of the measurements and calculations.

This book is therefore designed to help cardiologists, pulmonologists, and exercise physiologists keep pace with the expanding knowledge gained from computerized measurements of gas exchange during exercise. It serves as a guide for those who wish to use exercise testing to: (1) diagnose the pathophysiology of exertional dyspnea; (2) evaluate the severity of the patient's pathophysiologic features; (3) evaluate the effect of medical or surgical therapy; and (4) provide a physiologic basis for training strategies for rehabilitation or athletic performance. Thus, we have attempted to write a practical book, spanning the field of "exercise" from basic concepts in exercise physiology to the practical aspects of delivering a meaningful report to the patient's primary physician. By virtue of the detailed Appendices, it is also a source book for the technical aspects of measurement and calculation.

Because the first edition was used as a syllabus for semi-annual post-graduate courses on exercise testing and interpretation that we have given to visiting physicians, physiologists, and technicians over the past decade, the second edition has benefited by their comments and focused discussions. In addition, this second edition includes new knowledge and understanding gained from ongoing research. In summary, our goal was to write a comprehensive, practical, and current book for physiologists, physicians, and technicians interested in exercise physiology, pathophysiology, and testing.

Torrance, California

KARLMAN WASSERMAN
JAMES E. HANSEN
DARRYL Y. SUE
BRIAN J. WHIPP
RICHARD CASABURI

Acknowledgments

WE ARE extremely grateful to Marissa Salvatore and Leah Coone Kram for their editorial assistance and dedication and to Carol Brandon, Barbara Young, and Shirley Zagala for their accomplished secretarial support in the preparation of this book.

We are indebted to the many physicians who have participated in our semi-annual post-graduate course (practicum) in exercise testing, for which the first edition served as a syllabus. The second edition was stimulated by discussions with them and with current and former colleagues, as well as knowledge gained from new research. We hope that it closes the gap between physiologic knowledge and the application of cardiopulmonary exercise testing.

K.W. is especially indebted to his wife, Gail, for tolerating his diversions during innumerable nights and weekends while writing and editing this book.

K.W.
J.E.H.
D.Y.S.
B.J.W.
R.C.

Contents

Exercise Testing and Interpretation: An Overview

CHAPTER **1**

PHYSICAL EXERCISE requires the interaction of physiologic mechanisms that enable the cardiovascular and respiratory systems to support the increased energy demands of contracting muscles. Both systems are consequently stressed during exercise; their ability to respond adequately to this stress is a measure of their physiologic competence (or "health"). An appreciation of the normal response profiles of the gas transport systems that support cell respiration is essential to recognize the abnormal response patterns that characterize the many disease states that affect them.

Why Measure Gas Exchange to Evaluate Cardiovascular Function and Cellular Respiration?

The increased metabolic rate during exercise requires an appropriate increase in O_2 flow into the muscles. Simultaneously, the CO_2 produced by the muscles must be removed to avoid severe tissue acidosis with its adverse effects on cellular function. To satisfy the increased gas exchange needs of the muscle cell during exercise, precise coupling of the supporting physiologic mechanisms is required; this involves the lungs, the pulmonary circulation, the heart, and the peripheral circulation (Fig. 1-1). These physiologic processes must be efficiently integrated with the metabolic rate change to meet the demands of increased tissue O_2 supply and CO_2 elimination and also arterial blood gas homeostasis. Exercise testing offers the investigator the possibility of simultaneously studying the cellular, cardiovascular, and ventilatory systems responses under conditions of precisely controlled metabolic stress. Exercise tests in which gas exchange is not determined cannot realistically evaluate the ability of the cardiovascular and ventilatory systems to perform their common major function, i.e., gas exchange with cells.

Exercise testing with appropriate gas exchange measurements can also serve to grade the adequacy of cardiorespiratory function. This is of significant practical impact because of the increased number of therapeutic options now available for conditions that cause exercise limitation. Furthermore, the documentation and correct diagnosis of the pathophysiology of the cardiovascular and ventilatory systems are necessary preludes to the treatment and assessment of treatment of exercise limitation. For example, it is important to determine whether new medical, surgical, and rehabilitative procedures are effective interventions.

Moreover, an individual patient may have mixed defects (e.g., cardiac and respiratory), and consequently, it is often necessary to determine the relative contribution of each to the patient's symptoms before embarking on major therapeutic procedures directed at either one. Exercise testing can also provide vital information regarding the limits of systemic function before surgery or other therapy.

Cardiac Stress Testing and Pulmonary Stress Testing: A Fallacy

We would like to dispel a concept that has developed in American medicine, i.e., that there is cardiac stress testing and pulmonary stress testing. It is impossible to stress only the heart or only the lungs. Rather, as we have already pointed out, exercise requires the coordinated function of the heart, the lungs, and the peripheral and pulmonary circulations to achieve the cellular gas exchange required to live and work. Diseases of the heart cause both abnormal breathing and gas exchange responses; consequently, these abnormal responses can be used as indices to help identify heart disease. Similarly, abnormal cardiac responses can occur secondary to pulmonary disorders. To interpret exercise tests, physiologists and physicians must appreciate the inseparable and interactive roles of the cardiovascular and ventilatory systems in supporting cellular respiration and in generating energy for muscle contraction.

Normal Coupling of External to Cellular Respiration

Figure 1-1 schematizes the coupling of pulmonary to cellular respiration by the circulation. Obviously, the circulation must increase at a rate required to supply the cells with the oxygen needed. In fact, cardiac output has been shown to increase in proportion to the metabolic rate in normal subjects, with a slope relationship of cardiac output as a function of O_2 uptake of between 5 and 6 L per minute. Because 5 L of blood contain slightly less than 1 L of O_2, the normal circulatory response provides just enough O_2 to the cells to meet their requirement, leaving little in the venous effluent. Consequently, disease of the cardiovascular system is often characterized by the failure of O_2 uptake to increase appropriately for the work rate. This phenomenon is accompanied by a lactic acidosis.

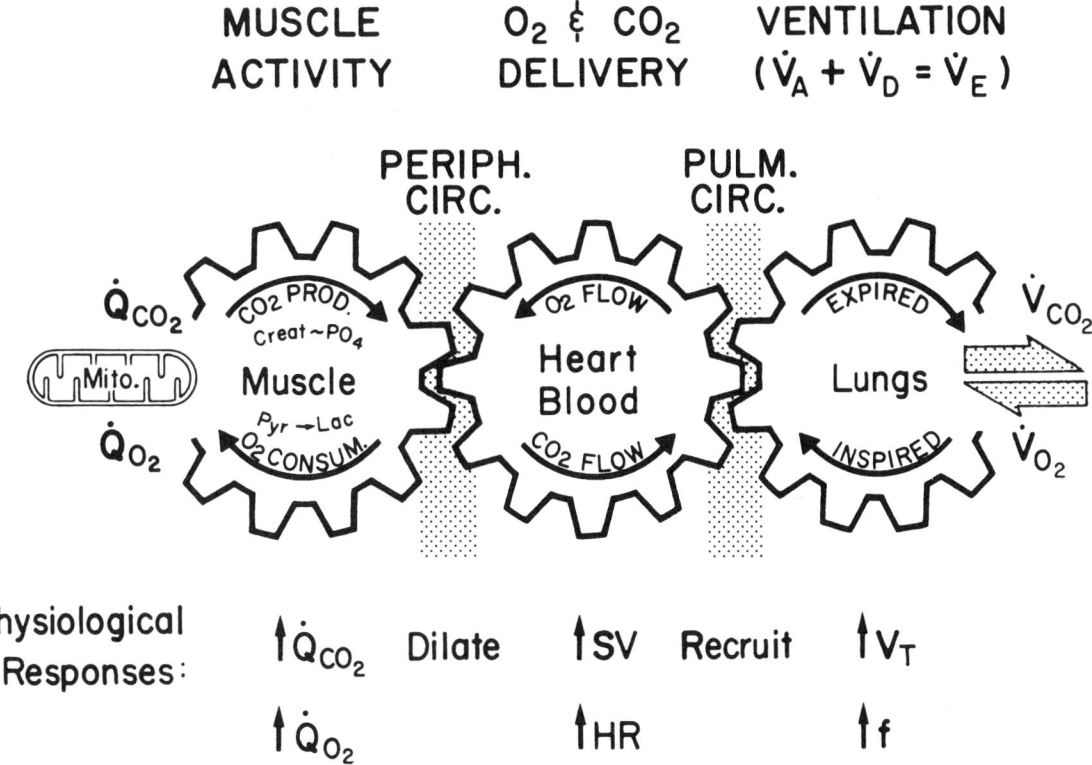

FIG. 1-1. A scheme illustrating the gas transport mechanisms for coupling cellular (internal) to pulmonary (external) respiration. The gears represent the functional interdependence of the physiologic components of the system. The large increase in O_2 utilization by the muscles ($\dot{Q}_{O_2}$) is achieved by increased extraction of O_2 from the blood perfusing the muscles, the dilatation of selected peripheral vascular beds, an increase in cardiac output (stroke volume and heart rate), an increase in pulmonary blood flow by recruitment and vasodilatation of pulmonary blood vessels, and finally, an increase in ventilation. O_2 is taken up ($\dot{V}_{O_2}$) from the alveoli in proportion to the pulmonary blood flow and degree of O_2 desaturation of hemoglobin in the pulmonary capillary blood. In the steady-state, $\dot{V}_{O_2} = \dot{Q}_{O_2}$. Ventilation (tidal volume (V_T) and breathing frequency (f)) increase in relation to the newly produced CO_2 ($\dot{Q}_{CO_2}$) arriving at the lungs and the drive to achieve arterial CO_2 and hydrogen ion homeostasis. These variables are related in the following way:

$$\dot{V}_{CO_2} = \dot{V}_A \cdot Pa_{CO_2}/P_B$$

where $\dot{V}_{CO_2}$ = minute CO_2 output, $\dot{V}_A$ = minute alveolar ventilation, Pa_{CO_2} = arterial CO_2 tension, and P_B = barometric pressure.

The representation of gears uniformly sized is not intended to imply equal changes in each of the components of the coupling. For instance, the increase in cardiac output is proportionally smaller than the increase in metabolic rate. This results in an increased extraction of O_2 from, and CO_2 loading into, the blood by the muscles. In contrast, at moderate work intensities, minute ventilation increases in approximate proportion to the new CO_2 brought to the lungs by the venous return. The development of metabolic acidosis, at heavy and very heavy work intensities, results in an increased ventilation to provide respiratory compensation for the metabolic acidosis.

For regulation of arterial pH, ventilation must increase linearly with the increase in CO_2 production; it must increase more when a lactic acidosis is superimposed on the respiratory acid (CO_2) load produced as a result of aerobic metabolism. Thus, the failure to provide an adequate increase in cardiac output, resulting in tissue hypoxia, also causes a steepening in the ventilatory response.[1] Failure of the ventilatory system to keep pace with the rate of CO_2 generated from aerobic metabolism causes a respiratory acidosis. Furthermore, failure to provide the additional increment in ventilation necessary to provide ventilatory compensation for the lactic acidosis of exercise induces a pronounced reduction in arterial pH.

Quantifying State and Time-Course of Cellular Respiration From Measurements of External Respiration

Physical activity is the major challenge to homeostasis of the cellular environment. Walking at a pace of 3 mph requires a 16- to 20-fold increase in O_2 consumption of the muscles of locomotion. The rate of acid production, in the form of CO_2, increases by a like amount. Despite these major acute changes in cellular respiration, external respiration increases with such precision that the blood is rearterialized with no or only minor changes in P_{O_2}, P_{CO_2}, and pH. Thus, blood recirculates to the highly metabolic muscle tissue in virtually the same aerated and acid-base state as existed at rest.[2-5] The normal subject is able to perform level walking (at typical rates of ambulation) without developing a metabolic acidosis.[2,4] This is because cellular respiration and external respiration, measured as O_2 uptake and CO_2 output, increase to steady-state, i.e., meet the entire energy demands of the task by wholly aerobic mechanisms. This steady-state occurs at approximately 3 minutes for O_2 uptake and 4 minutes for CO_2 output and ventilation.

The patterns of $\dot{V}O_2$ and $\dot{V}CO_2$ kinetics are characteristic, but different, for work rates in the range of work without and with a lactic acidosis (below and above the subject's anaerobic threshold, *AT*), as shown on the right side of Figure 1-2. The plots shown were obtained from 6-minute constant work rate tests and are the average of second-by-second responses to four identical cycle ergometer studies, interpolated from breath-by-breath measurements of $\dot{V}O_2$ and $\dot{V}CO_2$.[6]

To sustain the exercise, it is necessary to replenish adenosine triphosphate (ATP), which is the direct energy source for the muscle contraction, at rates commensurate with its utilization. This is predominantly an O_2 requiring process. At the start of upright exercise, there is an immediate increase in both $\dot{V}CO_2$ and $\dot{V}O_2$ lasting about 15 seconds (Fig. 1-2). This has been attributed to the rapid increase in pulmonary blood flow that accompanies the immediate increase in both stroke volume and heart rate.[6] The subsequent increase in $\dot{V}O_2$ by the lungs depends on the rate of hydrolysis of creatine~PO_4 and rephosphorylation of adenosine diphosphate (ADP) to ATP and on the change in O_2 stores, primarily in the venous circulation. The O_2 stores are finite and change only when the circulation is in a non-steady-state with respect to metabolic rate; in the steady-state, the O_2 stores are reduced but constant. Creatine ~PO_4 also decreases to a constant level within 2 to 3 minutes of exercise;[7] the level of ATP, however, remains essentially constant.[8] Because of the precise quantitative relationship between the O_2 consumed and the ~PO_4 produced,[9] the time-course of the changes in $\dot{V}O_2$ closely reflect the rate of ~PO_4 regeneration.

The initial changes in $\dot{V}CO_2$ are similar to those of $\dot{V}O_2$, i.e., during the first 15 seconds or so of exercise. In the following period, $\dot{V}CO_2$ rises more slowly than $\dot{V}O_2$ because of an increase in CO_2 stores. $\dot{V}CO_2$ typically remains less than $\dot{V}O_2$ in the steady-state of exercise below the *AT* because me-

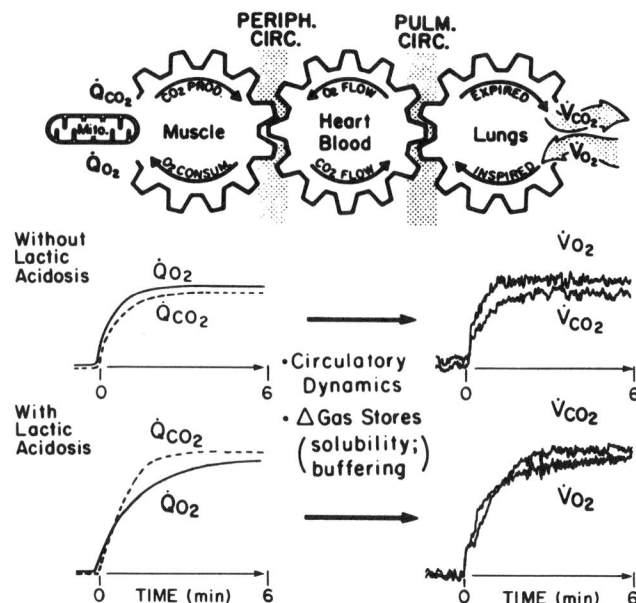

FIG. 1-2. Scheme of coupling of external to cellular respiration. Breath-by-breath data, interpolated second by second for 6 minutes of constant work-rate exercise for work with and without lactic acidosis, are shown on the right. Each study is an overlay of four repetitions to reduce random noise in the data and to enhance the physiologic events. Measurements of external respiration (right) can be used to reconstruct the changes in muscle cellular respiration (left). The factors that modulate the relationship between cellular respiration and external respiration are shown in the center. At the start of exercise there is normally a steep increase in both $\dot{V}O_2$ and $\dot{V}CO_2$ that plateaus for about 15 seconds as pulmonary blood flow accelerates because of a reflex increase in heart rate and stroke volume. A second factor that modulates gas exchange at the lungs is the solubility of CO_2 in the tissues. This is evidenced by a slower rise in $\dot{V}CO_2$ than $\dot{V}O_2$ at the airway (right). For work rates without a lactic acidosis, $\dot{V}O_2$ reaches a steady-state by 3 minutes and $\dot{V}CO_2$ by 4 minutes. For work rates with lactic acidosis, $\dot{V}O_2$ kinetics are slowed and may not reach a steady-state, whereas $\dot{V}CO_2$ kinetics remain virtually unchanged (see text for discussion of mechanisms). (The right side of this figure is drawn from data from Sietsema, K., Daly, J.A., and Wasserman, K.: Early dynamics of O_2 uptake and heart rate as affected by exercise work rates. J. Appl. Physiol., 67:2535–2541, 1989.)

tabolism in the steady state is solely aerobic. The ratio of increase in steady-state $\dot{V}CO_2$ relative to $\dot{V}O_2$ must define the respiratory quotient (RQ) of the muscle substrate.

When $\dot{V}O_2$ does not achieve a steady-state by 3 minutes, as illustrated by the measurements shown on the lower right of Figure 1-2, lactic acid increases in the body, i.e., the work rate is above the subject's *AT* and homeostasis is not achieved. $\dot{V}CO_2$ increases relative to $\dot{V}O_2$ when lactate increases because HCO_3^- is the principal buffer of the newly formed lactic acid; 22.3 ml of CO_2 are released for each millimole of HCO_3^- buffering lactic acid (derived from Avogadro's number whereby 1 mol or 6.02×10^{23} molecules of CO_2 occupies 22.3 L under standard conditions). Consequently, $\dot{V}CO_2$ rises to a level higher than $\dot{V}O_2$. In contrast to the slowing of $\dot{V}O_2$ kinetics for above AT work,[10] the $\dot{V}CO_2$ kinetics are similar for work rates below and above the AT. If the work rate is not too high above the AT, $\dot{V}O_2$ may reach a constant value before the subject fatigues. Otherwise, $\dot{V}O_2$ progressively increases until the subject is forced to stop from fatigue.

Patterns of Change in External Respiration (O_2 Uptake and CO_2 Output) as Related to Function, Fitness, and Disease

The changes in external ($\dot{V}O_2$ and $\dot{V}CO_2$) respiration needed to allow exercise energy output to increase are intimately and predictably linked to the increases in cellular respiration through the circulation. The contribution of aerobic and anaerobic metabolism can often be inferred from measurements of external respiration. Gas exchange kinetics differ in response to exercise depending on whether work is performed above or below the AT (Fig. 1-2). For work rates at which a lactic acidosis develops, the O_2 supply appears to be inadequate to meet the total O_2 need. Therefore, $\dot{V}O_2$ kinetics are affected, with a slow component in $\dot{V}O_2$ reflecting increased anaerobiosis. Complementing these changes in $\dot{V}O_2$ kinetics is an increase in $\dot{V}CO_2$ in excess of $\dot{V}O_2$ because of the CO_2 release from bicarbonate as it buffers lactic acid. When work is done in a truly homeostatic state, in which all the O_2 required by the muscle is provided to and utilized by the muscle, the $\dot{V}O_2$ kinetics are rapid and no lactic acidosis develops.

Individuals who are highly fit for endurance work do not develop a lactic acidosis until work rates become high. Their $\dot{V}O_2$ kinetics are relatively rapid, compared with less fit subjects, for work rates below the AT. $\dot{V}CO_2$ kinetics remain slightly slower than $\dot{V}O_2$ kinetics even in highly fit subjects, with the absolute $\dot{V}CO_2$ typically remaining below $\dot{V}O_2$. Circulatory disorders are associated with slow $\dot{V}O_2$ kinetics at relatively low work rates.

Factors Limiting Exercise

Symptoms that stop people from performing exercise are fatigue, dyspnea, and pain. In assessing cardiorespiratory function, the physiologic approach would be to stress large muscle groups while observing cardiovascular and ventilatory function. Exercise involving large muscle groups, such as walking, running, or cycling, is thought to be limited by O_2 transport.

FATIGUE

During large muscle group exercise, fatigue occurs when the $\dot{V}O_2$ requirement of the contracting muscle is not met by the O_2 transport system. Sullivan et al.[11] measured $\dot{V}O_2$ for the same submaximal work rate in patients with heart failure and in normal subjects. $\dot{V}O_2$ and therefore aerobic ATP production were reduced in the heart failure patients. When aerobic ATP production is below that required, the muscles reach a state in which their contractile behavior is eventually impaired, i.e., muscle fatigue.

Because a lactic acidosis accompanies an increased rate of anaerobic ATP production, it is tempting to attribute the fatigue to the intracellular consequences of the exercise lactic acidosis. The mechanisms of muscle fatigue under such conditions, however, remain a topic of debate. Low cellular pH, increased inorganic phosphate, impaired calcium release from the sarcoplasmic reticulum, and decreasing ATP have been proposed as mediators of fatigue. Thus, $\dot{V}O_2$ steady-state is delayed or not achieved for above AT exercise, as illustrated in the lower right panel of Figure 1-2. These slow kinetics predict that the subject will experience early fatigue for the exercise being performed.

DYSPNEA

The major function of the ventilatory control system during exercise appears to be to regulate arterial pH and to compensate for hypoxemia, should it occur. CO_2 reacts with water to become carbonic acid. If the CO_2 generated during aerobic ATP regeneration is not excreted by the lung as quickly as it is produced, arterial H^+ will increase. An additional source of H^+ at work rates above the AT is lactic acid. Because HCO_3^- is its primary buffer, CO_2 production increases as HCO_3^- buffers lactic acid. This additional CO_2 load, added to the aerobic CO_2 production and accompanied by a reduced blood HCO_3^- concentration, results in a disproportionate increase in H^+ with respect to the increase in $\dot{V}O_2$ or work rate. If the patient has impaired ventilatory capacity, he or she will be unable to regulate H^+. This may be expressed by the symptom of dyspnea.

Whereas normal sedentary subjects usually experience fatigue rather than dyspnea as a limiting factor while performing exercise involving large muscle groups, three types of normal subjects may experience dyspnea in response to exercise. Females may report dyspnea on exertion when they perform at the same work rate at which a male is asymptomatic. This is because they characteristically have about two thirds the ventilatory capacity of males of the same size. Moreoever, because of the reduction in maximal ventilatory capacity with aging, normal elderly people may experience exertional dyspnea. Finally, athletes with exceptionally high aerobic capacities may produce enough CO_2 combined with increased accumulation of lactic acid during high levels of exercise that they approach their ventilatory capacity.

PAIN

Pain in the chest or anginal referral areas is the most common symptom of patients with coronary artery disease. This is an expression of the inadequate O_2 supply to the myocardium relative to the myocardial O_2 demand. Reducing the O_2 demand by afterload reduction or increasing the O_2 supply by improving coronary perfusion can eliminate the pain, supporting the concept that the origin of the pain depends on the O_2 supply/demand balance.

Claudication also occurs because of an O_2 supply/demand imbalance to the exercising, ischemic extremity. Because walking at a normal pace requires an increase in O_2 utilization by the skeletal muscle of approximately 20-fold, the increase in the O_2 supply is critically important in order to perform normal ambulation without pain. If atherosclerotic changes in the conducting vessels to the lower extremity limit blood flow increase, this will be reflected in an O_2 supply/demand imbalance, slowed O_2 uptake kinetics,[12] and critically low levels of O_2 tension in the muscles.[13] Tissue hypoxia causes changes in cellular redox state and is accompanied by increased lactic acid and lactate/pyruvate ratio.[13] Thus, inadequate gas exchange in the claudicating legs appears to be the root cause of pain as it is with fatigue and dyspnea.

Evidence of Systemic Dysfunction Uniquely Revealed by Integrative Cardiopulmonary Exercise Testing

In medical practice, various levels of enthusiasm for use of integrative cardiopulmonary exercise testing prevail at the present time. In our experience, however, cardiopulmonary exercise testing has served uniquely to clarify mechanisms in pathophysiology and efficacy of treatment for which other technologies were less suitable. Several examples of clinical conditions in which integrative cardiopulmonary exercise testing has played a central, if not an essential role, are listed in the following paragraphs:

SEVERE PULMONARY VASCULAR DISEASE WITHOUT PULMONARY HYPERTENSION

Some patients with primary lung disease, particularly patients with interstitial lung disease, have a relatively large amount of pulmonary vascular disease. This limits the increase in pulmonary blood flow in response to exercise if the right ventricle does not hypertrophy sufficiently to overcome the increase in pulmonary vascular resistance.

The oxygen requirements of the tissues can only be met if left ventricular output is appropriate. If the right ventricular hypertrophy is inadequate to increase pulmonary blood flow during exercise to the extent required by the left side of the heart to support the O_2 needed to perform exercise, however, the O_2 uptake will increase more slowly than normal. The right ventricle does not hypertrophy to the same degree in all patients whose pulmonary vasculature is partially destroyed by lung disease. Some patients with lung disease have severe exercise limitation due to the inability to increase pulmonary blood flow. Yet they may have no electrocardiographic (ECG) or chest x-ray evidence of right ventricular hypertrophy or pulmonary hypertension. The entity of increased pulmonary vascular resistance limiting exercise performance, without increased pulmonary artery pressure, would not be recognized in clinical medicine if cardiopulmonary exercise testing were not performed on patients with this exercise-limiting pathophysiologic feature. Case 51 in Chapter 8 is a striking example of this entity.

FORAMEN OVALE PATENCY WITH DEVELOPMENT OF RIGHT TO LEFT SHUNT DURING EXERCISE

Because 25% of normal people have a potentially patent foramen ovale, the possibility exists that a right to left shunt may develop during exercise in 25% of patients who develop pulmonary vascular disease. During exercise, the increase in venous return will cause the right atrial pressure to increase if pulmonary vascular disease, with increased pulmonary vascular resistance, is present. When right atrial exceeds the left atrial pressure, right atrial blood flows through the patent foramen ovale and induces systemic hypoxemia. In this situation, the patient may have no or little hypoxemia at rest, but marked hypoxemia during exercise. Although measurements of arterial blood gases during air and O_2 breathing during exercise are necessary to support this diagnosis, it can easily be suspected during exercise from gas exchange measurements alone. An example of such a phenomenon is provided in case 61 of Chapter 8.

ATTRIBUTING EXERTIONAL DYSPNEA TO HYPOXEMIA

In many instances, patients with cardiorespiratory disorders develop hypoxemia during exercise, but one may be uncertain whether correcting the hypoxemia by O_2 breathing would alleviate or reduce their exercise-limiting symptoms. Exercise performance while breathing a high inspired O_2 gas mixture compared to an air-breathing exercise test will rapidly and objectively demonstrate whether hypoxemia contributes to exercise limitation or dyspnea. Because O_2 supplementation is expensive, but also rewarding when administered to the patient who would benefit from this treatment, it would be appropriate to use integrative cardiopulmonary exercise testing to obtain objective evidence that supplemental O_2 breathing would be of value. Only exercise testing provides this information, because no reliable algorithm exists that can be used to determine who would and who would not benefit from O_2 therapy. See cases 42, 55, and 56 in Chapter 8 as examples of the use of oxygen for diagnosis and treatment.

NONINVASIVE EVIDENCE OF DEVELOPMENT OF MYOCARDIAL DYSKINESIS DURING EXERCISE

At rest, the myocardium may be adequately perfused, so no abnormality in wall motion occurs. During exercise, however, left ventricular work is increased (increase in left ventricular pressure and heart rate) and coronary artery filling time (diastolic period) is decreased. Regions of the myocardium with reduced ability to increase blood flow may therefore experience an O_2 delivery/O_2 requirement imbalance. In these regions of the left ventricle, the rate of ATP production will be inadequate to sustain contraction. Thus, it will become dyskinetic with the part of the ventricular wall in which aerobic ATP production is normal. Stroke volume will therefore decrease at the work levels at which dyskinesis becomes manifest. This will often be reflected during exercise by (1) an abrupt slowing in oxygen uptake relative to the increase in work rate, (2) an acceleration of the heart rate increase relative to increasing $\dot{V}O_2$, and (3) ECG evidence of ischemia. Whereas myocardial dyskinesis can be observed during radionuclide imaging of the myocardium, the advantages of integrative cardiopulmonary exercise testing are that the dyskinesis of the myocardial wall can be correlated with the metabolic cost of exercise at all work levels tolerated, the procedure is noninvasive, it does not expose the patient to radiation, and it may be cost-saving. Results are especially valuable when accompanied by electrocardiographic abnormalities that suggest myocardial ischemia. Although it is not yet routinely applied for this purpose, integrative cardiopulmonary exercise testing may serve as an important screen of abnormality of left ventricular function. Cases 18 and 21 in Chapter 8 represent examples of this abnormality.

OCCUPATIONAL LUNG DISEASE AS A CAUSE OF EXERCISE LIMITATION

Most authorities agree that studies of resting lung function do not give reliable information with respect to whether this organ system is limiting during exercise. Moreover, the clinician assessing disability often misinterprets the organ system limiting exercise when integrative cardiopulmonary exercise testing is not part of the evaluation.[14] There is a distinct advantage, therefore, in doing integrative cardiopulmonary exercise testing as part of a disability evaluation work-up because objective answers can be obtained in distinguishing those people who have legitimate claims for disability benefits from those who do not.

The foregoing are only some clinical examples that illustrate the unique information revealed by integrative cardiopulmonary exercise testing. It is often the critical test needed to sort out the cause or causes of exercise limitation in patients with complex cardiovascular, respiratory, or metabolic disorders.

In summary, symptoms that limit exercise in patients can usually be detected by an abnormality in the gas transport processes that couple external to cellular respiration. Integrative exercise tests in which gas exchange is measured dynamically, rather than as a single steady-state measurement, can often identify the pathophysiology of reduced exercise tolerance. This functional diagnosis might even provide sufficient information for an anatomic diagnosis or, if not, may suggest other tests that would narrow the diagnostic choices.

When the cause of a patient's exercise intolerance is not clinically obvious, we believe that it is cost-effective to do an integrative cardiopulmonary exercise test before proceeding with invasive and expensive testing. It is possible that the economics of medicine will eventually dictate that integrative cardiopulmonary exercise testing, such as described in this book, be done as a first test in the work-up of the patient with exercise limitation of unknown etiology, rather than as the last test, as is common in this country today.

References

1. Wasserman, K., VanKessel, A., and Burton, G.G.: Interaction of physiological mechanisms during exercise. J. Appl. Physiol., 22:71–85, 1967.
2. Bouyhus, A., Pool, J., Binkhorst, R.A., and VanLeeuwen, P.: Metabolic acidosis of exercise in healthy males. J. Appl. Physiol., 21:1040–1046, 1966.
3. Holmgren, A., and McIlroy, M.B.: Effect of temperature on arterial blood gas tensions and pH during exercise. J. Appl. Physiol., 19:243–245, 1964.
4. Koyal, S.N., Whipp, B.J., Huntsman, D., Bray, G.A., and Wasserman, K.: Ventilatory responses to the metabolic acidosis of treadmill and cycle ergometry. J. Appl. Physiol., 40:864–867, 1976.
5. Barr, D.P., and Himwich, H.E.: Studies in the physiology of muscular exercise. III. Development and duration of changes in acid–base equilibrium. J. Biol. Chem., 58:539–555, 1923.
6. Sietsema, K., Daly, J.A., and Wasserman, K.: Early dynamics of O$_2$ uptake and heart rate as affected by exercise work rate. J. Appl. Physiol., 67:2535–2541, 1989.
7. Mahler. M.: First order kinetics of muscle oxygen consumption and an equivalent proportionality between $\dot{Q}o_2$ and phosphorylcreatine level. J. Gen. Physiol., 86:135–165, 1985.
8. DiPrampero, P.E., Davies, C.T.M., Cerretelli, P., and Margaria, R.: An analysis of O$_2$ debt contracted in submaximal exercise. J. Appl. Physiol., 29:547–551, 1970.
9. McGilvery, R.W.: Biochemistry: A Functional Approach, 3rd Ed. Philadelphia, W.B. Saunders, 1983, pp. 390–411.
10. Casaburi, R., Barstow, T.J., Robinson T., and Wasserman, K.: Influence of work rate on ventilatory and gas exchange kinetics. J. Appl. Physiol., 67:547–555, 1989.
11. Sullivan, M.J., Green, H.J., and Cobb, F.R.: Altered skeletal muscle metabolic response to exercise in chronic heart failure: relationship to skeletal muscle aerobic enzyme activity. Circulation, 84:1597–1607, 1991.
12. Meakins, J., and Long, C.N.H.: Oxygen consumption, oxygen debt and lactic acid in circulatory failure. J. Clin. Invest., 4:273–293, 1927.
13. Bylund-Fellenius, A.-C., Walker, P.M., Elander, A., Holm, S., Holm, J., and Schersten, T.: Energy metabolism in relation to oxygen partial pressure in human skeletal muscle during exercise. Biochem. J., 200:247–255, 1981.
14. Oren, A., Sue, D.Y., Hansen, J.E., Torrance, D.J., and Wasserman, K.: The role of exercise testing in impairment evaluation. Am. Rev. Respir. Dis., 135:230–235, 1987.

Physiology of Exercise

CHAPTER 2

9

THE PERFORMANCE OF muscular work requires the physiologic responses of the cardiovascular and ventilatory systems to be coupled with the increase in metabolic rate. Efficient coupling minimizes the stress to the component mechanisms supporting the energetics; that is, cellular respiratory requirements (internal respiration) can only be met by the interaction of physiologic mechanisms that link gas exchange between the muscle cells and the atmosphere (external respiration) (see Fig. 1-1). Inefficient coupling increases the stress to these systems, and when severe it can impair or limit work performance.

Normal gas exchange between the cells and the environment requires: (1) appropriate intracellular structure, energy substrate, and enzyme concentrations; (2) a heart capable of pumping the quantity of oxygenated blood needed to sustain energy production; (3) an effective system of blood vessels that can selectively distribute blood flow to match local tissue gas exchange requirements; (4) blood with normal hemoglobin of adequate concentration; (5) an effective pulmonary circulation through which the regional blood flow is matched to the appropriate ventilation; (6) normal lung mechanics and chest bellows; and (7) ventilatory control mechanisms capable of regulating arterial blood gas tensions and pH. The response of each of the coupling links in the gas exchange process is usually quite predictable and can be used as a frame of reference for evidence of impaired responses.

In this chapter, we review the essentials of skeletal muscle physiology, including the relationship of structure and function, cellular respiration, substrate metabolism, and the effect of an inadequate O_2 supply. After considering internal respiration, we examine the circulatory and ventilatory links between internal and external respiration. These links include the factors that determine the magnitude and time-course of the cardiovascular and ventilatory responses and how they are coupled with the metabolic stress of exercise.

Skeletal Muscle

MECHANICAL PROPERTIES

Human skeletal muscles consist of two basic fiber types (Types I and II), which are classified on the basis of both their contractile and their biochemical properties.[1] Type I (or "slow-twitch") fibers take a relatively long time to develop peak tension following their activation, i.e., some 80 msec,

compared to the 30-msec average for Type II (or "fast-twitch") fibers. The slower contractile properties of Type I fibers appear to result largely from the relatively low activity of the myosin adenosine triphosphatase (ATPase), the lower Ca^{++} activity of the regulatory protein troponin, and the slower rate of Ca^{++} uptake by sarcoplasmic reticulum. These same properties appear to confer a relatively high resistance to fatigue on the Type I fibers.

Biochemical differences between the two basic fiber types center chiefly on their capacity for oxidative and glycolytic activities. Type I fibers, being especially rich in myoglobin, are classified as red fibers, whereas Type II fibers, which contain considerably less myoglobin, are classified as white fibers. Type I slow-twitch fibers tend to have significantly higher levels of oxidative enzymes than Type II fast-twitch fibers, which typically have high glycolytic activity and enzyme profile. Type II fibers are further classified into Type IIa and Type IIb, based on the greater oxidative and lesser glycolytic potential of Type IIa fibers compared with Type IIb fibers. With respect to substrate stores, muscle glycogen concentration is, in fact, similar in both Type I and Type II fibers, but the triglyceride content is two to three times greater in Type I slow-twitch fibers. Evidence suggests that Type I slow-twitch fibers are more efficient than Type II fast-twitch fibers because they generate more work or develop more tension per unit of substrate energy utilized.[2]

Considerable potential for change exists in the enzyme concentrations of a particular fiber by specific training. For example, a fast-twitch fiber in an endurance-trained athlete could have higher concentrations of oxidative enzymes than slow-twitch fibers in a chronically sedentary subject.[3]

These structural and functional differences between fiber types depend to a large extent on the neural innervation of the fibers. A single motor neuron supplies numerous individual muscle fibers; this functional assembly is termed a "motor unit." These fibers are distributed throughout the muscle, rather than being spatially contiguous. Fibers comprising a motor unit are characteristically of the same "fiber type," and substrate depletion occurs uniformly within each fiber of the contracting unit.

Fiber type distribution within human skeletal muscle varies from muscle to muscle. For example, the soleus muscle typically has a much higher density of slow-twitch fibers (more than 80%) than the gastrocnemius muscle (about 50%) or the triceps brachii (about 20 to 50%). The vastus lateralis muscle (approximately 50% slow-twitch fibers) has been widely used for analysis of fiber type characteristics in man. The basic fiber type pattern of this muscle appears highly variable in different subjects. Endurance-trained athletes typically have a high percentage of slow-twitch fibers in this muscle (more than 90% not being uncommon) compared with untrained, control subjects (about 50%) or trained sprinters (20 to 30%).

Whereas basic fiber type pattern is genetically determined, it is greatly influenced by the neural characteristics of the efferent motor neuron. When the motor nerves innervating the fast flexor digitorum longus and the slow soleus muscles of the cat are cut and cross-spliced, the contractile and biochemical characteristics of the muscle begin to resemble the features of the muscle originally innervated by the nerve.[4] Thus, an important trophic influence on muscle function is conferred by its nerve supply. Training, however, does not cause significant interchanges between Type I and Type II fibers, but can cause changes within Type II fibers (e.g., from Type IIb to Type IIa).[5]

The pattern of activation of these fiber types depends on the form of exercise. For low-intensity exercise, Type I slow-twitch fibers tend to be recruited predominantly, whereas Type II fast-twitch fibers are recruited at higher work rates, especially at or above 70 to 80% of the maximal aerobic power.[6]

ENERGETICS

Skeletal muscle may be considered to be a machine that is fueled by the chemical energy of substrates derived from ingested food and stored as carbohydrates and lipids in the body. Although protein is a perfectly viable energy source, it is not used to fuel the energy needs of the body to any appreciable extent, except under conditions of starvation.

The free energy of the substrate (i.e., that fraction of the total chemical energy that is capable of doing work) is not used directly for muscle contraction. It must first be stored as the bond energy of adenosine triphosphate (ATP). The terminal phosphate bonds of this compound have a high free energy of hydrolysis (ΔG) and are designated "high-energy" phosphate bonds ($\sim PO_4$). Current estimates of ΔG per $\sim PO_4$, for physiologic conditions such as those occurring in contracting muscle, are as high as 12 to 14 kcal/mol. Muscle is ultimately, therefore, a digital device operating in discrete multiple units of $\sim PO_4$ energy, with one $\sim PO_4$ thought to be utilized per myosin cross-bridge linkage to and subsequent release from actin. The muscle uses this energy for the conformational changes externally manifested by shortening or increasing tension. Thus, muscular exercise depends on the intrinsic structural characteristics of muscle and on the body's systems that maintain an appropriate physico-chemical milieu for adequate ATP generation.

CELL RESPIRATION

Energy for muscular contraction is obtained predominantly by the oxidation of fuel in the mitochondria with a small additional amount from biochemical mechanisms in the cell cytoplasm (Fig. 2-1). This energy is used to form high-energy compounds, predominantly creatine phosphate and ATP, from which energy in the terminal phosphate bond can be made available for cellular reactions such as biosynthesis, active transport, and muscle contraction. Exercise entails an acceleration of the energy-yielding reactions in the muscles to produce $\sim PO_4$ at an increased rate for muscle contraction. This requires an increased utilization of O_2, to be matched by increased delivery of O_2 from the atmosphere to the mitochondrion and the simultaneous removal of CO_2, the major catabolic end-product of exercise.

Acetate, produced by the catabolism of carbohydrates, fatty acids, or (in nutritionally deficient states) amino acids, reacts with oxaloacetate in the mitochondrion, after esterification with coenzyme A (acetyl CoA), to form citrate in the Krebs or tricarboxylic acid (TCA) cycle (Fig. 2-1). Here the catabolic reactions result in CO_2 release and the transfer of hydrogen ions (protons) and their associated electrons to the mitochondrial electron transport chain, which then flow down an energy gradient; this results in ATP formation by oxidative phosphorylation of adenosine diphosphate (ADP). At the end of the electron transport chain, cytochrome oxidase catalyzes the reaction of each pair of protons and electrons with an atom of oxygen to form a molecule of water. For each pair of protons and electrons transferred, sufficient energy is released to form approximately three ATP from ADP, i.e., three if the electron transport process begins at nicotinamide adenine dinucleotide (NAD^+) but only two if it begins at flavin adenine dinucleotide (FAD^+) (Fig. 2-1).

Six ATP molecules are gained during the catabolism of glucose to pyruvate if the reduced nicotin-

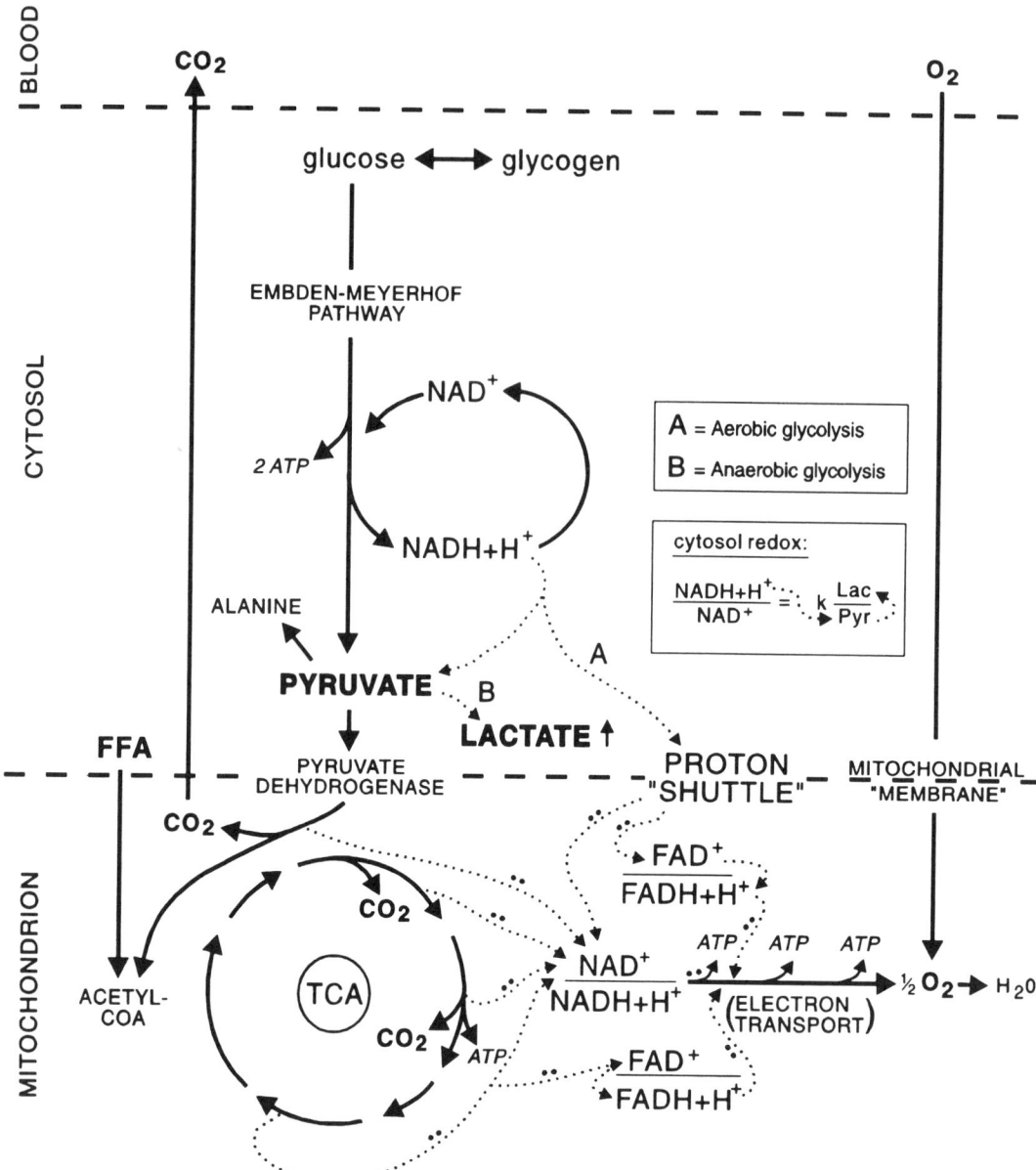

Fig. 2-1. Scheme of the major biochemical pathways for production of ATP. The transfer of H^+ and electrons to O_2 by the electron transport chain in the mitochondrion and the "shuttle" of protons from the cytosol to the mitochondrion (pathway A) are the essential components in aerobic glycolysis for the efficient utilization of carbohydrate substrate in regenerating ATP to replace that consumed by muscle contraction. Also illustrated is the important O_2 flow from the blood to the mitochondrion, without which the aerobic energy generating mechanisms within the mitochondrion would come to a halt. Pathway B would be capable of reoxidizing $NADH+H^+$ to NAD^+ with a net increase in lactic acid production (lactate accumulation) if the O_2 supply were inadequate to maintain pathway A. Lactate will increase relative to pyruvate as $NADH+H^+/NAD^+$ increases in the cytosol (see figure inset and text).

amide adenine dinucleotide ($NADH+H^+$) in the cytosol, formed during glycolysis, is reoxidized by the proton shuttle and FAD^+, i.e., pathway A of Figure 2-1.[7] The shuttle accepts hydrogen ions from the cytosolic $NADH+H^+$ and transfers them to mitochondrial coenzymes, NAD^+ or FAD^+, as illustrated in Figure 2-1. This method of regenerating oxidized NAD^+ in the cytosol maintains the cytosolic redox state and enables glycolysis to continue. Of the six ATP molecules

generated from glucose by this mechanism, two are formed in the cytosol by the Embden-Meyerhof (glycolytic) pathway and four in the mitochondrion during the coupled reoxidation of cytosolic $NADH+H^+$ by the mitochondrion, i.e., the mitochondrial membrane proton shuttle, and the cytochrome electron transport chain.[7] Because O_2 is the ultimate recipient of the protons generated by glycolysis and transported into the mitochondria, this glycolysis is aerobic (pathway A, Fig. 2-

1). It is the mechanism for glycolysis at low and moderate work intensities; this shuttle mechanism consequently regulates the cytosolic redox state.

The formation of acetyl CoA from pyruvate and its subsequent entry into the TCA cycle yields a total of 5 reduced mitochondrial NAD molecules, i.e., $NADH + H^+$. Because the reoxidation of each $NADH + H^+$ by the electron transport chain yields 3 ATP molecules, there is a net gain of 15 ATP. Two molecules of acetyl CoA are formed from each glucose molecule, however, so the total gain is 30 ATP from these reactions. When added to the 2 ATP gained from glycolysis and the 4 others obtained from reoxidation of cytosolic $NADH + H^+$ by the proton shuttle with the subsequent transfer of its protons and electrons to O_2 (Fig. 2-1), the total gain in ATP from the complete oxidation of glucose is 36. Because glycogen is the major carbohydrate source in the normally nourished person, however, an additional $\sim PO_4$ is obtained when a glycosyl unit is split from glycogen to form glucose-6 phosphate. Thus, 37 ATP molecules are obtained from each glycosyl unit. Because 6 molecules of O_2 are used for glucose oxidation and 36 high-energy phosphate bonds are formed, the $\sim PO_4:O_2 = 6$ for glucose (6.18 for glycogen). Six molecules of CO_2 and H_2O are catabolic end-products of these reactions.

Under conditions in which the mitochondrial proton shuttles fail to reoxidize the $NADH + H^+$, generated by glycolysis, at a rate sufficient to keep cytosolic $NADH + H^+/NAD^+$ normal (Fig. 2-1), the redox state of the cytosol is lowered. As $NADH + H^+$ accumulates in the cytosol at the expense of NAD^+, glycolysis would become inhibited if it were not for an alternate pathway capable of reoxidizing cytosolic $NADH + H^+$. Pyruvate can reoxidize the $NADH + H^+$ to NAD^+, but it is reduced to lactic acid in the process (pathway B, Fig. 2-1). This pyruvate oxidation of $NADH + H^+$ occurs without immediate use of O_2 and is thus termed anaerobic glycolysis. The substrate price for the production of energy from this reaction is expensive compared to the complete oxidation of glycogen to CO_2 and H_2O. The net gain in ATP is only 3 from each glycosyl unit instead of 37. For the same work rate, therefore, this pathway causes glycogen (and glucose) to be used at a considerably faster rate than in the totally aerobic state.[8,9] Moreover, the two lactic acid molecules formed from each glucose molecule or glycosyl

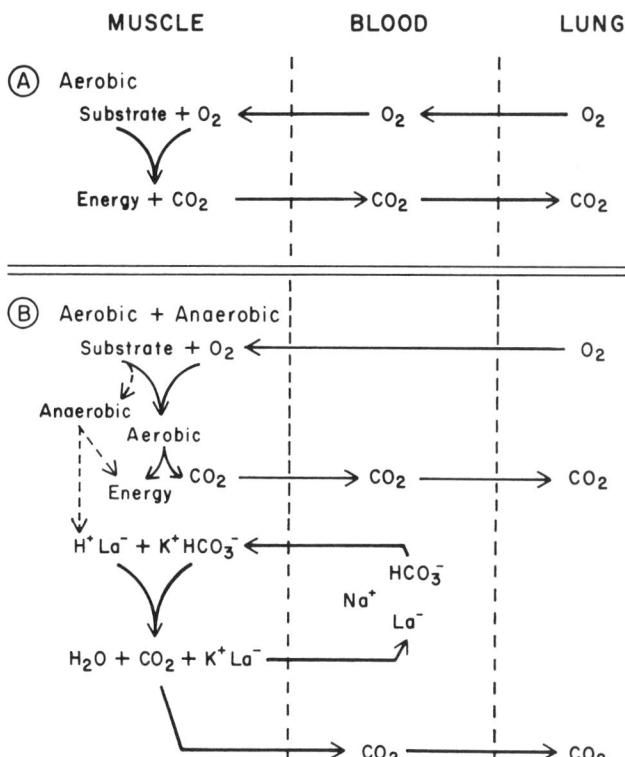

FIG. 2-2. Gas exchange during aerobic (A) and aerobic-plus-anaerobic (B) exercise. The acid-base consequence of the latter is a net increase in cell lactic acid production. The buffering of the accumulating lactic acid takes place in the cell at the site of formation, predominantly by bicarbonate. The latter mechanism increases the CO_2 production of the cell by approximately 22.3 ml per millimole of bicarbonate buffering of lactic acid. The increase in cell lactate and decrease in cell bicarbonate results in chemical concentration gradients causing lactate to be transported out of and bicarbonate to be transported into the cell.

unit cause a disturbance of acid-base balance in the cell and blood (Fig. 2-2).

That the *turn-on* of anaerobic ATP production does not signal the *turn-off* of aerobic ATP production deserves emphasis. Both aerobic and anaerobic mechanisms share in energy generation at high work rates, with the anaerobic mechanism providing an increasing proportion of energy as the work rate is increased.

SUBSTRATE UTILIZATION AND REGULATION

At this point, several terms need to be clarified for precision and to avoid possible confusion (see Fig. 1-1). The symbol $\dot{V}O_2$ indicates O_2 uptake by the lungs. It is distinguished from O_2 consumption by the cells, which is abbreviated $\dot{Q}O_2$. The abbreviation $\dot{V}CO_2$ indicates CO_2 output by the lungs, to distinguish it from CO_2 production by the cells, abbreviated $\dot{Q}CO_2$. Thus, the substrate mixture undergoing oxidation is characterized by the net rates of CO_2 yield or production ($\dot{Q}CO_2$) and O_2 utilization or consumption ($\dot{Q}O_2$). The ratio $\dot{V}CO_2/\dot{V}O_2$ as measured at the mouth (i.e., the gas exchange ratio, R) reflects $\dot{Q}CO_2/\dot{Q}O_2$, the metabolic respiratory quotient (RQ), *only* when there is a steady-state, i.e., CO_2 is not being added to or removed from the body CO_2 stores and the O_2 stores are constant, i.e., when $\dot{Q}CO_2 = \dot{V}CO_2$ and $\dot{Q}O_2 = \dot{V}O_2$.

During acute hyperventilation (resulting, for example, from acute hypoxia, pain, or anxiety, or of volitional origin), considerably more CO_2 is unloaded from the body CO_2 stores than O_2 is loaded into the O_2 stores. This is because hemoglobin is almost completely saturated with O_2 at the end of the pulmonary capillaries at sea level; on the other hand, appreciable amounts of CO_2 can be unloaded as alveolar ventilation is increased and Pa_{CO_2} is reduced. Thus, the gas exchange ratio, R, will exceed the metabolic RQ until a steady-state is again attained at the new level of ventilation. Similarly, during the acute metabolic acidosis of exercise, "extra" CO_2 is evolved when HCO_3^- buffers lactic acid (Fig. 2-2). This, too, will result in R's exceeding RQ until a new steady-state is attained (i.e., the CO_2 pool size is again constant although depleted), at which time R again equals RQ. Differences between R and RQ also occur during acute hypoventilation and recovery from metabolic acidosis, but in the opposite direction.

As seen in the following equations, carbohydrate (e.g., glycogen or glucose) is oxidized with RQ = 1.0 (i.e., 6 CO_2 produced/6 O_2 consumed) and has a ~PO_4:O_2 = 6.0 or 6.18, depending on whether glucose or glycogen is the substrate:

$$C_6H_{12}O_6 + 6\ O_2 \rightarrow 6\ CO_2 + 6\ H_2O + 36\ or\ 37\ ATP \quad (1)$$

Lipid (e.g., palmitate) is oxidized with RQ = 0.71 (i.e., 16 CO_2 produced/23 O_2 consumed) and has a ~PO_4:O_2 = 5.65 (i.e., 130 ATP/23 O_2):

$$C_{16}H_{32}O_2 + 23\ O_2 \rightarrow 16\ CO_2 + 16\ H_2O + 130\ ATP \quad (2)$$

Intermediate steady-state RQ values reflect different proportions of carbohydrate and fat utilized in the metabolic process (Fig. 2-3). For storage economy, fat is more efficient but for economy of O_2 utilization, carbohydrate is more efficient.

When a steady-state of gas exchange exists, R

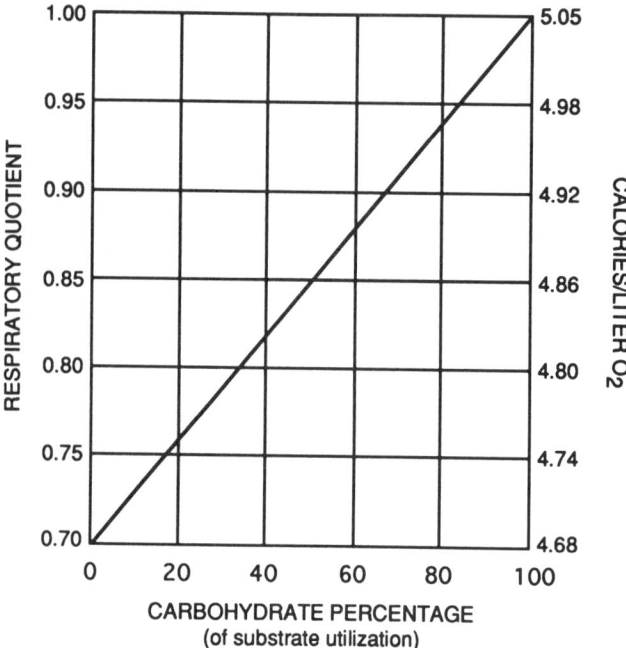

FIG. 2-3. The percentage of carbohydrate substrate in the diet estimated from the respiratory quotient measurement. The number of calories of energy obtained per liter of oxygen consumed for each combination is given on the right ordinate. (Plot of data from Lusk, G.: Science of Nutrition. Johnson Reprint Corp., New York, 1976, p. 65.)

provides an accurate reflection of RQ. During exercise, the muscle RQ can be estimated from the *increase* in $\dot{V}CO_2$ relative to the *increase* in $\dot{V}O_2$. It is apparent from gas exchange measurements that a greater proportion of carbohydrate is used for energy during muscular work than at rest. Because muscle RQ is approximately 0.95, on average,[10–13] total body RQ increases from a resting value of approximately 0.8 (on an average "Western diet") toward 0.95 during moderate exercise, depending on the work rate (Fig. 2-4). This indicates that about 85% of the substrate during exercise is derived from carbohydrate (Fig. 2-3). Whereas the fuel mixture for the total body derives proportionally more from carbohydrate than from lipid stores during exercise as work rate increases (Fig. 2-4), RQ decreases slowly over time during prolonged constant load exercise (Fig. 2-5). This reflects a reduction in the glycogen stores. When muscle glycogen becomes depleted, the exercising subject senses exhaustion.[14] Acute ingestion of glucose allows the work to continue.[15]

The rate of decrease in muscle glycogen during exercise can be slowed by raising blood glucose levels with a continued infusion of glucose.[16] The importance of muscle glycogen in work tolerance is well described by the experiments of Bergstrom

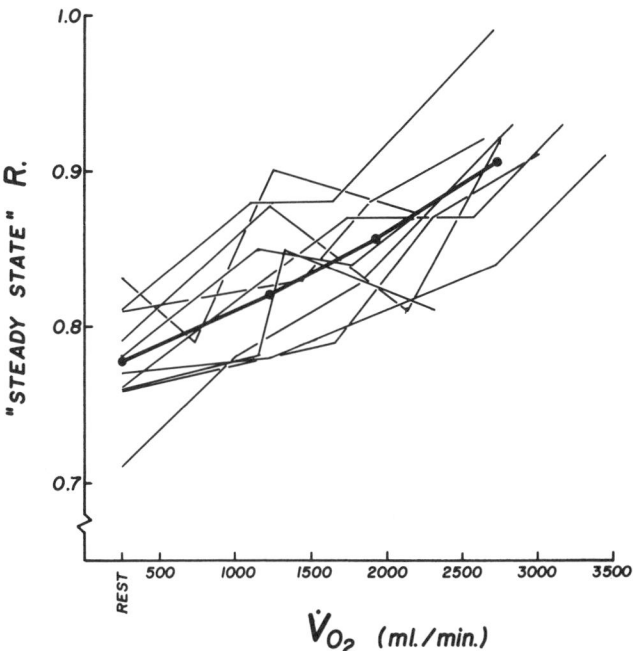

FIG. 2-4. The steady-state R (RQ) at various levels of exercise for the whole body determined as the ratio of steady-state $\dot{V}CO_2$ to $\dot{V}O_2$ for the levels of exercise indicated on the X-axis for 10 subjects. The heavy line is the average response.

et al.,[13] who demonstrated a high positive correlation between the tolerable duration of high-intensity work and the muscle glycogen content before exercise.

Physical fitness has been shown to affect the substrate utilization pattern by allowing a fitter subject to use a greater proportion of energy from fatty acids to perform a given level of work than an unfit one.[17] This glycogen-conserving consequence of fitness presumably allows more work to be performed before glycogen depletion and consequent exhaustion. The specific regulation of different substrates is considered in the following sections.

Carbohydrates

Skeletal muscle in man contains, on average, 80 to 100 mmol (15 to 18 g) glucose per kilogram of wet weight stored as glycogen. For the "standard" 70 kg man, this amounts to approximately 400 g of muscle glycogen. Note that this represents an estimate of the total skeletal muscle carbohydrate pool, whereas a contracting muscle can draw only on its own glycogen reserves and not on the pools in noncontracting muscles.

Normally, 5 to 6 g of glucose are available in the blood (100 mg/100 ml). Although muscle uptake of blood glucose increases considerably during exercise, the blood concentration does not fall except during prolonged work because of an increased rate of glucose release from the liver.

The liver represents a highly labile source of some 50 to 90 g of reserve glycogen. This glycogen is broken down into glucose and is released into the blood by glycogenolysis. Glucose can also be produced in the liver (gluconeogenesis) from lactate, pyruvate, glycerol, and alanine precursors. The rate of glucose release into the circulation depends on both the blood glucose concentration and a complex interaction of hormones such as insulin, glucagon, and the catecholamines epinephrine and norepinephrine.[18,19] As exercise intensity and duration increase, the circulating levels of catecholamines and glucagon increase. These increases release glucose from the liver, serving to maintain the level of blood glucose despite its increased utilization by the exercising

FIG. 2-5. Effect of exercise duration on the gas exchange ratio (R) for constant work rate exercise of moderate, heavy, and very heavy work intensity. Note that the gas exchange ratio is higher for the higher work intensities, but it declines with time after the initial increase. Results are those for a single subject.

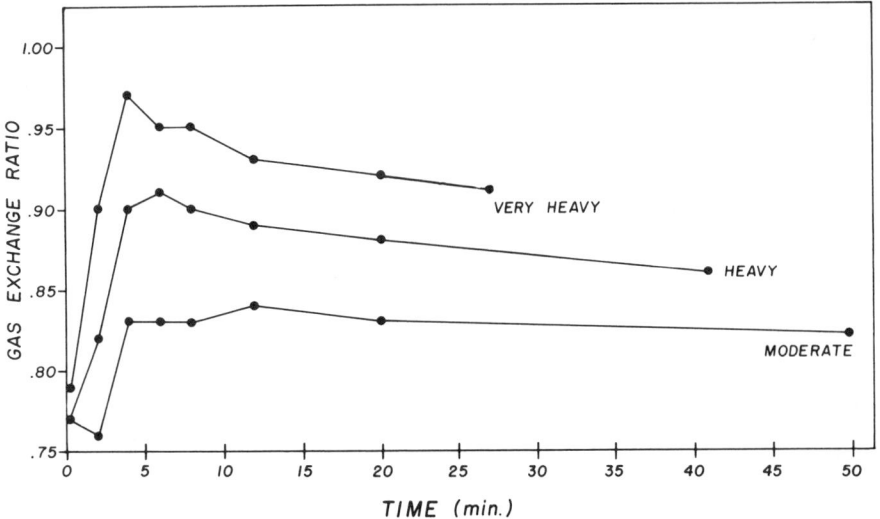

muscles. These regulatory processes maintain physiologically adequate concentrations of glucose except when muscle and liver glycogen stores become greatly depleted.

Lipids

Skeletal muscles have access to their own intramuscular store of lipids, averaging 20 g of triglycerides per kilogram of wet weight. This source has been shown to account for a considerable proportion of the total energy required by the muscles, depending on the duration of exercise and the rate of depletion of muscle glycogen.

Extramuscular lipid sources are also utilized during exercise. These derive from adipose tissue where triglycerides undergo hydrolysis to glycerol and free fatty acids (mainly palmitic, stearic, oleic, and linoleic acids). The fatty acids are transported in the blood, bound predominantly to albumin. The store of extramuscular lipid is large. In the "standard" 70 kg man, fat accounts for approximately 15 kg of triglycerides, equivalent to about 135,000 kcal of energy.

The sympathetic nervous system, along with catecholamines from the adrenal medulla, regulates adipose tissue lipolysis. Epinephrine and norepinephrine increase the local concentration of cyclic 3',5'-adenosine monophosphate (AMP) through activation of adenyl cyclase. This leads to increased rates of hydrolysis of the stored adipose tissue triglycerides. Other factors reduce the rate of adipose tissue lipolysis during exercise, including increased blood lactate and exogenous glucose loads.

The free fatty acids account for only a small proportion (usually less than 5%) of the total plasma fatty acid pool; the remainder are triglycerides. Resting plasma free fatty acid concentrations are approximately 0.5 mmol/L, rising during exercise to approximately 2 mmol/L. The turnover rate of the plasma free fatty acid pool is high, with a half-time of 2 to 3 minutes at rest and less during exercise. As a consequence, the flux of free fatty acids to the exercising muscle (i.e., plasma flow × plasma free fatty acid concentration) is an important determinant of skeletal muscle uptake.

The plasma concentration of free fatty acids does not increase, and may even decrease slightly, with physical training. Therefore, the increased proportional contribution of free fatty acid oxidation to exercise energetics, which is noted at a specific work rate after training, may reflect increased utilization from intramuscular sources. Adipose

tissue lipolysis does not appear to be enhanced by training and may even be depressed.

Amino Acid Metabolism

During exercise, the rate of release of intramuscular alanine increases appreciably but with little or no change in other amino acids.[20] The arterial concentration increases by as much as two-fold during severe exercise.[21] The source of the alanine released from muscle is predominantly from the transamination of pyruvate (derived from increased rates of carbohydrate metabolism). The amino groups are derived from the deamination of inosine monophosphate during purine nucleotide metabolism and by the branch-chain amino acids (valine, leucine, and isoleucine).

A highly linear relationship exists between the plasma concentrations of alanine and pyruvate at rest and during exercise. A decreased muscle release of alanine is observed in phosphorylase-deficient muscle (McArdle's syndrome) associated with the decreased output of pyruvate.[22] The alanine formed by transamination in muscle is transported in the blood to the liver where it serves as a precursor for gluconeogenesis. Thus, an alanine-glucose cycle is established between muscle and liver, with the carbon skeleton of alanine supporting hepatic glucose synthesis.

Oxygen Cost of Work

The O_2 cost of performing work depends on the work rate. Figure 2-6 shows the time course of O_2 uptake ($\dot{V}O_2$) from unloaded cycling for various levels of cycle ergometer exercise in a normal individual. Note that a steady-state is reached by 3 minutes up to a work rate of 150 watts (W). At higher work rates, $\dot{V}O_2$ continues to increase above the 3-minute value. The rate at which $\dot{V}O_2$ increases is greater, the higher the work rate, in this range of work not accompanied by a steady-state by 3 minutes.[23,24] The maximum $\dot{V}O_2$ for each of the work rates above 200 W was the same, thereby identifying the subject's $\dot{V}O_2$max. If the steady-state $\dot{V}O_2$ is measured for a range of cycle ergometer work rates below the subject's AT, such as shown for 50, 100, and 150 W in Figure 2-6, a linear relationship between $\dot{V}O_2$ and work rate is obtained (Fig. 2-7). The slope of this relationship is approximately the same for all normal people (approximately 10 ml/min/W). This means that work efficiency in man is relatively fixed for a

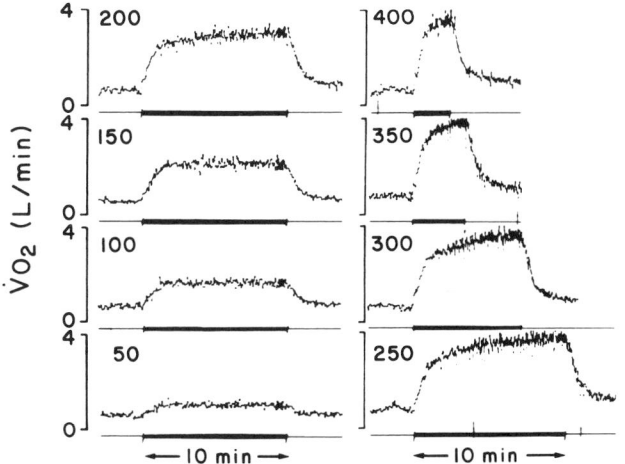

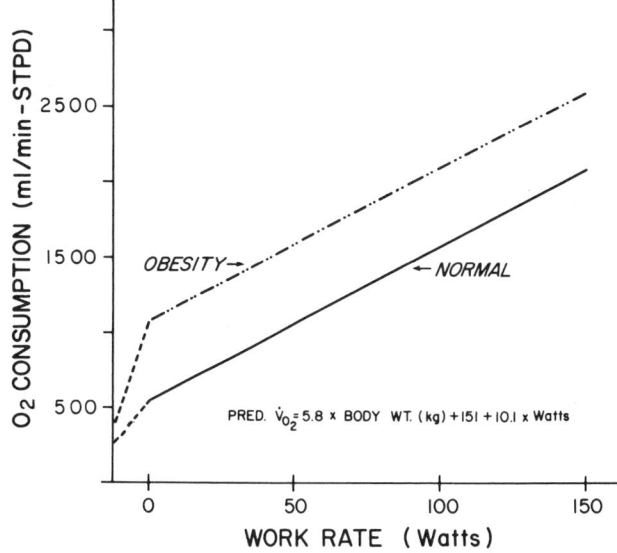

FIG. 2-6. Breath-by-breath time course of oxygen uptake for eight levels of constant work rate cycle ergometer exercise, starting from unloaded cycling. The work rate (watts) for each study is shown in the respective panel. The bar on the X-axis indicates the period of the imposed work rate. The $\dot{V}_{O_2}$ asymptote (steady-state) is significantly delayed for work above the anaerobic threshold. (From Whipp, B.J., and Mahler, M.: Dynamics of pulmonary gas exchange during exercise. *In* Pulmonary Gas Exchange. Vol. 2. Edited by J.B. West. New York, Academic Press, 1980, pp. 33–96.)

FIG. 2-7. The effect of work rate on steady-state oxygen consumption during cycle ergometer exercise. The oxygen consumption response in normal subjects is predictable for cycle ergometer work regardless of age, gender, or training. The predicting equation is given in the figure. In obese subjects, the oxygen requirement to perform work is displaced upward, the displacement dependent on body weight. (From Wasserman, K., and Whipp, B.J.: Exercise physiology in health and disease. Am. Rev. Respir. Dis., 112:219–249, 1975.)

given work task. Whereas the slope of the $\dot{V}_{O_2}$-work rate relationship is not affected by training, age, or gender, the position of the relationship depends on body weight. Obese subjects exhibit an upward displacement of approximately 5.8 ml/min/kg body weight.[25] On the cycle ergometer, this reflects the added work rate generated as a result of moving the heavier limbs. The effect of body weight on $\dot{V}_{O_2}$ is more pronounced on the treadmill because the work rate must be even greater to move the entire body.

WORK EFFICIENCY

Cycle ergometer work rate and the steady-state $\dot{V}_{O_2}$ measurement are commonly used interchangeably when describing the level of exercise being performed because work efficiency (caloric equivalent of the measured work ÷ caloric equivalent of the O_2 consumed for the measured work) varies only slightly from one individual to another.[26] Trained and untrained individuals, whether old or young, male or female, all have similar work efficiencies. This similarity reflects the basic biochemical energy-yielding reactions needed for muscle contraction. Care must be taken not to confuse changes in skill or motor efficiency due to practice, in the assessment of work efficiency, however. To measure work efficiency, one must use relatively simple tasks that do not

depend on technique and for which the work output can be measured, e.g., cycling.

To calculate muscle work efficiency, the caloric equivalent of the steady-state $\dot{V}_{O_2}$ (4.98 kcal/L $\dot{V}_{O_2}$ at RQ = 0.95; see Fig. 2-3) and the external power (0.014 kcal/min/W) for at least two *measured* work rates must be known. For lower extremity cycle ergometer work, normal subjects have an efficiency of approximately 28%.[25,27]

$\dot{V}_{O_2}$ UNSTEADY-STATE AS RELATED TO LACTATE INCREASE

The upward drift in $\dot{V}_{O_2}$ observed after 3 minutes during constant work rate exercise is only seen for work rates that are accompanied by a lactic acidosis.[23,24,28] The rate of rise in $\dot{V}_{O_2}$ in response to constant work rate exercise has been shown to correlate well with the increase in blood lactate.[24,28–30]

At least five mechanisms may contribute to the slow rise in $\dot{V}_{O_2}$ after 3 minutes of exercise: (1) progressive vasodilation to the local muscle units by metabolic vasodilators produced in response to relative O_2 lack, e.g., [H^+], thereby increasing O_2 flow and O_2 consumption at the O_2-deficient sites; (2) acidemia facilitating O_2 unloading from hemoglobin, thereby shifting the oxyhemoglobin dissociation curve downward and maintaining the capillary P_{O_2} at a functional level for diffusion transport; (3) the O_2 cost of conversion of lactate to glycogen in the liver, and possibly muscle, as the lactate concentration rises; (4) the increase in $\dot{V}_{O_2}$ needed to satisfy the increased work of the muscles of respiration and the heart at high ventilatory and cardiac output requirements; and (5) reduced muscular efficiency during heavy work either by recruiting more "fast-twitch" muscle fibers or by calling into play additional groups of muscles (such as more forceful pulling on the handlebars). Other mechanisms, such as increased catecholamine levels and increased body temperature at high work rates, could also add to the O_2 cost of heavy work. As discussed in the section of this chapter on gas exchange kinetics, the slow rise in $\dot{V}_{O_2}$ is strongly correlated with the blood lactate increase during exercise. The equation for the linear regression is similar among population groups, including patients with heart failure.

Lactate Increase and the Anaerobic Threshold

LACTATE INCREASE AS RELATED TO WORK RATE

Figure 2-8 shows the arterial blood lactate concentration as related to $\dot{V}_{O_2}$ in 3 groups of subjects

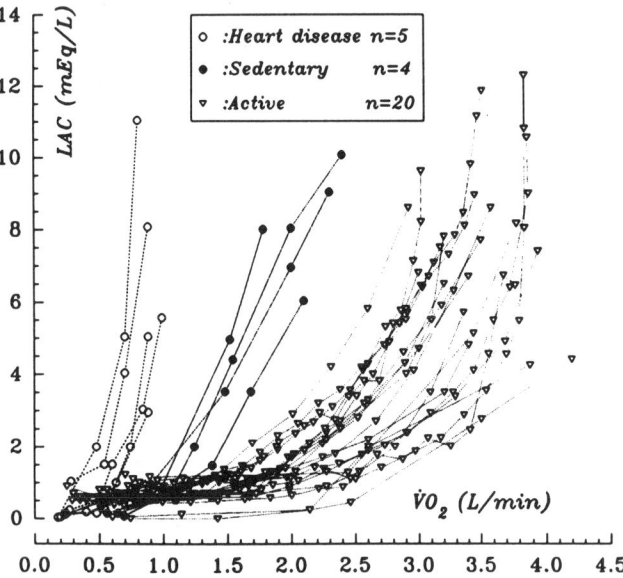

FIG. 2-8. Pattern of increase in arterial lactate in active and sedentary healthy subjects and in patients with heart disease as related to increasing exercise oxygen uptake ($\dot{V}_{O_2}$). Lactate (LAC) concentration rises from approximately the same resting value to approximately the same concentration at maximal exercise in each of the three groups. The fitter the subject for aerobic work, the higher the $\dot{V}_{O_2}$ before lactate starts to increase significantly above resting levels. (Modified from Wasserman, K., and Whipp, B.J.: Exercise physiology in health and disease. Am. Rev. Respir. Dis., 112:219–249, 1975.)

performing progressively increasing cycle ergometer work: normal subjects who are relatively active, sedentary normal subjects, and patients with heart disease. All show similar resting and low level exercise lactate concentrations. The pattern of lactate increase is the same for each group, but the $\dot{V}_{O_2}$ at which the lactate starts to increase differs. Lactate does not start to increase in subjects who are relatively physically active until $\dot{V}_{O_2}$ is increased to as much as 10 times the resting metabolic rate. In contrast, the $\dot{V}_{O_2}$ at which lactate starts to increase in sedentary subjects is about 4 times the resting level, equivalent to the $\dot{V}_{O_2}$ required for adults to walk at a normal pace. In cardiac patients with a low, symptom-limited maximum $\dot{V}_{O_2}$, arterial lactate increases at exceedingly low exercise levels. Activity that only doubles the resting metabolic rate can result in a marked increase in lactate. The $\dot{V}_{O_2}$ at which lactate starts to increase in normal subjects is, on average, about 50 to 60% of their $\dot{V}_{O_2}$max, although it may be considerably higher in aerobically fit subjects. Because of this variability in $\dot{V}_{O_2}$ at which lactate begins to increase, deriving a mean response profile from the responses of a group of subjects (even if normalized to $\dot{V}_{O_2}$max) will result in a spuriously curvilinear profile.

LACTATE INCREASE AS RELATED TO TIME

Work rate or power output is an absolute quantity of work performed per unit of time. A given work rate may be stressful for one individual, limiting the duration that the work could be sustained; it may not be detected as a significant stress by a more fit individual. Therefore, we use adjectives to describe the degree of physical stress, e.g., moderate, heavy, very heavy, based on the pattern of arterial lactate change, as suggested by Wells et al.,[31] because the magnitude of arterial lactate increase for a given work rate closely reflects the fitness of an individual for endurance (aerobic) exercise.[32]

For constant load cycle ergometer exercise, three patterns of arterial blood lactate concentration are observed (Fig. 2-9).[33] The first pattern is one in which either no increase in lactate is observed or lactate peaks early in exercise and then returns to its resting value as $\dot{V}_{O_2}$ reaches a steady-state. This is defined as moderate work intensity and implies that the work is not uncomfortable and hence can be sustained in a true steady-state. When arterial lactate increases and is maintained at higher than resting values by a balance between

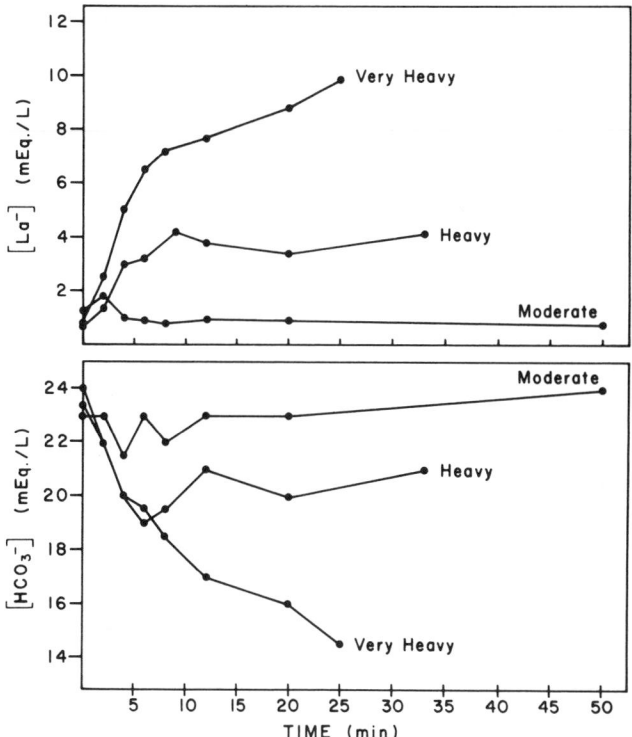

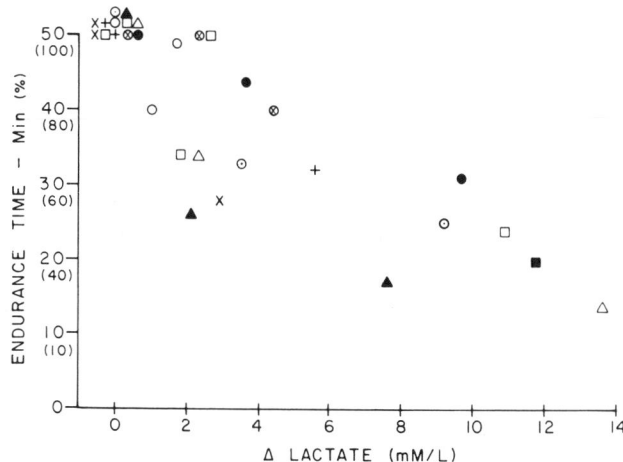

FIG. 2-10. The endurance time as related to the increase in arterial lactate (above the pre-exercise resting value) during the last minute of constant work rate cycle ergometer exercise. Data are from 30 experiments on 10 male subjects studied at 3 work rates, each for a target time of 50 minutes. Endurance time is reduced when lactate is increased. (From Wasserman, K.: The anaerobic threshold measurement to evaluate exercise performance. Am. Rev. Respir. Dis., 129(Suppl.):535–540, 1984.)

FIG. 2-9. Arterial lactate increase and bicarbonate decrease with time for moderate, heavy, and very heavy exercise intensities for a normal subject. Bicarbonate changes in opposite direction to lactate and in a quantitatively similar manner. Whereas the target exercise duration was 50 minutes for each work rate, the endurance time was reduced for the heavy and very heavy work rates.

sustained production and utilization, this is defined as heavy intensity exercise. This work can only be sustained for a limited duration, and a true steady-state does not exist, as evident from a continuously increasing minute ventilation and the development of a metabolic acidosis.[34] Exercise endurance is reduced, as shown in Figures 2-9 and 2-10.

When arterial lactate continues to increase throughout the exercise to the point of fatigue, this is termed very heavy work. At these work rates, arterial lactate typically continues to increase to levels > 5 mmol/L. The higher the lactate, the earlier the fatigue, whether arterial lactate is in the range of heavy or very heavy work intensity (Fig. 2-10).

THRESHOLD LACTATE INCREASE IN RESPONSE TO PROGRESSIVELY INCREASING WORK RATE

We tested both continuous exponential[35] and threshold[36] models extensively[37] to better understand the physiologic events that accompany the development of the highly reproducible lactic aci-

dosis engendered by heavy exercise. To obtain a better picture of the systematic pattern of the change in arterial lactate with increasing $\dot{V}O_2$, we plotted the arterial blood lactate and simultaneously measured $\dot{V}O_2$, after the $\dot{V}O_2$ scale was normalized for each subject to align the lactate threshold (LT) $\dot{V}O_2$ values,[37] for 17 physically active, healthy, young male subjects (Fig. 2-11). In this plot, the data points are distributed with the same deviation relative to the average curve as they were distributed in the individual curves for each subject. Because lactate increases steeply with little increase in $\dot{V}O_2$ as $\dot{V}O_2$max is approached, the data examined to address the question of model behavior for lactate increase are restricted to the region of interest, from resting lactate to that below an arterial lactate of 4.5 mmol/L. As illustrated in Figure 2-11 (upper panel), a mono-exponential model of lactate increase from rest as a function of $\dot{V}O_2$ does not describe the lactate data well. Lactate points fall above the exponential model curve at the low $\dot{V}O_2$ values, whereas in the region of $\dot{V}O_2$ just below that at which lactate starts to rise (identified as the threshold in the threshold model), the points fall below the exponential model curve. In contrast, the points distribute evenly around the two components of the threshold model (Fig. 2-11, lower panel).

Neither the threshold nor the mono-exponential model is a perfect fit for the lactate-$\dot{V}O_2$ relationship at all work levels, but analysis of the data

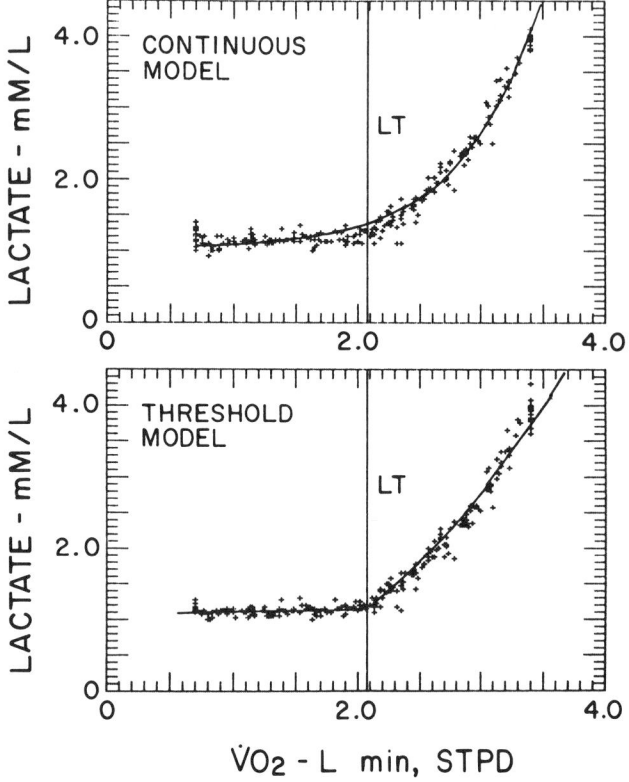

FIG. 2-11. The threshold behavior of arterial lactate increase as related to $\dot{V}O_2$ in response to exercise. Data are arterial lactate measurements from 17 active healthy subjects shown in Figure 2-8. Points only up to 4.5 mmol/L (the region of interest in evaluating threshold versus a continuous exponential model) are plotted. The vertical solid line shows the average threshold for the 17 subjects. The points for the individual subjects are plotted in the same relation to the threshold $\dot{V}O_2$ as existed in their individual plot. In the upper panel, the solid line describes the continuous exponential model. Lactate values fall above the exponential model line at the lowest $\dot{V}O_2$, whereas the lactate values are below the model curve in the region of the threshold. In contrast, the threshold model (solid lines, lower panel) is a better fit to the actual lactate measurements. Details of the mathematical analysis for a smaller number of subjects are presented in reference 37.

in the region of interest, i.e., below 4.5 mmol/L, clearly fits the threshold model better than the exponential model. Supporting the threshold model are numerous muscle biopsy studies showing that muscle lactate does not increase at mild to moderate work rates.[38–42] The $\dot{V}O_2$ at which lactate begins to increase in arterial blood lactate has been shown to be coincident with the lactate increase in the muscle.[38]

MECHANISMS OF LACTATE INCREASE

Overload of the Tricarboxylic Acid Cycle versus Change in Cytosolic Redox State

Lactate can accumulate in the muscle and blood during exercise if: (1) glycolysis proceeds at a rate

faster than pyruvate can be utilized by the tricarboxylic acid cycle of the mitochondria or (2) cytosolic $NADH + H^+$ cannot be reoxidized rapidly enough by the mitochondrial membrane proton shuttle-electron transport chain-cytochrome oxidase-O_2 pathway (see pathway A of Fig. 2-1). In this case, the cytosolic redox state is lowered, and reoxidation can take place by the reaction: pyruvate $+ NADH + H^+ \rightarrow$ lactate $+ NAD^+$ (see pathway B of Fig. 2-1). The first mechanism causes lactate to increase *as a result* of pyruvate increase, i.e., a mass action effect. The second mechanism occurs when the O_2 required by the exercising muscles cannot be supplied at a sufficiently rapid rate to reoxidize $NADH + H^+$ by pathway A. Thus, the cell redox state is lowered, forcing lactate to be *increased* relative to pyruvate.

Figure 2-12 shows a plot of the log-log transformation of arterial lactate, pyruvate, and lactate/pyruvate (L/P) ratio as a function of $\dot{V}O_2$ in one normal subject who was representative of the average response of 10 healthy subjects.[43] Below the *LT*, lactate increased by a few tenths of a millimole as pyruvate increased, but the L/P ratio did not increase until the *LT* was reached. Pyruvate also increased steeply, but not until the $\dot{V}O_2$ was well above that of the *LT*. Moreover, the rate of increase in pyruvate was always slower than for lactate. Consequently, the L/P ratio increased *at* the *LT* and continued to increase until $\dot{V}O_2$max. A similar phenomenon has been observed in the muscle cells of man.[44] The increase in the muscle L/P ratio was accompanied by an increase in the ADP/ATP

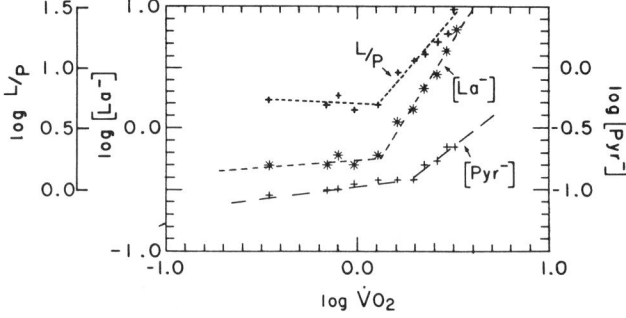

FIG. 2-12. Log lactate [La$^-$], log pyruvate [Pyr$^-$], and log lactate/pyruvate (L/P) ratio plotted against log $\dot{V}O_2$. The log-log transform of the lactate-$\dot{V}O_2$ and pyruvate-$\dot{V}O_2$ relationships allows easy detection of the lactate and pyruvate inflection points. The pyruvate inflection point generally is at a higher $\dot{V}O_2$ than the lactate inflection point. Because the prethreshold pyruvate slope is the same as the lactate slope, the L/P ratio does not increase until the lactate inflection point. (From Wasserman, K., Beaver, W.L., Davis, J.A., Pu, J.-Z., Heber, D., and Whipp, B.J.: Lactate, pyruvate, and lactate-to-pyruvate ratio during exercise and recovery. J. Appl. Physiol., 59:935–940, 1985.)

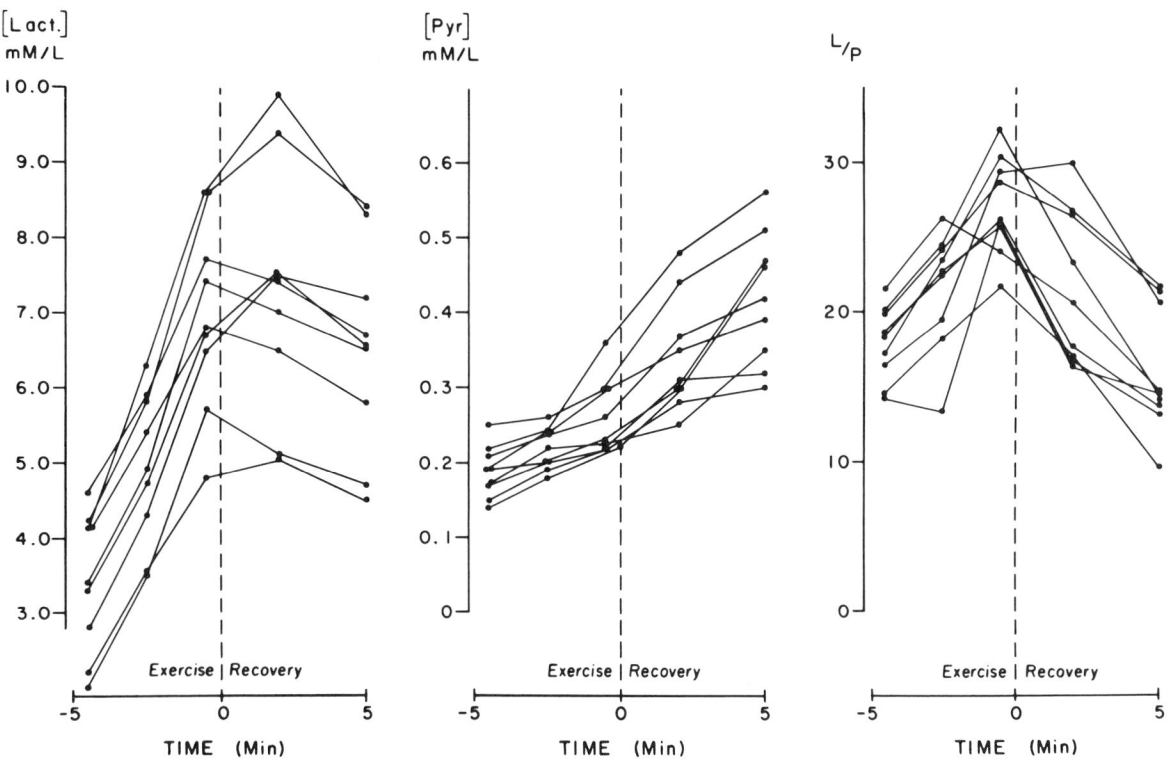

FIG. 2-13. Lactate (Lact), pyruvate (Pyr), and lactate-to-pyruvate (L/P) ratio during the last 5 minutes (highest three work rates) of exercise and the first 5 minutes of recovery. Studies show that lactate either increases or decreases slightly by 2 minutes of recovery. All subjects show a decrease by 5 minutes of recovery. In contrast, pyruvate continues to rise through the first 5 minutes of recovery. As a consequence, the L/P ratio decreases by 2 minutes and continues to decrease by 5 minutes of recovery toward the control values. (From Wasserman, K., Beaver, W.L., Davis, J.A., Pu, J.-Z., Heber, D., and Whipp, B.J.: Lactate, pyruvate, and lactate-to-pyruvate ratio during exercise and recovery. J. Appl. Physiol., 59:935–940, 1985.)

ratio.[44] This indicates that the increase in lactate is not simply a mass action phenomenon resulting from increased glycolysis and pyruvate concentration. Rather, the lactate increase results from a shift in equilibrium between lactate and pyruvate *as a result of* change in the $NADH + H^+/NAD^+$ ratio (cytosolic redox state) (see Fig. 2-1). Thus, reoxidation of cytosolic $NAD^+ + H^+$ appears to result from the conversion of pyruvate to lactate in contracting muscle cells with a falling redox state (see inset in Fig. 2-1). Simultaneously, reoxidation of cytosolic $NADH + H^+$ can take place, aerobically, in better oxygenated contracting muscle cells by pathway A (see Fig. 2-1). Because no O_2 is used in the reoxidation of pathway B (see Fig. 2-1), this glycolysis is *an*aerobic.

The reversal of the exercise-induced increase in the arterial L/P ratio is seen at the start of recovery (Fig. 2-13). The exercise-induced rise in arterial lactate continues into the recovery phase, but at a slowed rate; it subsequently starts to decrease.

Pyruvate concentration, on the other hand, actually increases more rapidly at the start of recovery. Thus, as soon as exercise stops (and the O_2 requirement decreases), the L/P ratio reverses, supporting the evidence obtained during exercise that the exercise-induced lactate increase is not simply a mass action effect consequent to pyruvate increase. The same reversal in L/P ratio, with lactate decreasing and pyruvate increasing at the start of recovery, takes place in the muscle cell.[45]

"Anaerobic Threshold" Concept: Role of O_2 and the Critical Capillary P_{O_2}

As blood flows from the arterial to the venous end of the capillary, P_{O_2} decreases (Fig. 2-14). Whereas mitochondria can respire and rephosphorylate ADP to ATP at a P_{O_2} of 1 mm Hg or less,[46] the capillary P_{O_2} needed to provide the pressure gradient for O_2 to diffuse from the red cell to the sarcoplasm to sustain muscle mitochondrial respira-

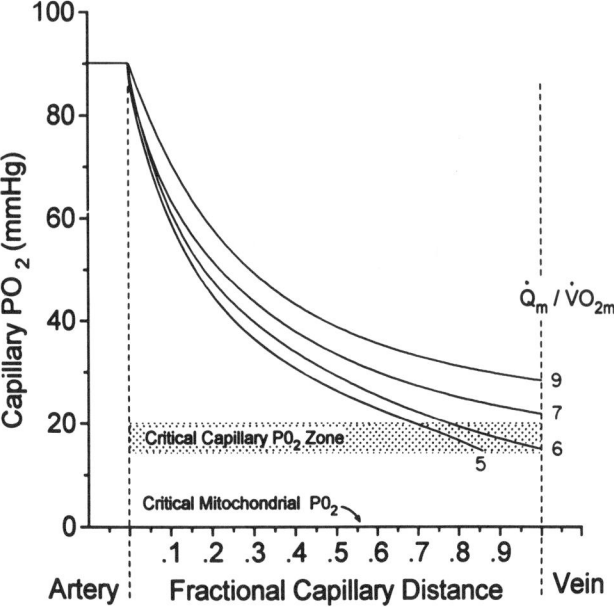

FIG. 2-14. Model of muscle capillary O_2 partial pressure along a representative muscle capillary during exercise. The model assumes a hemoglobin concentration of 15 g/dl, arterial P_{O_2} of 90 mm Hg, and a ratio of muscle blood flow ($\dot{Q}m$) to muscle $\dot{V}_{O_2}$ ($\dot{V}_{O_2}m$) of 6. Major points are that: (1) partial pressure difference between the O_2 source (capillary) and O_2 sink (mitochondrion), distance, area, and the diffusion coefficient of O_2 determine the mass transfer of O_2 (as dictated by Fick's law of diffusion); (2) capillary P_{O_2} is heterogeneous along the capillary bed despite a homogenous $\dot{Q}m/\dot{V}_{O_2}m$; (3) the end-capillary P_{O_2} (approximated by femoral vein P_{O_2} for leg exercise) is reduced to the critical capillary P_{O_2}, below which it cannot decrease further, because only one sixth of the O_2 entering the capillary remains at the end of the capillary; and (4) the Bohr effect, resulting from the exercise lactic acidosis, keeps P_{O_2} from potentially falling much below the critical capillary P_{O_2} toward the venous end of the capillary. Note that a global assessment of capillary P_{O_2} does not reflect the end-capillary P_{O_2}.

tion has been estimated to be 15 to 20 mm Hg.[47] This has been termed the "critical" capillary P_{O_2} because it represents the lowest capillary P_{O_2} that allows mitochondria to receive and consume O_2 during exercise. The major factors determining the P_{O_2} gradient between red cell and sarcoplasm are the resistances to O_2 diffusion by the red cell membrane, plasma, capillary endothelium, interstitial space, and sarcolemma.[47] The P_{O_2} gradient required for diffusion between the sarcoplasm and the mitochondrion is small because of the short distances for diffusion. In addition, the presence of myoglobin in the cell provides a capacitance function for mitochondrial respiration.

The capillary P_{O_2} must be heterogeneous, even if there were a single "ideal" blood flow/metabolic rate ratio in the muscle, because the blood enters the muscle with a $P_{O_2} = 90$ mm Hg (in a normal subject at sea level) and leaves the capillary bed

at a P_{O_2} approximately equal to the femoral vein P_{O_2} (Fig. 2-14). The "critical" capillary P_{O_2} would be the lowest P_{O_2} to which the end-capillary P_{O_2} could fall. The capillary P_{O_2} cannot decrease below this value because the mitochondrial P_{O_2} would be too low to sustain respiration. That the critical capillary P_{O_2} was reached would be evidenced by the failure of P_{O_2} to decrease further despite increasing work rate. Stringer et al.,[48] and Koike et al.,[49] demonstrated that femoral vein lactate starts to increase in the mid-range of a person's work capacity in normal subjects and in patients with cardiovascular disease, respectively (Fig. 2-15). The critical P_{O_2} value in these studies ranged between 15 and 20 mm Hg, in agreement with the estimates of Wittenberg and Wittenberg.[47]

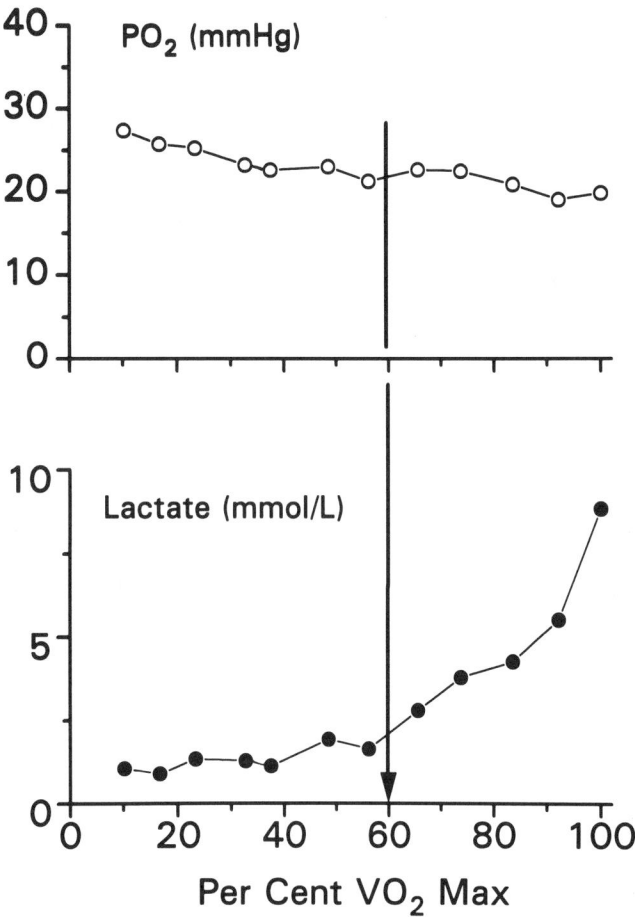

FIG. 2-15. Femoral vein P_{O_2} (mm Hg) and lactate (mmol/L) as a function of the percentage of $\dot{V}_{O_2}$max during a progressively increasing work rate test. The arrow indicates the lactate threshold (*LT*). Results are the average of five young, fit men. The standard deviations at rest (first point), *LT*, and highest $\dot{V}_{O_2}$ for P_{O_2} are 6.1, 2.4, and 3.3, respectively, and for lactate are 0.54, 0.37, and 2.9, respectively. (Modified from Stringer, W., Casaburi, R., French, W., Porszasz, J., and Wasserman, K.: The role of pH in maintaining muscle capillary P_{O_2} during heavy exercise. Am. Rev. Respir. Dis., 145:A881, 1992.)

To obtain this P_{O_2} at the end-capillary site, a blood flow of at least 6 L is needed to allow the muscles to consume 1 L of O_2 (leaving only one sixth of the arterial O_2 remaining at the venous end of the capillary), assuming a normal hemoglobin concentration and an alveolar P_{O_2} adequate to saturate the arterial hemoglobin to 95%. Figure 2-14 illustrates the change in P_{O_2} along the muscle capillary for various blood flow/metabolic rate ratios thought to be physiologic. This model allows for the Bohr effect resulting from aerobic metabolism (modelling decreasing pH in the capillary from aerobic CO_2 production), but not for anaerobic metabolism (lactic acidosis). A blood flow/O_2 consumption ratio of 5:1 would cause obligatory anaerobiosis and lactic acidosis because the P_{O_2} would fall below the critical level well before the blood had left the capillary. The model also illustrates how the lactic acidosis, which develops during heavy exercise, raises the end-capillary P_{O_2} through the accompanying increase in $[H^+]$ from lactic acid.

A lactic acidosis secondary to cellular hypoxia would be expected only if the critical capillary P_{O_2} were reached at the metabolic rate required to perform the exercise. Because the metabolic rate of the tissues other than the exercising muscles does not change from rest appreciably, it is safe to assume that the increase in $\dot{V}_{O_2}$ during leg cycling exercise is due to the increase in lower extremity muscle metabolism. Further, one can assume that femoral vein P_{O_2} and lactate closely approximate the end-capillary values. Figure 2-15, which is a plot of the average femoral vein P_{O_2} and lactate versus $\dot{V}_{O_2}$ for five normal subjects, demonstrates that capillary P_{O_2} falls to about 20 mm Hg at the $\dot{V}_{O_2}$ of the *LT* and does not decrease further despite increasing metabolic rate. The "floor" P_{O_2} must be the "critical" capillary P_{O_2} for the individual. Thereafter, femoral vein lactate increases without a further decrease in femoral vein P_{O_2}.

Figure 2-16 shows individual studies of femoral vein lactate versus P_{O_2} for normal subjects. Lactate does not start to increase until the "critical" capillary P_{O_2} is reached. The "critical" capillary P_{O_2} is reached and arterial lactate starts to increase

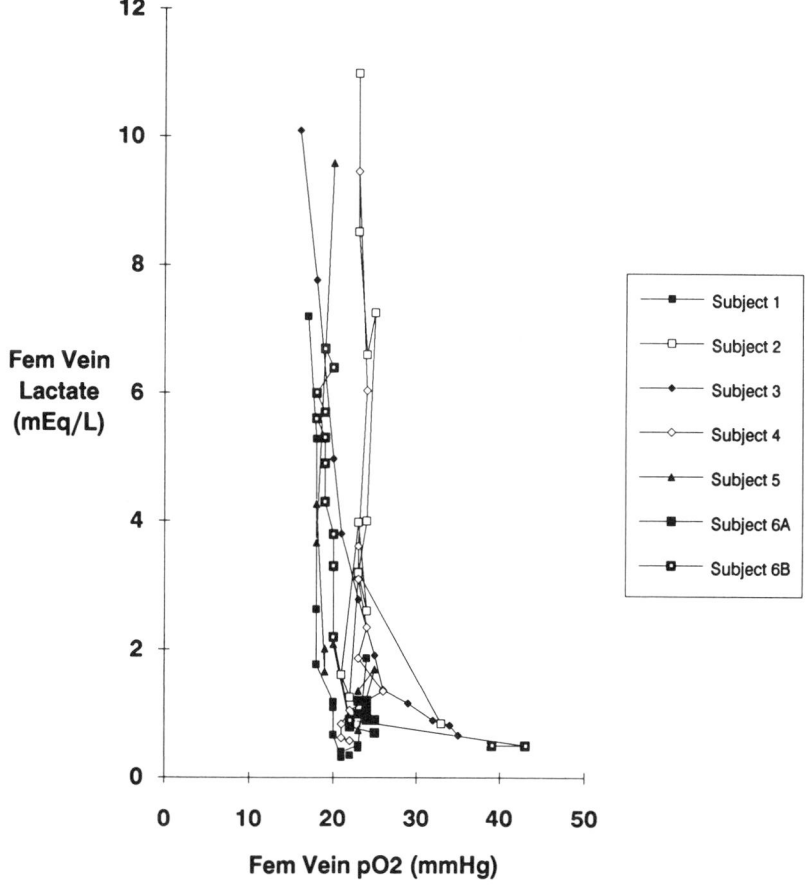

FIG. 2-16. Femoral vein lactate as a function of femoral vein P_{O_2} in 7 incremental exercise studies on 6 subjects. P_{O_2} decreased to an apparent "floor" value as work rate increased. Then lactate progressively increased with little further decrease in P_{O_2}. (Modified from Stringer, W., Casaburi, R., French, W., Porszasz, J., and Wasserman, K.: The role of pH in maintaining muscle capillary P_{O_2} during heavy exercise. Am. Rev. Respir. Dis., 145:A881, 1992.)

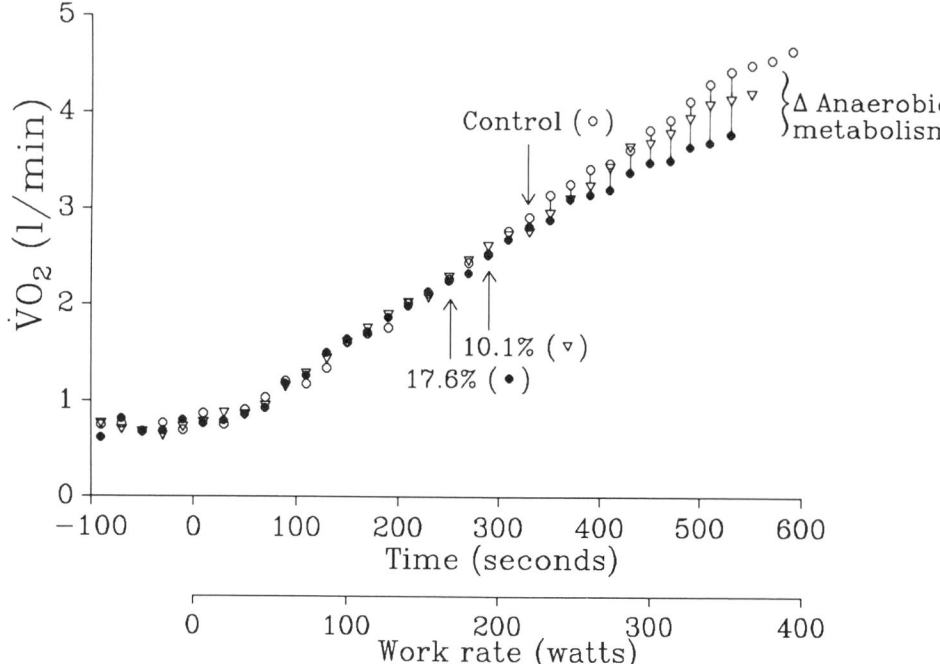

FIG. 2-17. $\dot{V}O_2$ response to three ramp tests (work rate increased at 40 W/min) during air breathing (control test) and air plus carbon monoxide breathing that resulted in HbCO levels of 10.1 and 17.6% in one subject. Points to the left of zero are measured during unloaded cycling. Each point is an average of 20 seconds of data. Arrows show time (and work rate) and $\dot{V}O_2$ of the anaerobic threshold[66] for the three tests. The area delineated by the bracket is the metabolic equivalent of the increased anaerobic metabolism caused when HbCO was increased to 17.6%. (From Koike, A., Weiler-Ravell, D., McKenzie, D.K., Zanconato, S., and Wasserman, K.: Evidence that the metabolic acidosis threshold is the anaerobic threshold. J. Appl. Physiol., 68:2521–2526, 1990.)

in the mid-range of a subject's work capacity, well below $\dot{V}O_2$max.

That lactate concentration and $\dot{V}O_2$ above the *LT* are O_2 transport dependent, but work below the *LT* is O_2 transport independent, is supported by studies in which carboxyhemoglobin (HbCO) was increased to approximately 10% and 20%.[29,50] These levels do not affect cellular respiration and ventilation at rest and low work rates.[51] The *LT* decreased, systematically, as HbCO concentration increased (Fig. 2-17).[50] Lactate increased in response to increased HbCO (10 and 20%) only for work rates above *LT* exercise.[29,52] Moreover, consistent with the concept that work above the *LT* is partially anaerobic is the finding that $\dot{V}O_2$ above the *LT*, but not below the *LT*, was reduced the higher the HbCO level (Fig. 2-17). Thus, a common statement in support of the argument that lactate increase has nothing to do with anaerobiosis, i.e., $\dot{V}O_2$ is not affected in the work rate range in which lactate is increased, is clearly incorrect.

The rate of anaerobic glycolysis is affected by blood oxygenation. Experimental observations demonstrate that blood lactate concentration can be reduced or increased as a result of changes in blood oxygenation.[8,29,52–54] For example, increasing blood O_2 content during exercise reduces arterial blood lactate, whereas reducing it increases blood lactate.[32,54] The diversion of pyruvate from glycolysis to the production of lactate results in accelerated use of carbohydrate stores.[8,9]

Sequential Contraction of Fiber Types

Another mechanism proposed for the increase in lactate during exercise is the increased contraction of Type IIb muscle fibers above the *LT*.[55] These fibers are known to contain high levels of glycogen, although no one has ever demonstrated that these fibers are activated at the *LT*. Furthermore, it would be necessary to demonstrate that Type IIb fibers have a redox state with a higher $NADH+H^+/NAD^+$ ratio and, therefore, a higher L/P ratio than Type I or Type IIa fibers. Additionally, no evidence suggests that activation of Type IIb fiber types is influenced by changes in oxygenation, as has been shown to affect arterial lactate concentration.

In summary, we find it difficult to account for the increase in lactate with an increase in L/P ratio, as seen in response to heavy exercise, by means of accelerated glycolysis, inadequate tricarboxylic acid cycle enzymes, or changes in the contracting muscle fiber type.

MECHANISMS OF BUFFERING THE EXERCISE-INDUCED LACTIC ACIDOSIS

Lactic acid is the predominant fixed acid produced during exercise. It has a pK of approximately 3.9 and therefore is essentially totally dissociated at the pH of the muscle cell (approximately 7.0). Because the H^+ produced as lactate accumulates must be buffered immediately on its formation,

CO_2 production by the cell must increase at a rate commensurate with the *rate* of HCO_3^- buffering of lactic acid. Thus, approximately 22.3 ml of CO_2 would be produced over that from aerobic metabolism for each millimole of lactic acid buffered by HCO_3^- (see Fig. 2-2). The increase in cell lactate and the decrease in cell HCO_3^- concentrations stimulate transmembrane exchange of these ions, with $[HCO_3^-]$ decreasing in the blood almost millimole for millimole with the increase in lactate concentration (Fig. 2-18).[33,56-60]

The mechanism for lactate movement out of the cell is primarily carrier mediated. The studies of Trosper and Philipson, working with cardiac sarcolemmal vesicles, suggest that transport is accelerated by the pH gradient across the sarcolemmal membrane.[61] At the cellular level, this is established primarily by the $[HCO_3^-]$ gradient because the intra- and extracellular fluid will have similar partial pressures of CO_2. Mainwood et al.[62] and Hirsche et al.[63] found that lactate efflux from muscle was highly influenced by the HCO_3^- concentration of the muscle perfusate. The reciprocal changes of lactate and HCO_3^- in the extracellular fluid during heavy exercise suggest that permeation of lactate across the sarcolemmal membrane is a coupled HCO_3^--lactate antiport carrier mechanism. Replacing the intracellular HCO_3^-, which is consumed when it buffers newly produced lactic

acid with HCO_3^- from the blood, minimizes the decrease in intracellular pH.

To better appreciate the dynamics of lactate and HCO_3^- movement between the cell and perfusing blood, arterial lactate and standard (Std) HCO_3^- were measured with a high temporal density (every 7.5 seconds during the first 3 minutes and then every 30 seconds during the remaining 3 minutes) during a 6-minute heavy and very heavy constant load exercise in 8 normal male subjects. Lactate started to increase at about 40 seconds and Std HCO_3^- started to decrease at about 50 seconds, on average (Fig. 2-19). Thereafter, lactate and Std HCO_3^- changed reciprocally. The simultaneous changes in Std HCO_3^- decrease and lactate increase for all arterial samples for heavy and very heavy exercise intensities for the 8 subjects, whose data contribute to the concentration-time plots shown in Figure 2-19, are shown in Figure 2-20. These studies show that the reciprocal changes in Std HCO_3^- and lactate anions are highly correlated after lactate increased about 0.5 and 1.0 mmol/L for heavy and very heavy intensity exercise, respectively.[57] This finding suggests that HCO_3^- buffers lactic acid in a stoichiometric manner, after non-HCO_3^- buffering of the equivalent of the first 0.5 to 1.0 mmol/L of net lactic acid production. The most likely mechanism for the consumption of the early hydrogen ions of lactate

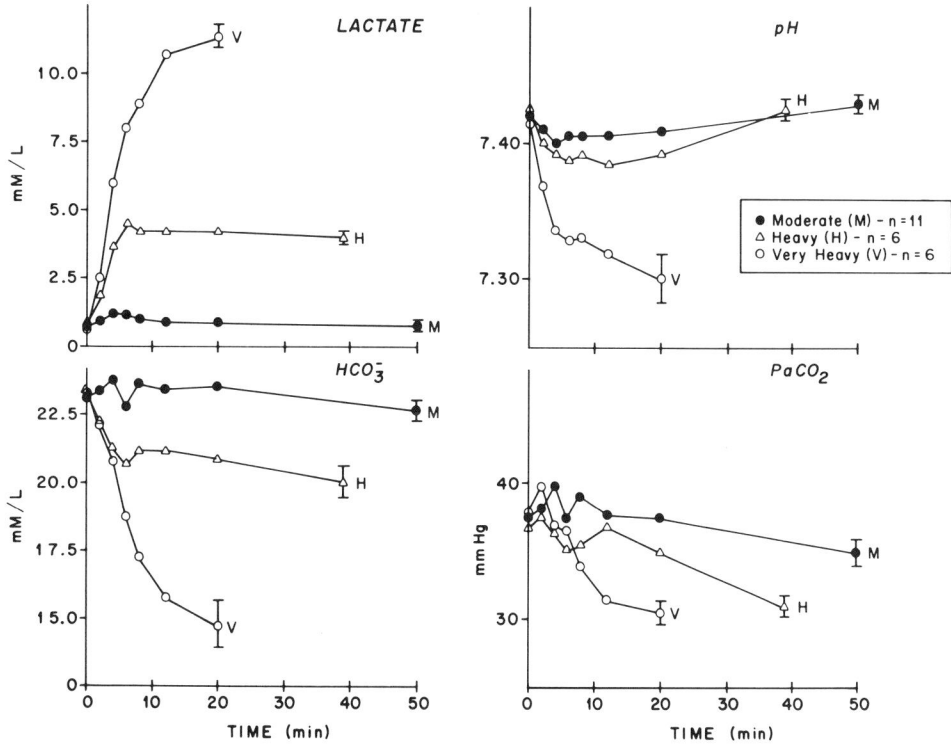

Fig. 2-18. Time course of change in arterial lactate, bicarbonate, pH, and Pa_{CO_2} for moderate, heavy, and very heavy exercise following the onset of constant load cycle ergometer exercise as related to time. Moderate exercise intensity (N = 11) refers to an increase in arterial lactate level of less than 0.8 mmol/L above rest. Heavy exercise intensity (N = 6) refers to an arterial lactate increase at the end of exercise of 2.5 to 4.9 mmol/L above that at rest. Very heavy intensity exercise (N = 6) refers to a lactate increase of 7 mmol/L or greater above that at rest at the end of exercise. (Data computed from subjects previously reported in Wasserman, K., VanKessel, A.L., and Burton, G.B.: Interaction of physiological mechanisms during exercise. J. Appl. Physiol., 22:71–85, 1967.)

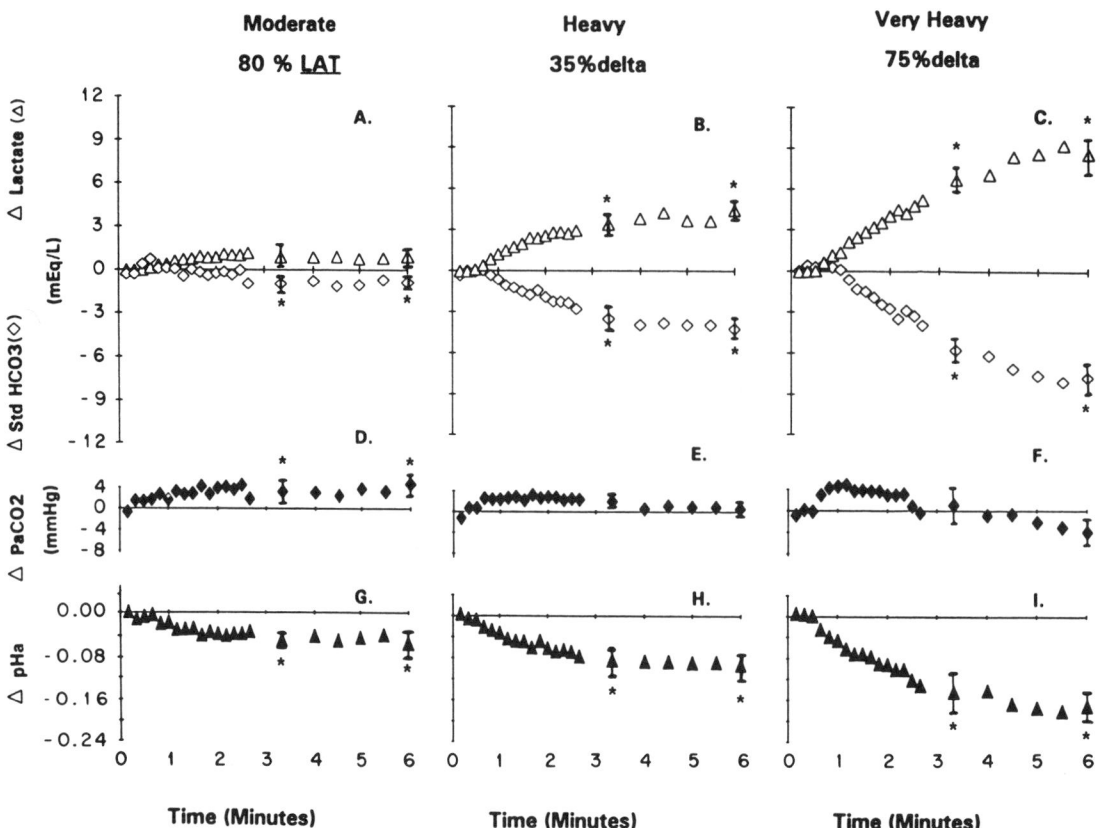

FIG. 2-19. Average responses to three exercise intensities displayed as change from resting measurements for arterial lactate, standard bicarbonate (Std HCO_3^-), Pa_{CO_2}, and pHa (n = 8 subjects). Resting values for all three exercise intensities for pHa, Pa_{CO_2}, Std HCO_3^-, lactate, and hemoglobin are 7.40 ± 0.03 (SD), 39.8 ± 3.1 mm Hg, 24.5 ± 1.3 mEq/L, 0.89 ± 0.47 mEq/L, and 14.2 g/dl, respectively. At selected times during exercise (3 and 6 minutes), SE (bars) and significant differences (*P < 0.05 from rest) are shown. (From Stringer, W., Casaburi, R., and Wasserman, K.: Acid-base regulation during exercise and recovery in man. J. Appl. Physiol., 72:954–961, 1992.)

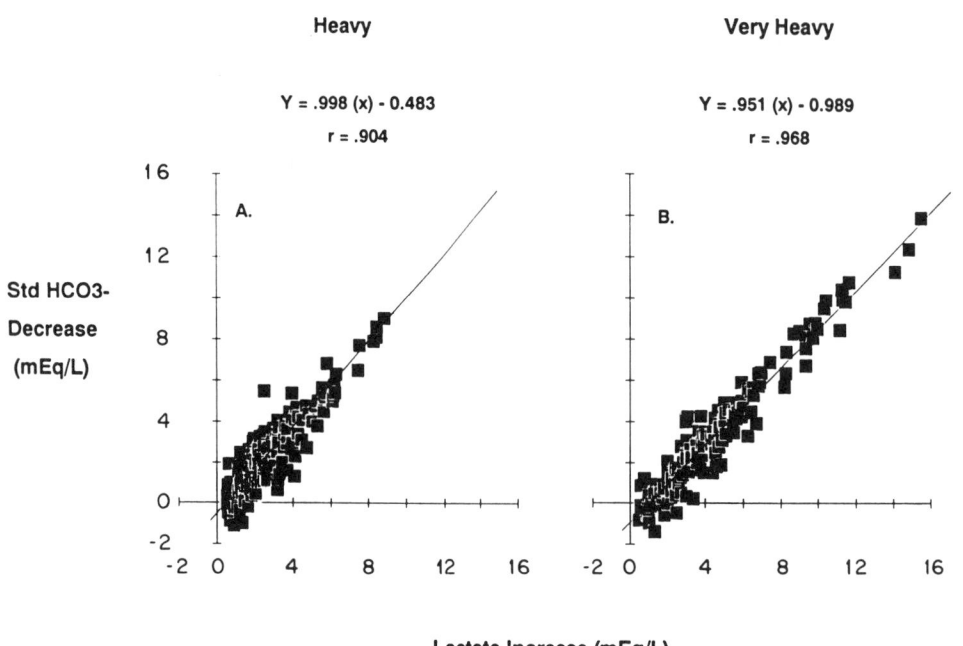

FIG. 2-20. Standard (Std) HCO_3^- decrease as a function of lactate increase from resting values for the heavy and very heavy work intensities shown in Figure 2-19. The fall in Std HCO_3^- is delayed until after lactate starts to increase (see regression equations). Thereafter, changes are approximately equal and opposite [heavy, n = 181: slope = 0.998 (CI 0.92 to 1.06), intercept = −0.48 (CI −0.71 to −0.26); very heavy, n = 141: slope = 0.951 (CI 0.92 to 0.98), intercept = −0.99 (CI −1.12 to −0.78)]. (From Stringer, W., Casaburi, R., and Wasserman, K.: Acid-base regulation during exercise and recovery in man. J. Appl. Physiol., 72: 954–961, 1992.)

is the hydrolysis of creatine phosphate, an early exercise event. When creatine phosphate hydrolyzes, the inorganic phosphate formed is in the dibasic form. This makes the cell more alkaline and therefore consumes H^+. An alternate mechanism might involve cellular buffers that have a pK at the pH of the cell water. Although they do not prevent the cell from becoming more acid, they slow the acid change resulting from a net increase in lactic acid production.

This initial non-bicarbonate buffering of H^+, followed by a stoichiometric buffering of lactic acid by HCO_3^-, was also shown during progressively increasing work rate.[56] Thus, the *LT*, i.e., the $\dot{V}O_2$ above which a sustained lactate increase occurs, slightly precedes the decrease in arterial Std HCO_3^-, i.e., the $\dot{V}O_2$ above which metabolic acidosis develops.

Anaerobic Threshold and its Related Parameters: The Lactate and Lactic Acidosis Thresholds

The $\dot{V}O_2$ at which arterial lactate and the L/P ratio increase is consistent for a given subject depending on fitness and the form of exercise. The $\dot{V}O_2$ at which this anaerobic supplementation of the aerobic energy exchange begins has been termed the anaerobic threshold (*AT*).[64]

The conceptual basis for the *AT* is: (1) the O_2 required by the metabolically active muscles can create an O_2 supply/demand imbalance so capillary PO_2 falls to its lowest value compatible with diffusion ("critical" capillary PO_2); this is reflected in a minimum end-capillary PO_2 and an increase in net lactic acid production as work rate is increased

above the level at which the "critical" capillary PO_2 is manifest (see Fig. 2-15); (2) the imbalance between the O_2 supply and O_2 requirement causes the proton scavenging mitochondrial membrane proton shuttle (see Fig. 2-1) to lose pace with the rate of $NADH + H^+$ production in the cytosol, resulting in a more-reduced cytosolic redox state; (3) when the redox state is lowered, pyruvate reacts with the increased $NADH + H^+$ and is reduced to lactate while regenerating NAD^+ and allowing glycolysis to continue (*LT*); (4) the accumulating lactic acid is immediately buffered, intracellularly, predominantly by HCO_3^- (see Fig. 2-2), generating additional CO_2; (5) HCO_3^- exchanges for lactate across the muscle cell membrane (see Fig. 2-2), causing arterial blood HCO_3^- to decrease as lactate increases (lactic acidosis threshold or *LAT*) (Fig. 2-21); and (6) the buffering and acid-base disturbances produce predictable changes in gas exchange (Fig. 2-22).

Because the *AT*, *LT*, and *LAT* are all part of the same phenomenon, from a practical point of view making the distinction only distinguishes the method of measurement and does not dispute the underlying mechanism, anaerobic metabolism, common to all three terms. While these terms are commonly used interchangeably, we regard the technically correct definitions to be as follows:

Anaerobic threshold (AT) is the exercise $\dot{V}O_2$ above which anaerobic high-energy PO_4 production supplements aerobic high-energy PO_4 production, with consequential lowering of the cytosolic redox state, increase in the L/P ratio, and a net increase in lactate production at the site of cellular anaerobiosis.

Lactate threshold (LT) is the exercise $\dot{V}O_2$ above

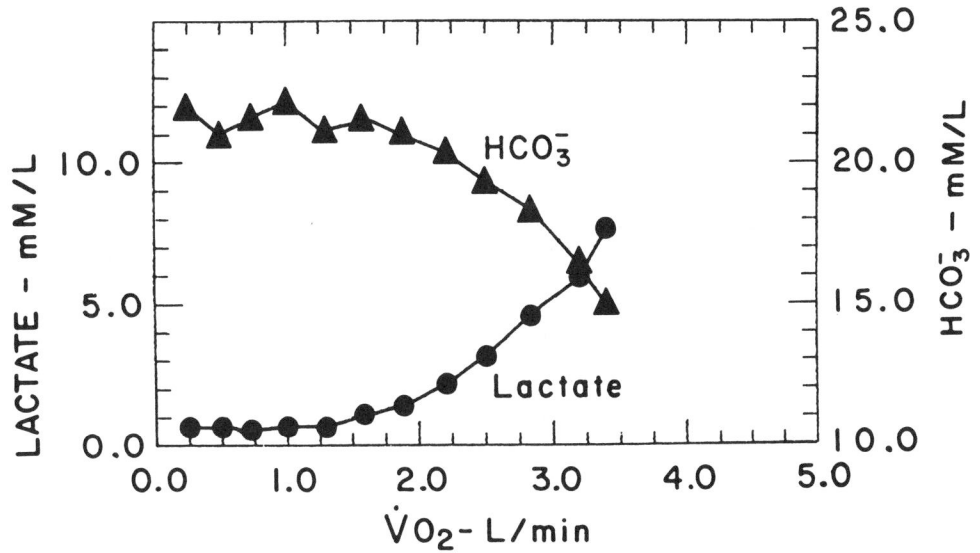

Fig. 2-21. The increase in arterial lactate and the decrease in standard HCO_3^- as related to the increase in O_2 uptake ($\dot{V}O_2$) during a progressively increasing work rate test on a cycle ergometer in a normal subject. (Modified from Wasserman, K., Beaver, W.L., Davis, J.A., Pu, J.-Z., Heber, D., and Whipp, B.J.: Lactate, pyruvate, and lactate-to-pyruvate ratio during exercise and recovery. J. Appl. Physiol., 59: 935–940, 1985.)

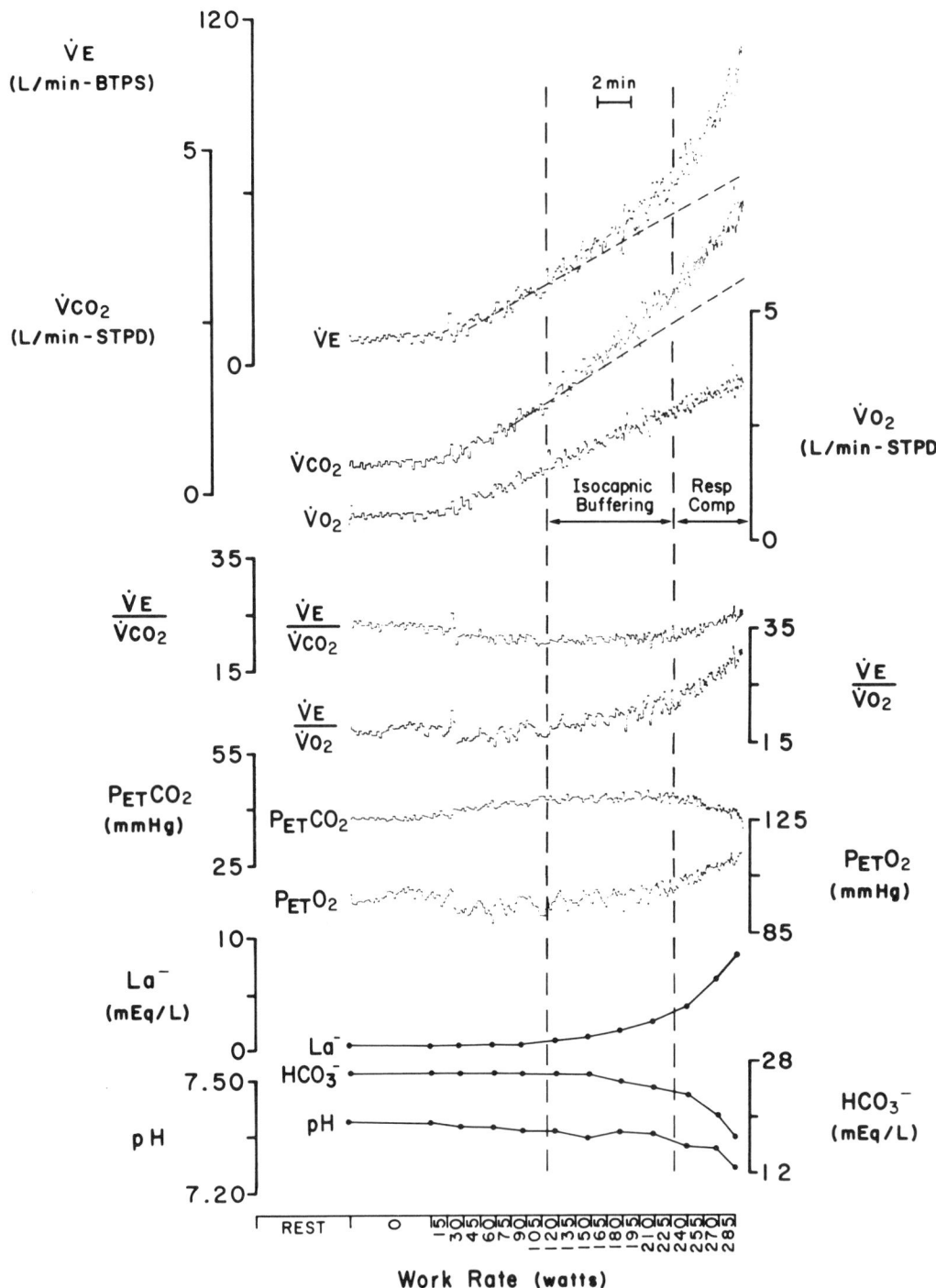

Fig. 2-22. Breath-by-breath measurements of minute ventilation ($\dot{V}E$), CO_2 output ($\dot{V}CO_2$), O_2 uptake ($\dot{V}O_2$), $\dot{V}E/\dot{V}CO_2$, $\dot{V}E/\dot{V}O_2$, PET_{CO_2}, PET_{O_2}, arterial lactate and bicarbonate, and pH for a 1-minute incremental exercise test on a cycle ergometer. The *LT* occurs when lactate increases (left vertical dashed line). This is accompanied by a fall in HCO_3^- (*LAT*) and generally an increase in $\dot{V}E/\dot{V}O_2$. "Isocapnic buffering" refers to the period when $\dot{V}E$ and $\dot{V}CO_2$ increase curvilinearly at the same rate without an increase in $\dot{V}E/\dot{V}CO_2$, thus retaining a constant PET_{CO_2}. After the period of isocapnic buffering, PET_{CO_2} decreases and $\dot{V}E/\dot{V}CO_2$ increases, reflecting ventilatory compensation for the metabolic acidosis of exercise.

which a net increase in lactate production is observed to result in a sustained increase in lactate concentration in the circulating blood.

Lactic acidosis threshold (LAT) is the exercise $\dot{V}O_2$ above which arterial Std HCO_3^- (the principal buffer of lactic acid) is observed to decrease because of a net increase in lactate production. During an incremental exercise test, this can be detected by an increase in CO_2 output above that which would be predicted from aerobic metabolism (because of dissociation of HCO_3^- as it buffers lactic acid).

EFFECT OF BUFFERING LACTIC ACID ON GAS EXCHANGE

Figure 2-22 shows the effect of an increasing work rate on ventilation and gas exchange for a cycle ergometer exercise test in which the work rate was incremented in 1-minute intervals, after a 4-minute warm-up period of pedalling without load. As the work rate is increased, $\dot{V}O_2$, $\dot{V}CO_2$, and $\dot{V}E$ rapidly enter a region in which they increase linearly until the exercise lactic acidosis develops. At work rates above the *LAT*, CO_2 output increases more rapidly than O_2 uptake because CO_2 generated by the bicarbonate buffering of lactic acid is added to the metabolic CO_2 production. This is the basis of the V-slope plot for measuring the AT^{66} (described later). Initially, $\dot{V}E$ increases proportionally with the increased CO_2 output (isocapnic buffering). Thus, $\dot{V}E$ retains a constant relationship with $\dot{V}CO_2$ ($\dot{V}E/\dot{V}CO_2$ appears constant or decreases slightly) while it increases relative to $\dot{V}O_2$ ($\dot{V}E/\dot{V}O_2$ increases) just above the *LAT* (Fig. 2-22). As the work rate is incremented further, $\dot{V}E$ starts to increase even more rapidly than CO_2 output (increase in $\dot{V}E/\dot{V}CO_2$), causing Pa_{CO_2} and PET_{CO_2} to decrease, thereby providing ventilatory compensation for the exercise-induced lactic acidosis. The increased hydrogen ion concentration stimulates arterial chemoreceptors, primarily the carotid

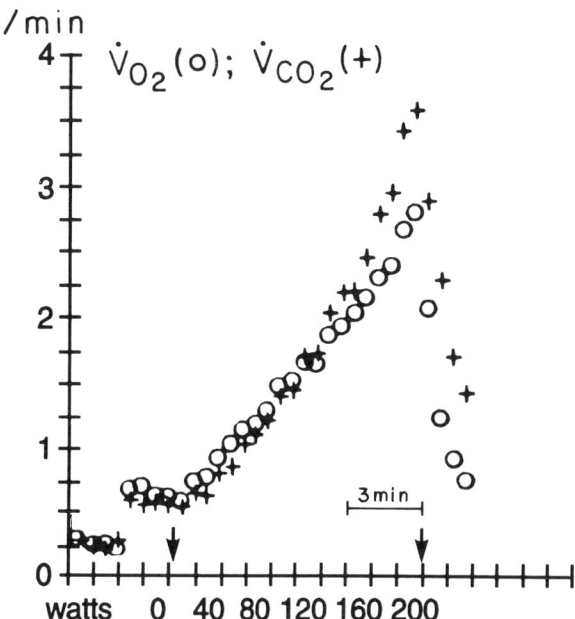

FIG. 2-23. $\dot{V}CO_2$ and $\dot{V}O_2$ as related to work rate for a 1-minute incremental (20 W/min) cycle ergometer exercise test. $\dot{V}CO_2$ starts to increase more steeply than $\dot{V}O_2$ as work rate is increased in the middle work rate range, reflecting buffering of lactic acid above the lactic acidosis threshold.

bodies, to increase ventilatory drive.[34] This mechanism reduces arterial P_{CO_2} and provides partial ventilatory compensation for the metabolic acidosis.[67] As seen in Figure 2-22, a major additional ventilatory drive (the nonlinear component of the $\dot{V}E$ increase) accompanies the metabolic acidosis. Table 2-1 contrasts the exercise responses for exercise above and below the *AT*.

Figure 2-2 shows the effect of buffering the cellular lactic acidosis with HCO_3^- on $\dot{V}CO_2$ relative to $\dot{V}O_2$. How $\dot{V}O_2$ and $\dot{V}CO_2$ increase as a function of work rate, as it is progressively increased, is shown in Figure 2-23. Plotting $\dot{V}CO_2$ as a function of $\dot{V}O_2$ (V-slope plot), from the results of a progressively increasing work rate test, demonstrates a break-point with a change in slope from slightly less than 1 to greater than 1 (Fig. 2-24). This slope

TABLE 2-1. *Differences in Response to Exercise for Constant Work Rates Below and Above the Anaerobic Threshold (AT)*

MEASUREMENT	BELOW *AT*	ABOVE *AT*
Exercise duration	Prolonged; limited by muscular and skeletal trauma or substrate, fluid balance, thermoregulation	Reduced; limited by "fatigue" or dyspnea
$\dot{V}O_2$, time to steady-state	< 3 min	> 3 min; steady-state may not occur
$\dot{V}CO_2$, time to steady-state	< 4 min	< 4 min
$\dot{V}E$, time to steady-state	< 4 min	> 4 min; steady-state usually does not occur
Pa_{CO_2}	constant	decreasing
pHa	approx. 7.4	metabolic acidosis

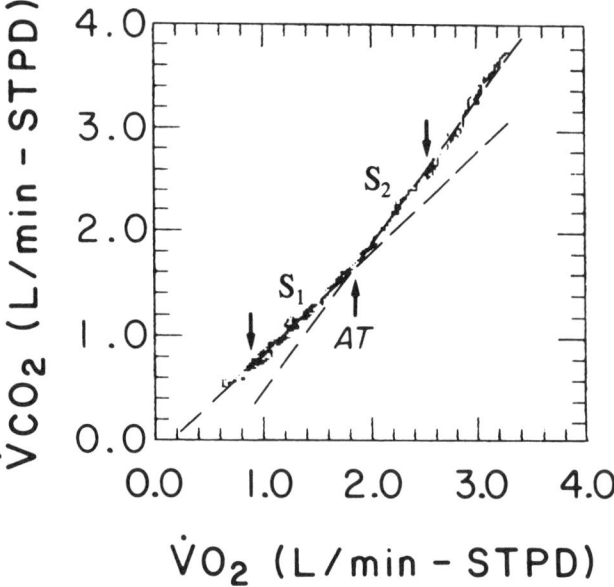

FIG. 2-24. CO_2 output ($\dot{V}CO_2$) as a function of oxygen uptake ($\dot{V}O_2$) during a progressively increasing work rate test demonstrating the transition from aerobic metabolism, in which $\dot{V}CO_2$ increases linearly with $\dot{V}O_2$ with a slope (S_1) slightly less than 1, to anaerobic plus aerobic metabolism, where the slope increases to a value greater than 1 (S_2). The steeper S_2 reflects the production of additional CO_2 from HCO_3^- buffering of lactic acid over that produced by aerobic metabolism. The intercept of S_1 and S_2 is the lactic acidosis threshold (*LAT*). Hyperventilation does not occur at the *LAT* during a progressively increasing work rate test and therefore does not contribute to the steepening of S_2. The lower downward arrow indicates where CO_2 stores are no longer increasing and calculation of S_1 starts. The upper downward arrow indicates the $\dot{V}O_2$ above which hyperventilation in response to metabolic acidosis starts. S_1 and S_2 are calculated from the data between these two arrows. (Modified from Beaver, W.L., Wasserman, K., and Whipp, B.J.: A new method for detecting the anaerobic threshold by gas exchange. J. Appl. Physiol., 60: 2020–2027, 1986.)

transition coincides with the *LAT* and is slightly higher than the *LT* for the reasons described in the section of this chapter on mechanisms of buffering the exercise-induced lactic acidosis.[66] The slope of the increase in $\dot{V}CO_2$ relative to $\dot{V}O_2$ below the threshold (S_1 in Fig. 2-24) has an average value of .95 with a small variation.[10,11] The transition to a slope greater than 1 (S_2 in Fig. 2-24) occurs, on average, in the mid-range of a healthy subject's aerobic capacity.

The intercept of S_1 and S_2 is the *LAT*, measured by gas exchange, and estimates the *AT*. The term *LAT* describes the biochemical event that causes the $\dot{V}CO_2$ versus $\dot{V}O_2$ slope to exceed 1, although the underlying mechanism is the lactic acidosis resulting from exercise above the *AT*. Hyperventilation (reduction in Pa_{CO_2} and increase in $\dot{V}E/\dot{V}CO_2$) rarely occurs at the *LAT*. As shown in Figure 2-22, when hyperventilation does occur during a progressively increasing work rate test, it does so at a higher $\dot{V}O_2$ (at the upper, downward directed arrow in Fig. 2-24). S_2 being steeper than 1 during the progressively increasing work rate test signifies that CO_2 is being released from cell HCO_3^- as it dissociates during the buffering of lactic acid (see Fig. 2-2).

S_1 has been found not to vary with the rate of increase in work rate.[10] S_2 becomes steeper the faster the work rate increase[10], however, presumably because of the faster rate of lactate formation relative to $\dot{V}O_2$ increase. The only factor that we have found to affect S_1 is glycogen depletion.[10] S_1 becomes more shallow under this condition, consistent with the lower respiratory quotient of the metabolic substrate. Figure 2-25 shows the simultaneous changes in arterial lactate, HCO_3^-, and CO_2 output as a function of $\dot{V}O_2$ during an incremental work rate test.

PHYSIOLOGIC CONSEQUENCES OF WORK ABOVE THE ANAEROBIC THRESHOLD

Table 2-1 contrasts the exercise responses for work above and below the *AT*. The *AT* appears to be the best discriminator of the highest work rate that can be endured for a prolonged period. Thus, a task performed below the *AT* can be sustained with relatively little stress to the subject. A task performed above the *AT* cannot be sustained as long as one performed below the *AT*; the higher the blood lactate in response to a constant work rate, the less is its tolerable duration (see Fig. 2-10). This is especially the case for work rates at which lactate continues to increase throughout the work.

Important functional adaptations affect mitochondrial O_2 supply when lactate accumulates. These include (1) vasodilatation in the vascular bed[68] and (2) a shift of the oxyhemoglobin dissociation curve to the right allowing O_2 to unload more readily from hemoglobin and O_2 extraction to increase.[69] Both mechanisms act locally to compensate for the O_2 availability-requirement imbalance.

Whereas net lactate production, through its H^+, stimulates breathing and may induce dyspnea in the ventilatorily limited subject, it may benefit the subject performing high-intensity exercise by facilitating oxyhemoglobin dissociation, thereby allowing increased O_2 extraction from blood.

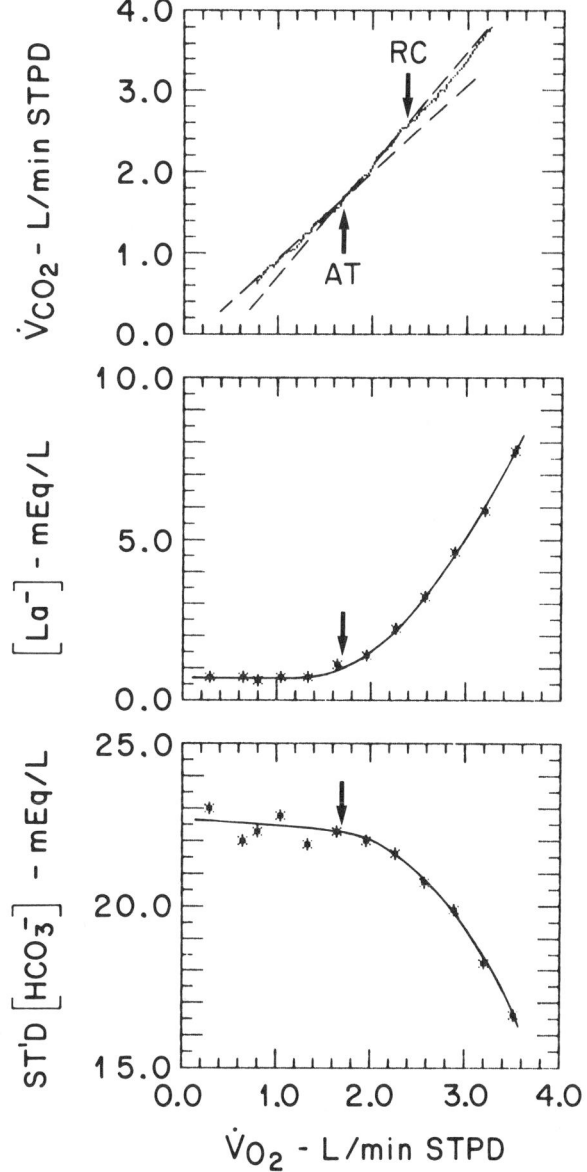

FIG. 2-25. Plots of arterial lactate and standard HCO_3^- concentrations and $\dot{V}CO_2$ as a function of $\dot{V}O_2$ for a single subject. Arrows indicate estimates of the anaerobic threshold (*AT*) from the $\dot{V}CO_2$ versus $\dot{V}O_2$ plot, which are seen to also represent reasonable estimates of lactate increase and HCO_3^- decrease versus $\dot{V}O_2$.

ESSENTIAL ROLE PLAYED BY LACTIC ACID DURING EXERCISE

A.V. Hill and associates[70] related blood lactate increase and subsequent removal of the O_2 debt. When the mechanism for glycolysis was worked out, and the recognition that three ATP molecules were generated from ADP during the anaerobic metabolism of one glycosyl component of glycogen to two lactate molecules,[71] it was generally appreciated that this mechanism spared molecular O_2. Perhaps the most important role that net lactic

acid accumulation plays during exercise, however, is in facilitating the dissociation of oxyhemoglobin, allowing the arterial-venous O_2 difference to increase normally when one performs heavy intensity work.

Earlier, we pointed out that capillary PO_2 reached a "critical" (floor) value at about the middle of a healthy subject's exercise capacity. Thus, further dissociation of oxyhemoglobin at work rates from the subject's middle to maximum work capacity does not take place by decreasing PO_2; it is approximately at this work rate that lactic acidosis develops. This would allow further oxyhemoglobin dissociation by the Bohr effect for exercise intensities above the *AT*.

Figure 2-26 illustrates the average of data from five subjects who exercised for 6 minutes at two work rates, the lower one just below the subject's *AT* and the higher one at a work rate above the *AT*. The femoral vein PO_2 values decreased to the same level (about 20 mm Hg) for both exercise intensities, showing that this is the critical capillary PO_2. Oxyhemoglobin saturation continues to decrease, however. The continued decrease in oxyhemoglobin saturation was parallel to and totally accounted for by the decrease in pH. It would therefore appear that because a critical capillary PO_2 is reached when one performs moderate work, it would not be possible to perform heavy work without a lactic acidosis. This may account for the marked exercise limitation of patients with McArdle's syndrome,[72] as well as the abnormally small oxyhemoglobin extraction in these patients.[73]

In the capillary, therefore, oxyhemoglobin dissociation during exercise depends primarily on two factors, decreasing PO_2 and increasing H^+. The first appears to play a more important role in oxyhemoglobin dissociation below the *LAT*, whereas the second has a major role above it (Fig. 2-27). By facilitating the unloading of O_2 from hemoglobin without reducing the capillary PO_2, the driving force for the mass flow of O_2 into the mitochondria is maintained. H^+ from lactic acid formation thus serves as a feedback adaptation to tissue hypoxia.

The biochemical interactions between capillary blood and muscle cell for optimizing the O_2 supply to mitochondria during heavy exercise are illustrated in Figure 2-28. At the arterial end of the capillary, oxyhemoglobin dissociates as the muscle consumes O_2, thereby reducing capillary PO_2. As PO_2 reaches its lower limit ("critical" capillary PO_2) for diffusion toward the venous end of the

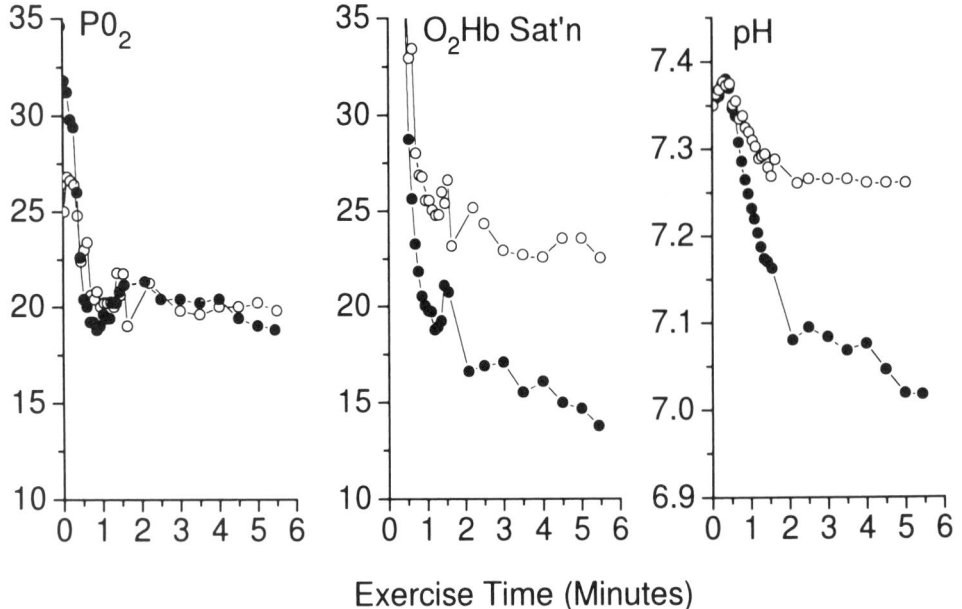

FIG. 2-26. Femoral venous P_{O_2}, oxyhemoglobin (HbO_2) saturation, and pH as related to time of exercise for two constant work rate tests, one below (open circles) and one above (solid circles) the lactic acidosis threshold (*LAT*). The data are the average of five subjects. The below and above *LAT* work rates averaged 113 and 265 W, respectively. Note that HbO_2 saturation is lower during the higher intensity exercise despite identical P_{O_2} values. This is related to the Bohr shift resulting from the lower pH in the high-intensity test. (From Stringer, W., Casaburi, R., French, W., Porszasz, J., and Wasserman, K.: The role of pH in maintaining muscle capillary P_{O_2} during heavy exercise. Am. Rev. Respir. Dis., 145:A881, 1992.)

capillary, lactic acid starts to increase in the cell. Capillary blood H^+ quickly increases because the lactic acid-producing cells produce extra CO_2 from HCO_3^- dissociation as well as CO_2 from aerobic metabolism. Simultaneously, capillary blood HCO_3^- is consumed (Fig. 2-28). Although the intracellular buffering of lactic acid by HCO_3^- minimizes the change in cell pH, it acidifies blood more

quickly than if a non-HCO_3^- buffer were to neutralize the cellular lactic acidosis. This is a most remarkable physiologic mechanism because the Bohr effect would not work as well with any other buffer. Thus, the lactic acidosis-facilitated oxyhemoglobin dissociation ensures a higher blood O_2 extraction and therefore a higher maximal $\dot{V}_{O_2}$ than would otherwise be possible.

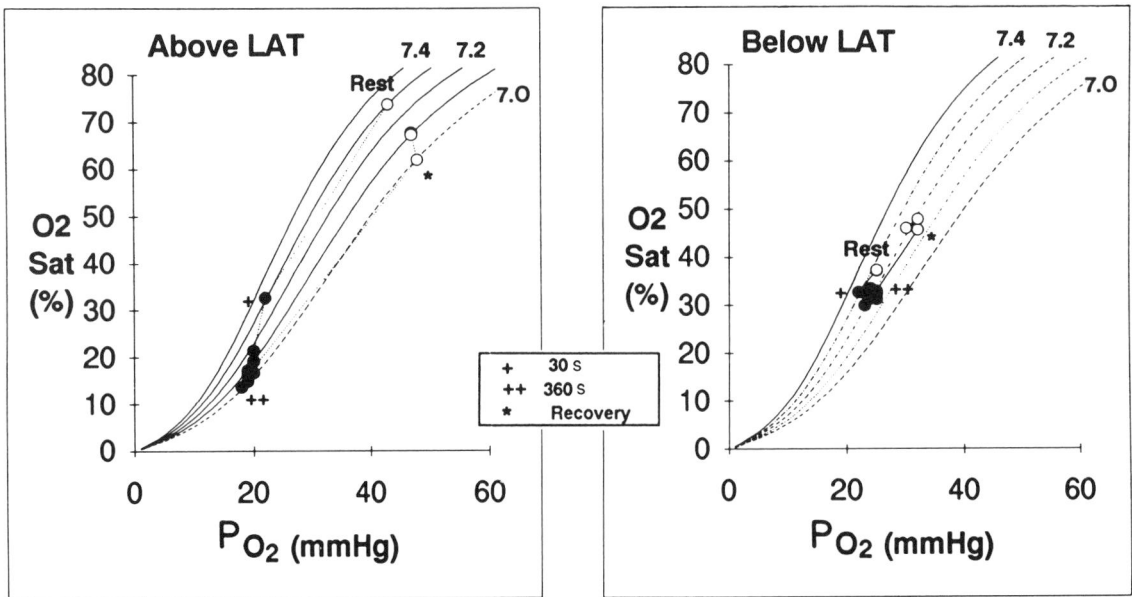

FIG. 2-27. Femoral vein oxyhemoglobin saturation, measured by co-oximetry, versus P_{O_2}, plotted on the lower part of the oxyhemoglobin dissociation curve (calculated from equations reported in reference 122), for a below and above lactic acidosis threshold (*LAT*) work rate for a normal subject. The measured pH agreed closely with the pH values indicated by the pH isopleths. Open circles represent rest and recovery values. (Data from Stringer, W., Casaburi, R., French, W., Porszasz, J., and Wasserman, K.: The role of pH in maintaining muscle capillary P_{O_2} during heavy exercise. Am. Rev. Respir. Dis., 145:A881, 1992.)

Metabolic-Cardiovascular-Ventilatory Coupling

ROLE OF CELLULAR RESPIRATION IN REGENERATING HIGH-ENERGY PHOSPHATE

Because increased rates of chemical energy utilization, in the form of high-energy phosphate ($\sim PO_4$), are needed for the muscle contraction of exercise, cellular O_2 consumption ($\dot{Q}O_2$) must increase in proportion to the rate of $\sim PO_4$ production needed to rephosphorylate ADP to sustain exercise, after the early utilization of creatine $\sim PO_4$ and O_2 stores. Creatine $\sim PO_4$ concentration rapidly decreases in proportion to the work rate performed,[74] and its concentration remains reduced as the work is sustained, returning to the pre-exercise resting level within the first few minutes of recovery.

The cardiovascular and the ventilatory systems have evolved to respond to the increased cellular O_2 requirement and to remove the major by-product of muscle bioenergetics, CO_2. Therefore, transfer of CO_2 and O_2 between the mitochondria and the outside environment requires a finely coordinated interaction of cardiovascular and ventilatory mechanisms geared to cellular metabolic activity.

A scheme describing the gas transport mechanisms for coupling cellular (internal) to pulmonary (external) respiration is shown in Figure 1-1. When exercise is initiated, high-energy phosphate bonds of pre-existing ATP split to support the immediate energy requirements of muscle contraction. The resulting ADP is rapidly rephosphorylated to ATP from creatine phosphate and the conversion of substrate energy to chemical energy ($\sim PO_4$), primarily in muscle mitochondria. Experimental evidence suggests that the increases in concentration of creatine, inorganic phosphate, and ADP in the muscle stimulate oxidative phosphorylation, thereby replenishing ATP.[46] This keeps the ATP relatively constant during exercise as the metabolic requirement approaches the subject's maximal exercise capacity. Only as maximal work rates are approached does ATP start to decrease and the less phosphorylated adenosine compounds increase.[44]

CARDIOVASCULAR TRANSPORT FUNCTION: OXYGEN SUPPLY

Cardiac output is increased at the start of exercise by increasing stroke volume and heart rate. Increased cardiac inotropy and increased venous re-

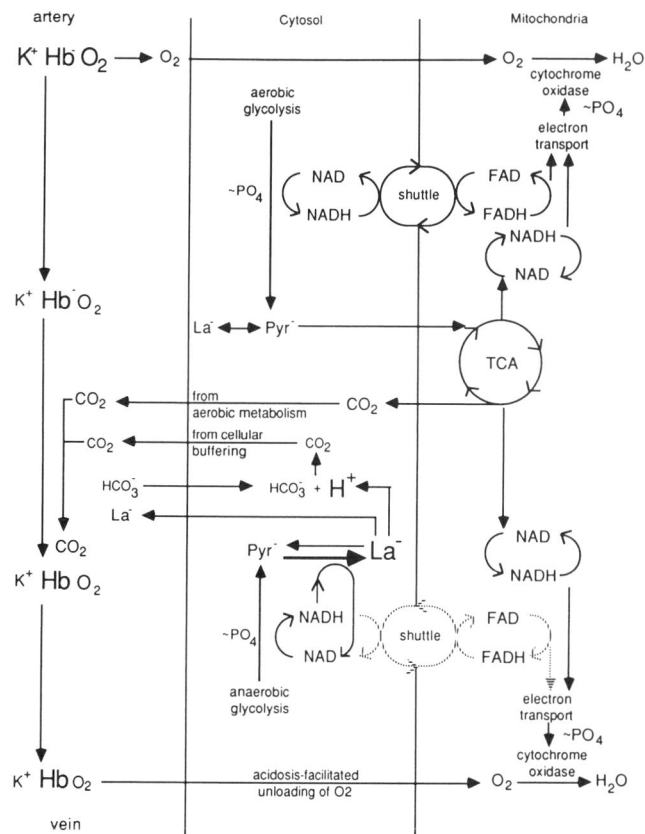

FIG. 2-28. Scheme dictating the changes in capillary oxyhemoglobin (HbO_2) saturation during transit from artery to vein during heavy intensity exercise. At the arterial end of the capillary, HbO_2 dissociates primarily because of a decrease in PO_2 as glycolysis proceeds aerobically, without increasing lactate, because the mitochondrial membrane proton shuttle regulates the cytosolic redox state (NADH/NAD). CO_2 is produced from aerobic metabolism, simultaneously, causing a reduction in pH, allowing further HbO_2 dissociation (Bohr effect). As the blood approaches the venous end of the capillary where the PO_2 is critically low (a PO_2 "floor"), the mitochondrial membrane proton shuttle fails to reoxidize NADH to NAD at an adequate rate. Thus, NADH/NAD increases, and accordingly, pyruvate is converted to lactate in proportion to the change in cell redox state. The effect is an increase in anaerobic glycolysis and cell lactate with a stoichiometric increase in hydrogen ion. The latter is immediately buffered by the bicarbonate buffer system in the cell, causing the consumption of cellular bicarbonate in proportion to the rate of lactate accumulation and additional cellular production of CO_2 to acidify the capillary blood further. In addition, the decreasing cellular HCO_3^- and increasing cellular lactate result in an intracellular-extracellular lactate and HCO_3^- exchange, as described in Figure 2-2. The sum of aerobically produced CO_2 and anaerobically produced CO_2 from HCO_3^- buffering of lactic acid, along with the decreasing blood bicarbonate, further acidifies the blood. This results in further Bohr effect dissociation of HbO_2. The lactic acidosis-facilitated dissociation of HbO_2 allows aerobic metabolism to proceed at a rate proportional to the rate of acidification of the blood and does not require a further reduction in capillary PO_2.

turn, secondary to external compression of veins by contracting muscles, increase stroke volume at the start of exercise.[75] As exercise continues, further increase in cardiac output is accomplished predominantly by increasing heart rate.

The pulmonary vascular bed dilates at the start of exercise in concert with the increase in right ventricular output and pulmonary artery pressure. This dilatation results in the perfusion of previously unperfused and underperfused lung units in the normal pulmonary vascular bed. A low pulmonary vascular resistance is essential for the normal exercise response of the left ventricle because, without it, the weakly muscled right ventricle could not readily pump the increased venous return through the pulmonary circulation to the left side of the heart to effect a normal cardiac output increase.

Because the cardiac output increase is disproportionately small compared to the increase in $\dot{V}O_2$, the extraction of O_2 from and the addition of CO_2 to the capillary blood by the muscles increase. Muscle blood flow increases in the muscle units with the highest metabolic activity.[76] Thus, the regional increase in blood flow appears to be matched to the increase in metabolic activity. Consequently, it is possible to extract over 85% of the O_2 going through the capillary bed of maximally working muscle.

The O_2 supply to the cells depends on five factors: (1) the partial pressure profile of O_2 in the capillary blood; (2) the hemoglobin concentration; (3) the cardiac output; (4) the distribution of perfusion to the tissues in need of O_2; and (5) the hemoglobin's affinity for O_2. The transport of O_2 from blood to mitochondria is dependent on maintaining an adequate diffusion gradient for O_2 as the blood travels through the contracting muscle. The PO_2 gradient at the arterial end of the capillary is high, but it decreases as it approaches the venous end, depending on the O_2 flow/metabolic rate ratio (see Fig. 2-14). Because the metabolic rate increases more than the O_2 flow, the venous O_2 content decreases during exercise, although its partial pressure may be maintained by a rightward shift of the oxyhemoglobin dissociation curve because of developing acidosis in the capillary (see Figs. 2-26 and 2-27).

Arterial PO_2

Mean arterial PO_2 (Pa_{O_2}) is a function of mean alveolar PO_2 (PA_{O_2}). For an idealized lung (all lung units having the same ventilation/perfusion ratio) where the gas exchange ratio is 0.8 and the Pa_{CO_2} is equal to 40, PA_{O_2} would equal approximately 100 mm Hg at sea level. Reductions in Pa_{O_2} relative to the ideal PA_{O_2} are due to one or more of the following mechanisms: (1) a right to

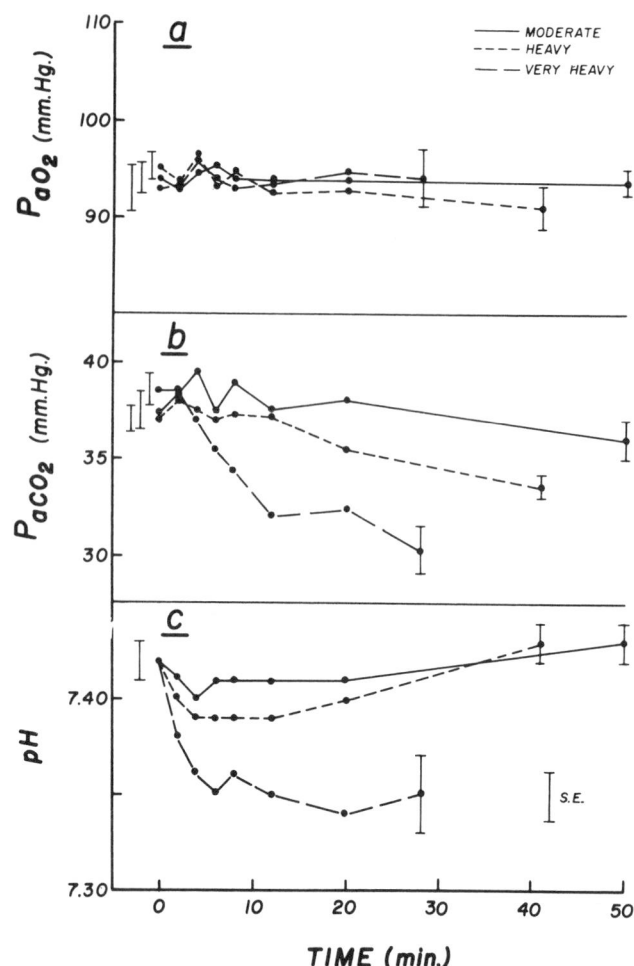

FIG. 2-29. Effect of prolonged constant work rate exercise of moderate, heavy, and very heavy work intensity on arterial blood gases and pH. Each point is the average of 10 subjects. (From Wasserman, K., VanKessel, A.L., and Burton, G.B.: Interaction of physiological mechanisms during exercise. J. Appl. Physiol., 22:71–85, 1967.)

left shunt; (2) O_2 diffusion disequilibrium at the alveolar-capillary interface; and (3) maldistribution of alveolar ventilation ($\dot{V}A$) with respect to lung perfusion ($\dot{Q}$). Normally, Pa_{O_2} is about 90 mm Hg (Fig. 2-29), and $P(A-a)_{O_2}$ is approximately 10 to 20 mm Hg during exercise.[33] This normal difference between the alveolar and arterial PO_2 is due to a small right to left shunt (possibly the thebesian blood vessels in the heart and the bronchial circulation) and the lack of total uniformity of $\dot{V}A/\dot{Q}$ within the lung. In highly fit subjects, however, diffusion impairments have also been demonstrated at high work rates.

Hemoglobin and Arterial O_2 Content

The arterial O_2 content depends on the arterial PO_2 and hemoglobin concentration. Because anemia results in a decreased blood O_2 content, it can compromise the supply of O_2 to the tissues during exercise. Any hemoglobin that is inactive (methemoglobin) or has carbon monoxide on the O_2-binding sites (as in cigarette smokers) also results in a reduced O_2 content. All the foregoing conditions result in a more rapid decrease in capillary P_{O_2} than normal, and the minimal capillary P_{O_2} needed for diffusion would occur earlier in the capillary for a given metabolic rate, or the blood flow/metabolic rate ratio of the muscle ($\dot{Q}m/\dot{V}_{O_2}m$) must increase.

Cardiac Output

The cardiac output obviously plays a key role in the O_2 supply to the cells. At the start of exercise in the upright posture, stroke volume increases virtually immediately,[77] the magnitude depending on the relative degree of the individual's fitness, age, and size.[75] In the exceptionally fit young person, the stroke volume can increase by as much as 100%; the increase is much smaller in less fit and elderly people. Further increases in cardiac output come about predominantly by increasing heart rate, i.e., heart rate usually increases linearly with $\dot{V}_{O_2}$. Although the stroke volume does not change after its initial increase or changes only slightly, the pattern of change in cardiac output with work rate can be inferred from the changing heart rate. The wide variation of absolute stroke volume among subjects of different fitness levels, however, precludes estimating the magnitude of the cardiac output change from heart rate measurements.

Distribution of Peripheral Blood Flow

During exercise, the fraction of the cardiac output diverted to the skeletal muscles increases, whereas the fraction perfusing organs such as the kidney, liver, and gastrointestinal tract decreases.[75] As the work rate is increased, the fraction of the cardiac output perfusing the exercising muscles normally increases. This redistribution in perfusion is apparently controlled by the autonomic nervous system and local metabolic factors such as increased $[H^+]$, P_{CO_2}, $[K^+]$, osmolarity, adenosine, temperature, and P_{O_2}.[68]

A useful noninvasive measurement for assessing perfusion redistribution is the $\dot{V}_{O_2}$/heart rate ratio (O_2-pulse). The O_2-pulse, calculated by dividing two noninvasive measurements, is equal to the product of stroke volume and arterial-mixed venous O_2 content difference ($C(a\text{-}\bar{v})_{O_2}$) as shown from analysis of the components of the Fick principle for cardiac output:

$$\text{cardiac output} = \dot{V}_{O_2}/C(a\text{-}\bar{v})_{O_2}$$

if heart rate (HR) $\times$ stroke volume (SV) is substituted for cardiac output in the foregoing equation, then:

$$\text{HR} \times \text{SV} = \dot{V}_{O_2}/C(a\text{-}\bar{v})_{O_2}$$

or, rearranging:

$$\dot{V}_{O_2}/\text{HR} = \text{SV} \times C(a\text{-}\bar{v})_{O_2}$$

The O_2-pulse is the amount of O_2 removed from each stroke volume. When both stroke volume and $C(a\text{-}\bar{v})_{O_2}$ reach their maxima, O_2 pulse will reach its maximum.

Oxyhemoglobin Dissociation in Tissue

The essential role of the Bohr effect on oxyhemoglobin dissociation was discussed earlier. Other factors considered here affect oxyhemoglobin dissociation.

Altered hemoglobin affinity for O_2, seen with abnormal hemoglobin or with altered acid-base balance, has little effect on arterial blood O_2 content in the patient with normal lungs at sea level. The position of the steep part of the oxyhemoglobin dissociation curve, commonly quantified by the P_{O_2} at an oxyhemoglobin saturation of 50% (P_{50}), affects the P_{O_2} for a given oxyhemoglobin saturation in the tissue capillaries, however. Genetic defects causing a shift of the oxyhemoglobin dissociation curve to the left (low P_{50}) can impair O_2 extraction by the exercising muscle because a "floor" P_{O_2} for diffusion is reached at a relatively high oxyhemoglobin saturation. This may induce polycythemia.[78] Hemoglobinopathies that shift oxyhemoglobin dissociation to the right (high P_{50}) allow O_2 to unload from hemoglobin more readily and are associated with anemia.[78] Shifts in P_{50} are common even in normal subjects. A rightward shift resulting from acidosis, increased temperature, or high levels of 2,3-diphosphoglycerate (2,3-DPG) favors diffusion of O_2 from the capillaries into the mitochondria. This contrasts with the leftward shift resulting from alkalosis, increased carboxyhemoglobin, or low 2,3-DPG concentration, where the O_2 diffusion gradient is reduced.

VENTILATORY COUPLING TO METABOLISM

The blood passing through the lungs must be rearterialized by: (1) eliminating the added CO_2; (2) replenishing O_2; and (3) achieving pH homeostasis. Minute ventilation ($\dot{V}E$) normally increases at a rate required to remove the added CO_2. In fact, the $\dot{V}E$ increase is generally so precise that arterial P_{CO_2} and pH are usually regulated at close to resting values throughout moderate exercise levels.[34] Above the *AT*, the metabolic acidosis stimulates ventilation further. At low and moderate work rates, the ventilatory increase is usually accomplished primarily by an increase in tidal volume and, to a lesser degree, breathing frequency (Fig. 2-30). Breathing frequency increases more significantly at work rates above the *AT*.

Carbon Dioxide Elimination

Like O_2 consumption, CO_2 production increases during exercise because of the increase in metabolic activity of the exercising muscles. The amount of CO_2 generated by this process is related to O_2 consumption by the RQ of the muscle substrate. As previously described, additional CO_2 is derived from bicarbonate buffering of lactic acid at work rates above the *AT*.

In contrast to tissue O_2 supply, the actual cardiac output needed for CO_2 elimination is not critical. CO_2 elimination is determined by the alveolar ventilation and the arterial (ideal alveolar) P_{CO_2} (Fig. 2-31). The cardiac output does determine the venous-arterial CO_2 content difference $C(\bar{v}\text{-a})_{CO_2}$ for a given metabolic (exercise) activity, however. The CO_2 content for a given venous (tissue) P_{CO_2} strongly depends on changes in buffer base and, to a lesser degree, on the O_2 content (Christiansen-Douglas-Haldane effect).[79] The O_2 content changes most in the lower work rate range (below the *AT*), whereas changes in buffer base are most pronounced in the heavy intensity range (above the *AT*) because of HCO_3^- buffering of lactic acid. Because these factors affect the position of the CO_2 dissociation curve, this compromises the accurate determination of the cardiac output from estimates of mixed venous P_{CO_2}, as is often done.

Determinants of the Ventilatory Requirement

The quantity of ventilation required to clear a given amount of CO_2 from the blood ($\dot{V}_{CO_2}$) depends on the CO_2 concentration in the alveolar gas ($F_{A_{CO_2}} = P_{A_{CO_2}}/P_B$). Mass balance considerations dictate that, in an idealized lung (gas concentrations are the same in all alveolar spaces because of uniform $\dot{V}A/\dot{Q}$), $\dot{V}_{CO_2} = \dot{V}A \times P_{A_{CO_2}}/P_B$. This is the alveolar ventilation equation in which $\dot{V}A$ represents the theoretic alveolar ventilation required for maximally efficient lungs to regulate Pa_{CO_2} (ideal alveolar P_{CO_2}) at a given $\dot{V}_{CO_2}$. This important relationship is plotted in Figure 2-31.

Not all respired air effectively ventilates the lungs because some must go to the conducting airways, uninvolved in gas exchange, and some to the nonperfused alveoli. The wasted fraction of the tidal volume (V_T) from the point of view of gas exchange, or the fraction of the tidal volume

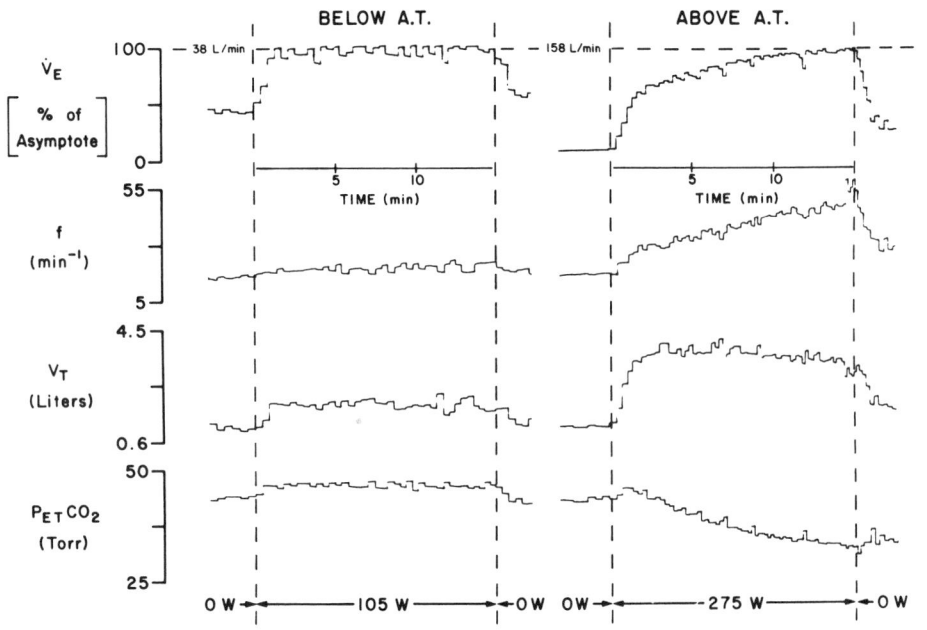

FIG. 2-30. Minute ventilation ($\dot{V}E$) plotted as a percentage of its asymptotic value, tidal volume (V_T), breathing rate (f), and end-tidal P_{CO_2} ($P_{ET_{CO_2}}$) for exercise below and above the anaerobic threshold in the same subject. The absolute values of minute ventilation are shown to the left of the vertical dashed line at the transition from unloaded cycling (0 W) to the indicated work rate. For the work rate below the anaerobic threshold, $\dot{V}E$, f, V_T, and $P_{ET_{CO_2}}$ reach a constant value after several minutes. For the work rate above the anaerobic threshold, $\dot{V}E$ and f continue to drift upward and $P_{ET_{CO_2}}$ downward (without a significant change or slight decrease in V_T), signifying the lack of ventilatory steady-state.

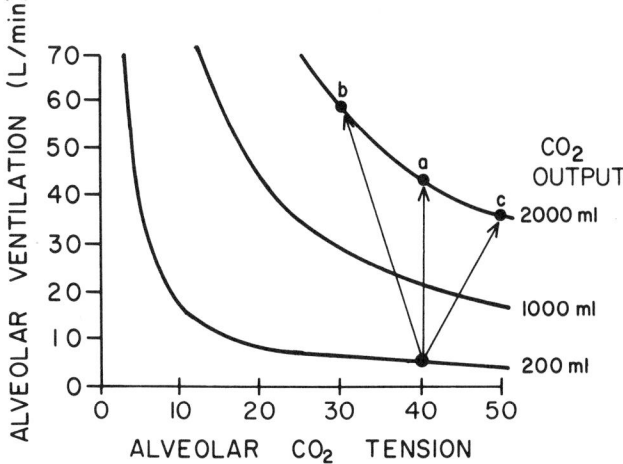

FIG. 2-31. Effect of changing arterial (ideal alveolar) P_{CO_2} during exercise on alveolar ventilation. The point on the CO_2 output isopleth of 200 ml/min represents the normal resting value. Points a, b, and c illustrate the alveolar ventilation for isocapnia, hypocapnia (-10 mm Hg), and hypercapnia ($+10$ mm Hg) for an exercise CO_2 output of 2000 ml/min. (From Wasserman, K.: Breathing during exercise. N. Engl. J. Med., 298:780–785, 1978.)

that is physiologic dead space (V_D), determines the difference between the actual volume of air respired during breathing ($\dot{V}_E$) and the theoretic alveolar ventilation, i.e., $\dot{V}_A = \dot{V}_E (1 - V_D/V_T)$. To determine the $\dot{V}_E$ needed to eliminate a given quantity of CO_2, substitute $\dot{V}_E (1 - V_D/V_T)$ for $\dot{V}_A$ in the alveolar ventilation equation given in the preceding paragraph and solve for $\dot{V}_E$. The resulting equation is:

$$\dot{V}_E \ (BTPS) = \frac{863 \times \dot{V}_{CO_2} \ (STPD)}{Pa_{CO_2} \times (1 - V_D/V_T)}$$

where 863 is the product of the barometric pressure, temperature, and water vapor correction, factors needed to express $\dot{V}_E$ at BTPS (body temperature, ambient pressure, saturated), $\dot{V}_{CO_2}$ at STPD (standard temperature and pressure, dry), and CO_2 as a partial pressure. From this equation it is evident that the quantity of breathing required for exercise is defined by three factors: (1) the $\dot{V}_{CO_2}$; (2) the level or *set-point* at which Pa_{CO_2} is regulated by the ventilatory control mechanisms; and (3) the V_D/V_T ratio. The influences of these three factors on $\dot{V}_E$ are illustrated in Figure 2-32. At work rates above the *AT*, $\dot{V}_E$ and $\dot{V}_A$ increase nonlinearly and steeply as $\dot{V}_{CO_2}$ increases because of the added ventilatory drive caused by metabolic acidosis. The quantitative interactions among $\dot{V}_{O_2}$, R, Pa_{CO_2}, V_D/V_T, and $\dot{V}_E$ are illustrated in Figure 2-33.

Acid-Base Regulation

Figures 2-18 and 2-19 show the acid-base changes in response to constant work rates of moderate, heavy, and very heavy intensity exercise. Because the end-products of the bioenergetic pathways for generating the $\sim PO_4$ for muscle contraction are acids, the volatile carbonic and the non-volatile lactic acid, ventilation must respond to this acid load if pH homeostasis of body fluids is to be preserved. Characteristically, below the *AT*, the arterial pH is regulated at resting levels or becomes slightly acid because of a small increase in Pa_{CO_2}.[67] For exercise above *AT*, the acidosis becomes more marked because of the net increase in lactic acid production. Thus, the pH reaction in response to exercise is normally acid, the ventilatory response not exceeding that needed to regulate pH. The ventilatory increase serves to constrain the fall in pH (see Fig. 2-22).

The recovery of pH following exercise is rapid, if the exercise is of moderate intensity (Fig. 2-34). At this exercise intensity, only the ventilatory excretion of the exercise-induced increase in CO_2 stores is required. If the exercise is of heavy or very heavy intensity, recovery of pH is slow because it is linked to the rate of regeneration of HCO_3^- which, in turn, depends on lactate catabolism.[34] In addition, in recovery, pH homeostasis seems to be an important determinant of ventilatory control. The reciprocal changes in arterial lac-

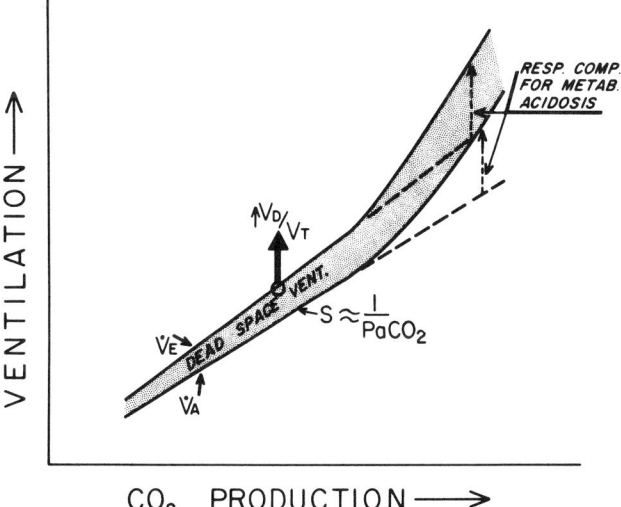

FIG. 2-32. Factors that determine alveolar and minute ventilation ($\dot{V}_A$ and $\dot{V}_E$, respectively) during exercise. V_D/V_T is the physiologic dead space/tidal volume ratio, and "S" is the slope (see "Determinants of the ventilatory requirement" for interpretation of this figure). (From Wasserman, K.: Breathing during exercise. N. Engl. J. Med., 298: 780–785, 1978.)

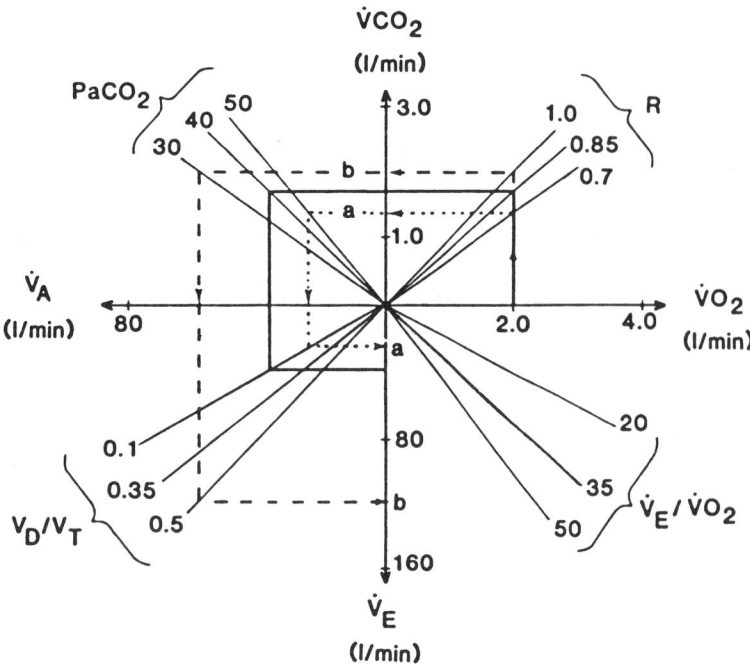

FIG. 2-33. Graphic display of the influence of the respiratory exchange ratio (R), arterial partial pressure of CO_2 (Pa_{CO_2}), and dead-space fraction of the breath (V_D/V_T) on ventilatory requirement ($\dot{V}_E$) for exercise with an O_2 consumption ($\dot{V}_{O_2}$) of 2 L/min (STPD). The ventilatory requirement can be significantly altered from the normal response (solid line), with a particular combination of determining variables leading to reduced (arrow a) or markedly high (arrow b) $\dot{V}_E$. $\dot{V}_A$ = alveolar ventilation. (From Whipp, B.J., and Pardy, R.L.: Breathing during exercise. In American Physiological Society. Handbook of Physiology. Section 3. Vol. III. Bethesda, MD, American Physiological Society, 1986, p. 605.)

tate and Std HCO_3^- during exercise and recovery are evident in Figures 2-18, 2-19, and 2-34.

Gas Exchange Kinetics

The $\dot{V}_E$, $\dot{V}_{O_2}$, or $\dot{V}_{CO_2}$ responses following the onset of constant work rate exercise from rest can be characterized by three time-related phases, as evident by the experimental data in Figure 2-35. The mechanisms of the gas exchange dynamics in response to exercise, as seen in Figure 2-35, are schematized in Figure 2-36. Phase I is the initial period, characterized by the immediate increase in gas exchange at the start of exercise. It lasts for

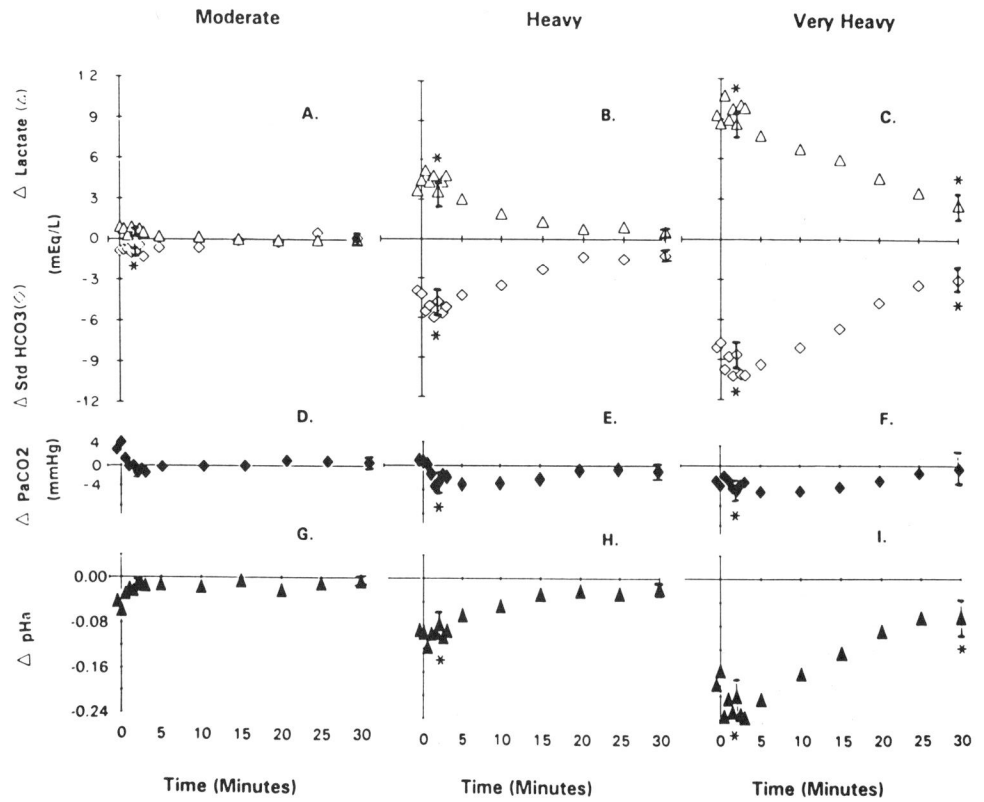

FIG. 2-34. ΔLactate and ΔStd HCO_3^- (A to C), ΔPa_{CO_2} (D to F), and ΔpHa (G to I) relative to resting values during 30 minutes of recovery from 6 minutes of moderate, heavy, and very heavy constant work rate exercise. Points are the average of 8 subjects. At selected times during recovery (2 and 30 minutes), SE and significant differences (*P < 0.05 from resting value) are provided. (From Stringer, W., Casaburi, R., and Wasserman, K.: Acid-base regulation during exercise and recovery in man. J. Appl. Physiol., 72:954–961, 1992.)

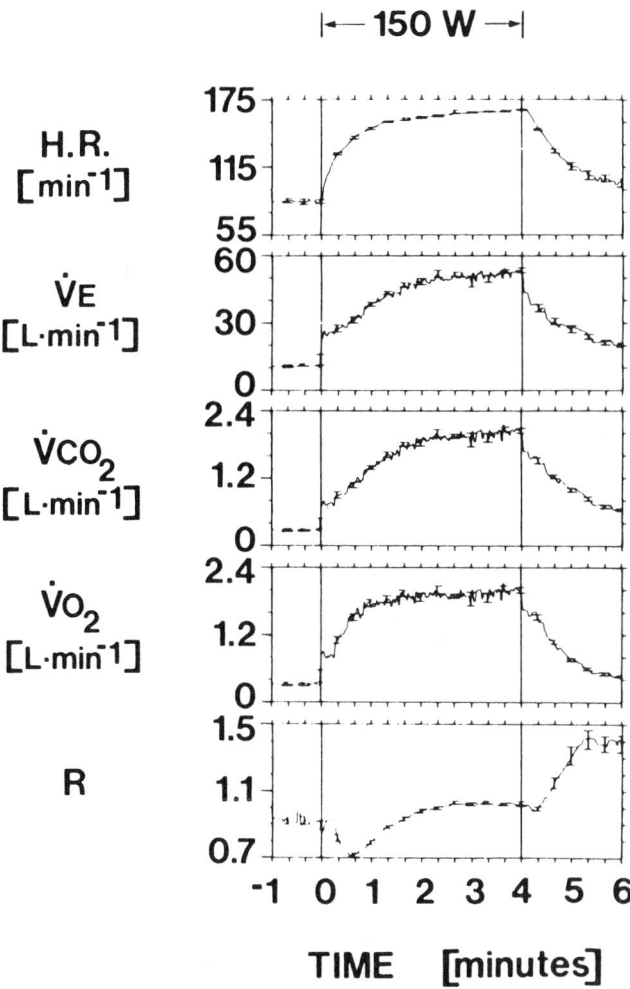

FIG. 2-35. Changes in ventilation and gas exchange during cycle ergometer constant work rate exercise starting from rest ("0" time) and ending at 4 minutes in a normal subject. This study is the average of six similar repetitions in which gas exchange was measured breath by breath. The vertical bars are the standard errors of the data. The abrupt increase in $\dot{V}E$, $\dot{V}CO_2$, and $\dot{V}O_2$ at the start of exercise ("0" time) is termed Phase I and is thought to be related, mechanistically, to the abrupt increase in cardiac output at the start of exercise. R is usually unchanged from rest for about 15 seconds. The start of Phase II is signalled by a decrease in R and is the period of exponential-like increase in $\dot{V}E$, $\dot{V}CO_2$, and $\dot{V}O_2$ to their asymptotes (Phase II). This is the period when increasing cellular respiration is reflected in lung gas exchange. R decreases transiently during Phase II because $\dot{V}O_2$ increases faster than $\dot{V}CO_2$ because of gas solubility differences in tissues. It usually then increases to a value higher than at rest because the RQ of the muscle substrate, being primarily glycogen, is higher than the average for the body, which depends on the RQ of the diet.

about 15 seconds. It is accounted for by the abrupt increase in pulmonary blood flow consequent to the increase in heart rate and stroke volume at the start of exercise, before blood from the exercising muscles has appeared in the lungs. Because the composition of this blood was determined under conditions of rest, R characteristically is the same

as that at rest (see Fig. 2-35). Phase II for $\dot{V}O_2$ lasts to about the third minute of exercise and reflects the changes in cellular respiration as blood in the muscles at the time of the start of exercise reaches the lungs. If the exercise is below the *AT*, a steady-state is achieved by 3 minutes (see Fig. 1-2). If above the *AT*, the steady-state is delayed or not achieved before the subject fatigues (see Figs. 1-2 and 2-6). Phase III starts at 3 minutes. Phase III can be used to determine whether the work rate is above or below the subject's *AT* and to ascertain the magnitude of the lactate increase (Fig. 2-37).[28,30]

OXYGEN UPTAKE KINETICS

In response to exercise, O_2 uptake from the lungs ($\dot{V}O_2$) reflects the O_2 consumed by the cells, excluding that provided by: (1) blood O_2 stores (oxyhemoglobin of the venous blood, physically dissolved O_2, and oxymyoglobin in muscles); (2) the O_2 equivalent of the decrease in muscle creatine $\sim PO_4$; and (3) O_2 spared by lactate accumulation in the body (11.2 ml of O_2 for each millimole of lactate when pyruvate, rather than the electron transport chain, reoxidizes cytosolic $NADH + H^+$ (see Fig. 2-1).

Gas stores in the lungs have little effect on $\dot{V}O_2$ kinetics because they do not change appreciably during exercise. The concentration of alveolar gas changes little, and rarely does the functional residual capacity (FRC) decrease as much as 1 L during exercise. Because 1 L contains 150 ml of O_2, an abrupt change in FRC at the start of exercise will have its primary impact on Phase I gas exchange.

The increase in $\dot{V}O_2$ is only transiently determined by the hemodynamic response to exercise (cardiac output and $C(a-\bar{v})O_2$). At the onset of moderate exercise, O_2 uptake from the lungs approximately doubles the resting $\dot{V}O_2$ and remains relatively unchanged during Phase I (first 15 seconds of exercise). If $C(a-\bar{v})O_2$ does not increase during Phase I, cardiac output can be inferred to have increased two-fold. Reporting on studies made during upright exercise that started from the motionless sitting position, Casaburi et al.[80] showed that about one third of the Phase I $\dot{V}O_2$ may be accounted for by the increase in $C(a-\bar{v})O_2$. This effect is apparently due to leg blood stasis because it disappears if stasis is prevented. The Phase I increase in $\dot{V}O_2$ noted in the upright position, in response to dynamic exercise from quiet rest, is greatly attenuated if exercise is performed

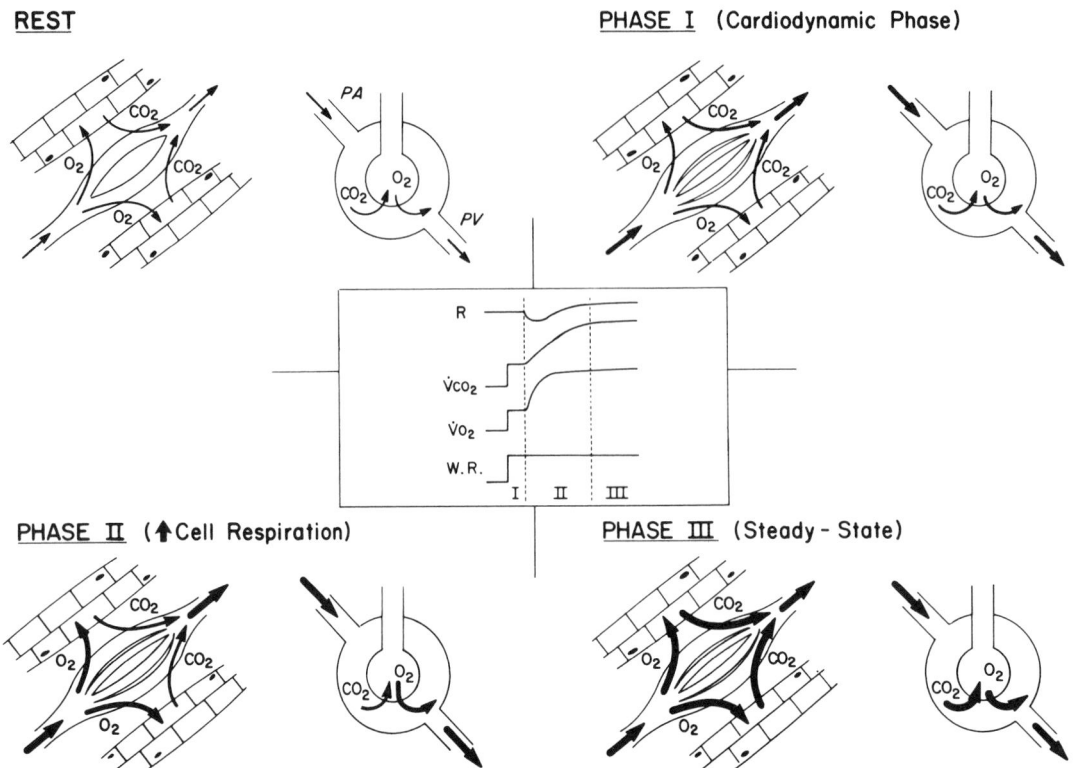

REST   PHASE I (Cardiodynamic Phase)

PHASE II (↑Cell Respiration)   PHASE III (Steady - State)

FIG. 2-36. Gas exchange at the lungs in response to constant work rate exercise (center diagram). Gas exchange at the cell (left side of each quadrant) couples to cardiorespiratory gas exchange (right side of each quadrant) through cardiovascular adjustments in the lungs and tissues. Phase I gas exchange is postulated to be caused by the immediate increase in cardiac output (pulmonary blood flow) at the start of exercise (cardiodynamic gas exchange). Phase II gas exchange reflects the decreased O_2 content and increased CO_2 content of the venous blood secondary to increased cell respiration as well as a further increase in cardiac output. (See the legend to Figure 2-35 for an explanation of the decrease in R during Phase II.) Eventually, a steady-state is reached between internal and external respiration (Phase III). PA = Pulmonary artery; PV = pulmonary vein; W.R. = work rate. (From Wasserman, K.: Coupling of external to internal respiration. Am. Rev. Respir. Dis., 129(Suppl.):S21-S24, 1984.)

in the supine position[81] or from prior mild exercise.[82]

During Phase II, $\dot{V}O_2$ increases as a single exponential with a time constant of approximately 30 seconds for a work rate below the *AT*.[83] If the exercise intensity is heavy or very heavy for a normal subject, or if the subject is so impaired that the cardiovascular response is inadequate to supply the total O_2 need, the increase in $\dot{V}O_2$ can be significantly slowed, and a steady-state is not achieved by 3 minutes (Figs. 1-2 and 2-38). In this metabolic state, lactate continues to increase until the $\dot{V}O_2$ reaches an asymptote.[84] A steady-state in $\dot{V}O_2$ is achieved and can be sustained only when all the cellular energy requirements are derived from reactions using O_2 transferred from the atmosphere.

O_2 Deficit

The O_2 deficit is traditionally computed as the difference between the total O_2 uptake and the prod-

uct of the steady-state $\dot{V}O_2$ and the exercise duration (Fig. 2-39). If the true steady-state value for $\dot{V}O_2$ is not reached at the time of cessation of work, however, the O_2 deficit will not be appropriately determined. A correct estimate of O_2 deficit can be obtained for work below the *AT* because a steady-state is readily achieved by 3 minutes.[85]

O_2 Debt

The total O_2 uptake in excess of the resting O_2 uptake during the recovery period is defined as the O_2 debt (Fig. 2-39).[70] Once $\dot{V}O_2$ reaches a steady-state during exercise, the debt no longer increases, regardless of the exercise duration.[86] In this instance, the O_2 debt is repaid within 5 minutes of recovery. If the work is above the *AT*, the O_2 debt can be high and may not be repaid for an hour or more. The size of the O_2 debt is linked to the increase in blood lactate concentration.[87] As long as the O_2 uptake fails to reach a steady-state and lactate continues to rise during constant work

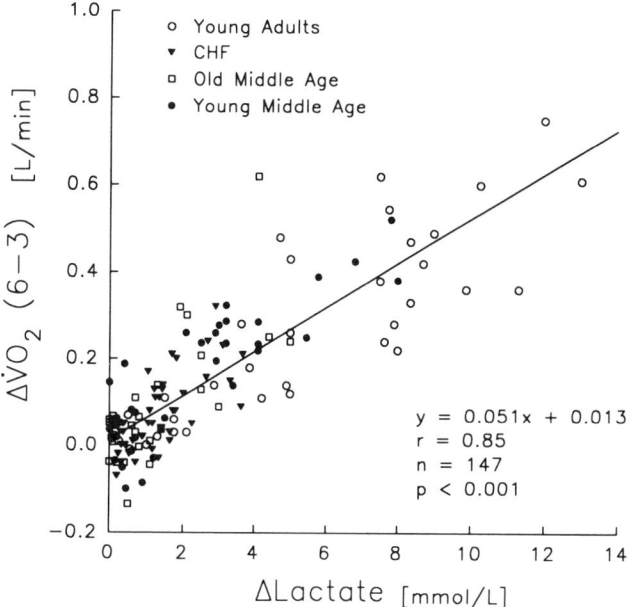

FIG. 2-37. Increase in blood lactate (above resting value) as related to the increase in oxygen consumption between 3 and 6 minutes of constant work rate exercise in normal young, young middle-aged, and late middle-aged adults and in patients with heart failure. Normally, $\dot{V}_{O_2}$ does not increase after 3 minutes when the work is performed below the anaerobic threshold ($\Delta\dot{V}_{O_2}(6-3) = 0$). (Data from references 28 and 30, with the data of late middle-aged adults added.)

rate exercise, the O_2 deficit and debt will continue to increase. For work levels at which a true steady-state in $\dot{V}_{O_2}$ can be achieved, the size of the O_2 debt approximates that of the O_2 deficit.[85]

If Phase I is a large fraction of the steady-state response for a given work rate, the O_2 deficit and debt will be small. In contrast, if Phase I is small, the O_2 deficit and debt will be relatively large. The O_2 deficit and debt will also be large if the Phase II $\dot{V}_{O_2}$ kinetics for a given work rate are slow. Because $\dot{V}_{O_2}$ kinetics are faster for the more fit subject, he or she will perform exercise more aerobically and will have a smaller O_2 deficit and debt for a given work rate.

CO_2 OUTPUT KINETICS

From approximately 15 to 40 seconds after the onset of constant work rate exercise, R pursues a downward course (see Fig. 2-35) because CO_2 produced from muscle metabolism increases slowly relative to O_2 consumption. This is attributed to the relatively high solubility of CO_2 in tissues compared to O_2. It subsequently increases to its new steady-state level as dictated by the ratio of the time constants of $\dot{V}_{CO_2}$ and $\dot{V}_{O_2}$. If a lactic acidosis occurs during the exercise, $\dot{V}_{CO_2}$ may increase faster than $\dot{V}_{O_2}$ because of the additional CO_2 formed as HCO_3^- dissociates during the buffering reaction (Fig. 2-40). This generally occurs after about 50 to 60 seconds of constant work rate exercise (Fig. 2-40).

Because of slower kinetics related to CO_2 solubility, the $\dot{V}_{CO_2}$ steady-state may not occur until approximately 4 minutes. $\dot{V}_E$ is similarly delayed because it follows $\dot{V}_{CO_2}$.[34]

If the work rate studied is below the AT, true homeostasis will occur in Phase III, and $\dot{V}_{O_2}$ and $\dot{V}_{CO_2}$ will achieve true steady-state values (see Fig. 1-2, upper panel and three lowest work rates in Fig. 2-38). For exercise above the AT, $\dot{V}_{O_2}$ does not achieve a steady-state by 3 minutes but continues to rise (see Fig. 1-2, lower panel and four highest work rates of Fig. 2-38). In contrast, the slow

FIG. 2-38. O_2 uptake ($\dot{V}_{O_2}$) and CO_2 output ($\dot{V}_{CO_2}$) as related to time at 7 different levels of work for a healthy subject. The 3 lowest work rates are below the subject's lactic acidosis threshold (LAT), whereas the 4 highest work rates are above it. The $\dot{V}_{O_2}$ continues to rise for the 4 work rates above the LAT, the rate of rise being more marked the higher the work rate. In contrast, the $\dot{V}_{CO_2}$ kinetics are relatively unchanging, reaching a constant level by 3 to 4 minutes in all 7 tests. (Modified from Casaburi, R., Barstow, T.J., Robinson, T., and Wasserman, K.: Influence of work rate on ventilatory and gas exchange kinetics. J. Appl. Physiol., 67:547–555, 1989.)

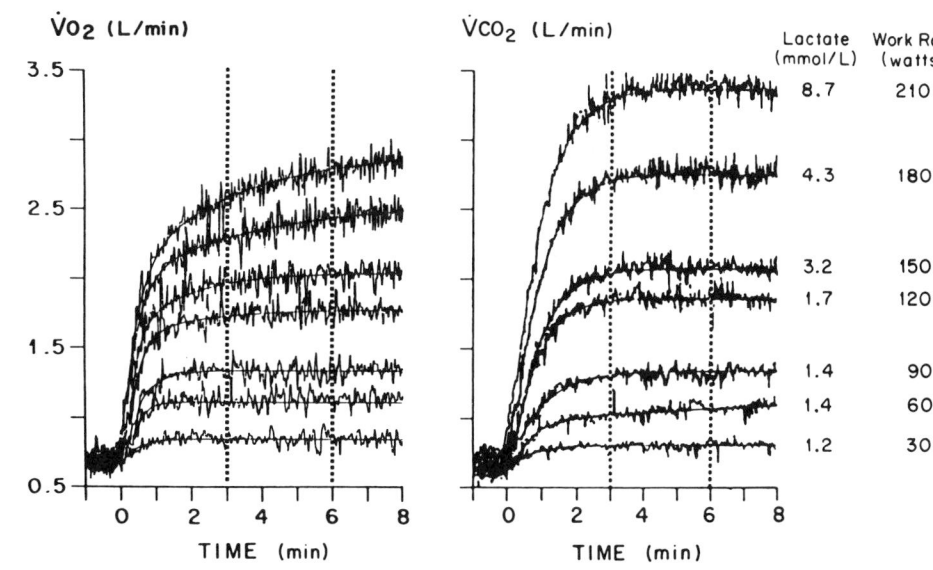

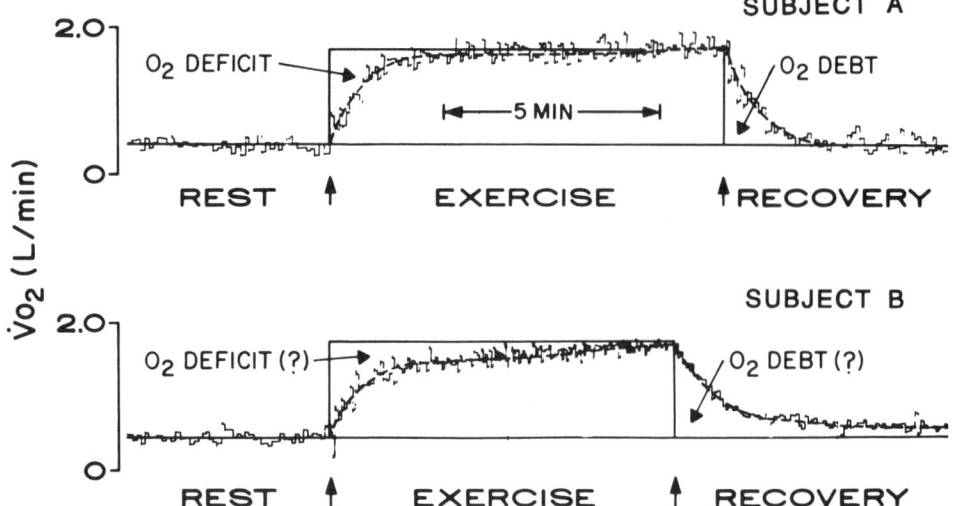

FIG. 2-39. O_2 uptake kinetics in response to constant work rate exercise of 100 W in two subjects at different levels of fitness. This figure illustrates the effect of fitness on O_2 deficit and O_2 debt. (See the text for precise definitions of O_2 deficit and O_2 debt.)

drift upward observed for $\dot{V}O_2$ is not observed for $\dot{V}CO_2$, and $\dot{V}CO_2$ increases to a higher value than $\dot{V}O_2$ (see Figs. 2-38 and 2-40).

Control of Breathing

OVERVIEW

Despite a manifold increase in CO_2 production and O_2 utilization during exercise, the ventilatory control mechanisms normally keep arterial PCO_2 and $[H^+]$ remarkably constant over a wide range of metabolic rates.[34,89] Ventilation appears to be coupled with CO_2 exchange during exercise. If $\dot{V}E$ did not increase appropriately for the increased rate of CO_2 production, a respiratory acidosis with associated disturbances in cellular function would result. Similarly, if ventilation increased proportionally more than the rate of CO_2 production, respiratory alkalosis would result and this would impair cellular function and O_2 unloading from hemoglobin in the muscles. In humans, exercise at moderate intensities usually is an isocapnic, isohydric, hypermetabolic state (see Figs. 2-18 and 2-19). A slight respiratory acidosis is transiently present in normal subjects because the ventilation increase lags behind the increase in CO_2 output.[90] A metabolic acidosis is normally present only for heavy or higher exercise intensities, because of increased blood lactate accumulation. Patients with abnormal respiratory mechanics or impaired chemoreceptor function, or normal subjects breathing through an apparatus that imparts a high resistive load, can develop a significant respiratory acidosis. Respiratory alkalosis does not typically de-

velop during exercise in normal subjects, however, and it is rarely seen in pathophysiologic states. Therefore, the physiologic mechanism(s) controlling breathing appear to operate with a small pH error to the acid side. The ventilatory control mechanism corrects this error by increasing ventilation and regulating $PaCO_2$. The $PaCO_2$ is rarely reduced in response to exercise except when the pH decreases because of metabolic acidosis.

Despite intensive research, no consensus exists on the mechanisms of respiratory control during exercise. The observation that arterial pH, PCO_2, and PO_2 are essentially unchanged during exercise of moderate exercise intensity has been difficult to explain mechanistically. Repeated efforts to discover chemoreceptors in locations where potential stimuli are available (e.g., pulmonary circulation or exercising limbs) to explain the exercise hyperpnea have been largely unsuccessful. The only chemoreceptors that have been clearly demonstrated to play a role in the hyperpnea of exercise are the carotid bodies.[91,92]

The following is a brief review of the mechanisms proposed to have a role in exercise hyperpnea (see the reviews by Whipp[89] and Wasserman, Whipp, and Casaburi[34] for more detailed discussions of this subject).

CORTICOGENIC OR CONDITIONED REFLEXES

The magnitude of the Phase I increase in $\dot{V}E$ varies appreciably from individual to individual, although high work rates generally result in only slightly further increases in Phase I over that ob-

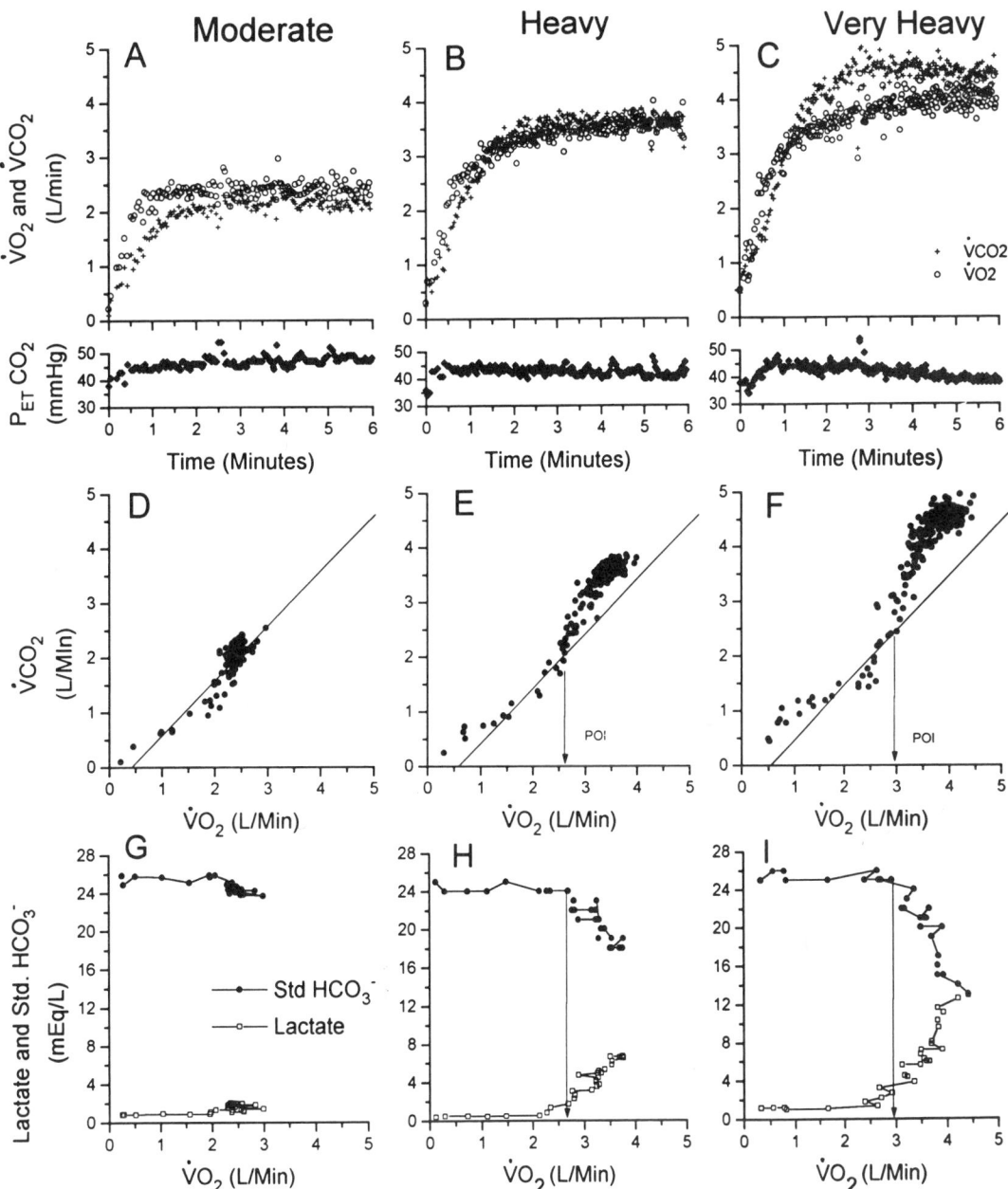

FIG. 2-40. O_2 uptake ($\dot{V}O_2$), CO_2 output ($\dot{V}CO_2$), and $P_{ET}CO_2$ plotted as a function of time (panels A, B, and C), and $\dot{V}CO_2$, arterial lactate, and standard (Std) HCO_3^- plotted as a function of $\dot{V}O_2$ (panels D to I) for constant work rate tests of moderate, heavy, and very heavy work intensity. Steepening of $\dot{V}CO_2$ relative to $\dot{V}O_2$ (arrow in panels E and F) occurs simultaneously with the increase in lactate and the decrease in standard HCO_3^- (arrow in panels H and I), reflecting the buffering of the lactic acid by HCO_3^-. (From Stringer, W., Wasserman, K., and Casaburi, R.: Lactic acidosis detection during constant work rate exercise from dynamic changes in $\dot{V}CO_2$ as a function of $\dot{V}O_2$. J. Appl. Physiol. Submitted for publication.)

served for the lightest loads. Consequently, for a mild work rate, the increase in $\dot{V}E$ during Phase I is a larger *fraction* of the total ventilatory response than that for a heavy work rate (Fig. 2-41). The magnitude of the increase in $\dot{V}E$ in Phase I is also not appreciably affected by different degrees of arterial oxygenation or in the absence of functioning carotid bodies. The ventilatory pattern increase after Phase I is greatly influenced by the

work rate in relation to the *AT* (see Fig. 2-30) and by the influence of carotid body chemosensitivity.

Anxiety might account for part of the rapid ventilatory increase at the start of exercise (Phase I) in some subjects. Krogh and Lindhard[93] suggested that the rapid $\dot{V}E$ increase at the start of exercise might originate from the cerebral cortex as a conditioned reflex. Eldridge et al.[94] and DiMarco et al.[95] obtained evidence from feline stud-

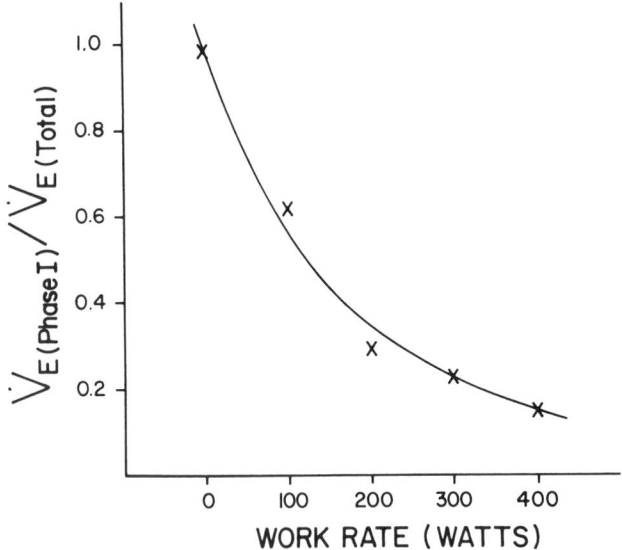

FIG. 2-41. The magnitude of the Phase I ventilatory response to exercise (from rest) as related to steady-state ventilation for various work rates. The higher the work rate, the smaller the fraction of the total ventilatory response attributable to Phase I.

ies suggesting that the ventilatory stimulus might involve hypothalamic mediation. The patterns of human ventilatory and gas exchange responses suggest that the sustained ventilatory response is predominantly metabolically coupled, however, and the initial ventilatory response might also be linked to the circulatory response to exercise.[34,81,96,97]

RESPIRATORY CENTER AND CENTRAL MEDULLARY CHEMORECEPTORS

The respiratory center includes collections of neurons in the brain stem that discharge rhythmically to stimulate motor neurons to the respiratory muscles. Medullary lesions associated with tumors, primary hypoventilation syndromes, or central respiratory depression associated with hypoxia-inducing pulmonary diseases can cause the respiratory pacemaker mechanisms to depend on peripheral chemoreceptor input for providing a controlled rhythmic output. Evidence that these pacemaker mechanisms may lose the required rhythmic discharge properties is the apnea produced by O_2 administration in some hypoxic patients.

The role of the medullary chemoreceptors in ventilatory control during exercise hyperpnea is unclear. Although these chemoreceptors respond to changes in pH and molecular CO_2, cerebrospinal fluid hypercapnia and acidosis do not occur during exercise. Moreover, the central chemoreceptors do not appear to respond to the acute exercise-induced metabolic acidosis.[67]

In patients with primary alveolar hypoventilation syndrome (patients with hypercapnia and a corresponding degree of hypoxemia with normal respiratory function who have a markedly diminished or absent ventilatory response to hypercapnia), the ventilatory response to exercise is diminished not only because they have hypercapnia at rest and exercise (high CO_2 set-point), but also because their arterial P_{CO_2} may increase further with exercise.[98] It is difficult to know, however, whether this occurs secondary to the central insensitivity to CO_2 or whether it is due to a failure of the respiratory center to integrate the afferent stimuli of exercise effectively to give an appropriate output.

CAROTID BODIES

Much has been learned about the role of carotid bodies during muscular exercise from studies on selected asthmatic patients who had both carotid bodies resected, but whose baroreceptors were left intact.[92,99] The ventilatory response to exercise was studied in these subjects when they: (1) were asymptomatic; (2) had normal, or near normal, respiratory function; and (3) had normal exercise tolerance. They manifested three major differences from normal subjects in their ventilatory responses to exercise: (1) the subjects without carotid bodies did not increase their ventilatory drive in response to hypoxia,[91] nor did they decrease their ventilatory drive in response to hyperoxia;[99] (2) they failed to develop ventilatory compensation for the exercise-induced metabolic acidosis[67] and consequently evidenced a greater acidemia during high-intensity exercise; and (3) their ventilatory increase during exercise was slow, causing a larger transient hypercapnia during Phase II than normally observed.[67]

Attenuating carotid body drive in normal subjects with altered acid-base status by breathing high O_2 slowed the Phase II ventilatory response.[100] The more baseline acidosis, the greater was the attenuation of the Phase II ventilatory response. Other studies on the short-term effect of hyperoxia during exercise on $\dot{V}_E$, while subjects breathed gases of varying $F_{I_{O_2}}$, support the concept that the carotid bodies have an important role in the normal ventilatory response to exercise.[101] Although the exact mechanisms mediating this response remain to be elucidated, several factors known to stimulate the carotid bodies increase during exercise. These include K^+, adenosine, osmolarity, catecholamines, and H^+. Whatever the precise integrative role of these mediators, their net effect is to contribute only approximately 20% to the exercise hyperpnea at normal levels of P_{O_2}. In hypoxia, however, the carotid bodies can account for more than 50% of the hyperpnea of exercise.

AORTIC BODIES

The aortic bodies seem to be unimportant as ventilatory chemoreceptors in man, in contrast to some other animal species (cats and dogs). Removal of the carotid bodies alone has been shown to eliminate the ventilatory responses to hypoxia and the acute metabolic acidosis of exercise.[67,91]

VAGAL REFLEXES

The lungs are richly innervated by branches of the vagus nerve. Whereas investigators have postulated that the vagus nerve might contribute importantly to the exercise hyperpnea, studies by Phillipson et al.[102] on the ventilatory response to exercise in awake dogs showed that vagal blockade, induced by bilateral cooling of the cervical vagus nerves, did not change the ventilatory response to exercise, although the breathing pattern was altered. These investigators concluded that the vagus nerves were not important in the overall ventilatory response to exercise at the exercise levels studied (up to $4 \times$ resting $\dot{V}_{O_2}$) in dogs.

MECHANORECEPTORS IN EXTREMITIES

To explain exercise hyperpnea, proprioceptors or muscle spindles in the exercising muscle had been postulated to play a major role in the genesis of exercise hyperpnea.[103] The principal argument for an appreciable role for the neural afferents from exercising muscles stems from the observation of a rapid increase in $\dot{V}_E$ at the start of exercise (Phase I) (see Fig. 2-35), in advance of the predicted arrival of the products of exercise metabolism in the central circulation.

Some neurophysiologic studies have helped to clarify the possible role of afferents from the exercising limb in exercise hyperpnea.[104] Studies in which the transmission of stimuli in large, myelinated fibers (e.g., transmitting proprioception) were interrupted[105] demonstrate that these recep-

tors play only a small role, if any. Hornbein et al.,[106] Hodgson and Mathews,[107] and Waldrop et al.,[108] using different approaches to stimulate the muscle spindles, demonstrated no significant role for these organs in exercise hyperpnea. Stimulation of the Type III and Type IV muscle afferents (i.e., unmyelinated or small-myelinated neurons) has been demonstrated to induce hyperpnea.[109] Studies have demonstrated that blocking their afferent transmission does not appreciably impair the hyperpnea, however.[110] This finding is consistent with work that demonstrates that the coupling of $\dot{V}_E$ to metabolic rate ($\dot{V}_{CO_2}$) is not abnormal in human patients with complete spinal cord transection who are caused to "exercise" by means of electrical stimulation of the leg muscles.[111,112] Even if ventilatory stimuli originating in the exercising muscles are active during exercise, however, the respiratory center is not stimulated with enough intensity by these signals to override the mechanisms that regulate arterial pH.

HEMODYNAMIC HYPERPNEA

Cardiovascular reflexes linked to the ventilatory control mechanism have been put forth as an alternative to mechanoreceptors in the extremities as an explanation for the rapid onset of exercise hyperpnea.[34,96,97,113] The abrupt increase in cardiac output and peripheral blood flow at the start of exercise could deliver increased quantities of blood to receptor sites downstream from the pulmonary capillaries, resulting in an increased P_{CO_2} and $[H^+]$ and decreased P_{O_2} at the sites of arterial chemoreceptors, if $\dot{V}_A$ did not keep pace with pulmonary blood flow increase. These changes could provide feedback stimuli to ventilation in less time than the circulation time between the muscles and arterial chemoreceptors. Casaburi et al.[80] showed that pulmonary artery O_2 saturation decreased within the first few seconds of the start of upright cycle ergometer exercise, much earlier than expected from the muscle capillary-pulmonary artery circulation time. This rapid appearance of highly desaturated venous blood at the pulmonary artery at the start of exercise was due to the abrupt increase in venous return at the start of exercise from the lower inferior vena cava. The blood from this site (dependent legs) is more desaturated and has a higher P_{CO_2} than mixed venous blood. Thus, at the start of lower extremity exercise in the upright position, this blood could be quickly injected into the pulmonary circulation by compression of the veins of the contracting muscles and increased abdominal pressure from the greater descent of the diaphragm. Both the rapid return of desaturated, high P_{CO_2} venous blood and the rapid immediate (Phase I) increase in ventilation are attenuated if the same cycling exercise is performed in the supine position so the legs and heart are at about the same level.[81,114]

The reason for linking the Phase I increase in $\dot{V}_E$ to the abrupt increase in cardiac output (cardiovascular reflex) rather than involving nonmetabolic neurogenic mechanisms is that two unlinked neurogenic mechanisms, one for blood flow and one for ventilation, would not likely produce the near-isocapnic hyperpnea so consistently observed from the start through the steady-state of moderate exercise. The control mechanism appears to account for the predictable regulation of pH in some way.

Dietary Substrate and the Physiologic Responses to Exercise

O₂ CONSUMPTION

Slightly more high-energy phosphate compounds are generated per molecule of O_2 utilized when carbohydrate is the substrate instead of fat

($\sim P{:}O_2$ = 6.0 and 5.65, respectively). Consequently, steady-state $\dot{V}_{O_2}$ should be slightly increased for a given work rate when fatty acids are the predominant substrate. The $\dot{V}_{O_2}$ required to perform cycle ergometer work after consuming a high-carbohydrate diet for 3 days as compared to a high-fat diet for a similar duration is shown in Figure 2-42. The $\dot{V}_{O_2}$ is slightly increased, as predicted, when the work task is performed with fatty acids as the dominant substrate as compared to carbohydrate.

HEART RATE

Because cardiac output increases linearly with $\dot{V}_{O_2}$, the higher $\dot{V}_{O_2}$ should predictably result in a higher cardiac output when fat, as compared to carbohydrate, is the dominant substrate. This is reflected in a slightly higher heart rate when fat, as compared to carbohydrate, is the dominant exercise substrate (Fig. 2-42).

CO₂ PRODUCTION

Whereas $\dot{V}_{O_2}$ and heart rate are less at a given work rate when carbohydrate is the major substrate, $\dot{V}_{CO_2}$ decreases when fat is the major

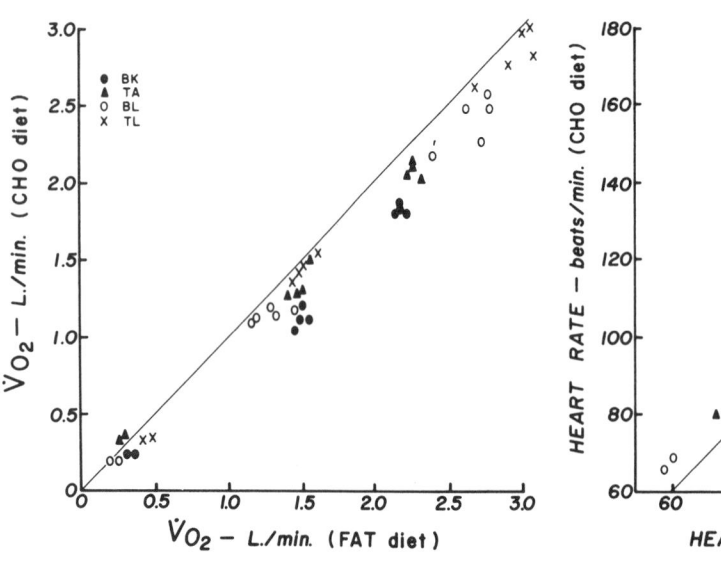

EFFECT OF DIET ON O₂ CONSUMPTION DURING EXERCISE

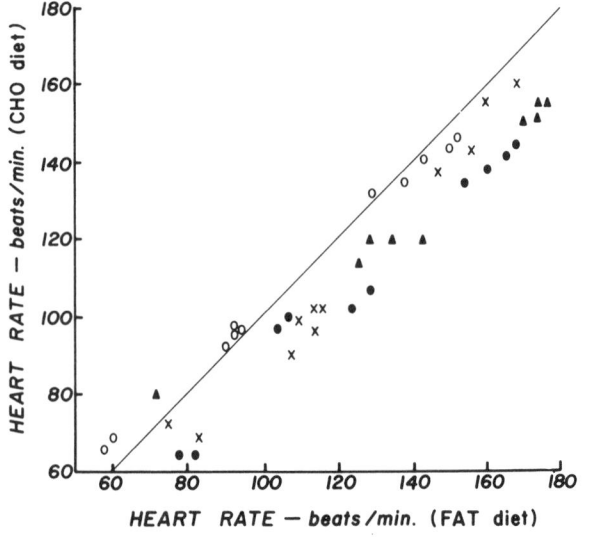

EFFECT OF DIET ON HEART RATE DURING EXERCISE

FIG. 2-42. Effect of dietary substrate on oxygen consumption and heart rate during exercise. Studies were done on four subjects at rest and at two levels of exercise after 3 days on a high-carbohydrate diet (RQ at rest = .97) and 3 days on a high-fat diet (RQ at rest = .75). The oxygen consumption is higher on the high-fat diet than on the high-carbohydrate diet during the performance of a given work rate. This is consistent with the biochemical evidence that the high-energy phosphate yield from carbohydrate is greater than that from fat for a given O_2 cost. Heart rate during exercise is also shown to be higher on the high-fat diet as compared to the high-carbohydrate diet, reflecting the link between oxygen consumption and cardiac output.

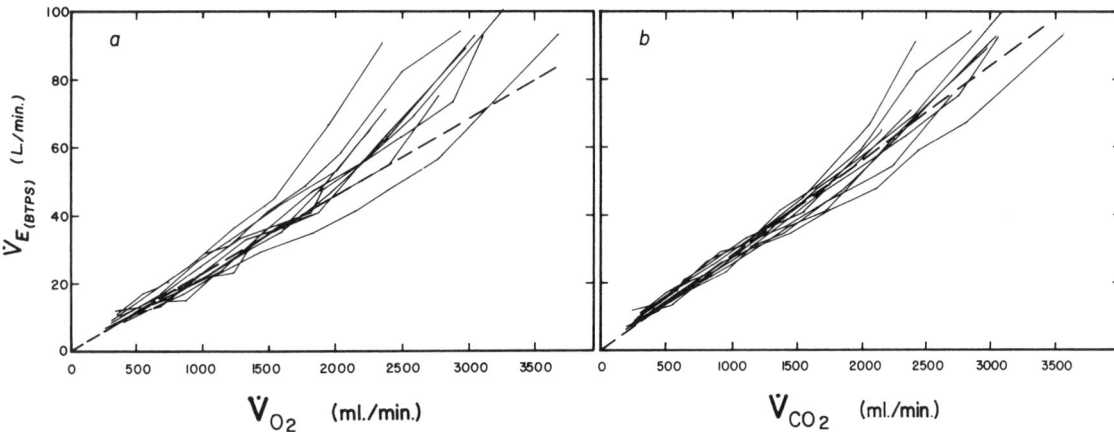

FIG. 2-43. Relationship between steady-state minute ventilation ($\dot{V}E$) and oxygen consumption ($\dot{V}O_2$) and CO_2 production ($\dot{V}CO_2$) in 10 normal subjects. The curvilinear increase in ventilation at high metabolic rates reflects respiratory compensation for the metabolic acidosis. The reduced dispersion noted in the correlation between $\dot{V}E$ and $\dot{V}CO_2$, as compared to $\dot{V}E$ and $\dot{V}O_2$, reflects the functional dependence of ventilation on CO_2 flow to the lungs and the effect of differences in RQ among the subjects. (From Wasserman, K., VanKessel, A.L., and Burton, G.B.: Interaction of physiological mechanisms during exercise. J. Appl. Physiol., 22:71–85, 1967.)

source of energy.[115,116] This may be predicted on the basis of the lower RQ for fat than for carbohydrate, although the effect is more striking at rest than during exercise. Thus, Sue et al.[115] found that a low-carbohydrate diet affected resting much more than exercise $\dot{V}CO_2$, RQ, or $\dot{V}E$. Apparently, the muscles are able to extract carbohydrate from a low carbohydrate diet, making the muscle substrate RQ higher than most other organs in the body. This enables the muscles to maintain the most efficient fuel possible for aerobic work (see Fig. 2-3), in contrast to other organs of the body.

MINUTE VENTILATION

$\dot{V}E$ has been shown to be less for a given work rate task with a predominant fat substrate, consistent with the hypothesis that the ventilatory control mechanisms appear to cause $\dot{V}E$ to change in proportion to CO_2 flow.[116] As with $\dot{V}CO_2$, however, the effect is more marked at rest than during exercise.[115] When $\dot{V}E$ is plotted against $\dot{V}CO_2$, the relationship is the same whether the RQ is high or low. Thus, a consistent relationship is observed among normal subjects when $\dot{V}E$ is plotted against $\dot{V}CO_2$ (Fig. 2-43). When $\dot{V}E$ is plotted against $\dot{V}O_2$, however, the responses among subjects are less consistent. The greater intersubject variability, with $\dot{V}O_2$ as the independent variable, is due to RQ differences among subjects; high RQ subjects have the steeper $\dot{V}E$ versus $\dot{V}O_2$ slope. The mechanism for the curvilinear steepening of $\dot{V}E$ at the higher metabolic rates is accounted for by the metabolic acidosis of heavy exercise and its ventilatory compensation as described in Figure 2-32.

Summary

Gas exchange during exercise should be considered from the standpoint of cellular respiration and how cardiovascular and ventilatory mechanisms are coupled to it. Not only does the magnitude of cellular respiration affect external respiration, but also the work rate above the subject's *AT* has a major influence on $\dot{V}E$. Work above the *AT* causes increased CO_2 and H^+ production, both having powerful effects on the ventilatory response to exercise. Moreover, gas exchange kinetics are altered and exercise endurance is reduced above the *AT*.

The physiologic responses to exercise are summarized in Figure 1-1. Approximately 28% of the calories generated during work are transformed into useful external work, whereas the remaining 72% are lost primarily as heat. The oxidative energy obtained from O_2 creditors (hemoglobin, myoglobin, creatine-$\sim PO_4$, and pyruvate conversion to lactate) varies with the work rate. At moderate work rates, however, the pyruvate-to-lactate mechanism contributes a small fraction of the credit, whereas for very heavy work rates, the pyruvate-lactate mechanism accounts for upwards of 80% of the total O_2 deficit.[33]

The peripheral blood flow distribution appears to depend on the work rate and local humoral factors that optimize the O_2 (blood) flow-metabolic rate relationship. Although cardiac output is linearly correlated with O_2 consumption, uniformity in the ratio of blood flow to O_2 consumption keeps the slope relatively low (approximately 6 L flow/L O_2 consumption) and causes the maximal O_2 extraction across the exercising extremity to be approximately 85% in the normal subject.

Minute ventilation is determined by the rate of CO_2 production, the physiologic dead space and the level at which arterial P_{CO_2} is regulated. Arterial P_{O_2} remains relatively constant during exercise, despite increasing $\dot{V}_{O_2}$.

Incremental exercise tests, which measure $\dot{V}_{O_2}$ and $\dot{V}_{CO_2}$ dynamically, allow detection of the *LAT*. Breath-by-breath measurements of $\dot{V}_{O_2}$ and $\dot{V}_{CO_2}$ during constant work rate exercise can also be used to determine whether exercise is being performed with or without a lactic acidosis and to estimate roughly the magnitude of the lactate increase and the exercise duration that might be tolerated at the work rate performed.

$\dot{V}_{O_2}$, $\dot{V}_{CO_2}$, and $\dot{V}_E$ abruptly increase at the start of exercise (Phase I). After the first 15 seconds of constant load exercise, $\dot{V}_{O_2}$, $\dot{V}_{CO_2}$, and $\dot{V}_E$ rise exponentially (Phase II) to a steady-state or an asymptote (Phase III). Their kinetics are influenced by cellular metabolism and the O_2 and CO_2 storage capacities in tissues. During Phases II and III, $\dot{V}_E$ follows closely the changing rate of CO_2 delivery to the lungs rather than the actual CO_2 produced or the O_2 consumed, if the exercise is performed without a lactic acidosis. $\dot{V}_E$ increases disproportionately to $\dot{V}_{CO_2}$ when the exercise induces a lactic acidosis.

Breath-by-breath gas exchange measurements also provide insight into mechanisms of respiratory control. This mechanism appears to be set to regulate arterial $[H^+]$ under a variety of conditions of exercise and recovery by regulating CO_2 excretion.

References

1. Saltin, B., and Gollnick, P.D.: Skeletal muscle adaptability: significance for metabolism and performance. *In* Handbook of Physiology. Section 10. Skeletal Muscle. Edited by L.D. Peachey. Bethesda, MD, American Physiological Society, 1983, p. 555.
2. Gibbs, C.L., and Gibson, W.R.: Energy production of rat soleus muscle. Am. J. Physiol., 223:874–881, 1972.
3. Henricksson, I., and Reitman, I.S.: Quantitative measures of enzyme activities in type I and type II muscle fibres of man after training. Acta Physiol. Scand., 97: 392–397, 1976.
4. Buller, A., Eccles, I., and Eccles, R.: Differentiation of fast and slow muscles in the cat hind limb. J. Physiol. (Lond.), 150:399–416, 1960.
5. Karlsson, J.: Introduction: basics in human skeletal muscles metabolism. Int. J. Sports Med., 2:1–5, 1982.
6. Essen, B.: Intramuscular substrate utilization. Ann. N.Y. Acad. Sci., 301:30–44, 1977.
7. Lehninger, A.L.: Biochemistry. New York, Worth, 1971, p. 407.
8. Cooper, D.M., Wasserman, D.H., Vranic, M., and Wasserman, K.: Glucose turnover in response to exercise during high- and low-$F_{I_{O_2}}$ breathing in man. Am. J. Physiol., 251:E209-E214, 1986.
9. Idstrom, J.P., Harihara Subramanian, V., Chance, B., Schersten, T., and Bylund-Fellenius, A.C.: Oxygen dependence of energy metabolism in contracting and recovering rat skeletal muscle. Am. J. Physiol., 248:H40-H48, 1985.
10. Cooper, C.B., Beaver, W., Cooper, D.M., and Wasserman, K.: Factors affecting the component of the alveolar CO_2 output-O_2 uptake relationship during incremental exercise in man. Exp. Physiol., 77:51–64, 1992.
11. Beaver, W.L., and Wasserman, K.: Muscle RQ and lactate accumulation from analysis of the $\dot{V}_{CO_2}$-$\dot{V}_{O_2}$ relationship during exercise. Clin. J. Sports Med., 1:27–34, 1991.
12. Clode, M., and Campbell, E.J.M.: The relationship between gas exchange and changes in blood lactate concentrations during exercise. Clin. Sci., 37:263–272, 1969.
13. Bergstrom, J., Hermansen, L., Hultman, E., and Saltin, B.: Diet, muscle glycogen and physical performance. Acta Physiol. Scand., 71:140–150, 1967.
14. Rosell, S., and Saltin, B.: Energy need, delivery, and utilization in muscular exercise. *In* The Structure and Function of Muscle. Vol.3. Edited by G.H. Bourne. New York, Academic Press, 1973.
15. Simonsen, E.: Depletion of energy yielding substances. *In* Physiology of Work Capacity and Fatigue. Edited by E. Simonsen. Springfield, IL, Charles C Thomas, 1971.
16. Ahlborg, B., Bergstrom, J., Ekelund, L.G., and Hultman, E.: Muscle glycogen and muscle electrolytes during prolonged physical exercise. Acta Physiol. Scand., 70:129–142, 1967.
17. Jones, N.L.: Exercise testing in pulmonary evaluation: rationale, methods, and the normal respiratory response to exercise. N. Engl. J. Med., 293:541–544, 1975.
18. Wasserman, D.H., Lickley, L.A., and Vranic, M.: Interactions between glucagon and other counter-regulatory hormones during normoglycemic and hypoglycemic exercise in dogs. J. Clin. Invest., 74:1404–1413, 1984.
19. Wasserman, D.H., and Cherrington, A.D.: Hepatic fuel metabolism during muscular work: role and regulation. Am. J. Physiol., 260:E811-E824, 1991.
20. Pozefsky, T., Felig, P., and Tobin, I.D.: Amino acid balance across tissues of the forearm in postabsorptive man: effects of insulin at two dose levels. J. Clin. Invest., 48:2273–2282, 1969.
21. Wahren, J.: Substrate utilization by exercising muscle in man. *In* Progress in Cardiology. Vol. 2. Edited by P.N. Yu and J.F. Goodwin. Philadelphia, Lea & Febiger, 1973, pp. 255–280.
22. Wahren, J., Felig, P., Havel, R.J., Jorfeldt, L., Pernow, B., and Saltin, B.: Amino acid metabolism in McArdle's syndrome. N. Engl. J. Med., 288:774–777, 1973.
23. Whipp, B.J., and Mahler, M.: Dynamics of pulmonary gas exchange during exercise. *In* Pulmonary Gas Exchange. Vol. 2. Edited by J.B. West. New York, Academic Press, 1980, pp. 33–96.

24. Whipp, B.J., and Wasserman, K.: Oxygen uptake kinetics for various intensities of constant load work. J. Appl. Physiol., 33:351–356, 1972.

25. Wasserman, K., and Whipp, B.J.: Exercise physiology in health and disease. Am. Rev. Respir. Dis., 112:219–249, 1975.

26. Astrand, P.O., and Rodahl, K.: Textbook of Work Physiology. 2nd Ed. New York, McGraw-Hill, 1977, pp. 393–411.

27. Whipp, B.J., and Wasserman, K.: Efficiency of muscular work. J. Appl. Physiol., 26:644–648, 1969.

28. Roston, W.L., Whipp, B.J., Davis, J.A., Effros, R.M., and Wasserman, K.: Oxygen uptake kinetics and lactate concentration during exercise in humans. Am. Rev. Respir. Dis., 135:1080–1084, 1987.

29. Koike, A., Wasserman, K., McKenzie, D.K., Zanconato, S., and Weiler-Ravell, D.: Evidence that diffusion limitation determines oxygen uptake kinetics during exercise in humans. J. Clin. Invest., 86:1698–1706, 1990.

30. Zhang, Y.Y., Wasserman, K., Sietsema, K.E., Barstow, T.J., Mizumoto, G., and Sullivan, C.S.: O_2 uptake kinetics in response to exercise: a measure of tissue anaerobiosis in heart failure. Chest, 103:735–741, 1993.

31. Wells, J.G., Balke, B., and Van Fossan, B.D.: Lactic acid accumulation during work: a suggested standardization of work classification. J. Appl. Physiol., 10:51–55, 1957.

32. Wasserman, K.: The anaerobic threshold measurement to evaluate exercise performance. Am. Rev. Respir. Dis., 129(Suppl.):535–540, 1984.

33. Wasserman, K., VanKessel, A.L., and Burton, G.B.: Interaction of physiological mechanisms during exercise. J. Appl. Physiol., 22:71–85, 1967.

34. Wasserman, K., Whipp, B.J., and Casaburi, R.: Respiratory control during exercise. In Handbook of Physiology, Vol. 2. Edited by N.S. Cherniack and J.G. Widdicombe. Bethesda, MD, American Physiological Society, 1986, pp. 595–619.

35. Hughson, R.H., Weisiger, K.W., and Swanson, G.D.: Blood lactate concentration increases as a continuous function in progressive exercise. J. Appl. Physiol., 62:1975–1981, 1987.

36. Beaver, W.L., Wasserman, K., and Whipp, B.J.: Improved detection of the lactate threshold during exercise using a log-log transformation. J. Appl. Physiol., 59:1936–1940, 1985.

37. Wasserman, K., Beaver, W.L., and Whipp, B.J.: Gas exchange theory and the lactic acidosis (anaerobic) threshold. Circulation, 81(Suppl. II): II-14-II-30, 1990.

38. Knuttgen, H.G., and Saltin, B.: Muscle metabolites and oxygen uptake in short-term submaximal exercise in man. J. Appl. Physiol., 32:690–694, 1972.

39. Jorfeldt, L., Juhlin-Dannfelt, A., and Karlsson, J.: Lactate release and relation to tissue lactate and human skeletal muscle during exercise. J. Appl. Physiol., 44:350–352, 1978.

40. Lindholm, A., and Saltin, B.: The physiological and biochemical response of standardlined horses to exercise of varying speed and duration. Acta Vet. Scand., 15:310–324, 1974.

41. Katz, A., and Sahlin, K.: Regulation of lactic acid production during exercise. J. Appl. Physiol., 65:509–518, 1988.

42. Chwalbinska-Moneta, J., Rogbergs, R.A., Costill, D.L., and Fink, W.J.: Threshold for muscle lactate accumulation during progressive exercise. J. Appl. Physiol., 55:1178–1186, 1983.

43. Wasserman, K., Beaver, W.L., Davis, J.A., Pu, J.-Z., Heber, D., and Whipp, B.J.: Lactate, pyruvate, and lactate-to-pyruvate ratio during exercise and recovery. J. Appl. Physiol., 59:935–940, 1985.

44. Bylund-Fellenius, A.C., Walker, P.M., Elander, A., Holm, S., Holm, J., and Schersten, T.: Energy metabolism in relation to oxygen partial pressure in human skeletal muscle during exercise. Biochem. J., 200:247–255, 1981.

45. Sahlin, K., Harris, R.D., Nylind, B., and Hultman, E.: Lactate content and pH in muscle samples obtained after dynamic exercise. Pflugers Arch., 367:143–149, 1976.

46. Chance, B., Mauriello, G., and Aubert, X.M.: ADP arrival at muscle mitochondria following a twitch. In Muscle as a Tissue. Edited by K. Rodahl and S.M. Horvath. New York, McGraw-Hill, 1962.

47. Wittenberg, B.A., and Wittenberg, J.B.: Transport of oxygen in muscle. Annu. Rev. Physiol., 51:857–878, 1989.

48. Stringer, W., Casaburi, R., French, W., Porszasz, J., and Wasserman, K.: The role of pH in maintaining muscle capillary P_{O_2} during heavy exercise. Am. Rev. Respir. Dis., 145:A881, 1992.

49. Koike, A., Wasserman, K., Taniguchi, K., Ohtomo, N., Hiroe, M., and Marumo, F.: The critical capillary P_{O_2} and the anarobic threshold during exercise in patients with cardiovascular diseases. Submitted for publication.

50. Koike, A., Weiler-Ravell, D., McKenzie, D.K. Zanconato, S., and Wasserman, K.: Evidence that the metabolic acidosis threshold is the anaerobic threshold. J. Appl. Physiol., 68:2521–2526, 1990.

51. Koike, A., Wasserman, K., Armon, Y., and Weiler-Ravell, D.: The work-rate-dependent effect of carbon monoxide on ventilatory control during exercise. Respir. Physiol., 85:169–183, 1991.

52. Vogel, J.A., and Gleser, M.A.: Effect of carbon monoxide on oxygen transport during exercise. J. Appl. Physiol., 32:234–239, 1972.

53. Yoshida, T., Udo, M., Chida, M., Ichioka, M., and Makiguchi, K.: Effect of hypoxia on arterial and venous blood levels of oxygen, carbon dioxide, hydrogen ions and lactate during incremental forearm exercise. Eur. J. Appl. Physiol., 58:772–777, 1989.

54. Lundin, G., and Strom, G.: The concentration of blood lactate acid in man during muscular work in relation to the partial pressure of oxygen of the inspired air. Acta Physiol. Scand., 13:253–256, 1947.

55. Ivy, J.L, Withers, R.T., Van Handel, P.J., Elger, D.H., and Costill, D.L.: Muscle respiratory capacity and fiber type as determinants of the lactate threshold. J. Appl. Physiol., 48:523–527, 1980.

56. Beaver, W.L., Wasserman, K., and Whipp, B.J.: Bicarbonate buffering of lactic acid generated during exercise. J. Appl. Physiol., 60:472–478, 1986.

57. Stringer, W., Casaburi, R., and Wasserman, K.: Acid-base regulation during exercise and recovery in man. J. Appl. Physiol., 72:954–961, 1992.

58. Owles, W.H.: Alterations in the lactic acid content of the blood as a result of light exercise, and associated changes in the CO_2-combining power of the blood and in the alveolar CO_2 pressure. J. Physiol. (Lond.), 69: 214–237, 1930.

59. Bouyhus, A., Pool, J., Binkhorst, R.A., and vanLeeuwen, P.: Metabolic acidosis of exercise in healthy males. J. Appl. Physiol., 21:1040–1046, 1966.

60. Yoshida, T., Udo, M., Chida, M., Makiguchi, K., Ichioka, M., and Muraoka, I.: Arterial blood gases, acid-base balance, and lactate and gas exchange variables during hypoxic exercise. Int. J. Sports Med., 10:279–285, 1989.

61. Trosper, T.L., and Philipson, K.D.: Lactate transport by cardiac sarcolemmal vesicles. Am. J. Physiol., 252: 483–489, 1987.

62. Mainwood, G.W., Worsley-Brown, P., and Paterson, R.A.: The metabolic changes in frog sartorius muscles during recovery from fatigue at different external bicarbonate concentrations. Can. J. Physiol. Pharmacol., 50: 143–155, 1971.

63. Hirsche, H., Hombach, V., Langhor, H.D., Wacker, U., and Busse, J.: Lactic acid permeation rate in working gastrocnemii of dogs during metabolic alkalosis and acidosis. Pflugers Arch., 356:209–222, 1975.

64. Wasserman, K., Whipp, B.J., Koyal, S.N., and Beaver, W.L.: Anaerobic threshold and respiratory gas exchange during exercise. J. Appl. Physiol., 35:236–243, 1973.

65. Patessio, A., Casaburi, R., Carone, M., Appendi, L., Donner, C.F., and Wasserman, K.: Comparison of gas exchange, lactate and lactic acidosis thresholds in COPD patients. Am. Rev. Respir. Dis., 148:622–626, 1993.

66. Beaver, W.L., Wasserman, K., and Whipp, B.J.: A new method for detecting the anaerobic threshold by gas exchange. J. Appl. Physiol., 60:2020–2027, 1986.

67. Wasserman, K., Whipp, B.J., Koyal, S.N., and Cleary, M.G.: Effect of carotid body resection on ventilatory and acid-base control during exercise. J. Appl. Physiol., 39: 354–358, 1975.

68. Duling, B.R.: Control of striated muscle blood flow. In The Lung: Scientific Foundations. Edited by Crystal, R.G. and J.B. West. New York, Raven Press, 1991, p. 1497.

69. Kilmartin, J.V., and Rossi-Bernardi, L.: Interaction of hemoglobin with hydrogen ions, carbon dioxide, and organic phosphates. Physiol. Rev., 53:836–890, 1973.

70. Hill, A.V., Long, C.N.H., and Lupton, H.: Muscular exercise, lactic acid, and the supply and utilization of oxygen. VI. The oxygen debt at the end of exercise. Proc. R. Soc. Lond., 97:127–137, 1924.

71. McGilvery, R.W.: Quantitative significance of lactate production. In Biochemistry: A Functional Approach. Philadelphia, W.B. Saunders, 1970, pp. 268–270.

72. McArdle, B.: Myopathy due to a defect in muscle glycogen breakdown. Clin. Sci., 10:13–35, 1951.

73. Lewis, S.F., and Haller, R.G.: The pathophysiology of McArdle's disease: clues to regulation in exercise and fatigue. J. Appl. Physiol., 61:391–401, 1986.

74. Mahler, M.: First order kinetics of muscle oxygen consumption and an equivalent proportionality between $\dot{Q}O_2$ and phosphorylcreatine level. J. Gen. Physiol., 86: 135–165, 1985.

75. Rowell, L.B.: Human Circulation Regulation During Physical Stress. New York, Oxford University Press, 1986, p. 215.

76. Guyton, A.C., Jones, C.E., and Coleman, T.G.: Cardiac output in muscular exercise. In Circulatory Physiology: Cardiac Output and its Regulation. Philadelphia, W.B. Saunders, 1973.

77. Loeppky, J.A., Greene, E.R., Hoekenga, D.E., Caprihan, A., and Luft, U.C.: Beat-by-beat stroke volume assessment by pulsed Doppler in upright and supine exercise. J. Appl. Physiol., 50:1173–1182, 1981.

78. Bunn, H.F., and Forget, B.G.: Hemoglobin: Molecular, Genetic and Clinical Aspects. Philadelphia, W.B. Saunders, 1986, pp. 595–616.

79. Christiansen, J., Douglas, C.G., and Haldane, J.S.: The absorption and dissociation of carbon dioxide by human blood. J. Physiol. (Lond.), 48:244–271, 1914.

80. Casaburi, R., Daly, J., Hansen, J.E., and Effros, R.M.: Abrupt changes in mixed venous blood gas composition following onset of exercise. J. Appl. Physiol., 67: 1106–1112, 1989.

81. Weiler-Ravell, D., Cooper, D.M., Whipp, B.J., and Wasserman, K.: Control of breathing at the start of exercise as influenced by posture. J. Appl. Physiol., 55: 1460–1466, 1983.

82. Whipp, B.J., Ward, S.A., Lamarra, N., Davis, J.A., and Wasserman, K.: Parameters of ventilatory and gas exchange dynamics during exercise. J. Appl. Physiol., 52: 1506–1513, 1982.

83. Casaburi, R., Barstow, T.J., Robinson, T., and Wasserman, K.: Influence of work rate on ventilatory and gas exchange kinetics. J. Appl. Physiol., 67:547–555, 1989.

84. Wasserman, K., Casaburi, R., Beaver, W.L., Roston, W.L., and Whipp, B.J.: Assessing the adequacy of tissue oxygenation during exercise. In New Horizons: Oxygen Transport and Utilization. Edited by C.W. Bryan-Brown and S.M. Ayres. Fullerton, CA, Society of Critical Care, 1987, pp. 109–144.

85. Whipp, B.J., Seard, C., and Wasserman, K.: Oxygen deficit-oxygen debt relationships and efficiency of anaerobic work. J. Appl. Physiol., 28:452–456, 1970.

86. Schneider, E.G., Robinson, S., and Newton, J.L.: Oxygen debt in aerobic work. J. Appl. Physiol., 25:58–62, 1968.

87. Margaria, R., Edwards, H.T., and Dill, D.B.: The possible mechanisms of contracting and paying the oxygen debt and the role of lactic acid in muscular contraction. Am. J. Physiol., 106:689–715, 1933.

88. Zhang, Y.Y., Sietsema, K.E., Sullivan, C.S., and Wasserman, K.: A method for measuring bicarbonate buffering of lactic acid during constant work rate exercise. Submitted for publication.

89. Whipp, B.J.: The control of exercise hyperpnea. In Regulation of Breathing. Edited by T. Hornbein. New York, Marcel Dekker, 1981, pp. 1069–1139.

90. Casaburi, R., Whipp, B.J., Wasserman, K., Beaver, W.L., and Koyal, S.N.: Ventilatory and gas exchange dynamics in response to sinusoidal work. J. Appl. Physiol., 42:300–311, 1977.

91. Lugliani, R., Whipp, B.J., Seard, C., and Wasserman, K.: Effects of bilateral carotid body resection on ventilatory control at rest and during exercise in man. N. Engl. J. Med., 285:1105–1111, 1971.

92. Wasserman, K., and Whipp, B.J.: The carotid bodies and respiratory control in man. In Morphology and Mechanisms of Chemoreceptors. Edited by A.S. Paintal. Delhi, Vallabhbhai Patel Chest Institute, 1976, pp. 156–175.

93. Krogh, A., and Lindhard, J.: The regulation of respiration and circulation during the initial stages of muscular work. J. Physiol. (Lond.), 47:112–136, 1913.

94. Eldridge, F.L., Millhorn, D.E., and Waldrop, T.G.: Exercise hyperpnea and locomotion: parallel activation from the hypothalamus. Science, 211:844–846, 1981.

95. DiMarco, A.F., Romaniuk, J.R., von Euler, C., and Yamamoto, Y.: Immediate changes in ventilation and respiratory pattern associated with onset and cessation of locomotion in the cat. J. Appl. Physiol., 343:1–16, 1983.

96. Wasserman, K., Whipp, B.J., and Castagna, J.: Cardiodynamic hyperpnea: hyperpnea secondary to cardiac output increase. J. Appl. Physiol., 36:457–464, 1974.

97. Jones, P.W., Huszczuk, A., and Wasserman, K.: Cardiac output as a controller of ventilation through changes in right ventricular load. J. Appl. Physiol., 53:218–224, 1982.

98. Lugliani, R., Whipp, B.J., Brinkman, J., and Wasserman, K.: Doxapram hydrochloride: a respiratory stimulant for patients with primary alveolar hypoventilation. Chest, 76:414–419, 1979.

99. Whipp, B.J., and Wasserman, K.: Carotid bodies and ventilatory control dynamics in man. Fed. Proc., 39:1628–1673, 1980.

100. Oren, A., Whipp, B.J., and Wasserman, K.: Effect of acid-base status on the kinetics of the ventilatory response to moderate exercise. J. Appl. Physiol., 52:1013–1017, 1982.

101. Griffiths, T.L., Henson, L.C., and Whipp, B.J.: Influence of inspired oxygen concentration on the dynamics of the exercise hyperpnea in man. J. Physiol. (Lond.), 380:387–403, 1986.

102. Phillipson, E.A., Hickey, R.F., Bainton, C.R., and Nadel, J.A.: Effect of vagal blockade on regulation of breathing in conscious dogs. J. Appl. Physiol., 29:475–479, 1970.

103. Dejours, P.: Control of respiration in muscular exercise. In Handbook of Physiology. Section 3. Vol. 1 Edited by W.O. Fenn and H. Rahn. Washington, D.C., American Physiological Society, 1964, pp. 631–638.

104. McCloskey, D.I., and Mitchell, J.H.: Reflex cardiovascular and respiratory responses originating in exercising muscle. J. Physiol. (Lond.), 224:173–186, 1972.

105. Kao, F.F.: An experimental study of the pathways involved in exercise hyperpnea employing cross-circulation techniques. In The Regulation of Human Respiration. Edited by D.J.C. Cunningham and B.B. Lloyd. Oxford, Blackwell Scientific Publications, 1961, pp. 461–502.

106. Hornbein, T.F., Sorenson, S.C., and Parks, C.R.: Role of

107. Hodgson, H.J.F., and Mathews, P.B.C.: The ineffectiveness of excitation of the primary endings of the muscle spindle by vibration as a respiratory stimulant in the decerebrate cat. J. Physiol. (Lond.), 194:555–563, 1968.

108. Waldrop, T.G., Rybicki, K., and Kaufman, M.P.: Chemical activation of group I and group II muscle afferents has no cardiorespiratory effects. J. Appl. Physiol., 56:1223–1228, 1984.

109. Kaufman, M.P., Waldrop, T.G., Rybicki, K.J., Ordway, G.A., and Mitchell, J.H.: Effects of static and rhythmic contractions on the discharge of group III and IV muscle afferents. Cardiovasc. Res., 18:663–668, 1984.

110. Fernandes, A., Galbo, H., Kjer, M., Mitchell, J.H., Secker, N.H., and Thomas, S.: Cardiovascular and ventilatory responses to dynamic exercise during epidural anaesthesia in man. J. Physiol. (Lond.), 420:281–293, 1990.

111. Brice, A.G., Forster, H.V., Pan, L.G., Funahashi, A., Hoffman, M.D., Murphy, C.L., and Lowry, T.F.: Is the hyperpnea of muscular contractions critically dependent on spinal afferents? J. Appl. Physiol., 64:226–233, 1988.

112. Adams, L., Frankel, H., Garlick, J., Guz, A., Murphy, K., and Semple, S.J.G.: The role of spinal cord transmission in the ventilatory response to exercise in man. J. Physiol. (Lond.), 355:85–97, 1984.

113. Innes, J.A., Solarte, I., Huszczuk, A., Yeh, E., Whipp, B.J., and Wasserman, K.: Respiration during recovery from exercise; effects of trapping and release of femoral blood flow. J. Appl. Physiol., 67:2608–2613, 1989.

114. Casaburi, R., Cooper, C., Effros, R.M., and Wasserman, K.: Time course of mixed venous oxygen saturation following various modes of exercise transition. FASEB J., 3:A849, 1989.

115. Sue, D.Y., Chung, M.D., Grosvenor, M., and Wasserman, K.: Effect of altering the proportion of dietary fat and carbohydrate on exercise gas exchange in normal subjects. Am. Rev. Respir. Dis., 139:1430–1434, 1989.

116. Brown, S.E., Wiener, S., Brown, R.A., Maratelli, P.A., and Light, R.W.: Exercise performance following a carbohydrate load in chronic airflow obstruction. J. Appl. Physiol., 58:1340–1346, 1985.

117. Lusk, G.: Science of Nutrition. Johnson Reprint Corp., New York, 1976, p. 65.

118. Wasserman, K.: Breathing during exercise. N. Engl. J. Med., 298:780–785, 1978.

119. Whipp, B.J., and Pardy, R.L.: Breathing during exercise. In American Physiological Society. Handbook of Physiology. Section 3. Vol. III. Bethesda, MD, American Physiological Society, 1986, p. 605.

120. Wasserman, K.: Coupling of external to internal respiration. Am. Rev. Respir. Dis., 129(Suppl.):S21–S24, 1984.

121. Stringer, W., Wasserman, K., and Casaburi, R.: Lactic acidosis detection during constant work rate exercise from dynamic changes in $\dot{V}CO_2$ as a function of $\dot{V}O_2$. Submitted for publication.

122. Severinghaus, J.W.: Simple accurate equations for human blood O_2 dissociation computations. J. Appl. Physiol., 46:599–602, 1979.

Measurements During Integrative Cardiopulmonary Exercise Testing

CHAPTER 3

EXERCISE TESTING PERMITS simultaneous evaluation of the ability of the cardiovascular and respiratory systems to perform their major function, i.e., gas exchange. This chapter describes measurements that can be used in the exercise laboratory to assess the physiologic responses to exercise. Because exercise requires an integrative cardiopulmonary response to support the change in muscle respiration to perform exercise, gas exchange measurements are fundamental to an integrative cardiopulmonary exercise test.

What is an Integrative Cardiopulmonary Exercise Test?

The primary function of the cardiovascular and pulmonary systems is to support cellular respiration. The success of the cardiovascular and pulmonary systems in meeting this function is reflected in the O_2 uptake ($\dot{V}O_2$) and CO_2 output ($\dot{V}CO_2$) in response to a specific work rate stimulus. An integrative cardiopulmonary exercise test can address many more questions than a test that only uses the electrocardiogram to address the presence or absence of coronary artery disease. While addressing the latter, the integrative exercise test also addresses questions about other disorders that may or may not accompany coronary artery disease. These questions are listed in Table 3-1,

along with the kinds of measurements that address each question. Because the considerations of integrative cardiopulmonary exercise testing are so broad, we expect that such a test, conducted at the beginning of a work-up of exercise limitation from any cause, could reduce the cost and time required to evaluate the patient.

When Should Integrative Cardiopulmonary Exercise Testing be Used?

1. When the cause of dyspnea or exercise limitation is uncertain, i.e., for differential diagnosis, integrative cardiopulmonary exercise testing can enable one to define the organ system whose response deviates most from normal and can thereby make further work-up more specific.
2. By providing an objective assessment of exercise capacity and impairment, cardiopulmonary exercise testing is of considerable, if not essential, value in disability evaluation.
3. Effective drug therapy and rehabilitation are best assessed by improved exercise capacity or improved efficiency in gas exchange between the muscle cells and the lungs; other measurements to assess effectiveness of

TABLE 3-1. *Questions Addressed by Cardiopulmonary Exercise Testing*

QUESTION	EXAMPLE OF DISORDER	MARKERS FOR ABNORMALITY
1. Is exercise capacity reduced?	Any disorder	Maximum $\dot{V}O_2$
2. Is the metabolic requirement for exercise increased?	Obesity	$\dot{V}O_2$-WR relationship
3. Is exercise limited by impaired O_2 flow?	Heart; peripheral vascular; pulmonary vascular; anemia; hypoxemia; carboxyhemoglobin	ECG; blood pressure; anaerobic threshold; blood lactate; HCO_3^-; $\Delta\dot{V}O_2/\Delta WR$; $\dot{V}O_2$/HR; HbCO
4. Is exercise limited by reduced ventilatory capacity?	Lung; chest wall	Breathing reserve; V_D/V_T
5. Is there an abnormal degree of ventilation-perfusion mismatching?	Lung; pulmonary circulation	$P(A-a)O_2$; $P(a-ET)CO_2$; V_D/V_T; $\dot{V}E/\dot{V}CO_2$
6. Is there a defect in muscle utilization of O_2 or substrate?	Muscle glycolytic or mitochondrial enzyme defect	$\dot{V}O_2$ and $\dot{V}CO_2$ kinetics, heart rate, blood lactate, lactate/pyruvate ratio
7. Is exercise limited by a behavioral problem?	Neurosis	Breathing pattern
8. Is work output reduced because of poor effort?	Poor effort with secondary gain	HRR; BR; peak R; $P(A-a)O_2$; $P(a-ET)CO_2$

Maximum $\dot{V}O_2$ = highest O_2 uptake measured; BR (breathing reserve) = maximum voluntary ventilation-ventilation at maximum exercise; $\Delta\dot{V}O_2/\Delta WR$ = increase in $\dot{V}O_2$ relative to increase in work rate; ECG (electrocardiogram); V_D/V_T = physiologic dead space/tidal volume ratio; BP (blood pressure); $P(A-a)O_2$ = alveolar-arterial PO_2 difference; HbCO = carboxyhemoglobin; $P(a-ET)CO_2$ = arterial-end tidal PCO_2 difference; HRR (heart rate reserve) = predicted maximum heart rate-maximum exercise heart rate; $\dot{V}E/\dot{V}CO_2$ = ventilatory equivalent for CO_2; Peak R = peak gas exchange ratio.

treatment are subordinate to the information provided by integrative cardiopulmonary exercise testing because they are indirect measures of treatment success.

4. Cardiopulmonary exercise testing has been shown to be of value for preoperative evaluation of risk for patients about to undergo major surgery;[1,2] such testing enables the examiner to evaluate the stress that the cardiopulmonary system can endure, and predictably, it is more informative than resting measures of function.

The measurements and functions that integrative cardiopulmonary exercise testing assess are summarized in Table 3-2. Fortunately, most are noninvasive and can be performed in modern car-

dioresipratory laboratories. The gas exchange variables that provide the most valuable information are described in this chapter, whereas methods of measurement, calculation, calibration, and accuracy are described in the Appendix.

Progressively Increasing Work Rate Exercise Testing

Measurements made during progressively increasing work rate exercise testing are useful because they enable the examiner to: (1) titrate the level of the subject's exercise limitation; (2) titrate the adequacy of the performance of various components in the external to internal gas exchange coupling; and (3) determine the organ system

TABLE 3-2. *Assessing Function With Physiologic Measurements*

MEASUREMENT	FUNCTION
Electrocardiogram	Myocardial O_2 availability-requirement balance
$\dot{V}O_2$	Cardiac output $\times$ $C(a-\bar{v})_{O_2}$
Maximum $\dot{V}O_2$	Highest $\dot{V}O_2$ achieved during presumed maximal effort for an incremental exercise test (specific for type of work), may or may not equal $\dot{V}O_2$ max
$\dot{V}O_2$max	Highest $\dot{V}O_2$ achievable as evidenced by failure of $\dot{V}O_2$ to increase despite increasing work rate (specific for type of work); highest cardiac output $\times$ $C(a-\bar{v})_{O_2}$
$\Delta \dot{V}O_2/\Delta WR$ during incremental exercise	Aerobic contribution to exercise (low value suggests high anaerobic contribution)
$\dot{V}O_2$ difference = Expected $\dot{V}O_2$ for maximum WR − maximum $\dot{V}O_2$	O_2 utilization below expected (inability to utilize O_2 normally) or above expected (exceptionally fit for the work task) at the maximum work rate performed by the subject
Cardiac output	Useful when related to vascular pressure
Anaerobic (Lactic Acidosis) Threshold *(AT or LAT)*	Highest $\dot{V}O_2$ that can be sustained without developing a lactic acidosis; important determinant of potential for endurance work (specific for form of work)
O_2 pulse ($\dot{V}O_2/HR$) = SV $\times$ $C(a-\bar{v})_{O_2}$	Product of SV and $C(a-\bar{v})_{O_2}$; under conditions when SV is constant, change in O_2 pulse is proportional to change in $C(a-\bar{v})_{O_2}$
HRR = predicted maximum HR − maximum exercise HR	Heart rate reserve at maximum exercise
Arterial pressure	Detecting systemic hypertension, ventricular outflow obstruction, or myocardial failure (pulsus alternans or decreasing pressure with increasing WR)
$\dot{V}E$ = $\dot{V}A$ + $\dot{V}D$	$\dot{V}D$ is increased at specific work rate due to mismatching of $\dot{V}A$ and $\dot{Q}$. $\dot{V}A$ is increased inversely with decrease in Pa_{CO_2} whether caused by a low CO_2 setpoint, metabolic acidosis, or hypoxemia.
BR = MVV − $\dot{V}E$ at maximum exercise or (MVV − $\dot{V}E$ at maximum exercise)/MVV	Breathing reserve; theoretical additional $\dot{V}E$ available at cessation of exercise
Exercise VD/VT	Measure of mismatching of ventilation and perfusion
$P(a-ET)_{CO_2}$	Detects high $\dot{V}A/\dot{Q}$ components of lung with mismatching of $\dot{V}A/\dot{Q}$
$P(A-a)_{O_2}$	Detects low $\dot{V}A/\dot{Q}$ components of lung with mismatching of $\dot{V}A/\dot{Q}$, diffusion defect, or right to left shunt
Expired flow pattern	Useful for indicating presence of significant airflow obstruction
VT/IC	Fraction of the inspiratory capacity used in breathing; high with restricted lung expansion
Immediate $\dot{V}O_2$ increase (Phase I) in response to constant WR	Ability to increase pulmonary blood flow at start of exercise
$\Delta \dot{V}O_2(6-3)$	Proportional to lactate increase; positive if work rate is above *LAT*
Abrupt change in $\dot{V}E$ and f during hyperoxic (100% O_2) switch	Contribution of the carotid body to ventilatory drive

WR = work rate; $\dot{V}E$ = minute ventilation; HR = heart rate; VD = physiological dead space; SV = Stroke volume; BR = breathing reserve; $C(a-\bar{v})_{O_2}$ = arterial-mixed venous O_2 content difference; MVV = maximal voluntary ventilation; HRR = heart rate reserve; VT = tidal volume; $\dot{V}D$ = physiological dead space ventilation per minute; IC = inspiratory capacity; $\dot{V}A$ = alveolar ventilation per minute; $\Delta \dot{V}O_2(6-3)$ = difference between $\dot{V}O_2$ at 6 and 3 minutes during constant work rate exercise.

whose response first becomes abnormal and the $\dot{V}O_2$ at which it occurs. These questions are best addressed during short (10-minute), progressive, non-steady-state exercise tests, rather than during a more prolonged exercise test with relatively long duration steps. Prolonged testing, which is more likely to fatigue the patient, is no more informative and limits the ability of the investigator to repeat testing to evaluate therapy. The relative merit of different protocols for exercise testing is discussed in greater detail in Chapter 5.

ELECTROCARDIOGRAM (ECG)

Because exercise causes the heart rate to increase and diastolic time to shorten, the time for coronary perfusion is decreased. Thus, coronary artery disease is more likely to be detected while exercising than during the resting state. The ECG is a valuable measure of the balance between myocardial O_2 availability and O_2 requirement for cardiac work. When the heart muscle contracts without adequate oxygen (ischemia), the muscle cells alter their ionic permeability, and the rate of reestablishing the normal ion gradients across the myocardial cell membrane slows after cardiac systole. Consequently, reestablishing the electrical membrane potential during repolarization is slowed in the ischemic areas of the myocardium. This causes the T wave and ST segments to change acutely when the O_2 requirement for the increased cardiac work of exercise exceeds its availability (Table 3-3). An increased frequency of ectopic beats as the work rate increases should also be considered pathologic and suggestive of myocardial ischemia. Some patients, however, manifest occasional premature ventricular or atrial contractions at rest that disappear or become less frequent during exercise. We regard these ectopic beats as benign and unrelated to a disturbance in the myocardial O_2 availability-requirement balance, because they are overridden by the sinus tachycardia of exercise.

In many instances, false-positive and borderline changes occur in the ECG when one relies solely on changes in the T wave and ST segments to detect myocardial ischemia. When these ECG changes are accompanied by myocardial dyskinesis, however, $\dot{V}O_2$ fails to rise appropriately with increasing work rate. Thus, a reduction in $\Delta\dot{V}O_2/\Delta WR$ accompanied by ECG changes consistent with myocardial ischemia, with or without angina, is more specific and suggestive of significant coronary artery disease. In addition, the diagnosis of ischemic heart disease becomes more likely when ECG changes occur in the presence of a fall in systemic blood pressure.

MAXIMAL OXYGEN UPTAKE ($\dot{V}O_2$max) AND MAXIMUM (PEAK) OXYGEN UPTAKE

The body clearly has an upper limit for O_2 utilization at a particular state of fitness or training. This is determined by the maximal cardiac output,[3] the potential for O_2 extraction by the exercising muscle,[4] and the ventilatory capacity.[5] Maximal aerobic power (i.e., maximal $\dot{V}O_2$ or $\dot{V}O_2$max) was originally defined as the $\dot{V}O_2$ at which performance of increasing levels of supramaximal work failed to increase $\dot{V}O_2$ further,[6] as illustrated in Figure 3-1A and shown experimentally in Figure 2-6. This upper limit in $\dot{V}O_2$ may also be determined in a progressively increasing exercise test, in which a plateau in $\dot{V}O_2$ is demonstrated despite further increases in the work rate. Thus, the maximal $\dot{V}O_2$ represents the *highest* $\dot{V}O_2$ attainable for a given form of exercise, as evidenced by a failure for $\dot{V}O_2$ to increase further despite an increase in work rate. Maximal $\dot{V}O_2$ should be contrasted with the maximum or peak $\dot{V}O_2$, which is simply the highest $\dot{V}O_2$ achieved for a given, presumed maximal exercise effort. In this instance, $\dot{V}O_2$ could potentially continue to increase with further increase in work rate. This value does not satisfy the foregoing definition of the *maximal* value. This distinction is diagrammed in Figure 3-1B. A plateau in $\dot{V}O_2$ during a progressively increasing work rate test provides the evidence necessary for the judgment that a maximal $\dot{V}O_2$ has, in fact, been attained.

The maximum $\dot{V}O_2$ may not equal the maximal $\dot{V}O_2$ ($\dot{V}O_2$max). In most normal subjects, however, progressively increasing work rate with the legs to the point of fatigue produces a maximum $\dot{V}O_2$ that closely approximates the predicted $\dot{V}O_2$max,[7] even when a plateau is not evident. A plateau in $\dot{V}O_2$ may also fail to occur during a progressively increasing work rate test when the subject stops exercising because of leg or chest pain, shortness of breath, mechanical limitation to breathing, or

TABLE 3-3. *Electrocardiographic Evidence of Myocardial Ischemia During Exercise (12 lead)*

ST segment depression
T wave changes
PVCs that appear during exercise

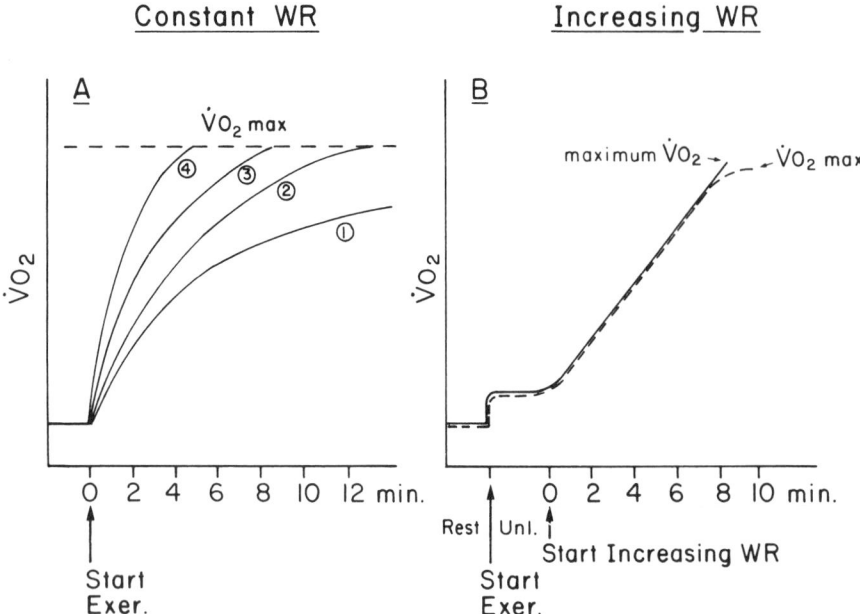

FIG. 3-1. Determining the maximal $\dot{V}_{O_2}$ ($\dot{V}_{O_2}$max) from supramaximal work rate tests (A). $\dot{V}_{O_2}$ measurements are related to time for progressively higher work rates. For work rate 1, the $\dot{V}_{O_2}$ asymptote is below $\dot{V}_{O_2}$max. Work rate 2 reaches a $\dot{V}_{O_2}$, which is the same as the $\dot{V}_{O_2}$ reached by work rates 3 and 4. Because the maximum $\dot{V}_{O_2}$ for work rates 2, 3, and 4 is the same despite increasing work rate, this identifies $\dot{V}_{O_2}$max for the form of work being studied. Distinguishing between $\dot{V}_{O_2}$max and maximum $\dot{V}_{O_2}$ from a maximal effort incremental exercise test is shown in B. When the subject's maximum tolerable work rate results in a flattening of the $\dot{V}_{O_2}$-work rate slope, this is the subject's maximal $\dot{V}_{O_2}$ or $\dot{V}_{O_2}$max. When the $\dot{V}_{O_2}$ does not slow its rate of rise with increasing work rate, but the subject has reached his or her maximum tolerable work rate, this is the highest or maximum $\dot{V}_{O_2}$ during the test.

lack of motivation. In these instances, the maximum $\dot{V}_{O_2}$ will be less than the predicted $\dot{V}_{O_2}$max.

In conditions in which O_2 flow to the tissues is impaired (e.g., cardiovascular disease, pulmonary vascular disease, and anemia) or O_2 utilization by the tissues (e.g., electron transport chain defect), reductions in the $\dot{V}_{O_2}$max and maximum $\dot{V}_{O_2}$ result. Note that at high exercise intensities, the $\dot{V}_{O_2}$ does not reflect all the high-energy phosphate expended by the subject. It does not account for the anaerobic (lactic acid generating) contribution to energy production, a progressively more important energy source as work rate increases.[8]

A progressively increasing work rate exercise test, as in Figure 3-1B, has several advantages: (1) the test starts out at relatively low work rates, so it does not require the application of great muscle force or a sudden, large cardiorespiratory stress; (2) the $\dot{V}_{O_2}$max or maximum $\dot{V}_{O_2}$ can be determined from a test lasting approximately 10 minutes; (3) the subject is stressed at relatively high work rates for only a few minutes; and (4) the $\dot{V}_{O_2}$-work rate relationship can be determined (cycle ergometry). To obtain the best data for interpreting the measured responses to a progressively increasing work rate exercise test, the work rate increments should be uniform in magnitude and duration. This means that the ergometer must be linear and accurately calibrated.

The maximum $\dot{V}_{O_2}$ is the first measurement to be examined because it establishes whether the patient's physiologic responses allow normal maximal aerobic function. Other measurements

are then used to differentiate the cause of any exercise limitation whether or not the subject reaches his or her predicted maximum $\dot{V}_{O_2}$.

OXYGEN UPTAKE AND WORK RATE

Although $\dot{V}_{O_2}$ measurements are made from respired gas measured at the mouth, they reflect O_2 utilization by the cells, including the muscle cells performing the work of exercise. The $\dot{V}_{O_2}$-work rate relationship describes how much O_2 is utilized by the exercising subject in relation to the quantity of external work performed. Thus, it gives important information concerning the coupling of external to cellular respiration, and we find it valuable to graph $\dot{V}_{O_2}$ as a function of work rate. Factors and mechanisms affecting $\dot{V}_{O_2}$ as a function of the work rate during exercise are described in the following sections (Fig. 3-2).

Pattern of Work Rate Increase and the $\dot{V}_{O_2}$ Response

$\dot{V}_{O_2}$ increases smoothly when cycle ergometer work rate is increased in a continuous ramp pattern or in equal steps of 1 minute's duration. This type of protocol has advantages in the ease with which the patient perceives the addition of work load during testing. Increasing work rate in 2- or 3-minute steps results in large abrupt changes in work rate, and the increase in $\dot{V}_{O_2}$ at each interval takes on a step appearance (Fig. 3-3).[9] Because the time constant for $\dot{V}_{O_2}$ at low work intensities is 35

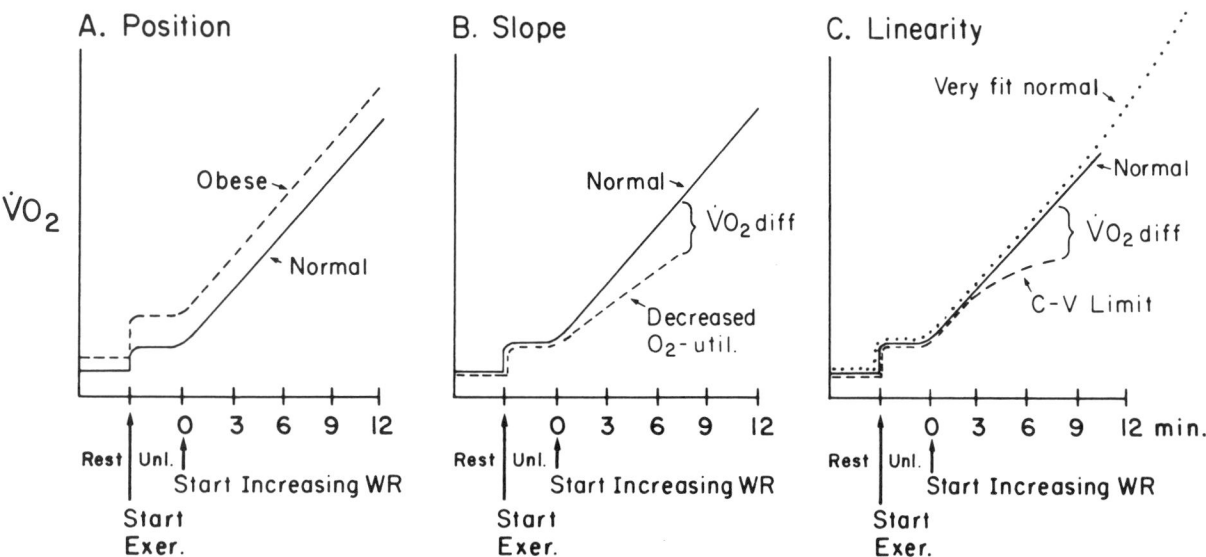

FIG. 3-2. Position displacement (A), slope (B), and linearity (C) of the $\dot{V}O_2$-work rate relationship. Obesity displaces the $\dot{V}O_2$-work rate relationship upward, but the slope is unchanged (A). A decreased slope of the $\dot{V}O_2$-work rate relationship (B) reflects inadequate O_2 availability to the exercising muscles, such as when peripheral blood flow is impaired. The linearity of the $\dot{V}O_2$-work rate relationship (C) can be altered in patients with cardiovascular diseases (slope becomes more shallow) because of impaired O_2 flow to the exercising muscles or in very fit people (slope becomes steeper; see text). The difference between the expected $\dot{V}O_2$ for the work rate performed and the actual $\dot{V}O_2$ at the maximum work rate of the subject is referred to as the $\dot{V}O_2$ difference.

to 45 seconds, steps at 1-minute increments give smooth increases in $\dot{V}O_2$, and the slope of increase $\dot{V}O_2$ with work rate can be calculated with either the ramp or 1-minute step increase.[9] For 3-minute step increases in work rate, the step appearance in $\dot{V}O_2$ is lost at the higher work intensity because of the slowing of $\dot{V}O_2$ kinetics as the subject approaches $\dot{V}O_2$max.[10] The loss of the step change in $\dot{V}O_2$ depends on fitness (Fig. 3-4).

Position Displacement of $\dot{V}O_2$ as a Function of the Work Rate

The position of the $\dot{V}O_2$-work rate relationship depends on body weight (see Fig. 3-2A). Obese subjects require increased $\dot{V}O_2$ to do a given amount of external work (see Chap. 2, "Oxygen cost of work"). Compared with a non-obese individual, the increase in $\dot{V}O_2$ caused by obesity during exercise is considerably greater than the increase in $\dot{V}O_2$ during rest. This is because of the added O_2 cost to move the limbs during cycling ergometry and the limbs and the body mass during treadmill exercise. From two separate studies of cycle ergometer exercise on adults, the $\dot{V}O_2$ during unloaded cycling at 60 rpm was displaced upward by an average of 5.8 ml/min for each kilogram of body weight.[11,12] Although upwardly displaced, the $\dot{V}O_2$-work rate relationship in obesity parallels that of the normal weight subject during

cycle ergometry. For treadmill exercise, a predictable adjustment for body weight is not possible because of complex mechanical factors such as the subject's varying center of gravity as the angle of the treadmill is changed and the variable length of the stride as the speed and grade are altered. These variables make it difficult to estimate the subject's actual power output during treadmill ergometry.

Slope of $\dot{V}O_2$ as a Function of Work Rate

The slope of $\dot{V}O_2$ as a function of work rate is important because it measures the aerobic work efficiency. The slope for the ramp or 1-minute incremental cycle ergometer progressively increasing work rate test has been found to be 10.2 ± 1.0 ml O_2/min/watt(W) for normal subjects by Hansen et al.[11] This is similar to the 10.1 ml O_2/min/W value previously obtained from steady-state measurements.[12] The slope of the $\dot{V}O_2$-work rate plot reflects the increased quantity of O_2 consumed per unit increase in work rate. If the muscles are unable to obtain the O_2 required because of inadequate O_2 delivery, then the slope would be shallower than normal (see Fig. 3-2B) and the predicted $\dot{V}O_2$max may not be reached. Although, theoretically, there may be several reasons for this slope to be reduced, including inadequate O_2 transport and limitation in O_2 diffusion from capil-

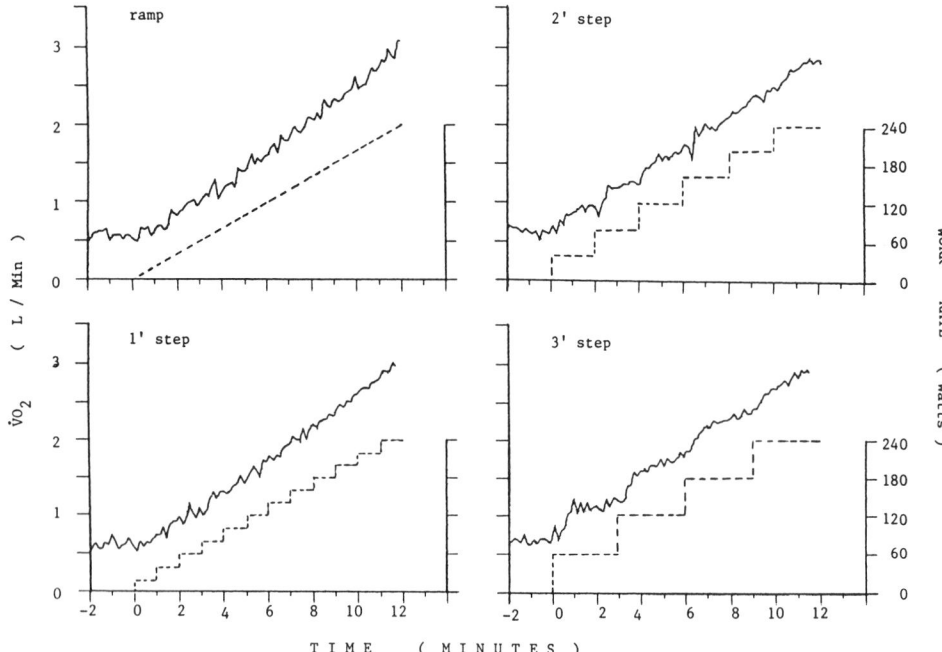

Fig. 3-3. $\dot{V}O_2$ response to four different protocols in a single subject ramp and 1-, 2-, and 3-minute steps. The dashed lines show the work rate and pattern of work rate increase with time. Data are the average of 9-second periods. (From Zhang, Y. Y., Johnson, M. C., II, Chow, N., and Wasserman, K.: Effect of exercise testing protocol on parameters of aerobic function. Med. Sci. Sports Exer., 23:625–630, 1991.)

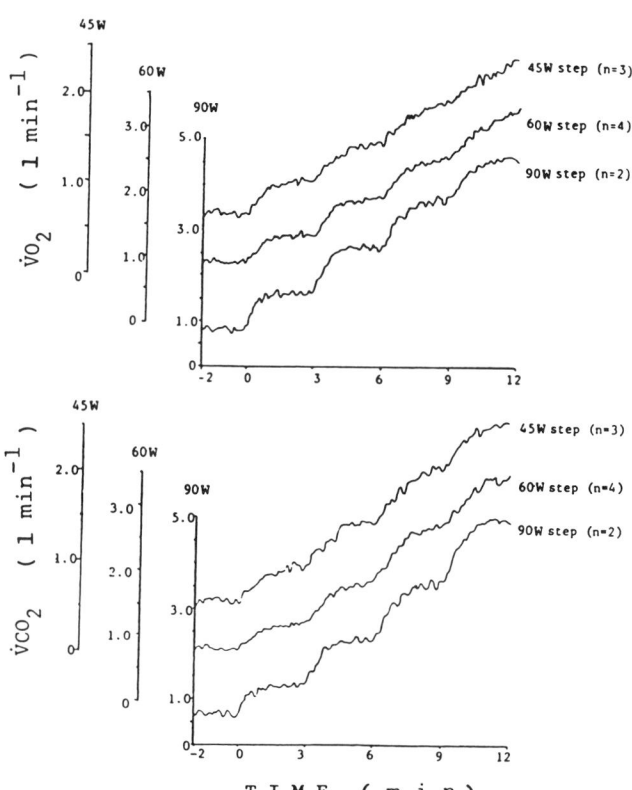

FIG. 3-4. The average time course of $\dot{V}O_2$ and $\dot{V}CO_2$ for each quarter of a subject's work capacity, assessed in 3-minute work rate steps, is shown for normal subjects at three fitness levels. The higher the step increases in work rate (90-, 60-, or 45-W steps), the greater the subject's fitness ($\dot{V}O_2$max). (From Zhang, Y. Y., Johnson M. C., II, Chow, N., and Wasserman, K.: The role of fitness on $\dot{V}O_2$ and $\dot{V}CO_2$ kinetics in response to proportional step increases in work rate. Eur. J. Appl. Physiol., 63:94–100, 1991.)

lary to mitochondria, a reduction is most likely to be evident in conditions of impaired or inadequate O_2 flow to the exercising extremities, such as in heart diseases or stenosis of the conducting vessels to the exercising muscles.

Linearity of $\dot{V}O_2$ as a Function of the Work Rate and the Rate at which Work Rate Is Increased

Because O_2 uptake kinetics are a more complex function of work rate than a single exponential at work rates above the anaerobic threshold (AT),[13–16] the slope of the $\dot{V}O_2$-work rate relationship is not necessarily constant as work rate is increased above the AT. If the size of the work rate increment is large relative to the subject's degree of fitness, then a relatively large proportion of energy generated would be anaerobic and the slope would be expected to become more shallow (Fig. 3-5, 60 W/min). In contrast, when the rate of increase in work rate is small, at least four factors can cause an augmented O_2 uptake and thereby cause the $\dot{V}O_2$-work rate slope to be steeper above the AT: (1) subjects often use additional muscle groups when performing heavy exercise, e.g., pulling on cycle handlebars to brace one's trunk on the ergometer as the pedals get harder to turn; this leads to additional and unmeasured arm work; (2) breathing work is increased nonlinearly as high levels of ventilation are reached, causing increased O_2 consumption by the breathing muscles; (3) significant lactate conversion to glycogen

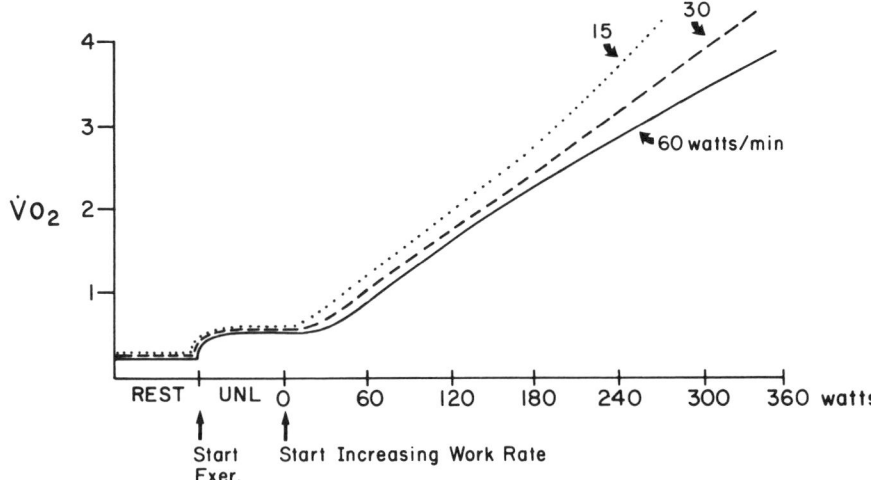

FIG. 3-5. Effect of work rate increment on the slope of the plot of $\dot{V}O_2$ versus work rate in a normal subject. A work rate increment for which the time from the start of the incrementing period to the maximum $\dot{V}O_2$ is between 8 and 12 minutes generally results in a linear $\dot{V}O_2$-work rate relationship to the subject's maximum. For work rate increments that are relatively large, causing the subject to fatigue in less than 8 minutes, $\dot{V}O_2$ may slow its rate of rise relative to work rate before the maximum $\dot{V}O_2$ is reached. In contrast, for relatively small work rate increments in which it takes 15 minutes or more before the subject fatigues, $\dot{V}O_2$ generally increases more steeply at high work rates. (Modified from Hansen, J.E., Casaburi, R., Cooper, D.M., and Wasserman, K.: Oxygen uptake as related to work rate increment during cycle ergometer exercise. Eur. J. Appl. Physiol., 57:140–145, 1988.)

(Cori cycle) by tissues actively involved in gluconeogenesis (liver) requires oxygen consumption to increase in those organs in which this reaction is occurring; and (4) anaerobic work is less efficient than aerobic work.

In view of the foregoing considerations, the finding of a deviation in the $\dot{V}O_2$-work rate slope above the *AT*, such as illustrated in Figure 3-5, is understandable. If the size of the work rate increment were relatively small for a fit subject, then the anaerobic contribution to energy generation (rate of lactate increase) at a given $\dot{V}O_2$ would be relatively small, and the factors noted previously would cause $\dot{V}O_2$ to rise more rapidly relative to the work rate[16,17] than that observed below the *AT*. In contrast, large work rate increments result in a sizable fraction of work done anaerobically above the *AT* (high rate of lactate increase), and $\dot{V}O_2$ would rise more slowly relative to work rate.[18] Thus, in the same subject, the $\dot{V}O_2$-work rate relationship above the *AT* can be more steep (small work rate increments) or less steep (large work rate increments), as compared to that observed below the *AT* (Fig. 3-5). Regardless of the increment used, however, the maximum $\dot{V}O_2$ is not affected to a significant degree. In general, work rate increments of 15 to 25 W per minute in normal men and 10 to 20 W in normal women give a similar rate of rise in $\dot{V}O_2$ both above and below the *AT*. A method for selecting the work rate increment for progressively increasing work rate exercise testing of normal subjects and patients is described in Chapter 5.

In disorders of the cardiovascular system, the linearity of the $\dot{V}O_2$-work rate relationship may be affected regardless of the rate at which work rate is increased (see Fig. 3-2C). The $\dot{V}O_2$ may increase normally as the work rate is increased at low levels, but $\dot{V}O_2$ may slow its rate of increase as the maximum $\dot{V}O_2$ is approached. This nonlinearity or decrease in slope of the $\dot{V}O_2$-work rate relationship is usually accompanied by a persistently steep $\dot{V}CO_2$-work rate slope, reflecting the CO_2 released from the HCO_3^- buffering of simultaneously generated lactic acid by anaerobiosis.[19,20] In this situation the subject's $\dot{V}O_2$max is clearly reduced.

Predicting $\dot{V}O_2$ or Mets from the Work Rate

Some laboratories estimate $\dot{V}O_2$ from work rate during exercise rather than directly measuring $\dot{V}O_2$. This practice is potentially inaccurate and should be discouraged. A unit called a "met" was derived from the average resting $\dot{V}O_2$ for a 70 kg, 40-year-old man. It is equal to 3.5 ml/min per kilogram of body weight. By assuming that a known fixed relationship exists during exercise between the ergometer work rate and the subject's $\dot{V}O_2$, some laboratories report an *estimate* of $\dot{V}O_2$ in milliliters per minute. After obtaining this derived $\dot{V}O_2$ and expressing it per kilogram of body weight, the $\dot{V}O_2$ is divided by 3.5 to obtain the number of mets performed by the subject.

Under certain conditions, however, $\dot{V}O_2$ cannot be accurately predicted from the estimated work rate for the reasons summarized in Table 3-4. For instance, if the ergometer is not accurately calibrated, the $\dot{V}O_2$ estimated could be in serious

TABLE 3-4. *When Work Rate Fails to Predict $\dot{V}_{O_2}$*

Faulty ergometer calibration
Steady-state not reached
Obesity
Valvular heart disease
Coronary artery disease
Cardiomyopathy
Peripheral vascular disease
Pulmonary vascular disease

error. In addition, if $\dot{V}_{O_2}$ is not in a steady-state, the $\dot{V}_{O_2}$ may be less or more than that extrapolated from the work rate (Fig. 3-5). Moreover, the $\dot{V}_{O_2}$ commonly does not increase linearly with increasing work rate in patients with cardiovascular diseases[21] (see Fig. 3-2 and the cardiovascular cases in Chap. 8). Thus, using work rate to estimate $\dot{V}_{O_2}$ or mets will lead to an overestimate in these patients. Finally, the correct body weight factor must be taken into account to estimate the $\dot{V}_{O_2}$. This factor is often ignored, or incorrect estimates of the effect of body weight on cycle ergometer $\dot{V}_{O_2}$ are used. Thus, the conversion of work rate to mets without actually measuring $\dot{V}_{O_2}$ is potentially highly inaccurate, particularly in patients, and this method should not be used.

Analysis of the $\dot{V}_{O_2}$-work rate relationship is of value only if the ergometer and the measurement system are accurately calibrated. Unfortunately, many cycle ergometers are not accurate, particularly over the low work rate range. We calibrate our cycle ergometer at regular intervals and have added a motor to the flywheel to obviate the initial work of overcoming the flywheel inertia (see Appendix). The accuracy and consistency of gas exchange measurements are also checked on a regular basis.

$\dot{V}_{O_2}$ DIFFERENCE

This term refers to the difference between the expected and measured $\dot{V}_{O_2}$ at the subject's maximum work rate (see Fig. 3-2). It is used to estimate the obligatory anaerobic component at the maximum work rate during a standardized incremental exercise test. The $\dot{V}_{O_2}$ difference calculation assumes that $\dot{V}_{O_2}$ increases relatively linearly with the work rate and that, at the subject's maximum work rate, there should be no difference between the expected $\dot{V}_{O_2}$ for that work rate and the measured $\dot{V}_{O_2}$, i.e., a $\dot{V}_{O_2}$ difference of zero. The expected $\dot{V}_{O_2}$ in milliliters per minute for cycle ergometry in which the work rate is increased in

ramp pattern or at 1-minute intervals is estimated from the equation:

$$\text{expected } \dot{V}_{O_2} \text{ (ml/min)} = \dot{V}_{O_2} \text{ unloaded}$$
$$+ 10.2 \text{ ml/min/W} \times (T \text{ min}$$
$$- 0.75 \text{ min}) \times S$$

where $\dot{V}_{O_2}$ unloaded is $\dot{V}_{O_2}$ measured after 3 minutes of unloaded pedalling, T is the total time in minutes of incremental work until maximum $\dot{V}_{O_2}$ is reached, 0.75 min is the time displacement between the start of the linear increase in work rate and the linear increase in $\dot{V}_{O_2}$ (estimated from normal subjects), i.e., the functional time constant for $\dot{V}_{O_2}$, and S is the slope of the work rate increment in watts per minute.

CARDIAC OUTPUT

Estimates of cardiac output during exercise are sometimes made with the indirect Fick method using measurement or estimation of $\dot{V}_{CO_2}$ and arterial P_{CO_2}, and mixed venous P_{CO_2} by the rebreathing method[22] (see Appendix). This method has multiple potential errors, however. First, estimation of arterial blood P_{CO_2} from alveolar or end-tidal P_{CO_2} measurements is unreliable, especially in patients.[23,24] Second, the assumption is made that mixed venous CO_2 content can be determined accurately from mixed venous P_{CO_2}. If the work is above the *AT*, however, the CO_2 content will be decreased for the same mixed venous P_{CO_2}[25] because of a shift downward in the subject's CO_2 dissociation curve. Third, the assumption is made that the CO_2 dissociation curve is linear, although in actuality it gets less steep the higher the P_{CO_2}.

If a catheter of the Swan-Ganz type is introduced into the pulmonary artery, the cardiac output can be determined by the direct Fick method. If a thermistor-tip catheter is used, a thermodilution curve can be obtained from the thermistor in the pulmonary artery, following the injection of iced saline into the lumen of the catheter opening into the right atrium. From this curve and the volume of iced saline injected, blood flow through the right atrium can be calculated.[26] Right heart catheterization is a significantly invasive measurement, however.

Cardiac output measurements tend not to be useful during exercise except when accompanied by simultaneous gas exchange or intravascular measurements. Pressure measurements are used with cardiac output to determine pulmonary vascular resistance or the degree of valvular stenosis. Cardiac output measurement may be useful when trying to assess whether the patient's reduced O_2 uptake is due to a low cardiac output. Cardiac output measurement, by itself, gives limited information, however. This is because the cardiac output measurement, even if accurate, does not reveal whether the cardiac output is adequate for the work rate performed. The major concern of exercise testing should be to determine whether the heart is capable of providing the exercise-stressed muscles with enough oxygen. To answer this important question, measurement of the *AT* during a progressively increasing work rate test is of greater theoretic and practical use. Similarly simultaneously measured $\dot{V}O_2$ and $\dot{V}CO_2$ kinetics in response to a constant work rate test can be used to determine whether the work rate is above the *AT* and by how much (see the section on *AT* determined from constant work rate tests in this chapter). These measurements are made noninvasively and, therefore, can be easily repeated.

ANAEROBIC (LACTATE, LACTIC ACIDOSIS) THRESHOLD (*AT, LT, LAT*)

The *AT* is defined as the level of exercise $\dot{V}O_2$ above which aerobic energy production is supplemented by anaerobic mechanisms and is reflected by an increase in lactate and lactate/pyruvate ratio in muscle or arterial blood (see Figs. 2-11 and 2-12). The biochemical and physiologic basis of the *AT* hypothesis and its relationship to lactate increase and the development of lactic acidosis are described in Chapter 2. The underlying mechanism for its measurement depends on the onset of anaerobic glycolysis leading to a net increase in lactic acid production (see pathway B of Fig. 2-1). At work rates below the *AT*, the muscle[27,28] and blood lactate/pyruvate[29] ratio is the same as at rest and no metabolic acidosis develops. Above the *AT*, a lactic acidosis develops. Thus, the threshold can be conceptually (anaerobic) or biochemically (lactate or lactic acidosis) defined. Like the $\dot{V}O_2$max, the threshold measurement is influenced by the size of the muscle groups involved in the activity.

Information Derived from the Anaerobic Threshold Measurement

Blood Lactate. There is a sustained increase in blood lactate and lactate/pyruvate ratio above the *AT*, i.e., *LT*.

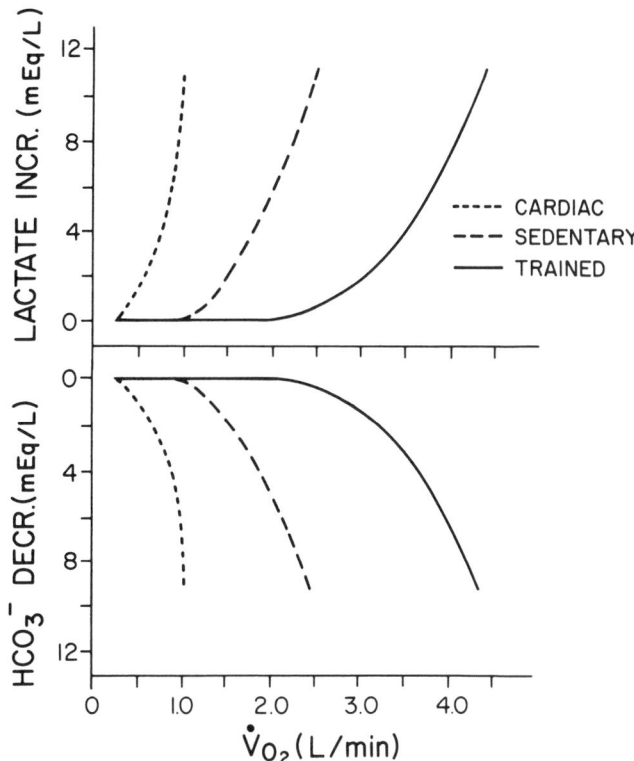

FIG. 3-6. Lactate increase and bicarbonate decrease during incremental exercise in trained and sedentary normal subjects and in patients with primary cardiac disease of class II severity as defined by the New York Heart Association Classification.[70] (From Wasserman, K.: *In* Physiologic basis of exercise testing. Pulmonary Diseases and Disorders. Edited by A.P. Fishman. New York, McGraw-Hill, 1980, pp. 337–347.)

$\dot{V}O_2$ *above which Lactic Acidosis Occurs (LAT).* Plasma bicarbonate decreases in a close reciprocal relationship with lactate increase (Fig. 3-6; also see Figs. 2-9, 2-19, and 2-21).

$\dot{V}O_2$ *above which There Is a Delay in Reaching a* $\dot{V}O_2$ *Steady-state.* The *AT* demarcates the work rate above which $\dot{V}O_2$ kinetics change. The steady-state in $\dot{V}O_2$, found to occur by 3 minutes when exercising at a constant work rate below the *AT*, is delayed for work rates above the *AT*. Thus, an increase in $\dot{V}O_2$ between the third and sixth minute of constant work rate exercise can be used as a marker to indicate that the work rate performed is above the subject's *AT*. $\Delta\dot{V}O_2(6–3)$ correlates with the magnitude of the lactate increase (see Fig. 2-37).

Work Rate above which $\dot{V}E$ Increases with Time. Ventilatory drive is stimulated by the metabolic acidosis resulting from lactate accumulation. $\dot{V}E$, primarily by increasing breathing frequency, increases as work rates above the *AT* are sustained (see Fig. 2-30). The rate of increase depends on the magnitude of the lactic acidosis and the work rate.

Sustainable Work Rate. To sustain exercise at a given work rate for a prolonged period of time without fatigue, exercise must be performed aerobically, i.e., below the *AT*. If the total high-energy phosphate ($\sim$P) required to perform the work cannot be supplied at an adequate rate by aerobic bioenergetic mechanisms and the $\sim$P reserve (preformed phosphocreatine and ATP), the muscles cannot sustain their contraction rate and fatigue must ensue. At work rates above *AT*, the greater the increase in arterial lactate, the less the endurance time. In an endurance cycling study of motivated young men, none could sustain pedalling for 50 minutes with an increase in lactate above 2.5 mmol/L (see Fig. 2-10). The higher the lactate concentration, the shorter the endurance time and the steeper the rate of increase of $\dot{V}_{O_2}$ during Phase III.[30]

Methods of Measurement

H^+ is produced, stoichiometrically, when lactate is produced in the cell. At the pH of cell water, virtually all this increased H^+ production must be buffered. The H^+ produced with the first 0.5 mmol/L increase in lactate appears to be buffered by non-HCO_3^- buffering mechanisms.[20,31] Above

that, HCO_3^- buffers the newly produced H^+ stoichiometrically.[20,31,32] Thus, an obligatory increase occurs in CO_2 production above that produced by aerobic metabolism at work rates above the *LAT*. It is relatively easy to detect the development of cellular lactic acidosis by measuring the rate of increase in $\dot{V}_{CO_2}$ relative to that of $\dot{V}_{O_2}$ during a progressively increasing exercise test. Beaver et al.[19] used a statistical regression method. Sue et al.[33] simplified the method, observing that the $\dot{V}_{CO_2}$ versus $\dot{V}_{O_2}$ relationship below the threshold had a slope consistently at or slightly less than 1.0, and that the slope changed to a value greater than 1.0 above the threshold.

A relatively short, progressive work rate test can rapidly determine the $\dot{V}_{O_2}$ at which lactic acidosis (*LAT*) develops when gas exchange is measured breath-by-breath, or as the average of several breaths, because the time delay is only a few seconds between the HCO_3^- buffering of lactic acid and the increase in CO_2 in the respired air. A flow diagram describing the sequence of gas exchange and ventilation changes in response to lactic acidosis for a progressively increasing work rate exercise test is shown in Figure 3-7.

V-slope method (Fig. 3-7, Mechanism I). Above the *LAT*, the net increase in lactic acid production results in an acceleration of the rate of increase

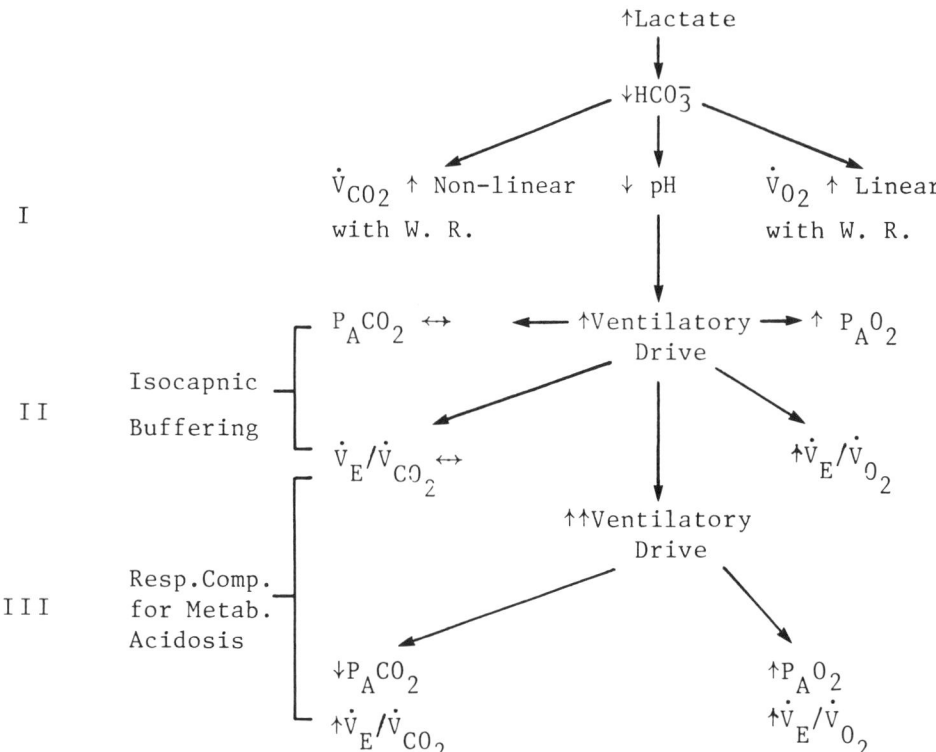

Fig. 3-7. Diagram of effects on gas exchange of increased lactate accumulation during a progressive incremental exercise test. Small arrows directed upward indicate increases, small arrows directed downward indicate decreases, and horizontal arrows indicate no change. Mechanism I describes gas exchange that results solely from buffering of newly formed lactic acid. Mechanism II describes changes in alveolar and end-tidal P_{CO_2} and P_{O_2} and ventilatory equivalents for O_2 and CO_2 that result from increased ventilatory drive consequent to CO_2 generated by buffering reaction. Mechanism III describes changes caused by further increase in ventilatory drive consequent to respiratory compensation for metabolic acidosis.

in $\dot{V}CO_2$ relative to $\dot{V}O_2$. When these variables are plotted against each other, the relationship is composed of two apparently linear components, the lower of which (S_1) has a slope of slightly less than 1.0, whereas the upper component (S_2) has a slope steeper than 1.0 (see Fig. 2-24). The intercept of these two slopes is the *LAT*, or the *AT* as measured by gas exchange. The increase in $\dot{V}CO_2$ in excess of that derived from aerobic metabolism must be generated from the buffering of lactic acid. This is an obligatory gas exchange phenomenon seen in all subjects who exercise to work levels above their *LAT*. This technique is referred to as the V-slope method because it relates the increase in volume of CO_2 output to O_2 uptake, as shown in Figure 2-24. S_1 and S_2 can be determined from statistically derived regression slopes of $\dot{V}CO_2$ versus $\dot{V}O_2$ in the respective regions of interest. The break-point or intercept of the two slopes can be selected by a computer program that defines the $\dot{V}O_2$ above which $\dot{V}CO_2$ increases faster than $\dot{V}O_2$, without hyperventilation. The values obtained by this method agree closely with the lactate and $[HCO_3^-]$ threshold.[19,33] If a patient develops a lactic acidosis with only slight activity, only S_2 may be evident; in this case, the *LAT*, and therefore the *AT*, will be less than the lowest exercise $\dot{V}O_2$.

Sue et al.[33] pointed out that because S_1 must have a slope value of 1.0 or less and S_2 a slope value of greater than 1.0, the break-point representing the *LAT* can be determined by placing a 45° right triangle on the $\dot{V}CO_2$ versus $\dot{V}O_2$ plot (plotted on equal scales). The $\dot{V}O_2$ at which the data points start to increase at an angle greater than 45° is the *LAT*. Whereas this method uses simultaneous measurements of $\dot{V}CO_2$ and $\dot{V}O_2$, it is independent of the subject's ventilatory response and insensitive to irregularities in breathing.

Ventilatory Equivalent Method (Fig. 3-7, Mechanism II). As the work rate is increased in a progressive exercise test (ramp or 1-minute steps), the linear pattern of increase in $\dot{V}CO_2$ and $\dot{V}E$ seen at low work rates (see Fig. 2-22) changes to a curvilinear pattern at high work rates while $\dot{V}O_2$ continues to increase relatively linearly. $\dot{V}E$ and $\dot{V}CO_2$ initially accelerate in a proportional manner above the *LAT*. Therefore, $\dot{V}E/\dot{V}O_2$ and $P_{ET}O_2$ increase, whereas $\dot{V}E/\dot{V}CO_2$ and $P_{ET}CO_2$ remain constant for a brief period (isocapnic buffering; see Figs. 2-22 and 3-8). Thus, hyperventilation occurs with respect to O_2 but not CO_2 as the *LAT* is exceeded. This isocapnic buffering period normally lasts at least 2 minutes. It is referred to as the isocapnic

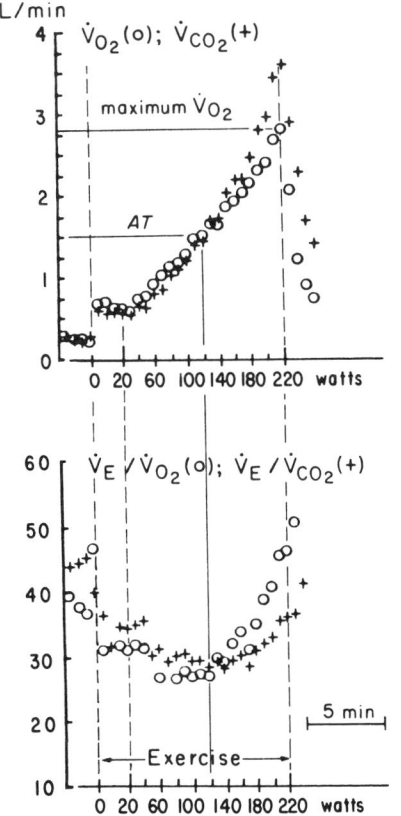

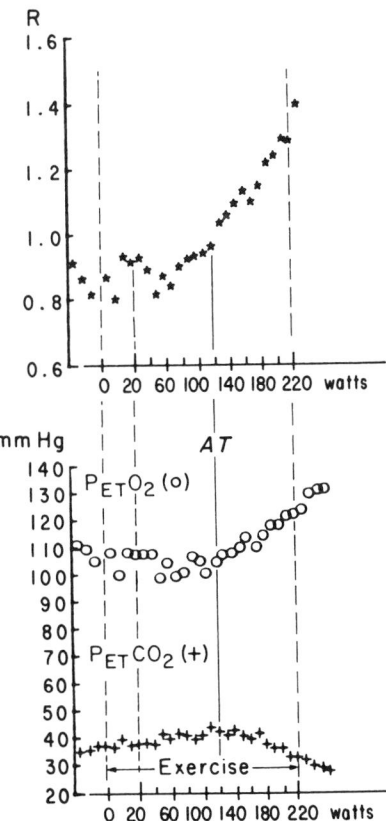

FIG. 3-8. Gas exchange for a normal subject during a 1-minute incremental exercise test. In each panel, the far-left dashed line indicates the start of unloaded cycling. The vertical dashed line second from the left indicates the start of the incremental period of exercise, and the right vertical dashed line indicates the end of exercise. The maximum $\dot{V}O_2$ is indicated. The anaerobic threshold (*AT*) is located where the $\dot{V}E/\dot{V}O_2$ curve inflects upward (vertical solid line). The nadir of the $\dot{V}E/\dot{V}CO_2$ curve does not occur until a higher work rate is reached and reflects the start of respiratory compensation for the metabolic acidosis. At the *AT*, $P_{ET}O_2$ increases, reflecting the hyperventilation with respect to $\dot{V}O_2$, whereas $P_{ET}CO_2$ does not start to decrease systematically until approximately 2 minutes later. At the *AT*, R increases more steeply, reflecting the increase in $\dot{V}CO_2$ relative to $\dot{V}O_2$.

buffering period because of the lack of hyperventilation with respect to CO_2 despite the development of metabolic acidosis.[34] The increase in $\dot{V}E/\dot{V}O_2$ without an increase in $\dot{V}E/\dot{V}CO_2$ is typical of buffering metabolic acid rather than other factors causing ventilation to increase out of proportion to CO_2 output, e.g., hypoxemia, pain, or psychogenic hyperventilation. When $\dot{V}E/\dot{V}O_2$ is observed to increase without a simultaneous increase in $\dot{V}E/\dot{V}CO_2$ during a progressively increasing work rate test, it is a specific gas exchange demonstration that the LAT has been surpassed.

One reason for increasing work rate relatively rapidly during the progressively increasing work rate test is to take advantage of the finding that the CO_2 contribution from buffering is observed only during the buffering process (the period of decreasing bicarbonate) and not after the lactate has been buffered. CO_2 generated from buffering is evident in the expired gas only during the period of lactate and HCO_3^- change.

As the work rate is increased further above the AT, the carotid bodies generally respond to the decreasing pH, and ventilatory stimulation is intensified (see Fig. 3-7, mechanism III, and Figs. 3-8 and 2-22). This causes Pa_{CO_2} to decrease, preventing pH from falling as much as would be predicted by the addition of lactic acid to a closed system. This ventilatory compensation for the lactic acidosis is reflected in an increase in $\dot{V}E/\dot{V}CO_2$ and a decrease in PET_{CO_2}, as well as by further increases in $\dot{V}E/\dot{V}O_2$ and PET_{O_2} (see Figs. 3-8 and 2-22). When ventilatory compensation for metabolic acidosis starts, the $\dot{V}O_2$ is well above the AT or LAT. This $\dot{V}O_2$ is sometimes referred to as the respiratory compensation point (RCP).

The AT is measured as a metabolic stress, i.e., in units of O_2 consumption and not work rate. In contrast to the RCP, it is unaffected by the rate with which the work rate is incremented[35,36] or by metabolic substrate.[37–39]

Improving Estimation of the Anaerobic Threshold

Occasionally, the AT cannot be reliably detected by the ventilatory equivalent method (see Fig. 3-7, mechanism II) because of atypical records caused by irregular breathing, an inappropriate rate of increase in work rate, suboptimal plotting scales, or a poor ventilatory response by the patient to the metabolic acidosis. To obviate these problems, one can measure blood lactate or standard bicarbonate directly. Beaver et al.[40] found that the lactate threshold (LT) during exercise can

be most reliably selected by plotting log blood lactate against log $\dot{V}O_2$. Similarly, the start of the $[HCO_3^-]$ fall, indicating the start of developing lactic acidosis (LAT), can be most reliably detected from a plot of log standard $[HCO_3^-]$ against log $\dot{V}O_2$.[31] A slight difference exists in the $\dot{V}O_2$ for these thresholds. LT precedes LAT, because of non-HCO_3^- buffering of the initial lactate increase.[20,31] Although we distinguish between LT and LAT for scientific correctness, the difference is not of clinical significance.

When the break-point between S_1 and S_2 is not clear using the V-slope method, it is likely that the CO_2 released from HCO_3^- buffering of lactic acid was small because work rate was increased too slowly during the progressively increasing work rate test,[41] or the patient could not produce lactic acid because of muscle phosphorylase deficiency (e.g., McArdle's syndrome).[42] In this instance, the test should be repeated with a faster rate of increase in work rate. If the break-point ($\dot{V}CO_2$ increasing faster than $\dot{V}O_2$) is still not observed, a deficiency in myophosphorylase should be considered.[42]

HEART RATE-OXYGEN UPTAKE RELATIONSHIP AND HEART RATE RESERVE

Cardiac output and heart rate normally increase linearly with $\dot{V}O_2$ during increasing work rate exercise[43] (Fig. 3-9). In many types of heart disease, the heart rate increase is relatively steep for the increase in $\dot{V}O_2$ because the stroke volume is low. In addition, in patients with coronary artery disease, $\dot{V}O_2$ commonly slows its rate of increase with work rate when the myocardium becomes ischemic, but heart rate typically continues to increase. Thus, the rate of increase in heart rate relative to $\dot{V}O_2$ becomes steeper, deviating from the linearity established at lower work rates (see Fig. 3-9). This implies that stroke volume is not being maintained and cardiac output increase is not keeping pace with the work rate increase. Although this curvilinear increase in the heart rate-$\dot{V}O_2$ relationship is not uniformly seen in patients with heart disease, it is a useful diagnostic observation and suggests a significant worsening in left ventricular function with increasing work rate.[44]

Pulmonary vascular disease is also associated with a steep heart rate response because venous return to the left side of the heart and, consequently, left ventricular output are reduced in this disorder. Patients with obstructive airway disease (OAD; see Fig. 3-9) commonly have a moderately

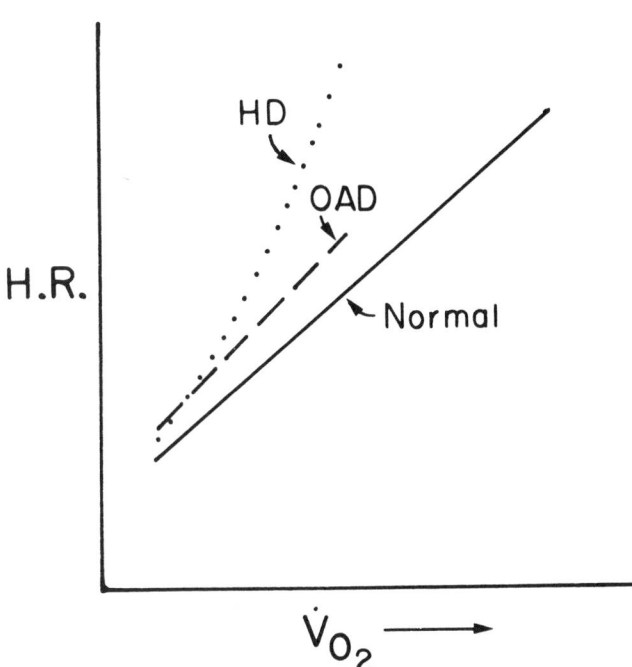

FIG. 3-9. Characteristic changes in heart rate (H.R.) relative to $\dot{V}O_2$ for normal subjects, for patients with chronic obstructive airway disease (OAD), and for those with heart disease (HD). The steeper heart rate-$\dot{V}O_2$ relationship for the patient with obstructive airway disease may reflect relative unfitness, whereas the relatively low maximum heart rate reflects respiratory limitation to the maximum level of exercise. The steepening heart rate-$\dot{V}O_2$ relationship in the patient with heart disease reflects the failure of $\dot{V}O_2$ to increase in response to the increasing work rate, as illustrated in Figure 3-2C.

TABLE 3-5. *Disorders Associated with Increased Heart Rate Reserve*

Claudication limiting exercise
Angina limiting exercise
"Sick sinus" syndrome
β-adrenergic blockade
Lung disease
Poor effort

tively small (less than 15 beats/min). It is also usually normal in patients with coronary artery and valvular heart disease and in patients with disorders of the pulmonary circulation. In contrast, patients with peripheral vascular disease and some patients with coronary artery disease may discontinue exercise because of pain before the maximal heart rate is reached. Patients with disorders of the conducting system of the heart, or sinoatrial node disease such as seen with certain cardiomyopathies, may also have a low maximum heart rate. Patients who take β-adrenergic blocking drugs or patients who are limited in exercise because of primary lung disease usually have a large heart rate reserve. Finally, those patients who make a poor effort have an increased heart rate reserve because they fail to stress their cardiovascular system at the time they stop exercising.

OXYGEN PULSE ($\dot{V}O_2/HR$)

The O_2 pulse is calculated by dividing the oxygen uptake by the heart rate. It is the volume of O_2 extracted by the peripheral tissues or the volume of O_2 added to the pulmonary blood per heart beat. This measurement is useful because it equals the product of stroke volume and the arterial-mixed venous O_2 difference ($C(a-\bar{v})_{O_2}$)(see Chap. 2 for a discussion of the distribution of peripheral blood flow). As the work rate is increased, the O_2 pulse increases (Fig. 3-10), primarily because of an increasing ($C(a-\bar{v})_{O_2}$). The upward displacement of the curve depends primarily on the size of the stroke volume. If the stroke volume is reduced, the $C(a-\bar{v})_{O_2}$ and, therefore, the O_2 pulse reach maximal values at a relatively low work rate, and the O_2 pulse has a low asymptote[45] (see the heart disease (HD) curve in Fig. 3-10). The maximum O_2 pulse is also low in anemia, high levels of carboxyhemoglobin, or severe arterial hypoxemia, all because of reduced arterial O_2 content.

The O_2 pulse measured breath-by-breath in the transition from rest to exercise and exercise to recovery also is informative. The immediate increase

elevated heart rate response at a given $\dot{V}O_2$ resulting from a reduced stroke volume. Heart rate increases linearly with work rate in this disorder, however. The maximum heart rate in the patient with ventilatory limitation is usually below the predicted value for the normal subject because the patient reaches the point of ventilatory limitation before the cardiovascular system is maximally stressed.[45]

The estimated *heart rate reserve* is an expression of the potential further heart rate increase at the end of a maximal effort progressively increasing work rate exercise test. We define this simply as the difference between the predicted maximal heart rate (see the section on maximal heart rate and heart rate reserve in Chapter 6) and the actual maximum exercise heart rate.

Although the predicted maximal heart rate has considerable variation, as determined from population studies, the heart rate reserve is still a useful concept for differential diagnosis. Table 3-5 lists disorders in which the heart rate reserve may be increased. Normally, the heart rate reserve is rela-

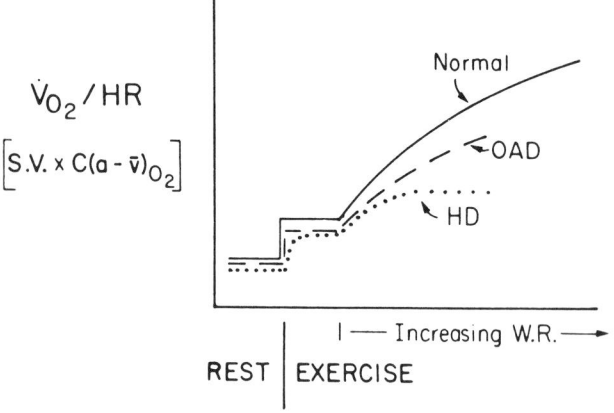

FIG. 3-10. Characteristic changes in $\dot{V}_{O_2}$/heart rate (HR) (O_2 pulse) as related to increase in work rate (W.R.). The $\dot{V}_{O_2}$/HR ratio is equal to stroke volume $\times$ C(a-$\bar{v}$)O_2. Thus, patients with low stroke volumes (e.g., heart disease [HD]) will tend to have low $\dot{V}_{O_2}$/HR values at maximal exercise. In contrast, patients with obstructive airway disease (OAD) have a pattern similar to that in normal subjects, although the values are lower at each work rate, reflecting the relatively low stroke volume in these patients.

in O_2 pulse at the start of exercise is dependent on the size of the stroke volume increase and the increase in C(a-$\bar{v}$)$_{O_2}$. The O_2 pulse decreases in the normal subject when stopping exercise; however, it commonly increases in patients with heart failure. The explanation for this paradoxical difference is that the afterload of the left ventricle is abruptly decreased when stopping exercise because of the rapid decrease in systemic arterial blood pressure. This allows improved ventricular ejection and increased stroke volume.[46]

ARTERIAL PRESSURE

Arterial pressure measurements, particularly when directly measured, are helpful in certain in-

stances. The normal responses of systolic, diastolic, and pulse pressures are described in Chapter 6, "Brachial artery blood pressure." The systolic pressure increases to a much greater degree than the diastolic pressure. The blood pressure changes are progressive with work rate. A decrease in systolic and pulse pressures with an increasing work rate suggests cardiac dysfunction. The development of a pulsus alternans may also be seen in patients with cardiomyopathies. Finally, the direct arterial pressure tracing, recorded at a fast speed, may provide evidence for ventricular outflow obstruction such as seen with aortic stenosis or hypertrophic cardiomyopathy.

BREATHING RESERVE

The breathing reserve is expressed either as the difference between the maximal voluntary ventilation (MVV) and the maximum exercise ventilation in absolute terms or this difference as a fraction of the MVV (see Table 3-2; Fig. 3-11). Except in extremely fit individuals who can attain high levels of $\dot{V}_E$, normal males have a breathing reserve of at least 15 L per minute or 10 to 40% of the MVV (Fig. 3-12).[47] A low breathing reserve is characteristic of patients with primary lung disease who have ventilatory limitation. The breathing reserve is high when cardiovascular diseases limit exercise performance.

TESTS OF UNEVEN $\dot{V}_A/\dot{Q}$

Wasted Ventilation and Dead Space/Tidal Volume Ratio

Alveolar ventilation is the theoretic ventilation required to eliminate the CO_2 produced by metabo-

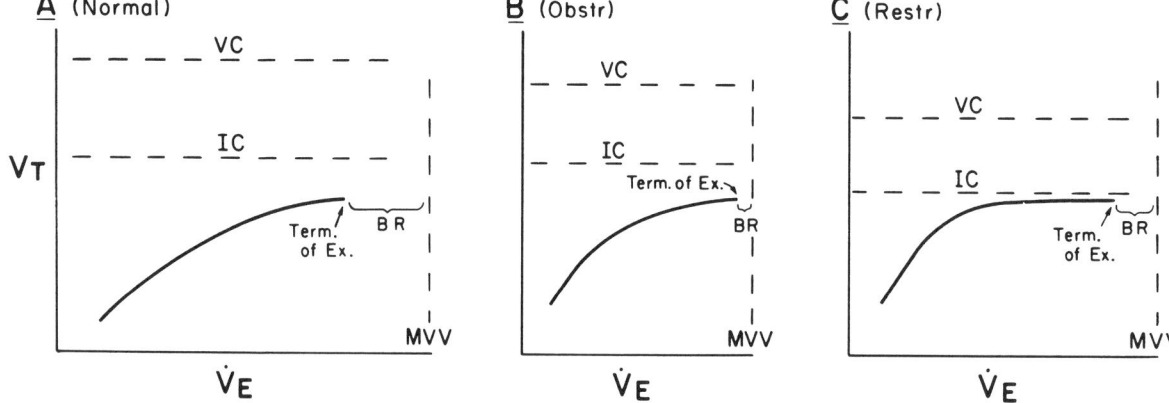

FIG. 3-11. Tidal volume as related to minute ventilation increase during incremental exercise testing in the normal subject (A) and in patients with obstructive (B) and restrictive (C) lung disease. The curve ends at the subjects' maximal exercise performance. The vertical dashed line indicates the subjects' MVV, and the distance between the highest $\dot{V}_E$ and MVV is the subjects' breathing reserve (BR). In the case of patients with obstructive lung disease, this is quite small. Although the V_T is always less than the vital capacity (VC) and inspiratory capacity (IC), it closely approximates the IC in restrictive lung diseases.

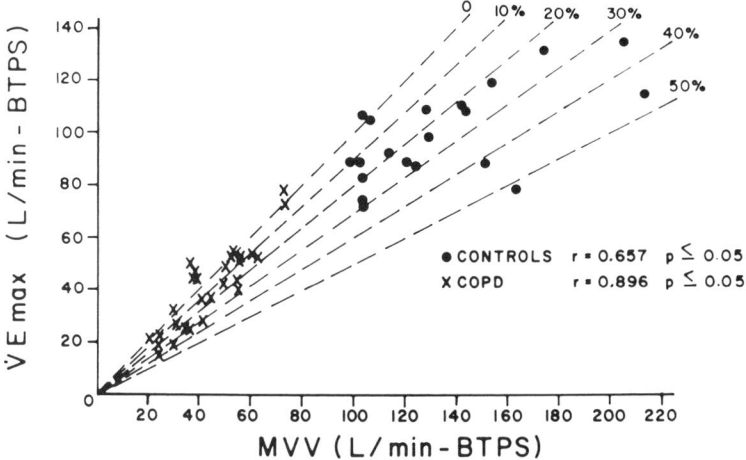

Fig. 3-12. Maximum exercise ventilation ($\dot{V}Emax$) as related to maximum voluntary ventilation (MVV) in patients with chronic obstructive pulmonary disease (COPD) and in normal subjects. The dashed-line isopleths indicate the percentage of breathing reserve.

lism at a given arterial ("ideal" alveolar) P_{CO_2}. The physiologic dead space ventilation is the difference between the minute ventilation and the alveolar ventilation. A valuable estimate of the degree of matching of ventilation to perfusion during exercise is the physiologic dead space/tidal volume ratio (V_D/V_T). The V_D/V_T is lowest when alveolar ventilation relative to perfusion is uniform.

At rest, the physiologic dead space volume is normally about one third of the breath. During exercise, it is reduced to about one fifth of the breath or even less (Fig. 3-13),[48] the major decrement occurring at the lowest work rates. In patients with pulmonary disorders in whom ventilation-perfusion relationships are uneven, however, or in patients with pulmonary vascular

disease whose alveoli are poorly or unperfused, the V_D/V_T is increased at rest and fails to decrease normally during exercise.

The V_D/V_T is a valuable measurement because it is typically abnormal in patients with primary pulmonary vascular disease or pulmonary vascular disease secondary to obstructive or restrictive lung disease. It is sometimes the only gas exchange abnormality evident during exercise testing.[24] Figure 3-13 illustrates the changes in V_D/V_T as the work rate is increased in the normal individual and in patients with alveolar ventilation-perfusion ratio ($\dot{V}A/\dot{Q}$) non-uniformity resulting from lung or pulmonary vascular diseases. In patients with non-uniform $\dot{V}A/\dot{Q}$, the V_D/V_T may be only slightly elevated at rest, but it remains relatively unchanged or even increases during exercise. Thus, exercise brings out the abnormality in ventilation-perfusion relationships.

When V_D/V_T is increased, $\dot{V}E$ is typically inordinately high for the work rate performed. $\dot{V}E$ may also be high in conditions in which the Pa_{CO_2} is relatively low (low CO_2 set-point), however, e.g., conditions associated with a chronic metabolic acidosis. In this setting, V_D/V_T will be normal if the lungs are normal, despite hyperventilation. Therefore, a high $\dot{V}E$ at a given work rate (high $\dot{V}E/\dot{V}O_2$) is indicative of either high V_D/V_T or hyperventilation. These pathophysiologic mechanisms can be differentiated if arterial P_{CO_2} is measured simultaneously with gas exchange.

Figure 3-14 shows the minute ventilation required for various metabolic rates ($\dot{V}_{CO_2}$) at designated values of Pa_{CO_2} and V_D/V_T. This plot is useful for demonstrating the relationships among $\dot{V}E$, Pa_{CO_2}, $\dot{V}_{CO_2}$, and V_D/V_T. It also serves as a nomogram for determining V_D/V_T when the three other variables are known.

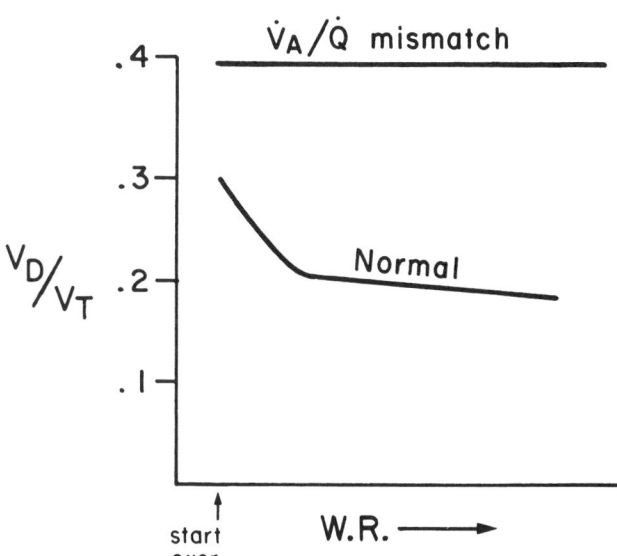

Fig. 3-13. The physiologic dead space/tidal volume ratio (V_D/V_T) during rest and at increasing work rate (W.R.) for the normal subject and for patients with ventilation-perfusion ($\dot{V}A/\dot{Q}$) mismatching.

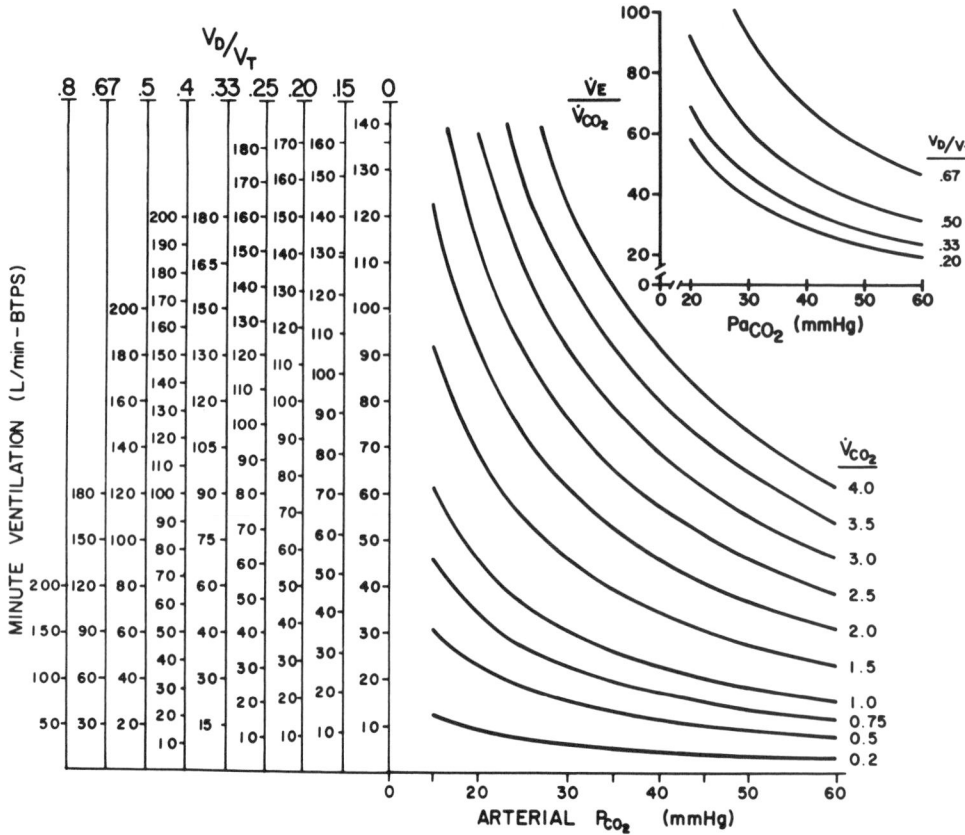

FIG. 3-14. Minute ventilation ($\dot{V}E$) required for various values of $\dot{V}CO_2$, as influenced by Pa_{CO_2} for various physiologic dead space/tidal volume (VD/VT) fractions. If any three of the foregoing values are known, the fourth might be determined. For instance, if $\dot{V}E$, $\dot{V}CO_2$, and Pa_{CO_2} are measured, then VD/VT can be determined from the ordinate that agrees with the measured $\dot{V}E$. The inset shows the effect of changing Pa_{CO_2} on the $\dot{V}E/\dot{V}CO_2$ ratio during exercise with a constant VD/VT. (From Wasserman, K., and Whipp, B.J.: Exercise physiology in health and disease. Am. Rev. Respir. Dis., 112:219–249, 1975.)

Arterial PO_2 (Pa_{O_2}) and Alveolar-Arterial PO_2 Difference ($P(A\text{-}a)_{O_2}$)

Normally, Pa_{O_2} does not decrease during exercise, and $P(A\text{-}a)_{O_2}$ remains under 20 mm Hg (Fig. 3-15A).[11,48,49] In patients with airway disease, a re-

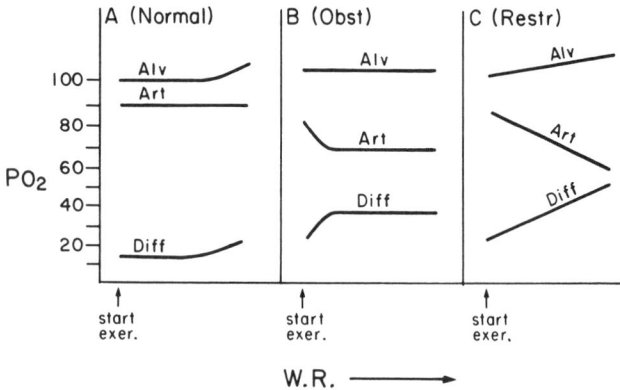

FIG. 3-15. Pattern of arterial and alveolar PO_2 and alveolar-arterial PO_2 differences in the normal subject (A) and in patients with obstructive (B) and restrictive (C) lung disease as related to increasing work rate.

duced Pa_{O_2} and an increased $P(A\text{-}a)_{O_2}$ during progressively increasing work rate exercise testing typically result from underventilation of regions of lung relative to their perfusion, i.e., low alveolar ventilation to perfusion ratio lung units (Fig. 3-16).[50,51] During exercise, when cardiac output increases, causing more desaturated blood to flow through low $\dot{V}A/\dot{Q}$ areas of the lungs, arterial hypoxemia becomes more marked. Fortunately, the small arteries leading to these poorly ventilated low $\dot{V}A/\dot{Q}$ areas of the lung constrict under the influence of decreasing alveolar PO_2.[52] This diverts blood flow to areas of relatively good ventilation and generally prevents hypoxemia from becoming progressive and marked as the work rate is increased (see Fig. 3-15B). Sometimes this mechanism fails, however, and hypoxemia worsens. Hypoxemia may also worsen in patients with obstructive lung disease when a potentially patent foramen ovale opens as right atrial pressure increases. This causes part of the venous return to shunt from right to left at the atrial level; 100% O_2 breathing is a simple, sensitive test to diagnose a

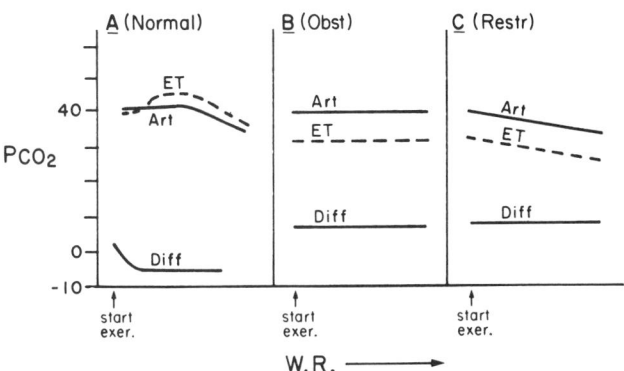

FIG. 3-16. Pattern of arterial and end-tidal P_{CO_2} values and arterial-end-tidal P_{CO_2} difference in the normal subject (A) and in patients with obstructive (B) and restrictive (C) lung disease as related to increasing work rate, all with normal resting Pa_{CO_2}.

right to left shunt that develops during exercise. For example, the Pa_{O_2} decreases 100 torr below normal for a 3 to 5% right to left shunt when breathing 100% O_2 during exercise.

Patients with pulmonary fibrosis or pulmonary vascular disease have a reduced pulmonary capillary bed. Therefore, when cardiac output increases, no alternative pathway for the increased blood flow exists other than through the same capillaries that are patent at rest. Therefore, these disorders are characteristically associated with exercise hypoxemia, which becomes systematically more pronounced as the work rate is increased (see Fig. 3-15C). This pattern of decreasing Pa_{O_2} and increasing $P(A-a)_{O_2}$ with increasing work rate reflects a decrease in residence time of red cells in the pulmonary capillaries when the pulmonary capillary blood volume is critically reduced. Thus, pulmonary capillary P_{O_2} does not have enough time to equilibrate with the alveolar P_{O_2}.

Pa_{O_2} might also decrease as the work rate is increased in conditions in which the alveoli are filled with material in which O_2 is relatively insoluble (e.g., as in pulmonary alveolar proteinosis). When the perfusion increases in these lung units, O_2 in the gas space fails to equilibrate with O_2 in the red cell, and hypoxemia becomes more marked as the blood flow increases (a diffusion defect). At rest, however, when pulmonary blood flow is low, Pa_{O_2} may be normal because red cell residence time in the pulmonary capillary is adequate.

When a patient hyperventilates, Pa_{O_2} may appear to be normal even in patients with pulmonary disease. Calculation of $P(A-a)_{O_2}$ may reveal abnormalities in blood oxygenation masked by hyperventilation. An abnormally elevated $P(A-a)_{O_2}$ is indicative of uneven $\dot{V}A/\dot{Q}$, a diffusion defect, and/or a right to left shunt.

Arterial-End-Tidal P_{CO_2} Difference $(P(a\text{-}ET)_{CO_2})$

Another valuable measurement that can be used as evidence of uneven $\dot{V}A/\dot{Q}$ or increased alveolar dead space is the $P(a\text{-}ET)_{CO_2}$[23,24,48] (Fig. 3-16). At rest, Pa_{CO_2} is approximately 2 mm Hg greater than $P_{ET_{CO_2}}$. During exercise, however, $P_{ET_{CO_2}}$ increases relative to Pa_{CO_2} (Fig. 3-16A and data in Chap. 6). The increase in $P_{ET_{CO_2}}$ comes about because of the increased rate of CO_2 delivery to the lung, associated with the high rate of CO_2 production during exercise. During exhalation, fresh air does not dilute the alveolar gas. Therefore, during this time alveolar P_{CO_2} approaches the venous P_{CO_2}. Direct measurements of instantaneously measured P_{CO_2} in the expired air show that the slope of P_{CO_2}, measured at the mouth, increases as work rate increases (Fig. 3-17). Because the $P_{ET_{CO_2}}$ is the highest P_{CO_2} in the alveolus during the respiratory cycle, and the arterial P_{CO_2} represents the average alveolar P_{CO_2}, $P_{ET_{CO_2}}$ is above the Pa_{CO_2} during exercise. In contrast, $P_{ET_{CO_2}}$ is normally less than the Pa_{CO_2} at rest because of the low resting rate of CO_2 production (see Figs. 3-16 and 3-17). Thus, $P(a\text{-}ET)_{CO_2}$ is slightly positive at rest but negative during exercise (on average, about -4 mm Hg). The slower the breathing rate, the higher the end-tidal P_{CO_2} relative to arterial P_{CO_2}.

If the $P(a\text{-}ET)_{CO_2}$ remains positive during exercise, this is evidence for decreased perfusion to ventilated alveoli (uneven $\dot{V}A/\dot{Q}$ with high $\dot{V}A/\dot{Q}$ units) (see Fig. 3-16 B and C). An extreme situation may be seen when CO_2-rich venous blood is diverted to the left side of the circulation without passing through the lungs during exercise (right to left shunt). In this case, Pa_{CO_2} is much higher than $P_{ET_{CO_2}}$ because the blood perfusing the lung is hyperventilated to compensate for the CO_2 load entering the arterial circulation through the shunt.[53] In this situation, $P(a\text{-}ET)_{CO_2}$ is markedly positive, the magnitude depending on the size of the right to left shunt.

Sue et al.[24] compared the resting D_{LCO} with arterial blood gases during maximal exercise in 276 male shipyard workers. Fourteen of 16 subjects with $D_{LCO} < 70\%$ had abnormal gas exchange, measured as an increase in $P(A-a)_{O_2}$, V_D/V_T, and $P(a\text{-}ET)_{CO_2}$, during exercise. Eighty-eight subjects had abnormal gas exchange with a normal D_{LCO}, however. Increases in V_D/V_T and $P(a\text{-}ET)_{CO_2}$ occur when there is a major component of uneven, high $\dot{V}A/\dot{Q}$ lung units. Both were usually abnormal in

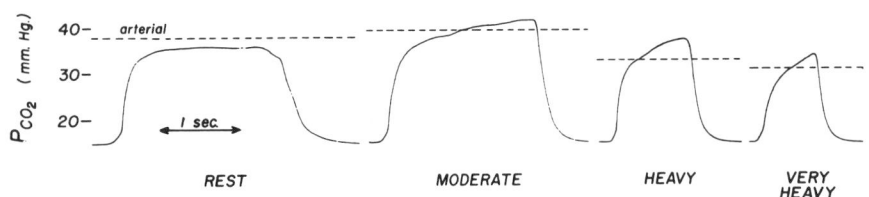

FIG. 3-17. Mean arterial (dashed lines) compared to instantaneous alveolar (solid lines) P_{CO_2} for the resting state and increasing intensities of exercise. The end-tidal P_{CO_2} is normally less than Pa_{CO_2} at rest but greater than Pa_{CO_2} during exercise. (From Wasserman, K., Van Kessel, A., and Burton, G.G.: Interactions of physiological mechanisms during exercise. J. Appl. Physiol., 22:71–85, 1967.)

the same subjects. In contrast, an increase in $P(A-a)_{O_2}$ is abnormal when there is a major component of uneven, low $\dot{V}_A/\dot{Q}$ lung units. An increased $P(a\text{-}ET)_{CO_2}$ and V_D/V_T occurred more frequently than an increased $P(A-a)_{O_2}$. When $P(A-a)_{O_2}$ was increased, $P(a\text{-}ET)_{CO_2}$ and V_D/V_T were also increased. In many instances, however, only $P(a\text{-}ET)_{CO_2}$ and V_D/V_T were abnormal.

Ventilatory Equivalents as Indices of Uneven $\dot{V}_A/\dot{Q}$

Because the measurements of V_D/V_T, $P(A-a)_{O_2}$, and $P(a\text{-}ET)_{CO_2}$ require arterial blood sampling, it is helpful to get a clue to a possible abnormality in $\dot{V}_A/\dot{Q}$ from noninvasive techniques. The nadir of the ventilatory equivalent for CO_2 or O_2 ($\dot{V}_E/\dot{V}_{CO_2}$ and $\dot{V}_E/\dot{V}_{O_2}$, respectively) can be used as a noninvasive guide to $\dot{V}_A/\dot{Q}$ unevenness during a progressively increasing work rate test. Normally, $\dot{V}_E/\dot{V}_{CO_2}$ and $\dot{V}_E/\dot{V}_{O_2}$ change as illustrated in Figure 3-18A. The $\dot{V}_E/\dot{V}_{O_2}$ normally decreases to its nadir at the lactic acidosis threshold (*LAT*), and the $\dot{V}_E/\dot{V}_{CO_2}$ decreases to its nadir when ventilatory compensation begins in response to metabolic (lactic) acidosis. The normal $\dot{V}_E/\dot{V}_{O_2}$ at the nadir is between 22 and 27 and $\dot{V}_E/\dot{V}_{CO_2}$ is between 26 and 30. Normal values for these ventilatory equivalents with a $P_{ET_{CO_2}}$ of approximately 40 mm Hg suggest a normal V_D/V_T and uniform matching of $\dot{V}_A$ to $\dot{Q}$ (see inset in Fig. 3-14). Elevated ventila-

tory equivalent values at the *AT* (Fig. 3-18 B and C) reflect either hyperventilation or an increase in V_D/V_T (uneven $\dot{V}_A/\dot{Q}$). Acute hyperventilation is supported by an R > 1. Hyperventilation can be clearly distinguished from increased V_D/V_T as a cause of high ventilatory equivalents only by measuring Pa_{CO_2} (see Fig. 3-14).

The ventilatory equivalents for O_2 and CO_2 can also be useful in providing evidence for insensitive chemoreceptors. In a progressive exercise test, the $\dot{V}_E/\dot{V}_{O_2}$ normally increases at work rates above the *AT*, the amount depending on the magnitude of the lactic acidosis and the sensitivity of the chemoreceptors in response to the acidosis (Fig. 3-18A). The subject with insensitive chemoreceptors may not reach the nadir for $\dot{V}_E/\dot{V}_{O_2}$ until the terminal work rate, and the value will be low.

Patients with chronic obstructive lung disease usually have uneven $\dot{V}_A/\dot{Q}$. Therefore, their $\dot{V}_E/\dot{V}_{O_2}$ is high (see Fig. 3-18B). Because of their mechanical limitation to breathing, however, they do not hyperventilate in response to metabolic acidosis. Thus, despite a metabolic acidosis, the $\dot{V}_E/\dot{V}_{CO_2}$ at the terminal work rate does not usually increase (see Fig. 3-18B).

ARTERIAL BICARBONATE AND ACID-BASE RESPONSE

Subjects making a maximal effort during a progressively increasing work rate exercise test nor-

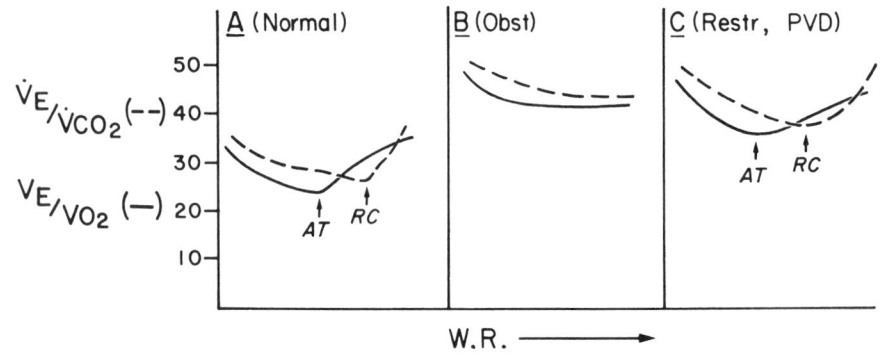

FIG. 3-18. Ventilatory equivalent for CO_2 ($\dot{V}_E/\dot{V}_{CO_2}$) and O_2 ($\dot{V}_E/\dot{V}_{O_2}$) for the normal subject (A) and for patients with obstructive (B) and restrictive or pulmonary vascular disease (C), as related to increasing work rate. The nadir in $\dot{V}_E/\dot{V}_{O_2}$ reflects the anaerobic threshold (*AT*), and the nadir of the $\dot{V}_E/\dot{V}_{CO_2}$ curve reflects the respiratory compensation point (RC).

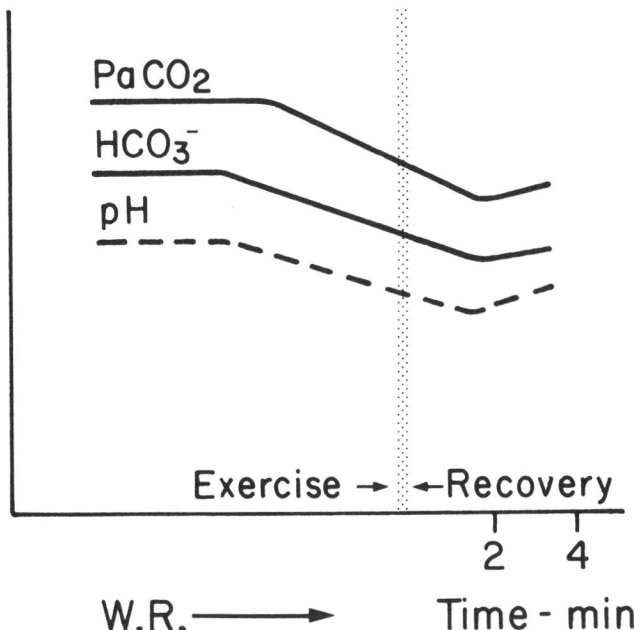

FIG. 3-19. Arterial P_{CO_2}, bicarbonate, and pH as related to increasing work rate and recovery. The stippled vertical bar indicates the point at which exercise stops. Note that the decrease in Pa_{CO_2} is delayed relative to the decrease in $[HCO_3^-]$ and pH (the period of isocapnic buffering). Also note that the P_{CO_2}, $[HCO_3^-]$, and pH continue to decrease in the recovery period with the lowest values at approximately 2 minutes of recovery.

mally develop a significant metabolic acidosis by the terminal work rate, even for an exercise testing protocol of relatively short duration (8 to 12 minutes), such as those used routinely in our laboratory (see Figs. 2-12, 2-22, and 3-19). The greatest reductions in arterial $[HCO_3^-]$ and pH are noted about 2 minutes after the cessation of the test, however (see Chaps. 6 and 8). We expect the $[HCO_3^-]$, after 2 minutes of recovery, to decrease at least 6 mmol/L below the resting value if the effort is good and the patient is not limited by a ventilatory disorder. The further decreases in arterial $[HCO_3^-]$ and pH during the immediate recovery period are probably secondary to the relatively slow decrease in perfusion to the most acidotic recovering muscles.

TIDAL VOLUME/INSPIRATORY CAPACITY RATIO (V_T/IC)

This ratio is usually abnormal in patients with restrictive lung diseases such as pulmonary fibrosis. Normally, V_T increases during exercise, but it rarely exceeds 80% of the inspiratory capacity (IC), measured during standard resting pulmonary function tests. Patients with restrictive lung diseases have a reduced IC, however, and so have a

limited ability to increase their V_T in response to exercise (see Fig. 3-11). The limited increase in V_T requires a high breathing rate to achieve the $\dot{V}_E$ needed for CO_2 elimination. Thus, in patients with pulmonary fibrosis, as the work rate is increased, the V_T/IC ratio reaches a value close to 1, V_T reaching an asymptote near the IC at a relatively low work rate. We routinely relate V_T to both the VC and the IC (see Chap. 8), but find the V_T/IC ratio to be more helpful than the V_T/VC ratio.

Constant Work Rate Exercise Testing

Whereas the absolute $\dot{V}_{O_2}$ required to perform a given work rate should be predictable from the principles established in Chapter 2, it is evident from Figure 1-1 that the ability to supply the O_2 needed to perform exercise depends on the cardiovascular response. In addition, the increase in $\dot{V}_{CO_2}$ depends on the rate of buffering of lactic acid by HCO_3^-, as well as the rate of aerobic metabolism measured as $\dot{V}_{O_2}$ (see Fig. 1-2).

Constant work rate tests permit the study of physiologic responses by specific organ systems to transport O_2 and CO_2. They also facilitate investigation of control mechanisms. All the measurements described for the increasing work rate exercise tests are equally applicable for the constant work rate tests. If the constant work rate performed has a $\dot{V}_{O_2}$ above the LAT, however, then $\dot{V}_{O_2}$ kinetics and the relationship between $\dot{V}_{O_2}$ and $\dot{V}_{CO_2}$ will change (see Fig. 1-2). These changes in kinetics reflect the patient's cardiovascular status during exercise at this work rate.

Research is ongoing to improve the method of quantifying gas exchange kinetics and the cardiovascular response to constant work rate exercise.

PHASE I OXYGEN UPTAKE

Normally, oxygen uptake abruptly increases at the start of exercise (Phase I) because of the immediate increase in blood flow through the lungs resulting from the increased venous return, enhanced cardiac inotropy, and increased heart rate (see Figs. 2-35 and 2-36). Increased pulmonary blood flow is the predominant mechanism accounting for the increase in $\dot{V}_{O_2}$ during the first 15 seconds of exercise. Under conditions in which pulmonary blood flow fails to increase abruptly at the start of exercise, the Phase I increase in oxygen uptake is attenuated.[54–57] This reduced Phase I increase in oxygen uptake may be found in disorders that limit the increase in pulmonary blood flow at the start of exercise.[55–57] On the other hand, a reduced ventilatory response in Phase I does not discernibly mask the normal rapid increase in $\dot{V}O_2$.[58]

OXYGEN UPTAKE KINETICS: IS THE WORK RATE PERFORMED ABOVE OR BELOW THE ANAEROBIC THRESHOLD?

After the immediate increase in $\dot{V}O_2$ and $\dot{V}CO_2$ (first 15 seconds of exercise) of a constant work rate test, $\dot{V}O_2$ and $\dot{V}CO_2$ increase as exponential functions (Phase II). Because of this, their rates of rise have been described by time constants, the time for 63% of the final response to be reached. Although this approach has been used by some investigators,[8,13–15,17] it is not a totally accurate measurement because $\dot{V}O_2$ has first order exponential kinetics only for work rates below the *AT*. Above the *AT*, the $\dot{V}O_2$ kinetics must be defined by at least two exponential functions, the second becoming more prominent the higher the work above the threshold.[14,15]

Mean Response Time

Sietsema et al.[59] performed multiple 6-minute constant work rate tests in normal subjects at work rates ranging from unloaded cycling to 150 W. These investigators assumed single exponential kinetics and calculated a *mean response time (MRT)*

for the data. The *MRT* measurement at the higher work rates allowed discrimination of the subject's fitness to perform a progressively increasing work rate test. Thus, the subjects with the highest $\dot{V}O_2max/kg$ body weight had the lowest *MRTs* for the 75-, 100-, and 150-W work rates (Fig. 3-20).

O_2 Deficit

From the studies of Sietsema et al.,[56,59] the less fit subjects have the higher O_2 deficit (see Chap. 2, "O_2 deficit"). Figure 3-21 shows the application of the measurements of oxygen uptake kinetics. For the same relatively low work rate (40-W cycling work), $\dot{V}O_2$ for a patient with chronic obstructive pulmonary disease (COPD) had a longer time constant than for a normal subject, matched for age and gender. When compared to the time constants for normal subjects at 50 W in Figure 3-20, it is evident that the consumption of oxygen by the exercising muscles is slow to increase in the patient with COPD. This indicates that the O_2 deficit is increased and implies the development of a lactic acidosis by the subject in response to the 40-W work rate.

Simultaneous $\dot{V}O_2$ and $\dot{V}CO_2$ Kinetics

For work below the *AT*, $\dot{V}CO_2$ rises slightly more slowly than $\dot{V}O_2$ during Phase II because of the relative high CO_2 solubility in muscle. This accounts for the transient decrease in R during the first minute of exercise, as shown in Figure 3-22.

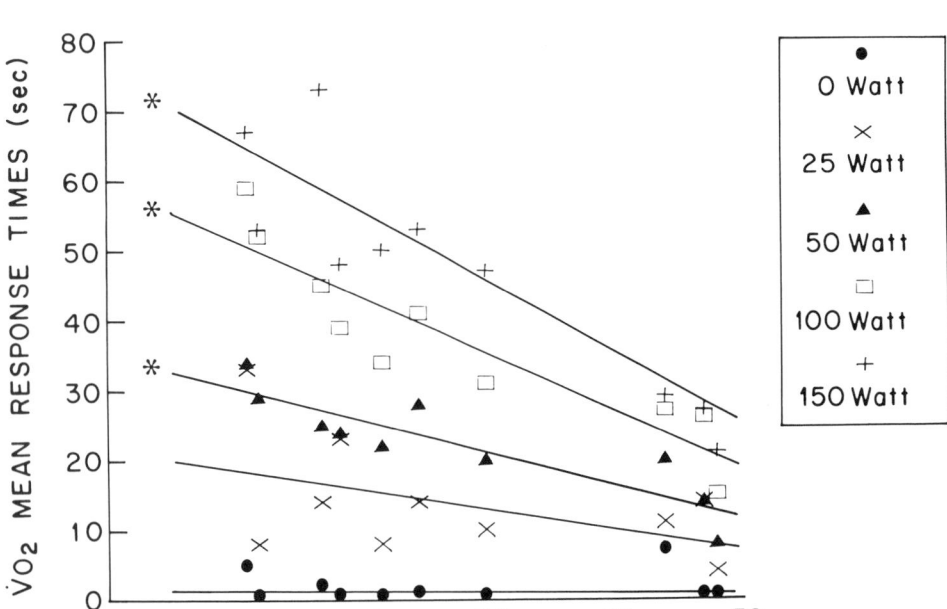

FIG. 3-20. Mean response times for O_2 uptake ($\dot{V}O_2$) as a function of fitness, characterized as maximum, or peak $\dot{V}O_2$ (ml/min/kg) for 10 normal subjects. Regression lines are drawn for data obtained at each of 5 work rates. The asterisk denotes a significant correlation between fitness and mean response time. (From Sietsema, K.E., Daly, J.A., and Wasserman, K.: Early dynamics of O_2 uptake and heart rate as affected by exercise work rate. J. Appl. Physiol., 67:2535–2541, 1989.)

Legend:
● 0 Watt
✕ 25 Watt
▲ 50 Watt
□ 100 Watt
+ 150 Watt

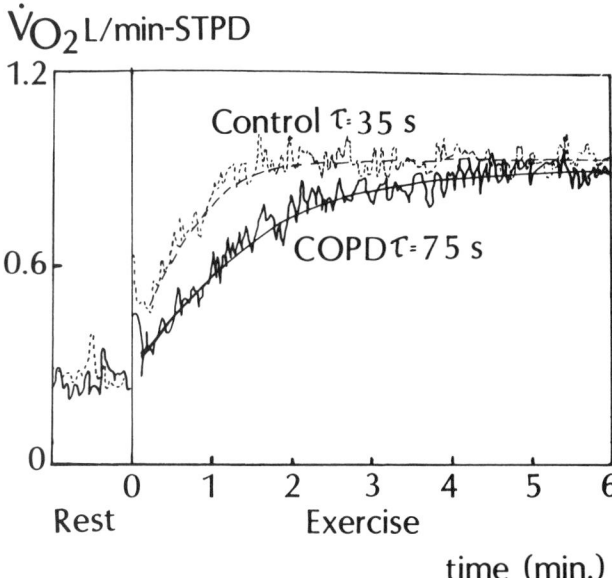

$\dot{V}O_2$ L/min-STPD

FIG. 3-21. Pattern of alveolar oxygen uptake ($\dot{V}O_2$) in a patient with chronic obstructive pulmonary disease (COPD) and a matched normal subject during the performance of 40-W cycle ergometer exercise. Note that $\dot{V}O_2$ during Phase I (the first 15 seconds of exercise) is less in this patient with COPD, and the rate of rise of $\dot{V}O_2$ to its asymptote during Phase II is also reduced, as shown by the longer time constant (T). (Data from Nery, L.E., Wasserman, K., Andrews, J.D., Huntsman, D.J., Hansen, J.E., and Whipp, B.J.: Ventilatory and gas exchange kinetics during exercise in chronic obstructive pulmonary disease. J. Appl. Physiol., 53:1594–1602, 1982.)

$\dot{V}CO_2$ increases more rapidly than $\dot{V}O_2$ after about 1 minute of constant work rate exercise, however, if the work rate is above the AT (see Fig. 1-2), accounting for the increase in the gas exchange ratio R shown in Figure 3-22 for the 100- and 150-W work rates. Thus, from the simultaneous analysis of $\dot{V}CO_2$ and $\dot{V}O_2$, it is possible to determine whether the work rate is accompanied by a lactic acidosis.

$\Delta\dot{V}O_2(6–3)$

Although $\dot{V}O_2$ after 3 minutes (Phase III) is constant when the exercise work rate is below the subject's AT, i.e., the subject is in metabolic homeostasis, $\dot{V}O_2$ has been shown to increase after 3 minutes, in proportion to the increase in lactate, for work rates above the AT.[14,30,60,61] The increase in oxygen uptake between 3 and 6 minutes of exercise ($\Delta\dot{V}O_2(6–3)$) can be determined by linear regression of the oxygen uptake between 3 and 6 minutes of exercise (Fig. 3-23). When $\Delta\dot{V}O_2(6–3)$ is correlated with the increase in lactate above rest, a good correlation is found for both patients and normal subjects (Fig. 3-24). The regression of the relationship goes through the origin, suggesting

that confounding factors other than lactate increase are relatively unimportant as the cause of $\Delta\dot{V}O_2(6–3)$ for above AT work.

Millimoles of HCO_3^- Buffering Lactic Acid

By measuring CO_2 output and O_2 uptake breath-by-breath for work above unloaded cycling exercise, Zhang et al.[62] demonstrated that the cumulative output of CO_2 progressively increases relative to the cumulative increase in O_2 uptake for constant work rate exercise associated with a lactic acidosis, in contrast to work for which a lactic acidosis was not found (Fig. 3-25). By multiplying $\dot{V}O_2$ by the muscle substrate respiratory quotient (approximately 0.95), the aerobic CO_2 production was calculated by Zhang et al.[62] The difference between the total CO_2 output and the aerobic CO_2 output should represent the CO_2 output from buffering lactic acid plus CO_2 from hyperventilation, if any (Fig. 3-25). The latter was found to account for only about 6% of the excess CO_2 over that derived from aerobic metabolism in the subjects who hyperventilated in response to the exercise-induced lactic acidosis at 6 minutes of exercise (50% of the subjects). When the number of millimoles of CO_2 output derived from the buffering of lactic acid at 6 minutes of constant work rate exercise was calculated, this quantity correlated closely with the lactate increase determined from antecubital vein blood sampled 2 minutes into recovery (Fig. 3-26). This method, therefore, describes a noninvasive estimate of the *magnitude* of lactate increase during constant work rate exercise.

Combining Measurements Reflecting Anaerobic Metabolism and Lactic Acid Buffering

When a subject exercises at a constant work rate below the AT, $\dot{V}O_2$ reaches a steady-state within 3 minutes (see Fig. 2-38). This means that cellular oxidative mechanisms are satisfied solely by atmospheric O_2 and that Phase II (the component that reflects decreasing mixed venous oxygen content and increasing cardiac output) has been completed. In a steady-state below the AT, no anaerobic mechanisms support bioenergetics, and the O_2 debt has reached a maximum.[63] Constant work rate exercise performed at a level above the AT results in a delay or an inability to reach a constant $\dot{V}O_2$, however (see Fig. 2-38). As reported previously, $\dot{V}O_2$ continues to increase even after 3 minutes, the rate depending on the fractional distance

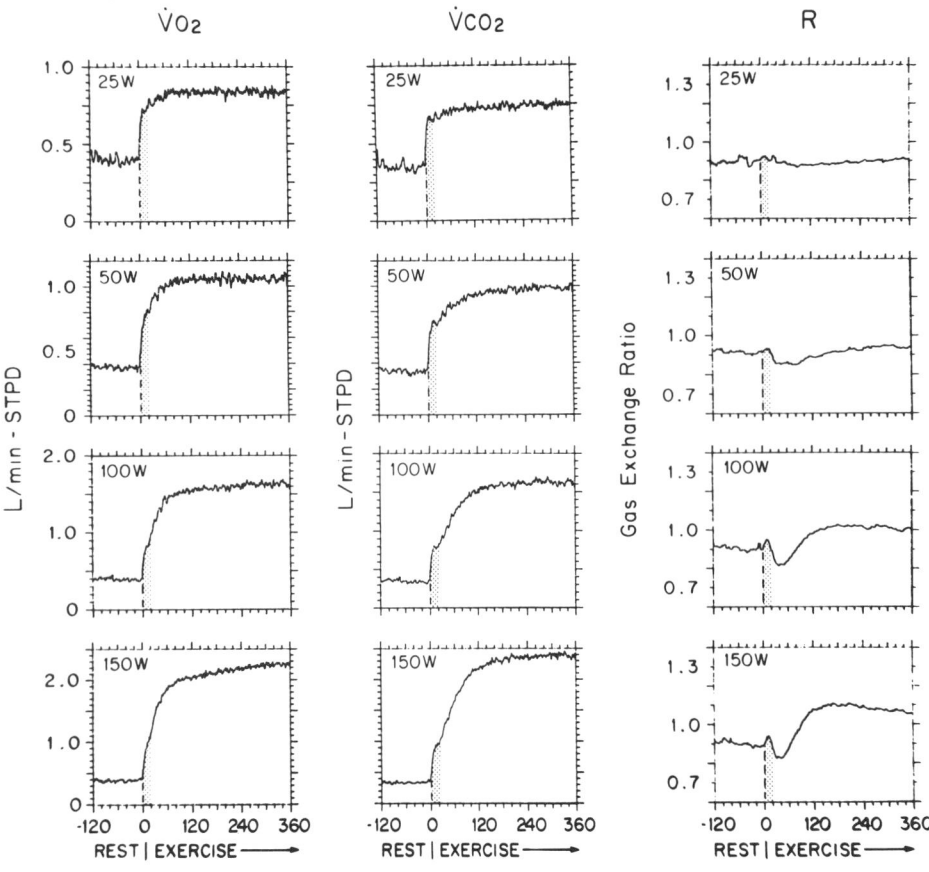

FIG. 3-22. $\dot{V}O_2$, $\dot{V}CO_2$, and gas exchange ratio (R) for 25-, 50-, 100-, and 150-W work in a normal subject. To reduce random noise, the subject performed each work rate on different days, six times. The data were then time averaged to enhance the physiologic responses and to reduce noise. (Data from Sietsema, K.E., Daly, J.A., and Wasserman, K.: Early dynamics of O_2 uptake and heart rate as affected by exercise work rate. J. Appl. Physiol., 67: 2535–2541, 1989.)

between AT and $\dot{V}O_2$max (Fig. 3-27). Thus, to determine whether a specific work rate is above the AT, measurement of $\dot{V}O_2$ at 3 and 6 minutes during a 6-minute constant work rate test is helpful. If the 6-minute $\dot{V}O_2$ is greater than the 3-minute $\dot{V}O_2$, then the work rate will be above the AT. The

$\Delta\dot{V}O_2(6-3)$ correlates well with the lactate increase, as shown in Figure 3-24.

Measurement of $\dot{V}CO_2$ simultaneously with $\dot{V}O_2$ provides added confirmation of the work rate with respect to the AT. If $\dot{V}CO_2$ is greater than $\dot{V}O_2$ at 3 minutes of exercise (before significant hyperven-

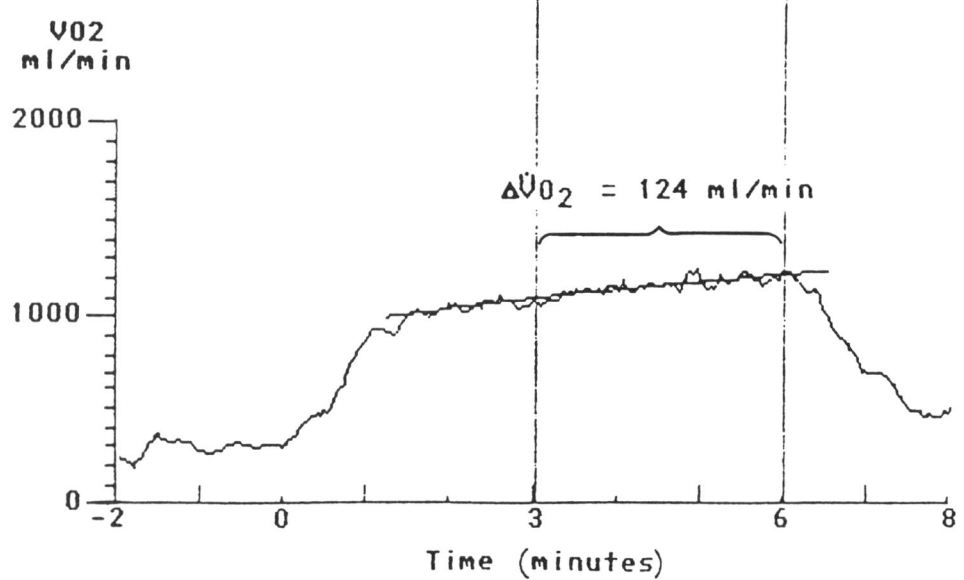

FIG. 3-23. Method illustrating the measurement of the difference in oxygen uptake ($\dot{V}O_2$) between 6 and 3 minutes ($\Delta\dot{V}O_2$ (6–3)) of constant work rate exercise in a patient with cardiac disease (70 W). The straight line drawn on the plot between 3 and 6 minutes was determined by the best least square fit for the breath-by-breath data. The difference in $\dot{V}O_2$ at the 6- and 3-minute points is calculated from the 3- and 6-minute intercepts of the linear regression of the data between 3 and 6 minutes.

tilation), this indicates that the work performed is above the *AT* (see Chap. 2).

Expiratory Flow Pattern

The expiratory flow pattern can be useful in detecting airway obstruction during exercise. The normal expiratory flow pattern has its peak close to the middle of expiration. The expiratory flow pattern of the patient with obstructive airway disease has an early peak and appears trapezoidal because exhalation is sustained until the next inspiration is initiated. Thus, expiration is abruptly terminated without an end-expiratory pause (Fig. 3-28). This pattern can normalize in asthmatics after bronchodilators are given (Fig. 3-28). Although the expiratory flow pattern gives only qualitative evidence of airflow obstruction during exercise, it is obtained simply by recording expired airflow with a pneumotachometer. More complex approaches, such as flow-volume analysis and increase in functional residual capacity, might add further information on disturbances in lung mechanics during exercise.

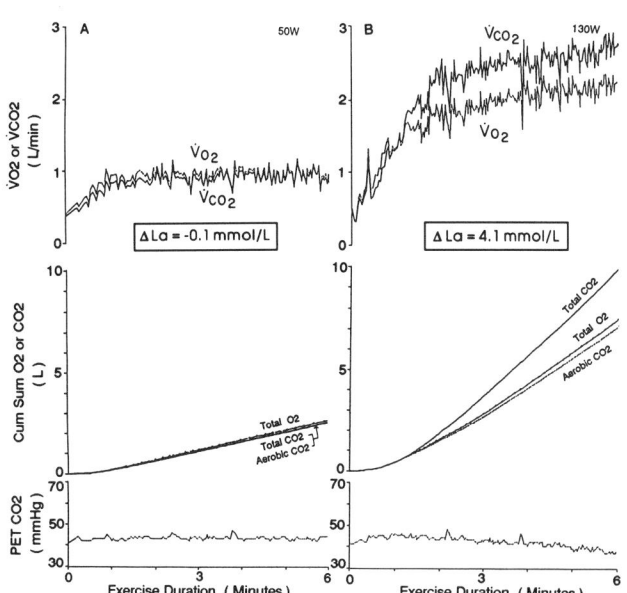

FIG. 3-25. Breath-by-breath changes in $\dot{V}_{O_2}$, $\dot{V}_{CO_2}$, total or accumulated O_2 uptake (cum sum O_2), total or accumulated CO_2 output (cum sum CO_2), aerobic CO_2 output ($\dot{V}_{O_2} \times 0.95$), and $P_{ET_{CO_2}}$ in response to 50-W (panel A) and 130-W (panel B) work rate tests for one subject. The difference between the accumulated total CO_2 output and aerobic CO_2 output is the accumulated buffer CO_2 output. In panel A, the total and aerobic cum sum CO_2 curves overlap and cannot be distinguished. The antecubital vein lactate at the end of 6 minutes of exercise for each study is shown. (From Zhang, Y.Y., Sietsema, K.E., Sullivan, C.S., and Wasserman, K.: A method for measuring bicarbonate buffering of lactic acid during constant work rate exercise. Submitted for publication.)

Carotid Body Contribution to Ventilation

Several techniques[64,65] have been proposed to study the contribution of the carotid bodies to the ventilatory response to breathing stimuli. We find a modified Dejours test,[66] performed during moderate constant work rate exercise,[67,68] to be informative and applicable to patients with lung diseases. In the steady-state of an air breathing exercise test, the surreptitious switch to 100% oxygen results in an almost immediate decrease in ventilation (within one or two breaths) if the carotid bodies actively contribute to ventilatory drive. By continuously monitoring ventilation breath-by-breath, the magnitude of the decrement in ventilation can be measured (Fig. 3-29). Ventilation decreases to a nadir by 15 seconds. This decrease reflects the carotid body contribution to the ventilatory drive and can be expressed as a percentage of the pre-O_2 breathing ventilation. Once the nadir is reached, ventilation starts increasing back toward its control value despite continued breathing of 100% O_2, but usually not reaching it. The

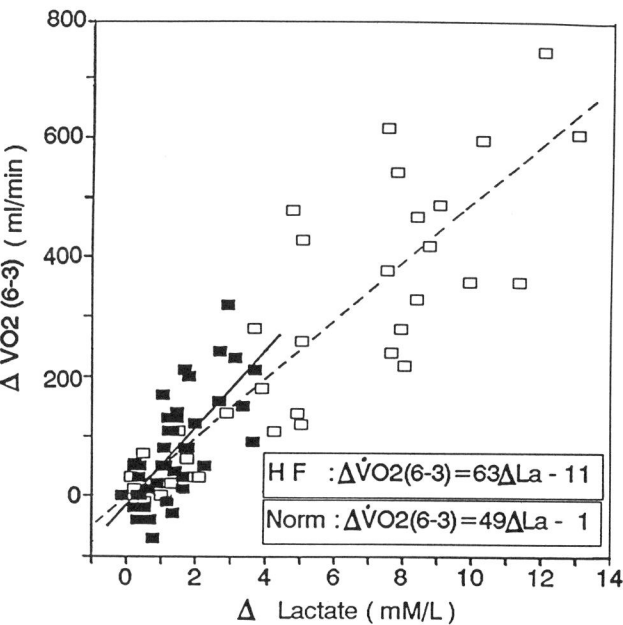

FIG. 3-24. Degree of unsteady-state in oxygen uptake ($\dot{V}_{O_2}$), expressed as the increase in $\dot{V}_{O_2}$ between 3 and 6 minutes ($\Delta\dot{V}_{O_2}(6-3)$), as a function of the increase in blood lactate above rest in normal subjects (open squares) and in patients with heart failure (solid squares). The blood was sampled from the antecubital vein at 2 minutes of recovery (exercise) as well as at rest. Neither the slopes nor the intercepts of the regression equations differed significantly between the two groups. (Data from references 30 and 60.)

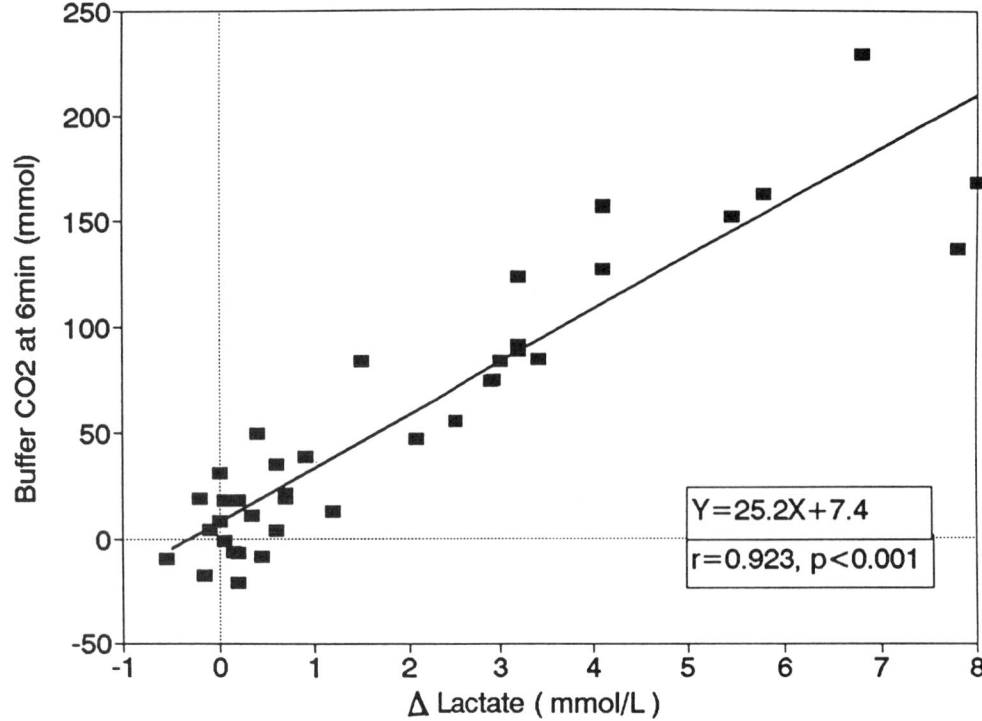

FIG. 3-26. Buffer CO_2 (mmol) as a function of the increase in blood lactate concentration (La) at the end of 6 minutes of exercise. (From Zhang, Y.Y., Sietsema, K.E., Sullivan, C.S., and Wasserman, K.: A method for measuring bicarbonate buffering of lactic acid during constant work rate exercise. Submitted for publication.)

most likely explanation for this rebound in $\dot{V}E$ is the stimulus to ventilation caused by the increase in Pa_{CO_2}. That is, whereas hyperoxia continues to inhibit carotid body drive to ventilation, the increase in P_{CO_2} resulting from the transient ventilatory decrease stimulates the central chemoreceptors. Thus, part of the carotid body contribution to ventilatory drive is masked if ventilation is not measured dynamically breath-by-breath.

The modified Dejours test is done rapidly, lasting only about 1 to 2 minutes of exercise, and is safe. It can be performed at work rates below or above AT to determine the separate contribution of the exercise-induced lactic acidosis to ventilatory control.

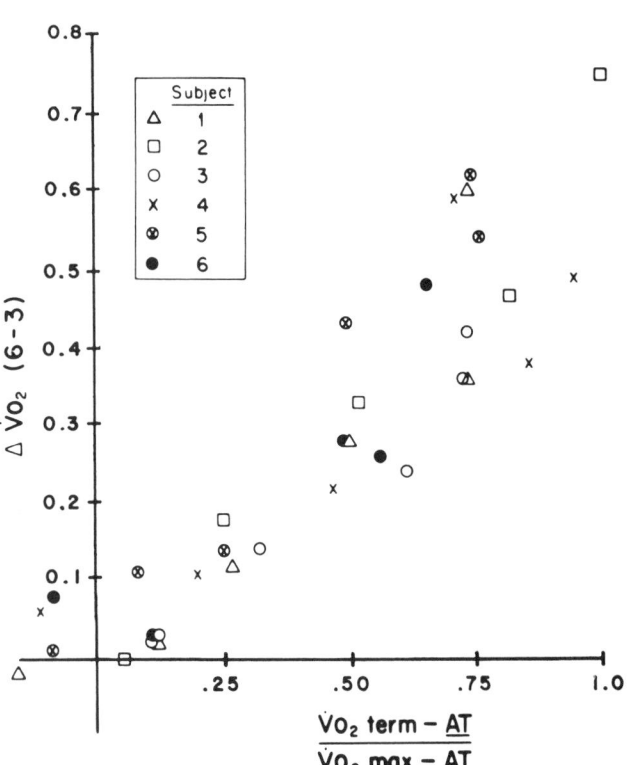

FIG. 3-27. Difference between 6- and 3-minute $\dot{V}O_2$ for constant work rate exercise ($\Delta\dot{V}O_2(6-3)$) as related to the fraction of the distance between the $\dot{V}O_2$max and the AT of the difference between the $\dot{V}O_2$ asymptote at the termination of exercise ($\dot{V}O_2$term) and the AT. (Modified from Roston, W.L., Whipp, B.J., Davis, J.A., Effros, R.M., and Wasserman, K.: Oxygen uptake kinetics and lactate concentration during exercise in man. Am. Rev. Respir. Dis., 135:1080–1084, 1987.)

EXPIRATORY FLOW DURING EXERCISE

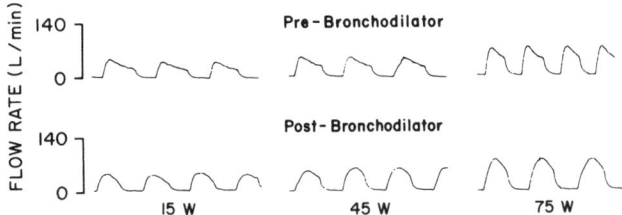

FIG. 3-28. Expiratory flow pattern in an asthmatic subject at increasing work rates before and after bronchodilator therapy. (From Brown, H.V., Wasserman, K., and Whipp, B.J.: Strategies of exercise testing in chronic lung disease. Bull. Eur. Physiopathol. Respir., 13: 409–423, 1977.)

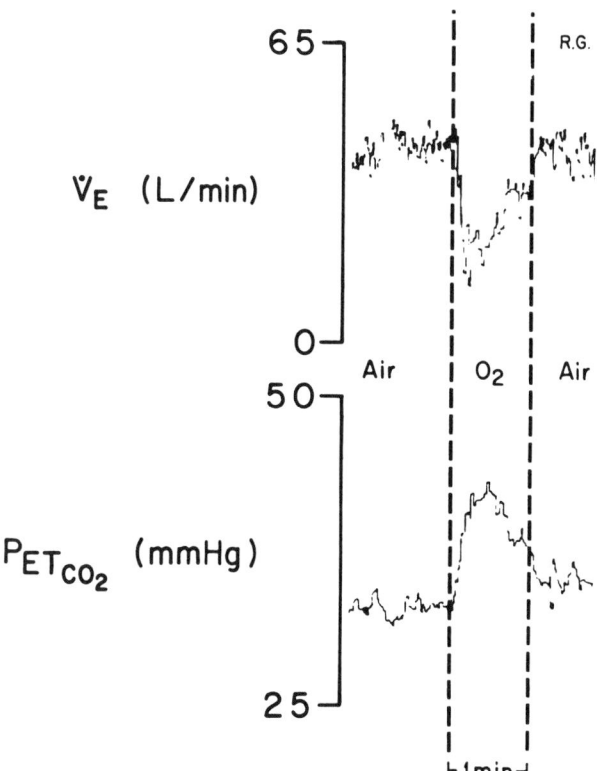

FIG. 3-29. Illustration of a safe test for assessing carotid body contribution to ventilation during exercise. The study is that of a patient with pulmonary alveolar proteinosis with a Pa_{O_2} of 54 during exercise. A work rate is selected at which the patient can perform without difficulty and for which a steady-state in ventilation is reached by 4 to 5 minutes. When $\dot{V}E$ is constant, the inspired gas is switched from air to 100% oxygen for 1 minute. $\dot{V}E$ decreases to a nadir within several breaths, and as a consequence, $P_{ET_{CO_2}}$ rises. After 15 seconds, $\dot{V}E$ spontaneously starts to rebound toward the air-breathing value because of CO_2 stimulation of central chemoreceptors. By 45 seconds, $\dot{V}E$ becomes relatively constant at a reduced value, and $P_{ET_{CO_2}}$ levels off at an elevated value as compared to the control period. Thus, three phases in ventilation are observed when switching to 100% oxygen breathing: the first 15 seconds when the carotid bodies are attenuated maximally; the period between 15 and 45 seconds, which shows a rebound in $\dot{V}E$ presumably caused by the increase in arterial P_{CO_2}; and the period after 45 seconds when $\dot{V}E$ and $P_{ET_{CO_2}}$ reach constant values. The abrupt changes in $\dot{V}E$ in response to the O_2 switch and return to air breathing reflect the rapid control exerted by the carotid bodies in the regulation of ventilation. (From Wasserman, K., Whipp, B.J., and Davis, J.A.: Respiratory physiology of exercise: metabolism, gas exchange, and ventilatory control. In International Review of Physiology III. Vol. 23. Edited by J.G. Widdicombe. Baltimore, University Park Press. 1981, pp. 149–211.)

Summary

Changes in O_2 uptake and CO_2 output by the lungs reflect changes in cell respiration induced by exercise. Cardiac output and ventilation modulate the changes in cell respiration seen at the airway in health and disease. Measurements that assess these functions following controlled work rate perturbations define the physiologic state of the organ systems that participate in gas transport. Defects in the coupling of external to internal respiration result in gas exchange abnormalities characteristic of the limiting organ system. For example, whereas diseases of the heart, the lungs, and the peripheral and pulmonary circulations all result in demonstrable abnormalities in gas exchange, each type of disorder manifests specific and relatively unique abnormalities that are amplified by exercise testing. The effect of various disease states on these measurements is described in Chapter 4.

References

1. Older, P., Smith, R., Courtney, P., and Hone, R.: Preoperative evaluation of cardiac failure and ischemia in elderly patients by cardiopulmonary exercise testing. Chest. 104:701–704, 1993.
2. Smith, T.P., Kinasewitz, G.T., Tucker, W.Y., Spillers, W.P., and George, R.B.: Exercise capacity as a predictor of post-thoracotomy morbidity. Am. Rev. Respir. Dis., 129:730–734, 1984.
3. Andersen, P., and Saltin, B.: Maximal perfusion of skeletal muscle in man. J. Appl. Physiol., 366:233–249, 1985.
4. Vogel, J.A., and Gleser, M.A.: Effect of carbon monoxide on oxygen transport during exercise. J. Appl. Physiol., 32:234–239, 1972.
5. Whipp, B.J., and Ward, S.A.: Coupling of ventilation to pulmonary gas exchange during exercise. In Exercise: Pulmonary Physiology and Pathophysiology. Edited by B.J. Whipp and K. Wasserman. New York, Marcel Dekker, 1991, pp. 271–307.
6. Taylor, H.L., Buskirk, E., and Henschel, A.: Maximal oxygen intake as an objective measure of cardiorespiratory performance. J. Appl. Physiol., 8:73–80, 1955.
7. Cooper, D.M., Weiler-Ravell, D., Whipp, B.J., and Wasserman, K.: Aerobic parameters of exercise as a function of body size during growth in children. J. Appl. Physiol., 56:628–635, 1984.
8. DiPrampero, P.E.: Energetics of muscular exercise. Rev. Physiol. Biochem. Pharmacol., 88:143–222, 1981.
9. Zhang, Y.Y., Johnson, M.C., II, Chow, N., and Wasserman, K.: Effect of exercise testing protocol on parameters of aerobic function. Med. Sci. Sports Exerc., 23:625–630, 1991.
10. Zhang, Y.Y., Johnson, M.C., II, Chow, N., and Wasserman, K.: The role of fitness on $\dot{V}O_2$ and $\dot{V}CO_2$ kinetics in response to proportional step increases in work rate. Eur. J. Appl. Physiol., 63:94–100, 1991.
11. Hansen, J.E., Sue, D.Y., and Wasserman, K.: Predicted values for clinical exercise testing. Am. Rev. Respir. Dis., 129:S49–S55, 1984.
12. Wasserman, K., and Whipp, B.J.: Exercise physiology in health and disease. Am. Rev. Respir. Dis., 112:219–249, 1975.
13. Linnarsson, D.: Dynamics of pulmonary gas exchange and heart rate changes at start and end of exercise. Acta Physiol. Scand., 415(Suppl. 1):5–68, 1974.

14. Whipp, B.J., and Wasserman, K.: Oxygen uptake kinetics for various intensities of constant load work. J. Appl. Physiol., 33:351–356, 1972.

15. Barstow, T.J., Casaburi, R., and Wasserman, K.: Oxygen uptake kinetics and the O_2 deficit as related to exercise intensity and blood lactate. J. Appl. Physiol., 75:755–762, 1993.

16. Whipp, B.J., and Mahler, M.: Dynamics of gas exchange during exercise. In Pulmonary Gas Exchange. Vol. II. Edited by J.B. West. New York, Academic Press, 1980.

17. Hesser, C.M., Linnarsson, D., and Bjurstedt, H.: Cardio-respiratory and metabolic responses to positive, negative and minimum-load dynamic leg exercise. Respir. Physiol., 30:51–67, 1977.

18. Haouzi, P., Fukuba, Y., Casaburi, R., Stringer, W., and Wasserman, K.: O_2 uptake kinetics above and below the lactic acidosis threshold during sinusoidal exercise. J. Appl. Physiol. In press.

19. Beaver, W.L., Wasserman, K., and Whipp, B.J.: A new method for detecting the anaerobic threshold by gas exchange. J. Appl. Physiol., 60:2020–2027, 1986.

20. Stringer, W., Casaburi, R., and Wasserman, K.: Acid-base regulation during exercise and recovery in man. J. Appl. Physiol., 72:954–961, 1992.

21. Koike, A., Hiroe, M., Adachi, H., Yajima, T., Nogami, A., Ito, H., Takamoto, T., Taniguchi, K., and Marumo, F.: Anaerobic metabolism as an indicator of aerobic function during exercise in cardiac patients. J. Am. Coll. Cardiol., 20:120–126, 1992.

22. Jones, N.L., and Campbell, E.J.M.: Clinical Exercise Testing. Philadelphia, W.B. Saunders Company, 1982, pp. 130–138.

23. Jones, N.L., McHardy, C.J.R., and Naimark, A.: Physiological dead space and alveolar-arterial gas pressure differences during exercise. Clin. Sci., 31:19–29, 1966.

24. Sue, D.Y., Oren, A., Hansen, J.E., and Wasserman, K.: Diffusing capacity for carbon monoxide as a predictor of gas exchange during exercise. N. Engl. J. Med., 316:1301–1306, 1987.

25. Rubin, S.A., and Brown, H.V.: Ventilation and gas exchange during exercise in severe chronic heart failure. Am. Rev. Respir. Dis., 129(Suppl.):S63-S64, 1984.

26. Weisel, R.D., Berger, R.L., and Hechtman, H.B.: Measurement of cardiac output by thermodilution. N. Engl. J. Med., 292:682–684, 1975.

27. Bylund-Fellenius A.-C., Walker, P.M., Elander, A., Holm, S., Holm, J., and Schersten, T.: Energy metabolism in relation to oxygen partial pressure in human skeletal muscle during exercise. Biochem. J., 200:247–255, 1981.

28. Sahlin K., Katz, A., and Henriksson, J.: Redox state and lactate accumulation in human skeletal muscle during dynamic exercise. Biochem. J., 245:551–556, 1987.

29. Wasserman, K., Beaver, W.L., Davis, J.A., Pu, J.-Z., Heber, D., and Whipp, B.J.: Lactate, pyruvate, and lactate-to-pyruvate ratio during exercise and recovery. J. Appl. Physiol., 59:935–940, 1985.

30. Roston, W.L., Whipp, B.J., Davis, J.A., Effros, R.M., and Wasserman, K.: Oxygen uptake kinetics and lactate concentration during exercise in man. Am. Rev. Respir. Dis., 135:1080–1084, 1987.

31. Beaver, W.L., Wasserman, K., and Whipp, B.J.: Bicarbonate buffering of lactic acid generated during exercise. J. Appl. Physiol., 60:472–478, 1986.

32. Osnes, J.-B., and Hermansen, L.: Acid-base balance after maximal exercise of short duration. J. Appl. Physiol., 32:59–63, 1972.

33. Sue, D.Y., Wasserman, K., Moricca, R.B., and Casaburi, R.: Metabolic acidosis during exercise in patients with chronic obstructive pulmonary disease. Chest, 94:931–938, 1988.

34. Wasserman, K.: Breathing during exercise. N. Engl. J. Med., 298:780–785, 1978.

35. Davis, J.A., Whipp, B.J., Lamarra, N., Huntsman, D.J., Frank, M.H., and Wasserman, K.: Effect of ramp slope on determination of aerobic parameters from the ramp exercise test. Med. Sci. Sports Exerc., 14:339–343, 1982.

36. Buchfuhrer, M.J., Hansen, J.E., Robinson, T.E., Sue, D.Y., Wasserman, K., and Whipp, B.J.: Optimizing the exercise protocol for cardiopulmonary assessment. J. Appl. Physiol., 55:1558–1564, 1983.

37. Yoshida, T.: Effect of dietary modifications on lactate threshold and onset of blood lactate accumulation during incremental exercise. Eur. J. Appl. Physiol., 53:200–205, 1984.

38. McClellan, T.M., and Gass, G.C.: The relationship between ventilation and lactate threshold following normal, low and high carbohydrate diets. Eur. J. Appl. Physiol., 58:568–576, 1989.

39. Cooper, C.B., Beaver, W., Cooper, D.M., and Wasserman, K.: Factors affecting the components of the alveolar CO_2 output-O_2 uptake relationship during incremental exercise in man. Exp. Physiol., 77:51–64, 1992.

40. Beaver, W.L., Wasserman, K., and Whipp, B.J.: Improved detection of the lactate threshold during exercise using a log-log transformation. J. Appl. Physiol., 59:1936–1940, 1985.

41. Wasserman, K.: Determinants and detection of anaerobic threshold and consequences of exercise above it. Circulation, 81(Suppl. VI):VI-29-VI-39, 1987.

42. Riley, M., Nicholls, P., and Patterson, V.H.: Anaerobic threshold: the problem of McArdle's disease. J. Appl. Physiol., 75:745–754, 1993.

43. Donald, K.W., Bishop, J.M., Cumming, C., and Wade, O.L.: The effect of exercise on the cardiac output and central dynamics of normal subjects. Clin. Sci., 14:37–73, 1955.

44. Koike, A., Itoh, H., Taniguchi, K., and Hiroe, M.: Detecting abnormalities in left ventricular function during exercise by respiratory measurement. Circulation, 80:1737–1746, 1989.

45. Nery, L.E., Wasserman, K., French, W., Oren, A., and Davis, J.A.: Contrasting cardiovascular and respiratory responses to exercise in mitral valve and chronic obstructive pulmonary diseases. Chest, 83:446–453, 1983.

46. Koike, A., Itoh, H., Doi, M., Taniguchi, K., Marumo, F., Umehara, I., and Hiroe, M.: Beat-to-beat evaluation of cardiac function during recovery from upright bicycle ex-

ercise in patients with coronary artery disease. Am. Heart J., 120:316, 1990.

47. Sue, D.Y., and Hansen, J.E.: Normal values in adults during exercise testing. Clin. Chest Med., 5:89–97, 1984.

48. Wasserman, K., Van Kessel, A., and Burton, G.G.: Interactions of physiological mechanisms during exercise. J. Appl. Physiol., 22:71–85, 1967.

49. Whipp, B.J., and Wasserman, K.: Alveolar-arterial gas tension differences during graded exercise. J. Appl. Physiol., 27:361–365, 1969.

50. West, J.B.: Ventilation/Perfusion and Gas Exchange. Oxford, Blackwell Scientific Publications, 1965, p. 8.

51. Farhi, L.E.: Ventilation perfusion relationship and its role in alveolar gas exchange. In Advances in Respiratory Physiology. Edited by C. Caro. London, Edward Arnold, 1966, p. 177.

52. Fishman, A.P.; Hypoxia on the pulmonary circulation: how and where it acts. Circ. Res., 38:221–231, 1976.

53. Sietsema, K.E., Cooper, D.M., Perloff, S.K., Child, J.S., Rosove, M.H., Wasserman, K., and Whipp, B.J.: Control of ventilation during exercise in patients with central venous-to-systemic arterial shunts. J. Appl. Physiol., 64:234–242, 1988.

54. Weiler-Ravell, D., Cooper, D.M., Whipp, B.J., and Wasserman, K.: The control of breathing at the start of exercise as influenced by posture. J. Appl. Physiol., 55:1460–1466, 1983.

55. Nery, L.E., Wasserman, K., Andrews, J.D., Huntsman, D.J., Hansen, J.E., and Whipp, B.J.: Ventilatory and gas exchange kinetics during exercise in chronic obstructive pulmonary disease. J. Appl. Physiol., 53:1594–1602, 1982.

56. Sietsema, K.E., Cooper, D.M., Rosove, M.A., Perloff, J.K., Child, J.S., Canobbio, M.M., Whipp, B.J., and Wasserman, K.: Dynamics of oxygen utpake during exercise in adults with cyanotic congenital heart disease. Circulation, 73:1137–1144, 1986.

57. Sietsema, K.E.: Oxygen uptake kinetics during exercise in patients with pulmonary vascular disease. Am. Rev. Respir. Dis., 145:1052–1057, 1992.

58. Weissman, M.L., Jones, P.W., Oren, A., Lamarra, N., Whipp, B.J., and Wasserman, K.: Cardiac output increase and gas exchange at the start of exercise. J. Appl. Physiol., 52:236–244, 1982.

59. Sietsema, K.E., Daly, J.A., and Wasserman, K.: Early dynamics of O_2 uptake and heart rate as affected by exercise work rate. J. Appl. Physiol., 67:2535–2541, 1989.

60. Zhang, Y.Y., Wasserman, K., Sietsema, K., Ben-Dov, I., Barstow, T., Mizumoto, G., and Sullivan, C.: O_2 uptake kinetics in response to exercise. Chest, 103:735–41, 1993.

61. Wasserman, K., Casaburi, R., Beaver, W.L., Roston, W.L., and Whipp, B.J.: Assessing the adequacy of tissue oxygenation during exercise. In New Horizons: Oxygen Transport and Utililization. Edited by C.W. Bryan-Brown and S.M. Ayres. Fullerton, CA, Society of Critical Care, 1987, pp. 109–144.

62. Zhang, Y.Y., Sietsema, K.E., Sullivan, C.S., and Wasserman, K.: A method for measuring bicarbonate buffering of lactic acid during constant work rate exercise. Submitted for publication.

63. Schneider, E.G., Robinson, S., and Newton, J.L.: Oxygen debt in aerobic work. J. Appl. Physiol., 25:58–62, 1968.

64. Rebuck, A.S., and Slutsky, A.S.: Measurement of ventilatory responses to hypercapnia and hypoxia. In Regulation of Breathing. Edited by T.F. Hornbein. New York, Marcel Dekker, 1981, pp. 745–772.

65. Severinghaus, J.W.: Proposed standard determination of ventilatory responses to hypoxia and hypercapnia in man. Chest, 70(Suppl.):129–131, 1976.

66. Dejours, P.: Control of respiration by arterial chemoreceptors. Ann. N.Y. Acad. Sci., 109:682–695, 1963.

67. Whipp, B.J., and Wasserman, K.: Carotid bodies and ventilatory control dynamics in man. Fed. Proc., 39:2668–2673, 1980.

68. Springer, C., Cooper, D.M., and Wasserman, K.: Evidence that maturation of the peripheral chemoreceptors is not complete in childhood. Respir. Physiol., 74:55–64, 1988.

69. Hansen, J.E., Casaburi, R., Cooper, D.M., and Wasserman, K.: Oxygen uptake as related to work rate increment during cycle ergometer exercise. Eur. J. Appl. Physiol., 57:140–145, 1988.

70. Pardee, H.E.B., DeGraff, A.G., Della Chapelle, C.E., Eggleston, C., Kossman, C.E., Maynard, E., Schwedel, J.B., Stewart, H.J., and Wright, I.S.: Functional capacity Classification of patients. In Nomenclature and Criteria for Diagnosis of Diseases of the Heart and Blood Vessels. 5th Ed. New York, New York Heart Association, 1953, p. 81.

71. Brown, H.V., Wasserman, K., and Whipp, B.J.: Strategies of exercise testing in chronic lung disease. Bull. Eur. Physiopathol. Respir., 13:409–423, 1977.

72. Wasserman, K., Whipp, B.J., and Davis, J.A.: Respiratory physiology of exercise: metabolism, gas exchange, and ventilatory control. In International Review of Physiology III. Vol. 23. Edited by J.G. Widdicombe. Baltimore, University Park Press. 1981, pp. 149–211.

Pathophysiology of Disorders Limiting Exercise

CHAPTER 4

MANY DISORDERS INTERFERE with the normal metabolic-cardiovascular-ventilatory coupling needed for exercise. These include primary disorders of hemoglobin, the peripheral circulation, the heart, the pulmonary circulation, the lungs, the chest wall, respiratory control, and metabolic pathways in bioenergetics (Fig. 4-1). Individually or in combination, these disorders limit exercise by causing symptoms of dyspnea, fatigue, and/or pain. Table 4-1 lists the most common disorders and the pathophysiologic features causing exercise limitation. Pathophysiologic mechanisms contributing to the exercise intolerance of each of these disorders and useful measurements for distinguishing them are described in this chapter.

Obesity (Table 4-2)

Whereas the obese subject has some increase in resting metabolic rate ($\dot{V}O_2$) relative to lean body mass, the increase is more marked during dynamic exercise (see Fig. 3-2). More energy is needed to move heavy legs in cycling exercise or the large body mass while ambulating (internal work) in addition to that needed to perform external work. As adipose tissue is added to the body, commensurate growth of the heart and blood vessels to meet this abnormally elevated metabolic requirement of muscular activity does not occur. Consequently, for the obese individual to do any form of physical work, there must be greater than normal cardiovascular and ventilatory responses.

Constraints are imposed on the maximal performance of the cardiovascular and ventilatory systems by obesity, however, especially in the extremely obese subject. Because of the large mass,

resting cardiac output per kilogram of lean body weight is already high. During exercise, the further increase in cardiac output is limited.[1] The added mass on the chest wall and the constraining pressure from the abdomen effectively "chest strap"[2-5] the patient and cause the resting end-expiratory lung volume (FRC) to be reduced (in extreme cases, close to the residual volume).[6] This can lead to atelectasis of peripheral lung units and results in hypoxemia at rest. In addition, pulmonary vascular resistance can be increased, primarily as a result of pulmonary insufficiency, but also possibly from mechanical kinking of blood vessels at low lung volume. Thus, cor pulmonale may be present.

The increased O_2 cost of performing mechanical work is predictable and well worked out for cycle ergometer work.[7,8] The $\dot{V}O_2$-work rate relationship is displaced upward, depending on the degree of obesity, but without a discernable change in slope (see Fig. 3-2). The effect of adipose tissue distribution in the body, i.e., legs or trunk, on $\dot{V}O_2$ has not been investigated.

The maximum $\dot{V}O_2$ and AT are low when related to body weight, but they are usually normal when related to height[8] and lean body mass.[9] Because of the high metabolic cost to do even modest work, an active obese subject may have good cardiovascular fitness. Thus, the actual $\dot{V}O_2$max, based on height or lean body weight, may be greater than that predicted for a normal, sedentary subject. The hypoxemia commonly present at rest, resulting from atelectasis of peripheral lung units, improves during exercise, presumably because the deep breathing reexpands the atelectic lung units. It is the only pulmonary condition in which arterial oxygenation improves during exercise. Ventilation-perfusion relationships are usually normal during exercise. Thus, exercise V_D/V_T, $P(A-a)_{O_2}$, and $P(a-ET)_{CO_2}$ values are normal.

Peripheral Vascular Diseases (Table 4-3)

Because of the reduced diameter of, and pathologic changes in, the conducting arteries to the limbs, peripheral vascular diseases impair the ability to increase blood flow appropriately during exercise, allowing O_2 flow to match the O_2 requirement (see Fig. 2-14) necessary for exercise to be performed totally aerobically. The failure of the O_2 supply to the exercising muscles to meet the high O_2 requirement may result in a reduced

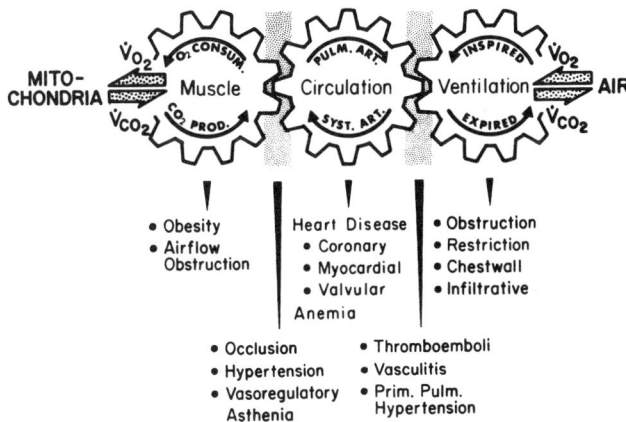

FIG. 4-1. Sites of interference in the metabolic-cardiovascular-ventilatory coupling for various disease states.

TABLE 4-1. *Disorders and Mechanisms Impairing Work Tolerance*

DISORDER	PATHOPHYSIOLOGY	PRIMARY LIMITATION
Obesity	Increased metabolic requirements; cardiorespiratory restriction	Low cardiorespiratory reserve
Peripheral vascular disease	Prevents normal vasodilation	Impaired muscle O_2 supply
Heart disease	Limited cardiac output (stroke volume) increase	Low tissue O_2 delivery
Pulmonary vascular occlusion	Limited cardiac output increase; decreased efficiency of gas exchange	Impaired tissue O_2 delivery; increased ventilatory requirement
Ventilatory Disorders		
Obstructive lung disease	Increased airway resistance; abnormal $\dot{V}_A/Q$	Reduced ventilatory capacity; increased ventilatory requirement
Restrictive lung disease	Reduced lung compliance; decreased efficiency of gas exchange; exercise-induced hypoxemia	Reduced ventilatory capacity; increased ventilatory requirement; low tissue O_2 delivery
Chest wall disease	Decreased chest wall compliance; respiratory muscle weakness	Reduced ability to breathe
Defects in hemoglobin content and quality	Reduced blood O_2 capacity	Impaired tissue O_2 delivery
Smoking	Increased carboxyhemoglobin, hypertension, increased airway resistance	Low tissue O_2 delivery, reduced ventilatory capacity
Metabolic acidosis	Reduced buffering capacity; low Pa_{CO_2} setpoint	Increased ventilatory requirement
Muscle and Musculoskeletal abnormalities		
Neuromuscular disease, arthritis	Musculoskeletal coupling inefficiency; inflammation	Reduced mechanical efficiency; pain
Myophosphorylase deficiency (McArdle's Syndrome)	Deficiency in carbohydrate substrate; lacks the ability to support metabolism with anaerobiosis	Pain
Electron transport defect	Inability to use O_2 to oxidize substrate; low work rate metabolic acidosis	Fatigue
Miscellaneous		
Anxiety reaction	Hyperventilation with respiratory alkalosis; regular breathing; breath-holding spells	Shortness of breath
Malingering	Irregular breathing; respiratory alkalosis; no or little metabolic acidosis	Secondary gain

$\Delta\dot{V}_{O_2}/\Delta$work rate ($\Delta\dot{V}_{O_2}/\Delta WR$) ratio at even low work levels. Although a compensatory increase in mitochondrial number in the ischemic muscle may occur, it is inadequate to make up for the deficiency in O_2 flow.[10] Consequently, the ischemic muscles produce lactic acid. Leg pain and fatigue at relatively low work rates accompany this condition. When the lactic acidosis is evident in the cen-tral circulation, breathing is further stimulated. If the patient also has lung disease, dyspnea may be an important symptom.

The maximum $\dot{V}_{O_2}$ and the lactic acidosis threshold are reduced. Because lactate may not enter the central circulation in a detectable quantity because of reduced muscle perfusion, evidence of systemic lactic acidosis will not be as evident as that in the ischemic muscles.

Many patients with peripheral vascular disease have excessively elevated blood pressure responses for the low work rate performed. The

TABLE 4-2. *Discriminating Measurements during Exercise in Obesity**

High O_2 cost to perform external work
Upward displacement of $\dot{V}_{O_2}$-work rate relationship
Maximum $\dot{V}_{O_2}$/body weight and AT/body weight are low
Maximum $\dot{V}_{O_2}$/height and AT/height are normal or high if life style is active
Normal to high O_2 pulse when $\dot{V}_{O_2}$max predicted from height
Low Pa_{O_2} at rest that normalizes during exercise
Normal V_D/V_T
Commonly, failure to develop ventilatory compensation for metabolic acidosis

* See Table 3-2 for a definition of symbols.

TABLE 4-3. *Discriminating Measurements during Exercise in Peripheral Vascular Disease**

Low $\Delta\dot{V}_{O_2}/\Delta WR$
Low maximum $\dot{V}_{O_2}$
Low AT
Leg pain
May have abnormal increase in blood pressure

* See Table 3-2 for a definition of symbols.

heart rate at maximum exercise is usually relatively low because the patient stops exercise from claudication at a work rate too low to provide a maximal cardiac stimulus.

Heart Diseases

Because gas transport is the major and most immediate role of the cardiovascular system, cardiac dysfunction of all four primary types (i.e., coronary artery, cardiomyopathic, valvular, and congenital) will cause changes in the pattern of $\dot{V}O_2$, $\dot{V}CO_2$, and heart rate in response to exercise.

In nearly all heart defects, the increase in HR as a function of $\dot{V}O_2$ is steeper than normal. This reflects the increased dependence on heart rate to increase cardiac output, because stroke volume is reduced consequent to the disease. Although the heart rate-$\dot{V}O_2$ relationship is usually relatively steep in heart disease, exceptions occur in which the heart rate response to exercise is inappropriately low. These include patients taking β-adrenergic blocking drugs and some patients with cardiomyopathies whose sinoatrial node fails to respond appropriately with tachycardia to the low cardiac output state.

Because of the relatively low cardiac output response, mixed venous oxygen reaches its lowest value, and the arterial-mixed venous oxygen difference $(C(a-\bar{v})O_2)$ its highest value, at a low work rate.[11] Consequently, the O_2 pulse $(C(a-\bar{v})O_2 \times SV)$ reaches a constant value that is low and occurs at an unusually low work rate compared to normal (Fig. 4-2). The $\Delta\dot{V}O_2/\Delta WR$ commonly becomes shallow near the maximum work rate (see Fig. 3-2C), reflecting an increased proportion of anaerobic metabolism because of limited O_2 transport.

Patients with heart diseases develop metabolic acidosis at low work rates; this may become chronic and evident at rest and is accompanied by a low Pa_{CO_2}.[12] This disorder necessitates a high minute ventilation that becomes more marked the higher the work rate (see Chap. 2, "Determinants of the ventilatory requirement"). The work of Rubin and Brown suggests that some patients with congestive heart failure develop mismatching of ventilation relative to pulmonary perfusion resulting in an increased VD/VT and a further increase in the breathing requirement to maintain blood pH homeostasis.[13] The chronic metabolic acidosis and its acute exacerbation during exercise, and any accompanying increase in VD/VT, may be significant contributors to the symptom of dyspnea in patients with chronic heart failure.

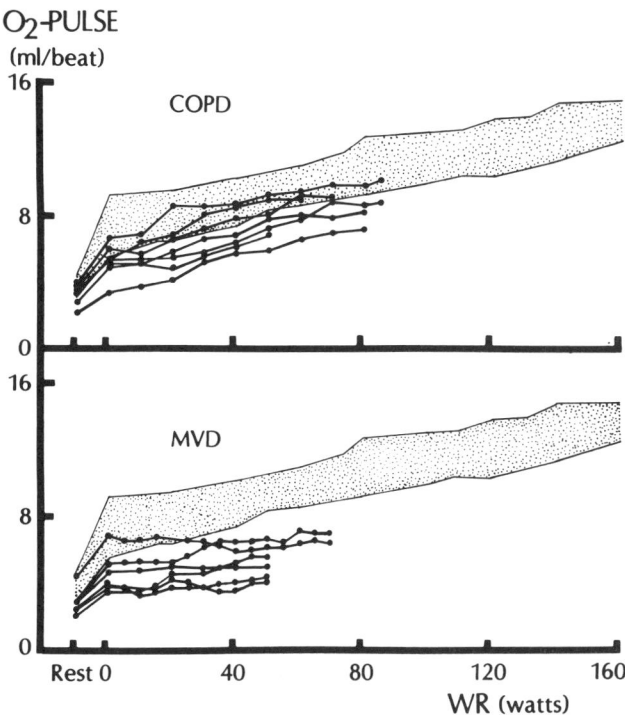

FIG. 4-2. O_2-pulse response to incremental exercise in patients with chronic obstructive pulmonary disease (COPD) (upper panel) and mitral valve disease (lower panel) compared with the range of values of a control group (stippled area). (From Nery, L.E., Wasserman, K., French, W., Oren, A., and Davis, J.A.: Contrasting cardiovascular and respiratory responses to exercise in severe chronic obstructive pulmonary disease. Chest, 83:446–453, 1983.)

Constant work rate tests are helpful for evaluating the cardiovascular response to specific levels of exercise. If the work rate is above the lactic acidosis threshold, $\dot{V}O_2$ will not reach a steady-state by 3 minutes. The magnitude of the increase in $\dot{V}O_2$ between 3 and 6 minutes $(\Delta\dot{V}O_2(6–3))$ is related to the exercise lactic acidosis (see Fig. 3-24).

Immediately after exercise, the O_2 pulse commonly increases in all cardiac disorders. This paradoxical increase may be due to an immediate increase in stroke volume in these patients at the start of recovery because of the abrupt decrease in left ventricular afterload when exercise stops.[14]

CORONARY ARTERY DISEASE (TABLE 4-4)

Although mild coronary artery disease may only be manifested in the laboratory by electrocardiographic (ECG) changes at high work rates, more significant coronary artery disease will cause the maximum $\dot{V}O_2$ and the AT to be reduced. Patients with coronary artery disease may or may not experience chest pain. ECG changes consistent with ischemia occur when the exercise-induced in-

TABLE 4-4. *Discriminating Gas Exchange Measurements during Exercise in Coronary Artery Disease**

$\Delta\dot{V}_{O_2}/\Delta WR$ normal at low work rates, but may break sharply, becoming more flat as work rate is increased towards maximum; usually accompanied by ECG evidence of ischemia; chest pain is sometimes absent
Low maximum $\dot{V}_{O_2}$
Low maximal O_2 pulse
Heart rate-$\dot{V}_{O_2}$ relationship becomes abnormally steep as maximum $\dot{V}_{O_2}$ is approached
High breathing reserve
Metabolic acidosis at end exercise
Immediate post-exercise O_2 pulse increase

* See Table 3-2 for a definition of symbols.

crease in myocardial oxygen requirement is not met by the myocardial oxygen supply. Development of increasingly frequent ectopic beats during exercise, as the work rate is increased, may also result from myocardial ischemia.

Characteristically, the $\Delta\dot{V}_{O_2}/\Delta WR$ is normal at low work rates of an incremental exercise test but may decrease sharply when the ECG becomes abnormal, whether or not angina is present. The slope of rise in $\dot{V}_{O_2}$ versus work rate may become more shallow, but $\dot{V}_{CO_2}$ continues to increase when the ECG changes. When myocardial ischemia occurs, heart rate as a function of $\dot{V}_{O_2}$ usually becomes steeper, and the O_2 pulse fails to increase further and is below the predicted maximal value. These changes are likely due to the decrease in stroke volume secondary to dyskinesis of the left ventricular wall in the region of ischemia.

MYOPATHIC HEART DISEASE (TABLE 4-5)

Because patients with cardiomyopathies have difficulty in transporting oxygen to the skeletal muscle, the increase in skeletal muscle $\dot{V}_{O_2}$ relative to the increase in work rate is usually slower than

TABLE 4-5. *Discriminating Gas Exchange Measurements during Exercise in Myopathic Heart Disease**

$\Delta\dot{V}_{O_2}/\Delta WR$ may *gradually* slow toward $\dot{V}_{O_2}$max
Low maximum $\dot{V}_{O_2}$
AT frequently low
Low maximal O_2 pulse
Steep but linear increase in HR-$\dot{V}_{O_2}$ relationship with sometimes low maximal HR
Development of oscillatory breathing and $\dot{V}_{O_2}$ pattern of 45- to 90-second periods at low WR; oscillatory pattern is less evident as peak WR is reached; O_2 pulse increases immediately post-exercise
Slow $\dot{V}_{O_2}$ kinetics and high $\Delta\dot{V}_{O_2}(6-3)$ above *AT* during constant work rate test

* See Table 3-2 for a definition of symbols.

normal. This slowing is gradual in patients with cardiomyopathies, in contrast to the abrupt slowing of $\dot{V}_{O_2}$ increase relative to work rate in coronary artery disease. The failure to transport O_2 at the rate needed to regenerate the ATP used for muscular contraction makes it impossible to sustain muscular contraction, i.e., the muscle fatigues. This physical sign is also sensed by the patient as a symptom.

The maximal $\dot{V}_{O_2}$ is reduced consequent to the low cardiac output response to exercise. The anaerobic threshold is also commonly reduced. The maximum O_2 pulse is low because of the reduced stroke volume. The heart rate increase is steep relative to the increase in $\dot{V}_{O_2}$. The maximal heart rate may be reduced in these patients, however, because their myopathy is commonly accompanied by chronotropic incompetence.

Exercise brings out an interesting oscillatory pattern with a period of 45 to 90 seconds in $\dot{V}_{O_2}$, $\dot{V}_{CO_2}$, and $\dot{V}_E$. This pattern is usually reduced as peak work rate is approached. Of the oscillatory variables, $\dot{V}_{O_2}$ leads the other changes and is of greatest amplitude relative to the mean value.[15] This suggests that the circulatory output itself is oscillatory.

VALVULAR HEART DISEASE (TABLE 4-6)

Because the stroke volume is reduced in patients with valvular heart disease, the increase in $\dot{V}_{O_2}$ relative to increase in work rate is usually low, i.e., low $\Delta\dot{V}_{O_2}/\Delta WR$. Both the *AT* and the $\dot{V}_{O_2}$max are reduced. The O_2 pulse is reduced and reaches a plateau value at a relatively low work rate (Fig. 4-2). Heart rate increases steeply relative to $\dot{V}_{O_2}$, with a maximal heart rate achieved at a relatively low work rate.

CONGENITAL HEART DISEASE (TABLE 4-7)

Constant work rate tests are of particular value in patients with congenital heart disease. Because

TABLE 4-6. *Discriminating Gas Exchange Measurements in Valvular Heart Disease**

$\Delta\dot{V}_{O_2}/\Delta WR$ commonly low and may gradually decrease
Low maximum $\dot{V}_{O_2}$
Low *AT*
Low and unchanging O_2 pulse
Steep linear increase in HR-$\dot{V}_{O_2}$ relationship
Slow $\dot{V}_{O_2}$ kinetics and high $\Delta\dot{V}_{O_2}(6-3)$ during constant work rate test

* See Table 3-2 for a definition of symbols.

TABLE 4-7. *Discriminating Gas Exchange Measurements during Exercise in Congenital Heart Disease**

Low maximum $\dot{V}O_2$

Low *AT*

Phase I $\dot{V}O_2$ reduced when accompanied by increased pulmonary vascular or valvular resistance

Slow $\dot{V}O_2$ kinetics and high $\Delta\dot{V}O_2(6-3)$ during constant work rate test

Immediate hyperpnea and decrease in P_{ETCO_2} in cyanotic type; magnitude of increase in $\dot{V}E$ and decrease in P_{ETCO_2} related to size of right to left shunt

Immediate worsening of hypoxemia at start of exercise in cyanotic type

* See Table 3-2 for a definition of symbols.

TABLE 4-8. *Physiologic Findings during Exercise in Diseases of the Pulmonary Circulation**

High $\dot{V}E$ at submaximal work rates

High V_D/V_T

High $P(a\text{-}ET)_{CO_2}$

Pa_{O_2} decreases as WR is increased

$P(A\text{-}a)_{O_2}$ increases with increasing WR

Low maximum $\dot{V}O_2$

Low *AT*

$\Delta\dot{V}O_2/\Delta WR$ more shallow toward maximum WR

Low O_2 pulse

* See Table 3-2 for a definition of symbols.

the increase in $\dot{V}O_2$ is dependent on pulmonary blood flow, the ease with which the right ventricle can increase blood flow through the lungs can be measured from the oxygen uptake kinetics. Thus, patients with pulmonary outflow obstruction or patients with a right to left shunt fail to increase pulmonary blood flow appropriately at the start of exercise. Consequently, the Phase I increase in $\dot{V}O_2$ is reduced or absent.[16] Phase II kinetics are also inappropriately slow, and the magnitude of Phase II becomes a relatively large portion of the total oxygen requirement at low work rates. The slow Phase II kinetics are measured as a long time constant.[16] They are also reflected in a slowly increasing $\dot{V}O_2$ between 3 and 6 minutes of exercise (high $\Delta\dot{V}O_2(6-3)$). As in other cardiovascular disorders, the maximal $\dot{V}O_2$ and *AT* are reduced.

A markedly elevated ventilatory response is noted, particularly in patients with cyanotic congenital heart disease.[17] In this disorder, the blood flowing through the lungs is hyperventilated to compensate for the blood that bypasses the lungs and enters the left side of the circulation through the right to left shunt. Hyperventilation of the blood passing through the lungs results in an immediate decrease in end-tidal P_{CO_2} at the start of exercise, and this decrease is sustained until the start of recovery. The arterial P_{CO_2} and pH remain relatively unchanged in patients with a right to left shunt, whereas the P_{O_2} decreases.[17] The unchanged acid-base status suggests that the respiratory control mechanism is set to regulate pH in this population of patients.

Pulmonary Vascular Diseases (Table 4-8)

Diseases of the pulmonary circulation, such as pulmonary emboli and idiopathic pulmonary vascular occlusion, characteristically cause reduced perfusion to ventilated alveoli. Consequently, alveoli with unoccluded capillaries must accept a greater than normal perfusion and must be ventilated to a proportionately greater degree than normal to remove the metabolic CO_2 and to maintain Pa_{CO_2} (pH) at a normal level. The overventilation of the poorly perfused alveoli is wasted (alveolar dead space). Because minute ventilation is the sum of the "ideal" or effective alveolar ventilation and the physiologic dead space ventilation, minute ventilation is increased in patients with pulmonary vascular diseases at rest and to a greater degree during exercise. The increased dead space ventilation results in a high V_D/V_T and a persistently positive $P(a\text{-}ET)_{CO_2}$.

Arterial hypoxemia, which worsens as the work rate is increased, is a common occurrence in patients with pulmonary vascular diseases, even when Pa_{O_2} is normal at rest. Several mechanisms may play a role. First, if the time available for diffusion equilibrium of O_2, already shortened by the reduced size of the functional capillary bed, is further shortened by the exercise-induced increase in pulmonary blood flow, equilibration of alveolar and end-capillary P_{O_2} is less likely to occur. Consequently, Pa_{O_2} decreases as work rate is increased.

Another cause of hypoxemia during exercise in patients with increased pulmonary vascular resistance is the development of a right to left shunt resulting from the opening of a potentially patent foramen ovale. Approximately 20% of the population is thought to have an "unsealed" foramen ovale. This is normally of no importance because left atrial pressure is higher than right atrial pressure. Consequent to high and fixed pulmonary vascular resistance, pulmonary artery pressure increases during exercise when right ventricular output increases. If the right ventricle cannot pump the venous return into the pulmonary circu-

TABLE 4-9. *Discriminating Measurements during Exercise in Patients with Obstructive Lung Disease**

Low maximum $\dot{V}O_2$
High VD/VT
High $P(a\text{-}ET)CO_2$
High $P(A\text{-}a)O_2$
Low breathing reserve
Increased O_2 cost of work
Lactic acidosis at low work rates
Failure to develop respiratory compensation for metabolic acidosis
High heart rate reserve
Abnormal (trapezoidal) expiratory flow pattern

* See Table 3-2 for a definition of symbols.

lation as fast as it is delivered (right ventricular failure), right ventricular end-diastolic pressure and, therefore, right atrial pressure will rise. If the right atrial pressure exceeds that of the left atrium, some of the right atrial flow will pass through the unsealed foramen ovale, creating a right to left shunt only during exercise. The development of a right to left shunt can easily be identified by repeating the exercise test while the subject breathes 100% oxygen. If this shunt develops, the arterial PO_2 should decrease well below the predicted (> 600 mm Hg) during O_2 breathing. The Pa_{O_2} will decrease 100 mm Hg during exercise for a right to left shunt equal to 3 to 5% of the cardiac output, depending on the mixed venous saturation, in the arterial PO_2 range above 150 mm Hg.

Finally, hypoxemia from low $\dot{V}A/\dot{Q}$ lung units is common in acute pulmonary embolism, but it is a less important cause of arterial hypoxemia in patients with chronic pulmonary vascular occlusive disease. In patients with pulmonary vascular occlusive disease, high $\dot{V}A/\dot{Q}$ lung units predominate and do not cause hypoxemia.

Pulmonary vascular occlusions cause a hemodynamic stenosis in the central circulation, making it difficult for the right ventricle to deliver blood to the left atrium at a rate sufficient to meet the increased cardiac output needed for exercise. Because the cardiac output increase in response to exercise is reduced, the maximum $\dot{V}O_2$, AT, and O_2 pulse are reduced in patients with pulmonary vascular disease, similar to that seen in patients with primary heart disease. Thus, physiologic measurements during exercise are particularly helpful in diagnosing chronic pulmonary vascular occlusive disease. The abnormalities are those associated with a low cardiac output state and disturbances in gas exchange, especially during exercise.

Ventilatory Disorders

OBSTRUCTIVE LUNG DISEASES (TABLE 4–9)

Here we consider patients with chronic airflow obstruction (CAO), including emphysema, chronic bronchitis, bronchial asthma, and mixtures of these three disease entities. The symptom that limits exercise in the patient with obstructive pulmonary disease is almost always dyspnea. This is because of the difficulty in achieving the ventilation needed to eliminate the additional CO_2 generated during exercise at the level of Pa_{CO_2} regulated by the patient and because many of these patients are highly sedentary and develop a lactic acidosis at a relatively low work rate (Table 4-10).

Figure 4-3 conceptualizes the pathophysiologic features leading to dyspnea in patients with CAO. The two major contributing factors are the decreased ventilatory capacity and the increased ventilatory requirement. In emphysema, the decreased ventilatory capacity is due to increased airflow obstruction combined with reduced lung elastic recoil, whereas in chronic bronchitis and asthma, the decreased ventilatory capacity is due to increased airway resistance.

TABLE 4-10. *Effect of Airway Obstruction due to Emphysema on Average Blood Lactate Concentration, Minute Ventilation, and Work Rate at an O_2 Consumption of Approximately 1.0 L/min*

FEV_1 (L)	$\dot{V}O_2$ (L/min STPD)	WR (Watts)	$\dot{V}E$ (L/min BTPS)	$\dot{V}E/\dot{V}O_2$	La (mmol/L)	La/$\dot{V}O_2$
1.02	0.90	35	35	39	3.03	3.37*
1.80	1.05	34	36	34	2.95	2.80†
Normal	~1.00	50	25	25	< 1.00	< 1.00‡

* Data from ref. 18.
† Data from ref. 19.
‡ Data from ref. 7.
FEV_1 = forced expiratory volume in 1 second; WR = work rate; $\dot{V}E$ = minute ventilation; La = blood lactate concentration; STPD = standard temperature and pressure, dry; BTPS = body temperature, ambient pressure, saturated.

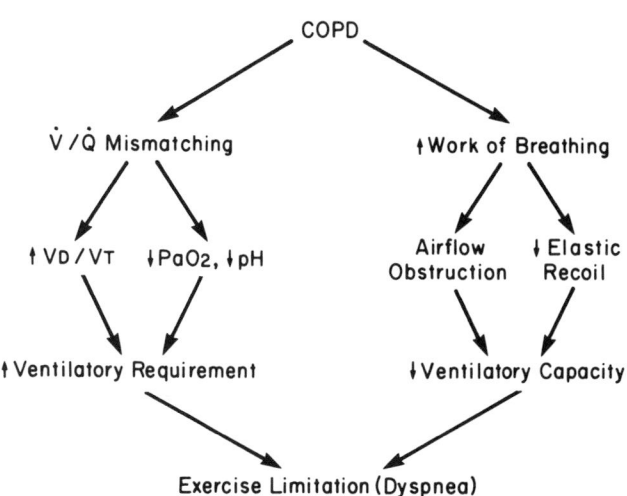

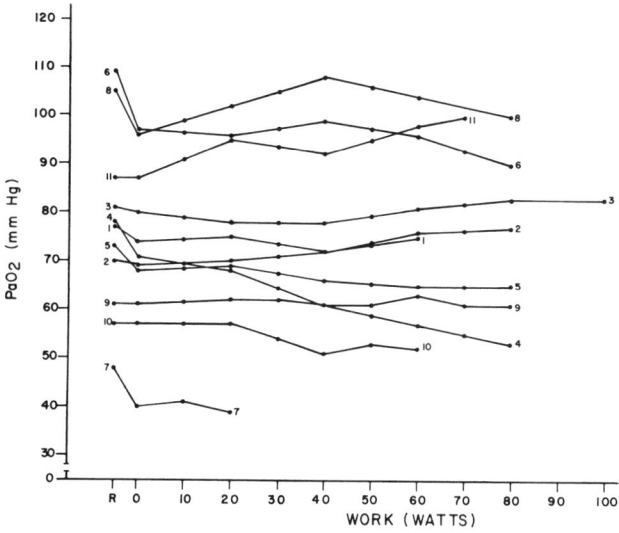

FIG. 4-3. Factors that play a role in exercise limitation and dyspnea in patients with chronic obstructive pulmonary disease (COPD). These patients have both an increase in ventilatory requirement to perform exercise and a reduction in ventilatory capacity. See text for a detailed discussion of each of the factors shown. $\dot{V}_A/\dot{Q}$ = ventilation-perfusion ratio; VD/VT = dead space-tidal volume ratio.

FIG. 4-5. Pa_{O_2} as related to increase in work rate for the same 11 patients shown in Figure 4-4 (each point is a different work rate). The numbers on each curve identify the patient and allow cross-correlation with each patient's Pa_{CO_2} shown in Figure 4-4.

The increased ventilatory requirement in patients with CAO is primarily due to inefficient ventilation of the lungs consequent to the mismatching of ventilation to perfusion; i.e., certain regions of the lungs are hypoventilated, whereas others are hyperventilated. This has the effect of increasing the fraction of the breath that is wasted (increases VD/VT), thereby requiring an increased ventilation to eliminate the CO_2 produced by the patient to maintain the P_{CO_2} at its set-point (see Fig. 2-32).

Hypoxemia results from the underventilation of perfused lung units. Despite increasing ventilatory drive through the carotid body chemoreceptors,[20] the hypoxic stimulus rarely is sufficient to induce a respiratory alkalosis in these patients. In addition, ventilatory compensation for the exercise-induced lactic acidosis rarely occurs in these

patients (see Fig. 3-18 and cases of patients with CAO in Chap. 8). With severe airway obstruction, Pa_{CO_2} often rises and respiratory acidosis worsens.[12]

As shown in Figure 4-4, ambulatory patients with stable obstructive lung disease regulate Pa_{CO_2} at a reasonably constant level despite increasing work rates. Although regulation of Pa_{O_2} is less precise in these patients (Fig. 4-5), it usually does not fall to extremely low levels, even at the patient's maximum work rate. The shape of the oxyhemoglobin dissociation curve generally allows arterial O_2 content to be maintained at satisfactory levels despite a moderate decrease in Pa_{O_2}.

The alveolar-arterial P_{O_2} difference $(P(A-a)_{O_2})$ is usually increased as a consequence of the perfusion of relatively poorly ventilated airspaces. The

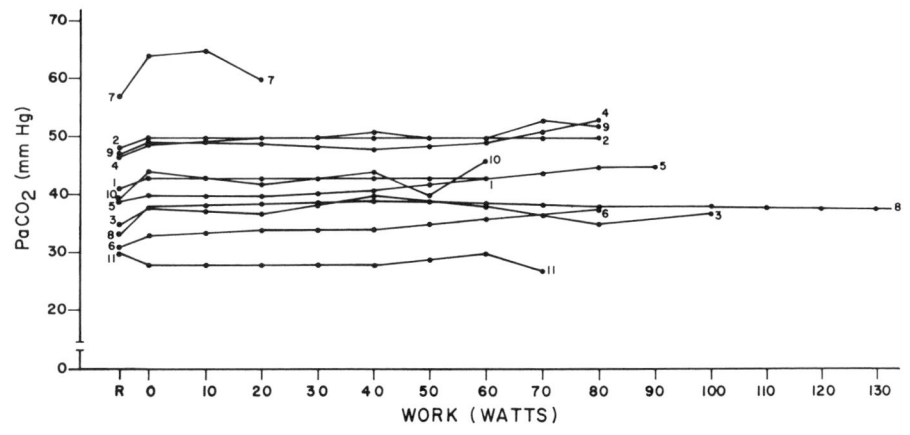

FIG. 4-4. Pa_{CO_2} as related to work rate in 11 patients with stable chronic airflow obstruction (each point is a different work rate). The numbers on each curve identify the patient.

increase in $P(A\text{-}a)_{O_2}$ is usually not systematic with increasing work rate, as in patients with primary pulmonary vascular disease or pulmonary fibrosis. The arterial-end-tidal P_{CO_2} difference $(P(a\text{-}ET)_{CO_2})$ is also increased, reflecting mismatching of ventilation to perfusion. $P(a\text{-}ET)_{CO_2}$ remains relatively constant and elevated as work rate is increased, rather than decreasing and becoming negative as in normal subjects.

Although one may predict that the O_2 cost of work will be increased in patients with CAO, this has been difficult to demonstrate. That these patients do have an increased metabolic cost becomes evident, however, when one examines the work that could be performed for a given $\dot{V}_{O_2}$ (Table 4-10). We found that the work output was reduced at a $\dot{V}_{O_2}$ of 1 L/min in two studies on patients with CAO. Moreover, patients with CAO develop a lactic acidosis at a relatively low work rate[18,19] (Table 4-10). This is most likely due to the sedentary life style of these patients. When training these patients, their lactate level for a given work rate decreases, and the ventilatory requirement for exercise decreases.[19]

Dyspnea depends on a balance between how much air must be breathed to keep pace with metabolism and how much can be breathed. Patients with CAO must breathe more to maintain blood gases and pH, but they cannot breathe as much as a normal subject. The maximal voluntary ventilation (MVV) is a reasonable resting measure of the patient's ventilatory capacity. Work tasks requiring ventilation rates in excess of this value cannot be sustained. Thus, the breathing reserve, defined as the difference between the MVV and $\dot{V}_E$ at the maximum level of exercise that the subject could perform (MVV − $\dot{V}_{Emax}$), is decreased to values close to zero in patients with CAO (Fig. 4-6), in contrast to the large ventilatory reserve found in most normal subjects[21–23] and in patients with heart disease at the end of exercise.

Whereas the maximum $\dot{V}_{O_2}$ is reduced in patients with uncomplicated obstructive lung disease, the $\dot{V}_{O_2}$-work rate relationship, in response to a progressively increasing work rate test, usually does not approach a plateau, as is commonly seen in patients with circulatory limitation. This is because ambulatory patients with stable obstructive lung disease are usually more limited in their ability to eliminate CO_2 (ventilatory limitation) than in their ability to make O_2 available to the mitochondria.

Often, these patients develop a lactic acidosis at relatively low work rates because of the relatively

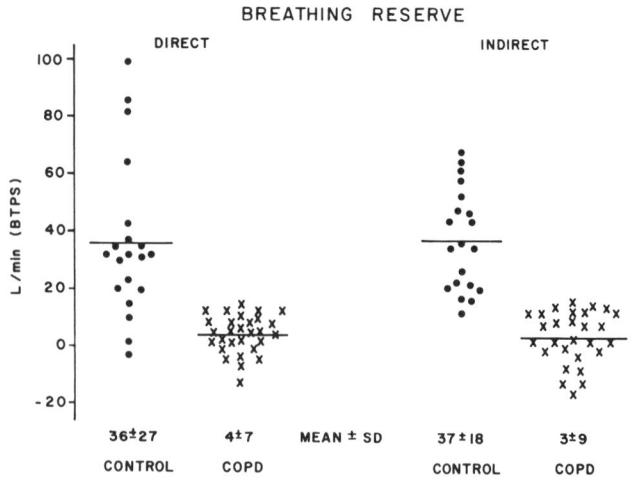

FIG. 4-6. Breathing reserve (MVV − maximum $\dot{V}_E$) for a group of normal subjects and a group of patients with stable chronic obstructive pulmonary disease (COPD). The values under each column show the mean ± standard deviation. Measurements are made using the directly measured MVV and the indirectly measured MVV calculated by multiplying FEV_1 by 40. Note that the breathing reserve in patients with COPD is small and the standard deviation is narrow, reflecting the importance of airflow limitation in determining exercise intolerance.

untrained state of these patients (Table 4-10). Patients with severe airflow obstruction may not be able to exercise sufficiently to reach their AT, however, and they may not develop a lactic acidosis during exercise.

The heart rate at maximum work rate is generally low (high heart rate reserve) (Fig. 4-7), but it can be increased if the patient's maximum work rate can be improved through O_2 breathing or bronchodilatation. In contrast to cardiac disorders, O_2-pulse generally continues to rise normally with increasing work rate, although the final absolute values are reduced (see Fig. 4-2).

Examining the expiratory flow pattern can be useful. Typically, as shown in Figure 3-28, it has an early expiratory peak and then a sustained expiratory flow until the point of inhalation, giving the recorded pattern a trapezoidal appearance. No apneic pause occurs at the end of exhalation, as in the normal subject.

RESTRICTIVE LUNG DISEASES (TABLE 4-11)

Pulmonary fibrosis develops from chronic lung inflammation.[24] The pathologic features are usually nonuniform, so some acini, including their blood supply, are completely replaced by scar tissue, whereas neighboring units are less or uninvolved but may undergo compensatory hyperinflation. The net effect is a reduction in the total number of

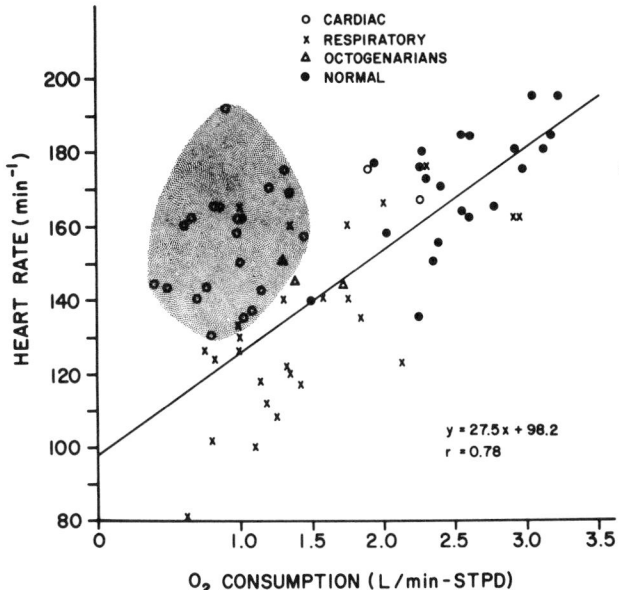

FIG. 4-7. Heart rate at maximal exercise for normal subjects, octogenarians, and patients with chronic respiratory disease or cardiac disease. The normal subjects reach a higher maximum heart rate and $\dot{V}O_2$. Note that the octogenarians fall on the same slope as the younger normal subjects, although their maximum heart rate and maximum oxygen uptake are less. Similarly, the patients with respiratory defects have a still lower maximum oxygen uptake and heart rate. The cardiac patients (stippled area) have a higher maximum heart rate relative to the maximum O_2 uptake than that of the other subjects. (From Wasserman, K., and Whipp, B.J.: Exercise physiology in health and disease (state of the art). Am. Rev. Respir. Dis., 112:219–249, 1975.)

functioning acini and, consequently, a relatively noncompliant, small lung.[25] Whereas both the total lung capacity and its subcompartments are reduced, the predominant reduction is that of the inspiratory capacity. Thus, the extent to which the tidal volume can increase with exercise is limited, and the patient must increase breathing frequency to a value higher than normal to achieve the ventilatory requirement for exercise. Consequently, the V_T/IC ratio is high and approaches 1, and the breathing frequency at maximum exercise often exceeds 50 breaths/min in patients with restrictive

TABLE 4-11. *Discriminating Measurements during Exercise in Patients with Restrictive Lung Diseases**

Low maximum $\dot{V}O_2$
High V_T/IC
Breathing frequency > 50 at max WR
Low breathing reserve
High V_D/V_T
High $P(a\text{-}ET)CO_2$
Pa_{O_2} decreases and $P(A\text{-}a)_{O_2}$ increases as WR is increased
$\Delta\dot{V}O_2/\Delta WR$ is reduced

* See Table 3-2 for a definition of symbols.

lung diseases. Ventilation at the maximum work rate may approach the indirect MVV.

Early in the pathophysiologic development of the interstitial lung diseases, it appears as though the pulmonary capillary bed is functionally reduced and fails to increase in response to exercise. This restricted capillary bed results in a shortened red cell transit time in the pulmonary capillaries as the exercise work rate is increased. The progressive reduction of the red cell residence time in the pulmonary capillary, as work rate and cardiac output increase, results in a systematic decrease in Pa_{O_2} similar to that seen in pulmonary vascular disease. This systematic change in Pa_{O_2} is usually not seen in obstructive lung disease. Low $\dot{V}A/\dot{Q}$ ratios might also contribute to the hypoxemia in patients with pulmonary fibrosis.[26] The ventilatory response of patients with pulmonary fibrosis is steep, partially because of a reduced Pa_{CO_2} set-point, but mainly because of an increased V_D/V_T. Worsening hypoxemia as the work rate is increased, elevated dead space ventilation caused by nonuniform ventilation-perfusion ratios, and a rapid, shallow breathing pattern contribute to dyspnea, which is the primary symptom of patients with restrictive lung disorders.

Pulmonary alveolar proteinosis is a good example of exercise hypoxemia that is primarily due to a diffusion defect.[27] This disease results in alveolar filling by a semi-solid proteinaceous material. Pulmonary fibrosis is minimal or nonexistent. Frequently, the vital capacity and total lung capacity are only slightly reduced, and FEV_1 is normal. Because the mean path length from lung gas to capillaries is increased considerably in this disorder by a medium unfavorable for permeation by O_2, this diffusion barrier limits the mass flow of O_2 into the pulmonary capillaries for hemoglobin to become normally saturated with O_2. During exercise, when red cell transit time in the capillary bed is reduced and its residence time shortened, less time is available for diffusion equilibrium. Thus, hypoxemia and increasing $P(A\text{-}a)_{O_2}$ take place during exercise, becoming progressively more abnormal as the work rate is increased.[27] The prominent feature of this disorder is a systematic decrease in Pa_{O_2} with increasing metabolic stress.

CHEST WALL (RESPIRATORY PUMP) DEFECTS (TABLE 4-12)

Defects of the respiratory pump include muscle weakness, chest deformities, rigidity of the thoracic cage (as in ankylosing spondylitis), and mus-

TABLE 4-12. *Discriminating Measurements during Exercise in Patients With Chest Wall Defects**

Low maximum $\dot{V}O_2$
High VT/IC
High breathing frequency
Normal $\Delta \dot{V}O_2 / \Delta WR$
Low breathing reserve
High heart rate reserve
Normal PaO_2

See Table 3-2 for a definition of symbols.

cle and motor nerve disorders. Patients with these disorders, like those with restrictive pulmonary disorders, have a limited ability to increase VT. Although their lungs are essentially normal, the maximal intrapleural pressure available to expand the lungs is insufficient to allow VT to increase normally as the work rate is increased. Therefore, to obtain the increase in $\dot{V}E$ required for work, these patients must predominantly increase breathing frequency.

The reduced maximum $\dot{V}O_2$ defines the degree of exercise limitation. The $\dot{V}O_2$ increases normally with increasing work rate. Because the lung parenchyma is essentially normal, PaO_2 is usually normal and does not decrease as the work rate is increased. The breathing reserve is low at the termination of exercise, however, a characteristic of conditions in which the breathing mechanics limit maximal exercise performance. In contrast, heart rate reserve is high because the reduction in maximal work rate results from breathing limitation.

Defects in Hemoglobin Content and Quality (Table 4-13)

Because we have been focusing on defects of the O_2 transport system that might result in exertional dyspnea, it is appropriate to consider changes in the properties of blood that might impair O_2 delivery to the mitochondria. The patient with a reduced O_2 carrying capacity commonly has a relatively high cardiac output, with a higher than ex-

TABLE 4-13. *Discriminating Measurements during Exercise in Patients With Anemias, HbCO, and Conditions Associated With a Low P_{50}**

Low maximum $\dot{V}O_2$
Low *AT*
Low O_2 pulse
Normal VD/VT, $P(a\text{-}ET)CO_2$ and $P(A\text{-}a)O_2$

See Table 3-2 for a definition of symbols.

pected heart rate for a given work rate, i.e., a relative tachycardia. The stroke volume is normal or even increased, in contrast to patients with cardiac diseases and disorders of the pulmonary circulation, disorders in which stroke volume is reduced. Because the arterial O_2 content is low, the potential for the arterial-venous O_2 difference to increase in response to exercise is limited, and the maximum O_2 pulse is reduced. As in other disorders of O_2 flow, the maximum $\dot{V}O_2$ and *AT* are likely to be reduced. Measurements that reflect ventilation-perfusion mismatching are normal.

ANEMIA

Anemia, of course, results in a reduced O_2 carrying capacity. This compromises O_2 delivery to the mitochondria because the capillary PO_2 falls more rapidly than normal (see Fig. 2-14) as blood travels from artery to vein. Thus, the diffusion gradient of O_2 from the blood to the mitochondria might reach critically low levels before the blood exits from the capillaries of the exercising muscle, thereby requiring anaerobic mechanisms for ATP generation at lower work rates than normal (see Fig. 2-1). Subjects with anemia commonly experience breathlessness with increased ventilatory drive during exercise. Whereas the O_2 content is low, the arterial PO_2 is not reduced. Because the carotid bodies respond to arterial PO_2 and not O_2 content,[20] the reduced O_2 content is not itself the cause of the increased ventilatory drive and therefore the symptom of breathlessness. More likely, the breathlessness and increased ventilatory drive with exercise in the more anemic patient are the consequence of the metabolic acidosis that accompanies the patient's low anaerobic threshold. The acidemia results in an increased ventilatory drive (mediated by the carotid bodies) and a relatively high minute ventilation at a low maximum work rate.

HEMOGLOBINOPATHIES

Conditions that cause a leftward shift in the oxyhemoglobin dissociation curve (reduced P_{50}), such as hemoglobinopathies, a decrease in 2,3-DPG, such as a defect in red cell metabolism, an increase in carboxyhemoglobin, or increased glycosylated hemoglobin, such as found in the poorly controlled diabetic, should result in a low capillary blood PO_2 for a given $\dot{V}O_2$ and capillary oxyhemoglobin saturation.[28] Thus, during exercise the PO_2

difference between capillary and mitochondrion may reach its critical value, below which it cannot fall despite an increased bioenergetic demand for O_2, at a reduced work rate. Thus, the O_2 flow through the muscle would not provide all the O_2 needed by the mitochondria. Consequently, the mitochondrial membrane proton shuttle (see Fig. 2-1) would not reoxidize $NADH + H^+$ rapidly enough to maintain the normal redox state of the cytosol. Exercise studies on a group of these patients support the concept that these disorders lead to anaerobic glycolysis and increased net lactate production at reduced work rates.[29]

CARBOXYHEMOGLOBINEMIA

Cigarette smoking adversely affects exercise tolerance by its effects on the blood, the cardiovascular system, and the lungs. Carboxyhemoglobinemia results in a reduced O_2 carrying capacity without the reduced blood viscosity found in anemia. When carboxyhemoglobin level is increased, arterial oxygen content is reduced, causing a leftward shift of the oxyhemoglobin dissociation curve. This reduces the maximum $\dot{V}O_2$ and AT.[30–32] Heart rate, blood pressure, and the double product (heart rate × systolic blood pressure) are increased when one performs exercise immediately after smoking.[32] Ventilation-perfusion relationships become abnormal, as evident from the increased $P(a\text{-}ET)_{CO_2}$ during exercise. The effect of short-term smoking on airway resistance was not detected in the same normal young male subjects who had acute cardiovascular changes and changes consistent with worsened $\dot{V}A/\dot{Q}$ matching, however.

Chronic Metabolic Acidosis (Table 4-14)

Chronic metabolic acidosis can result from poorly controlled diabetes, chronic renal failure with a renal tubular acidosis, chronic heart failure, or ingestion of certain drugs, such as a carbonic anhydrase inhibitor (acetazolamide) in the treatment of glaucoma. These conditions reduce blood $[HCO_3^-]$. This causes the arterial P_{CO_2} to be regulated at a low set-point.[33,34] Consequently, for a given work rate, the ventilatory requirement is relatively high (see Fig. 2-31) and leads to an apparent increase in "sensitivity" of the respiratory control mechanisms (i.e., high $\Delta\dot{V}E/\Delta\dot{V}O_2$).

The presence of a chronic metabolic acidosis before exercise begins is evident from the resting arterial blood gases. The $[HCO_3^-]$ and Pa_{CO_2} are reduced; pH is only slightly reduced or normal. A high resting ventilation for the metabolic rate necessarily accompanies a low Pa_{CO_2}. During exercise, $\dot{V}E$ increases proportionally with the increase in CO_2 production. Because the slope of the $\dot{V}E$-$\dot{V}_{CO_2}$ relationship is steeper the lower the Pa_{CO_2}, the effect of the metabolic acidosis on ventilation is amplified progressively as work rate is increased (see Fig. 2-31). For example, if the Pa_{CO_2} is maintained at 30 mm Hg during exercise, the ventilatory equivalent for CO_2 will be approximately 40 L of ventilation per liter of CO_2 output, in contrast to 30 L in subjects with normal lungs and V_D/V_T maintaining Pa_{CO_2} at 40 mm Hg (see Fig. 3-14). Without measuring arterial blood gases, a relatively steep slope relationship between $\dot{V}E$ and $\dot{V}_{CO_2}$ (an elevated ventilatory equivalent for CO_2) during exercise (with R in the normal range) signifies either chronic hyperventilation or increased V_D/V_T. Arterial blood gas and pH measurements differentiate these two potential causes of the high ventilatory response.

By itself, chronic metabolic acidosis is not a prominent cause of dyspnea, but in conjunction with other diseases such as obstructive airways disease, it may lower the CO_2 set-point to such a marked degree that the ventilatory requirement to perform a given work rate may exceed the subject's MVV. In this case, the dyspnea sensation would be high. Correction of the metabolic acidosis might reduce the ventilatory requirement below the subject's MVV and relieve the dyspnea sensation.

Muscle Disorders and Endocrine Abnormalities

Little information is available concerning the metabolic cost of exercise in patients with muscle disorders. Because of reduced motor efficiency, patients with neuromuscular disorders with accom-

TABLE 4-14. *Discriminating Measurements during Exercise in Patients With a Chronic Metabolic Acidosis**

Low $[HCO_3^-]$
Steep $\dot{V}E/\dot{V}_{CO_2}$ relationship
Normal $P(A\text{-}a)_{O_2}$ and $P(a\text{-}ET)_{CO_2}$
Normal V_D/V_T

* See Table 3-2 for a definition of symbols.

panying spasticities and motor incoordination presumably have an increased O_2 requirement for performing physical work. We have not had the opportunity to evaluate these patients in the exercise laboratory.

Certain muscle enzyme deficiencies limit exercise performance. For example, patients with inability to use muscle glycogen because of myophosphorylase deficiency (McArdle's syndrome)[35] are unable to exercise to work levels that require anaerobic mechanisms to supplement the energy generated by aerobic mechanisms. These patients experience severe muscle pain when attempting to exercise at levels that normally induce a lactic acidosis. The $\dot{V}_{O_2}$-work rate relationship (work efficiency) appears to be normal for work rates below the level that induces pain in these patients.[36] These patients are limited in their maximum work capacity to work rates predicted to be the anaerobic threshold of normal sedentary subjects. Thus, their maximum $\dot{V}_{O_2}$ is of the order of 1 L/min. Their ventilatory response to exercise is normal,[37] although it has also been reported to be high.[38] The heart rate and cardiac output responses of these patients are inordinately high for the metabolic rate, and the arterial-venous O_2 difference at maximal work rate is low.[39] Investigators have suggested that the latter is due to failure to extract O_2 normally, because of the reduced Bohr effect consequent to the failure to increase skeletal muscle lactic acid and reduce capillary pH to the level needed for normal O_2 extraction.[40]

Patients with electron transport chain defects develop a lactic acidosis at exceptionally low work rates.[41] As in patients with myophosphorylase deficiencies, however, the gas exchange abnormalities accompanying these metabolic defects have not been well studied.

Diabetes mellitus affects large arteries (atherosclerosis), small blood vessels, and capillaries. When the disease is poorly controlled, diabetic patients also have a leftward shift in the oxyhemoglobin dissociation curve (glycosylated hemoglobin). Any one of these abnormalities could reduce the AT and $\dot{V}_{O_2}$max. Studies in diabetic children suggest that the AT and maximum $\dot{V}_{O_2}$ are reduced even when the patient's diabetes is under good control.[42–44]

The ventilatory response to exercise has been demonstrated to be increased and the Pa_{CO_2} reduced in women during the progestational phase of the menstrual cycle.[45,46] The effect of this increased ventilatory drive on maximal exercise performance in women is unknown.

Anxiety and Malingering

Anxiety reactions occasionally cause dyspnea during exercise. One manifestation of anxiety is intense hyperventilation with development of severe respiratory alkalosis. The hyperventilation pattern is unique in that the breathing frequency is regular. In addition, the tachypnea starts abruptly, as though "switched on," rather than gradually, as is normally seen during progressive exercise. Hyperventilation might actually start at rest, in anticipation of the exercise.

Another manifestation of an anxiety reaction described as shortness of breath may, in fact, be irregular breathing or breath-holding. Observing the behavior pattern and the patient's facial expression may be helpful in detecting this problem.

It is important to distinguish malingering for secondary gain from other disorders. An exercise test in which both heart rate reserve and breathing reserve are high and the AT is not reached argues in favor of poor effort. A sustained increase in R above 1.0 will not be evident and arterial blood measures will not demonstrate a significant lactic acidosis. The breathing pattern may be irregular, with short periods of tachypnea alternating with bradypnea causing wide swings in Pa_{CO_2} and $P_{ET_{CO_2}}$ unrelated to the changing work rate.

Defect Combinations

A patient's symptoms may be more marked than predicted from the non-exercise assessment of the severity of the patient's disease. Such may be the case when the primary disease is combined with a second disease, or a complicating habit (smoking), or use of a drug that affects ventilatory drive directly or indirectly through a metabolite (e.g., H^+). Thus, patients with coronary artery disease who have hypertension or who smoke might be less symptomatic if their blood pressure were under adequate control or if they did not smoke. Patients with chronic airflow obstruction may be more symptomatic if they also have chronic metabolic acidosis or obesity. Because coronary artery disease and chronic airflow obstruction are so common, both defects may be present in the same patient and may therefore make the patient's symptoms more pronounced than if the two diseases did not coexist. Cardiopulmonary exercise tests, with and without treatment, e.g., O_2 enrichment or vasodilator drugs, are probably the best way to identify which disease is the primary contributor to the patient's symptoms, as well as to provide a noninvasive, relatively inexpensive method to assess therapy.

Summary

The major function of the cardiovascular and ventilatory systems is gas exchange between the cells and the atmosphere. Therefore, impairments in cardiovascular and respiratory function are most apparent during exercise because cell respiration is stimulated and defects are amplified. Because each component of the gas transport system that couples external to internal respiration has a different role, the pattern of the gas exchange abnormality differs according to the pathophysiology. Recognition of these differences allows the examiner to distinguish the limiting organ system in the patient experiencing exercise intolerance. Thus, whereas primary heart disease and primary lung disease both cause a reduction in work capacity, the patterns of the gas exchange response differ. For instance, in primary heart disease, the $\dot{V}O_2$ at the maximum work rate performed tends to be low and the slope of the $\dot{V}O_2$-work rate relationship commonly decreases. Concurrently, the heart rate-$\dot{V}O_2$ relationship is steep, the O_2 pulse is low and unchanging, the breathing reserve is high, and the heart rate reserve is relatively low. In contrast, in the patient with obstructive lung disease, the $\dot{V}O_2$-work rate relationship usually increases linearly with a normal $\dot{V}O_2$-heart rate relationship, but the breathing reserve is low and the heart rate reserve is high. Patients with pulmonary vascular disease and peripheral vascular disease manifest a still different set of abnormalities. By making measurements that address the gas transport function of each site in the coupling of external to cellular respiration, it is possible to deduce the physiologic status of each component.

References

1. Alexander, J.K., Amad, K.H., and Cole, V.W.: Observations on some clinical features of extreme obesity, with particular reference to circulatory effect. Am. J. Med., 32:512–524, 1962.
2. Bates, D.V., Macklem, P.T., and Christie, R.J.: Respiratory Function in Disease. 2nd Ed. Philadelphia, W.B. Saunders, 1971, pp. 100–101.
3. Gilbert, R., Sipple, J.H., and Auchincloss, J.H.: Respiratory control and work or breathing in obese subjects. J. Appl. Physiol., 16:21–26, 1961.
4. Sharp, J.G., Henry, J.P., Sweany, S.K., Meadows, W.R., and Pietras, R.J.: The total work of breathing in normal and obese men. J. Clin. Invest., 43:728–739, 1964.
5. Cherniack, R.M.: Respiratory effects of obesity. Can. Med. Assoc. J., 80:613–616, 1959.
6. Ray, C.S., Sue, D.Y., Bray, G., Hansen, J.E., and Wasserman, K.: Effects of obesity on respiratory function. Am. Rev. Respir. Dis., 128:501–506, 1983.
7. Wasserman, K., and Whipp, B.J.: Exercise physiology in health and disease (state of the art). Am. Rev. Respir. Dis., 112:219–249, 1975.
8. Hansen, J.E., Sue, D.Y., and Wasserman, K.: Predicted values for clinical exercise testing. Am. Rev. Respir. Dis., 129:S49-S55, 1984.
9. Buskirk, E., and Taylor, H.L.: Maximal oxygen intake and its relation to body composition, with special reference to chronic physical activity and obesity. J. Appl. Physiol., 11:72–78, 1957.
10. Bylund-Fellenius, A.C., Walker, P.M., Elander, A., Holm, S., Holm, J., and Schersten, T.: Energy metabolism in relation to oxygen, partial pressure in human skeletal muscle during exercise. Biochem. J., 200:247–255, 1981.
11. Weber, K.T., and Janicki, J.S.: Cardiopulmonary Exercise Testing: Physiological Principles and Clinical Applications. Philadelphia, W.B. Saunders, 1986, p. 183.
12. Nery, L.E., Wasserman, K., French, W., Oren, A., and Davis, J.A.: Contrasting cardiovascular and respiratory responses to exercise in severe chronic obstructive pulmonary disease. Chest, 83:446–453, 1983.
13. Rubin, S.A., and Brown, H.V.: Ventilation and gas exchange during exercise in severe chronic heart failure. Am. Rev. Respir. Dis., 129(Suppl.):S63-S64, 1984.
14. Koike, A., Itoh, H., Dai, M., Taniguchi, K., Marumo, F., Umehara, I., and Hiroe, M.: Beat-to-beat evaluation of cardiac function during recovery from upright bicycle exercise in patients with coronary artery disease. Am. Heart J., 120:316–323, 1990.
15. Ben-Dov, I., Sietsema, K.E., Casaburi, R., and Wasserman, K.: Evidence that circulatory oscillations accompany ventilation oscillations during exercise in patients with heart failure. Am. Rev. Respir. Dis., 145:776–781, 1992.
16. Sietsema, K.E., Cooper, D.M., Rosove, M.A., Perloff, J.K., Child, J.S., Canobbio, M.M., Whipp, B.J., and Wasserman, K.: Dynamics of oxygen uptake during exercise in adults with cyanotic congenital heart disease. Circulation, 73:1137–1144, 1986.
17. Sietsema, K.E., Cooper, D.M., Perloff, S.K., Child, J.S., Rosove, M.H., Wasserman, K., and Whipp, B.J.: Control of ventilation during exercise in patients with central venous-to-systemic arterial shunts. J. Appl. Physiol., 64:234–242, 1988.
18. Cooper, C.B., Daly, J.A., Burns, M.R., et al.: Lactic acidosis contributes to the production of dyspnea in chronic obstructive pulmonary disease. Am. Rev. Respir. Dis., 143:A80, 1991.
19. Casaburi, R., Patessio, A., Ioli, F., et al.: Reductions in exercise lactic acidosis and ventilation as a result of exercise training in obstructive lung disease. Am. Rev. Respir. Dis., 143:9–18, 1991.

20. Comroe, J.H.: The peripheral chemoreceptors. *In* Handbook of Physiology. Section 3. Respiration. Edited by W.O. Fenn and H. Rahn. Washington, D.C., American Physiological Society, 1964, pp. 557–583.
21. Brown, H.V., and Wasserman, K.: Exercise performance in chronic obstructive pulmonary diseases. Med. Clin. North Am., 65:525–547, 1981.
22. Bye, P.T.P., Farkas, G.A., and Roussos, C.H.: Respiratory factors limiting exercise. Am. Rev. Physiol., 45:439–451, 1983.
23. Pierce, A.K., Luterman, D., Loundermilk, J., Blomquist, G., and Johnson, R.L., Jr.: Exercise ventilatory patterns in normal subjects and patients with airway obstruction. J. Appl. Physiol., 25:249–254, 1968.
24. Fulmer, J.D.: An introduction to the interstitial lung diseases. Clin. Chest Med., 3:457–473, 1982.
25. Keogh, B.A., Lakatos, E., Price, D., and Crystal, R.G.: Importance of the lower respiratory tract in oxygen transfer. Am. Rev. Respir. Dis., 129(Suppl.):S76-S80, 1984.
26. Wagner, P.D., Dantzker, D.R., Dueck, R., de Polo, J.R., Wasserman, K., and West, J.B.: Distribution of ventilation-perfusion ratios in patients with interstitial lung disease. Chest, 69:256–257, 1976.
27. Wasserman, K. and Mason, G.R.: Pulmonary alveolar proteinosis. *In* Textbook of Respiratory Medicine. Edited by J.F. Murray and J.A. Nadel. Philadelphia, W.B. Saunders, 1988, pp. 1535–1548.
28. Bunn, H.F., and Forget, B.G.: Hemoglobinopathy due to abnormal oxygen binding. *In* Hemoglobin: Molecular, Genetic and Clinical Aspects. Philadelphia, W.B. Saunders, 1986, pp. 595–622.
29. Butler, W.M., Spratling, L.S., Kark, J.A., and Shoomaker, E.B.: Hemoglobin Osler: report of a new family with exercise studies before and after phlebotomy. Am. J. Hematol., 13:293–301, 1982.
30. Pirnay, S., Dujardin, J., Deroanne, R., and Petit, J.M.: Muscular exercise during intoxication by carbon monoxide. J. Appl. Physiol., 31:573–575, 1971.
31. Vogel, J.A., and Gleser, M.A.: Effect of carbon monoxide on oxygen transport during exercise. J. Appl. Physiol., 32:234–239, 1972.
32. Hirsch, G.L., Sue, D.Y., Wasserman, K., Robinson, T.E., and Hansen, J.E.: Immediate effects of cigarette smoking on the cardiorespiratory responses to exercise. J. Appl. Physiol., 58:1975–1981, 1985.
33. Oren, A., Wasserman, K., Davis, J.A., and Whipp, B.J.: The effect of CO_2 set-point on the ventilatory response to exercise. J. Appl. Physiol., 51:185–189, 1981.
34. Jones, N.L., Sutton, J.R., Taylor, R., and Toews, J.: Effect of pH on cardiorespiratory and metabolic responses to exercise. J. Appl. Physiol., 43:959–964, 1977.
35. McArdle B.: Myopathy due to a defect in muscle glycogen breakdown. Clin. Sci., 10:13–35, 1951.
36. Davis, J.A., Wasserman, K., and Andersen, T.: O_2 consumption as related to work-rate in McArdle's syndrome. Unpublished observations.
37. Riley, M., Nugent, A.-M., Steele, I.C., Bell, N., Trimble, E.R., Nicholls, D.P., and Patterson, V.H.: Gas exchange during exercise in McArdle's disease. J. Appl. Physiol., 75:745–754, 1993.
38. Haller, R.G., and Lewis, S.F.: Abnormal ventilation during exercise in McArdle's syndrome: modulation by substrate availability. Radiology, 36:716–719, 1986.
39. Lewis, S.F., and Haller, R.G.: The pathophysiology of McArdle's disease: clues to regulation in exercise and fatigue. J. Appl. Physiol., 61:391–401, 1986.
40. Wasserman, K., Hansen, J.E., and Sue, D.Y.: Facilitation of oxygen consumption by lactic acidosis during exercise. News Physiol. Sci., 6:29–34, 1991.
41. Bogaard, J.M., Scholte, H.R., Busch, H.F.M., Stam, H., and Versprille, A.: Anaerobic threshold as detected from ventilatory and metabolic exercise responses in patients with mitochondrial respiratory chain defect. Adv. Cardiol., 35:135–145, 1986.
42. Berger, M., Berchtold, P., Cuppers, H.J., Drost, H., Kley, H.K., Muller, W.A., Wiegelmann, W., Zimmerman-Telschow, H., Gries, F.A., Kruskemper, H.L., and Zimmerman, H.: Metabolic and hormonal effects of muscular exercise in juvenile type diabetics. Diabetologia, 13:355–365, 1977.
43. Rubler, S., and Arvan, S.: Exercise testing in young asymptomatic diabetic patients. Angiology, 27:539–548, 1976.
44. Storstein, L., and Jervell, J.: Response to bicycle exercise testing in long-standing juvenile diabetes. Acta Med. Scand., 205:277–280, 1979.
45. Skatrud, J.B., Dempsey, J.A., and Kaiser, D.G.: Ventilatory response to medroxyprogesterone acetate in normal subjects: time course and mechanism. J. Appl. Physiol., 44:939–944, 1978.
46. Lahiri, S., and Gelfant, R.: Mechanisms of acute ventilatory responses. *In* Regulation or Breathing. Part II. Edited by T. Hornbein. New York, Marcel Dekker, 1981, p. 820.

Protocols for Exercise Testing

THE OBJECTIVE OF clinical exercise tests should be to learn the maximum about the patient's pathophysiologic causes of exercise limitation (1) with the greatest accuracy, (2) with the least stress to the patient, and (3) in the shortest period of time. The optimal examination allows the simultaneous evaluation of the adequacy of the muscles, heart, lungs, and peripheral and pulmonary circulations to meet the gas exchange requirements of exercise. The test should enable the investigator to distinguish disorders in these systems from inadequate effort, obesity, anxiety, or unfitness. For the differential diagnosis of exercise limitation caused by cardiovascular or respiratory disease, relatively complete gas exchange measurements should be made. Exercise with large muscle groups is needed to stimulate internal respiration sufficiently to stress the cardiovascular and pulmonary systems adequately; therefore, either a cycle ergometer or a treadmill should be used for testing. Isometric exercise is of limited value because it is largely anaerobic, providing little information about the ability of the cardiovascular and respiratory systems to support the energy requirements of exercise. The protocol selected for exercise testing depends on the purpose of the test. For instance, if one is certain that the only possible cause of the patient's symptoms is coronary artery disease, then monitoring the electrocardiogram (ECG) with 12 leads using the Bruce,[1] Naughton,[2] or Ellestad[3] protocol is satisfactory. The criteria for diagnosing myocardial ischemia secondary to coronary artery disease are extensively described elsewhere.[3] If one is less certain that the exclusive cause of the patient's dysfunction is coronary artery disease, however, then a more comprehensive examination is needed. The protocol that we find most useful in providing a diagnosis of the pathophysiology of exercise limitation is a cycle ergometer test in which the work rate is increased by a uniform amount each minute or less (incremental test), as described in the following sections of this chapter.

Description and Use of Incremental Work Rate Tests

With the advent of rapidly responding gas analyzers and computers, it has become feasible to obtain a large amount of accurate metabolic, ventilatory, and circulatory data in a brief period of time with minimal stress and maximal safety to the pa-

tient. The following is a detailed description of our testing procedures.

PREPARING THE PATIENT

Instructions to Patient

At the time of scheduling, the patient is advised to wear comfortable clothes and low heel or athletic shoes, to adhere to his or her usual medical regimen, to eat a light meal no less than 2 hours before arrival, and to avoid cigarettes and coffee for at least 2 hours.

Initial Physician Evaluation

While the exercise system is being calibrated by the technician, the physician takes a history from the patient with particular emphasis on medications, tobacco use, accustomed activity levels, and the presence of angina pectoris or other exercise-induced symptoms. The physician examines the patient with particular attention to the heart, lungs, and peripheral pulses, determines blood pressure from each arm, and obtains an accurate shoeless height and weight.

Informed Consent

The patient is told that he or she will be asked to make a maximal effort but is advised that exercise can be stopped at any time. The patient is advised of potential discomforts and risks associated with the procedure and the kinds of information that will be obtained. Finally, the patient is encouraged to ask questions about the testing before giving written consent.

Resting Respiratory Function

Recent spirometric data are accepted unless the patient has variable obstructive lung disease or performed erratically when spirometry was last obtained. Under these conditions, the vital capacity (VC), inspiratory capacity (IC), forced expiratory volume in 1 second (FEV_1), and maximal voluntary ventilation (MVV) are obtained when the patient arrives at the exercise laboratory for testing. The American Thoracic Society has published detailed instructions for performing spirometric testing.[4] The direct MVV is calculated from a 12-second maneuver of rapid and deep breathing; the indirect MVV is calculated by multiplying the FEV_1 by 40.[5] The MVV values are needed for measurement of the exercise breathing reserve. In patients with severe interstitial lung disease, the indirect MVV is often more appropriate to use than the direct MVV if the direct MVV maneuver had been performed at extremely high breathing frequencies unattainable during cycle or treadmill exercise. On the other hand, in patients with inspiratory obstruction, neuromuscular disorders, and severe obesity, the direct MVV should be used even if considerably less than the indirect MVV. In patients with poor spirometric efforts, the indirect MVV is usually more appropriate.

Equipment Familiarization

If the treadmill is used, time is provided for practice trials, so the patient can get on and off the moving treadmill belt with confidence. If the cycle is used, the seat height is adjusted so the legs are nearly completely extended when the pedals are at their lowest point. Because a mouthpiece is in the patient's mouth during testing, the patient is taught to use the signal "thumbs up" if everything is satisfactory and "thumbs down" if he or she is experiencing any unexpected difficulty. The patient is advised to point to the site of discomfort if chest pain or pressure (possible symptoms of angina pectoris) or leg pain is experienced. The code of finger signals for intensity is: the index finger if mild, two fingers if moderate, and three fingers if severe. In our laboratory we stop the exercise with a signal of moderate chest discomfort.

The mouthpiece and noseclip are tried. The patient is advised that it is acceptable to swallow with the mouthpiece in place or moisten the inside of the mouth with the tongue. The accumulation of large quantities of saliva in the vicinity of the gas sampling tube orifice can lead to plugging of the tube and erroneous gas concentration measurements. This problem can be minimized by having the gas sampling tube enter the breathing valve-mouthpiece assembly from above with the sampling tube tip free of the inner surface and by incorporating a saliva trap into the mouthpiece assembly.

Exercise ECG

Silver/silver chloride ECG electrodes with circumferential adhesive provide good electrical contact. For 12-lead tracings, the "arm" electrodes are placed at the lateral and superior corners of the scapulae, and the "leg" electrodes are placed near the right and left inferior rib margins between the mid-clavicular and anterior axillary lines (Fig. 5-1). (Lower positions increase signal artifact, especially in obese patients.) V1 and V2 positions are moved one interspace caudad, whereas V3 through V6 positions are in their usual locations. The three electrodes for the oscilloscope monitor may be positioned as depicted in Figure 5-1.

Arterial Catheter

If the study requires arterial blood sampling, a catheter is inserted into one of the radial or brachial arteries using the Seldinger technique (see Appendix E for detailed description of how to place the catheter).[6] It is important to check radial and ulnar artery pulsations before and after cathe-

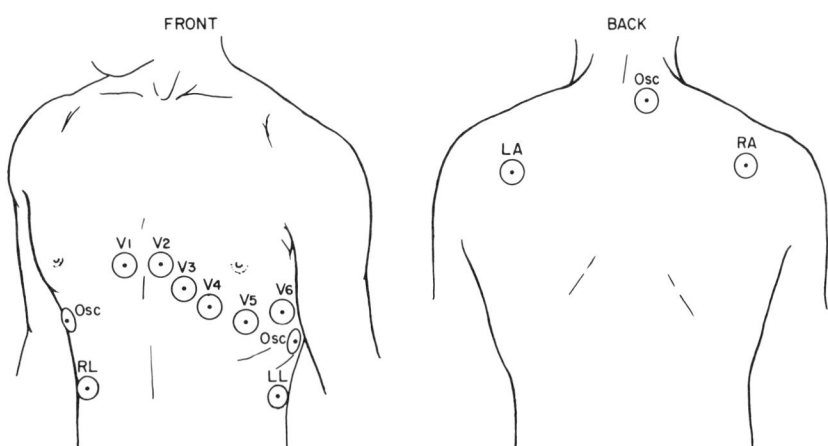

FIG. 5-1. ECG lead placement for upright ergometry. The V1 and V2 electrodes are placed more caudad than usually done for supine tracings, whereas V3, V4, V5, and V6 are in their usual locations. The "arm" electrodes (LA and RA) are placed posterior to the shoulders, whereas the "leg" electrodes (LL and RL) are placed anterolaterally near the lower rib margins. The three oscilloscope (OSC) electrodes are placed separately to minimize electrical interference.

ter insertion. The catheter is attached to a stopcock and a miniature blood pressure transducer via a continuous flush device that provides a slow infusion of a heparinized saline solution (10 units/ml). When one uses a brachial artery catheter, the catheter should be long enough (20 to 25 cm) so that its hub can be brought around to the lateral aspect of the lower part of the upper arm (Fig. 5-2). The transducer is positioned on the upper arm at a height corresponding to the fourth interspace of the mid-clavicular line (mid-atrial level when the patient is upright). To avoid spurious dilution of the blood specimen with heparinized saline, about 0.5 ml of blood is discarded before collecting each arterial blood sample (usually by letting the blood flow into gauze under arterial pressure before the syringe is connected to the stopcock). Each sample is collected for approximately 20 seconds, so its

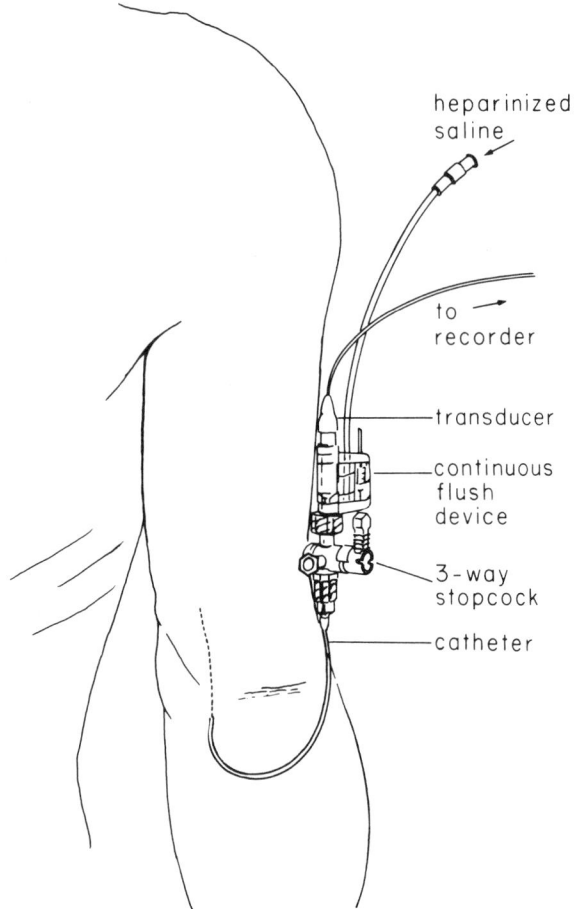

heparinized saline

to recorder

transducer

continuous flush device

3-way stopcock

catheter

FIG. 5-2. Brachial artery catheter placement. A 25-cm polyvinyl catheter has been placed percutaneously in the left brachial artery. The dressings have been removed to show catheter placement. The hub of the catheter connects to a continuous flush device, a three-way stopcock, and a transducer, the last located on the lateral arm parallel to the fourth intercostal space in the mid-clavicular line (at the mid-atrial level in the sitting position).

gas tensions are representative of the mean arterial value and minimally influenced by ventilatory variations in alveolar gas tensions. Immediately after sampling, the catheter lumen is flushed with heparinized saline. If an arterial catheter is not inserted, arterial O_2 saturation can be estimated with a calibrated pulse oximeter as an index of blood oxygenation (see Appendix C).

TESTING

Measurements at Rest

An arterial blood specimen is obtained with the patient in the sitting position before he or she is moved to the ergometer, to avoid effects on the breathing pattern induced by the mouthpiece. A noseclip is put on the patient and is checked for leaks, and the mouthpiece is inserted. In our laboratory, we frequently continuously record expiratory and inspiratory airflow, O_2 and CO_2 tension at the mouthpiece, oximetry, and a single-lead ECG on a multi-channel recorder. Heart rate (HR), breathing frequency (f), $\dot{V}_E$, $\dot{V}_{O_2}$, $\dot{V}_{CO_2}$, R, $P_{ET_{CO_2}}$, $P_{ET_{O_2}}$, and O_2 pulse ($\dot{V}_{O_2}$/HR) are printed out breath-by-breath or every quarter to half minute by averaging an integral number of whole breaths. These may be plotted out after the test, as shown in Chapter 8. If an arterial catheter has been placed, arterial blood pressure is recorded continuously and arterial blood is sampled for blood gases, pH, lactate, co-oximetry, and hematocrit values at rest. If an arterial catheter is not used, blood pressure is obtained with a pressure cuff and pulse oximeter values are recorded. A 12-lead ECG is obtained with the subject in the supine position and again while on the ergometer before exercise.

Unloaded Exercise

When an electromagnetically braked cycle ergometer is used, to overcome the inertia of the cycle flywheel, an accessory motor[7] can be used to rotate the flywheel at a rate of slightly over 60 rpm while the patient's feet are motionless on the pedals. As soon as the patient starts pedalling, the accessory motor is turned off. This is particularly helpful for testing patients with limited strength in their legs. At a verbal signal, the patient begins 3 minutes of unloaded pedalling. The patient is advised to look at the rpm meter and to maintain a cycling speed of 60 rpm. A metronome may be used to assist the patient in maintaining cadence, i.e., one leg stroke for each beat of the metronome. A 12-lead ECG, blood pressure measurement, and, if the patient has an arterial catheter, a blood sample are obtained near the end of the 3 minutes of unloaded pedalling.

Incremental Exercise

Measurements are continued while the work rate is increased continuously (ramp)[8] or by a uniform amount each minute until the patient is limited by symptoms or is unable to continue safely (Fig. 5-3). An increment rate of 5, 7, 10, 15, 20, 25, or 30 watts(W) per minute is selected, depending on the expected performance of the patient (see later). A 12-lead ECG and arterial samples for blood gas and pH measurement are ordinarily obtained every 2 minutes. The technician and physician work cooperatively in observing the patient's facial expression, checking the blood pressure and ECG recordings for untoward changes and arrhythmias, looking for leaks at the nose or mouthpiece, observing for signals from the patient, and verbally encouraging the patient to maximize his or her performance. The resistance of the cycle is removed if the patient evidences distress, if there is a fall in mean blood pressure greater than 10 mm Hg, if a significant arrhythmia develops, or if the patient has ST segment depression of 3 mm or greater. The exercise is also terminated if the patient is unable to maintain cycling frequency above 40 rpm. If practical, an arterial blood sample is obtained during the last half minute of exercise.

Recovery

The patient respires through the mouthpiece during 2 minutes of recovery. In the immediate post-exercise period, the patient is advised to continue to pedal at a slow frequency with no load on the ergometer. This prevents the precipitous fall in blood pressure that is occasionally experienced when vigorous exercise is abruptly terminated. A final arterial blood sample is obtained at 2 minutes of recovery.

Special Protocol for Very Infirm or Very Obese Patients

When we expect patients to have an extremely severe exercise limitation, we frequently use the following special protocol in which, after the rest period, the external work load is incremented less rapidly than usual in the initial portion of the test. For the first 3 minutes of unloaded pedalling, the

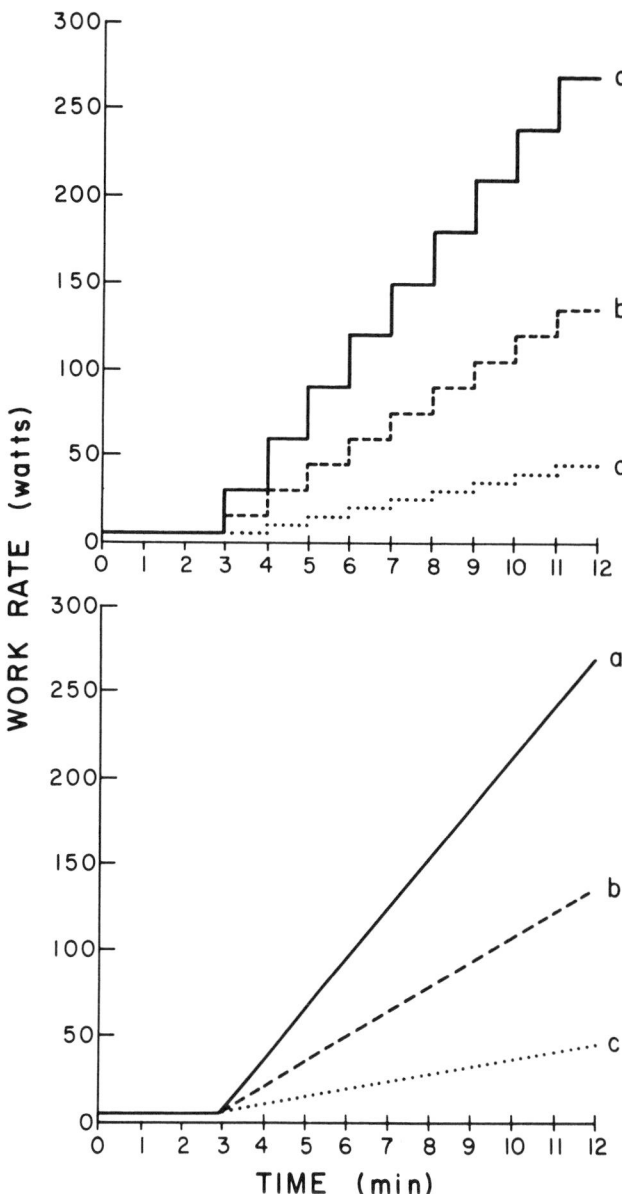

FIG. 5-3. One-minute incremental (upper) and ramp incremental (lower) protocols for cycle ergometry. In both cases, the subject initially cycles for 3 minutes of unloaded pedalling. In the example shown, the work rate is incremented 30 (a), 15 (b), or 5 (c) W per minute depending on the height, age, gender, and health of the subject. The increment is added at the start of each minute for the 1-minute test, whereas the increment is completed at the end of each minute for the ramp test. Larger or intermediate increments can also be used. The cycle is returned to the unloaded setting when the cycling frequency cannot be maintained over 40 rpm or when the physician or subject decides to terminate the incremental exercise.

patient cycles at 20 rpm, for the fourth minute at 40 rpm, and for the fifth minute at 60 rpm, all with the accessory motor rotating the flywheel at a speed of slightly over 60 rpm so the exercise is truly unloaded. In the sixth minute, the accessory motor is turned off while the patient continues pedalling at 60 rpm. Starting with the seventh minute, the work rate is increased by 5 to 10 W per minute. This protocol allows the accumulation of more data at a very low metabolic rate and frequently allows delineation of very low *LAT* values, which are otherwise unmeasureable. This is especially true in patients with very obese legs, in whom unloaded pedalling at 60 rpm may cause the $\dot{V}O_2$ to exceed 1.0 L per minute. We do not insist that the patient cycles smoothly at 20 and 40 rpm; intermittent movement of the pedals is satisfactory.

IMMEDIATE POST-EXERCISE CARE

Immediately after removal of the mouthpiece, the physician questions the patient in a non-leading fashion about what symptoms caused him or her to stop exercise. A series of questions may be required to assess just what the patient means by his or her statement of limiting symptoms. It is important to differentiate calf from thigh pain and to determine the exact character of any chest discomfort.

If, on review of the data, it appears that the test was terminated prematurely because of insufficient effort, a repeat test after a recovery period of 30 to 45 minutes may be indicated. For instance, if the patient made an insufficient effort, as suggested by the combination of high breathing and HR reserves, a low R, and only a slight fall in bicarbonate, the test bears repeating with greater encouragement from the examiner. The blood analysis values are also reviewed before the residual blood in the syringes is discarded to allow remeasurement of any questionable blood values.

If the test is satisfactory and does not need to be repeated, the arterial catheter is removed, keeping direct pressure over the puncture site in the brachial artery for at least 5 minutes. When the pressure is removed, the site is inspected carefully for evidence of external or internal bleeding. With adequate pressure and observation after removal of the catheter, hematomas can be avoided. With any evidence of bleeding, pressure is continued for at least another 3 minutes. A light dressing covered with a tight elastic bandage is then applied to the puncture site, and the peripheral pulses are checked. The patient is advised not to use that arm for heavy exercise for the next 24 hours. The dressing and elastic bandage can be removed by the patient after several hours have elapsed.

FINAL REPORT

In our laboratory, after entry of blood gas and blood pressure values, the computer produces graphic and tabular displays of the results of the exercise study similar to those shown in Chapter 8. Others may prefer a different format. The physician's final report should include: (1) a short clinical history; (2) a description of the procedure; (3) subjective and objective observations concerning the patient's performance during testing; (4) tabular and graphic displays (usually one page each) of the exercise responses; (5) a summary table with measurements of resting and maximum exercise respiratory and cardiovascular variables; (6) copies of the ECG, expiratory flow, or blood pressure tracings if abnormal; and (7) an interpretation.

CRITIQUE OF 1-MINUTE INCREMENTAL TEST

Duration of Test and Incremental Size

Balke and colleagues introduced the use of 1-minute incremental treadmill tests for the study of fitness in a large military population.[9,10] Although Balke initially used a 1% increment in grade per minute with a constant treadmill speed of 3.3 mph, he also used a 2% increment in grade every minute. Several investigators, including Consolazio,[11] Jones,[12] and Spiro,[13] and their colleagues, used the cycle ergometer with the work rate increment increased by an equal amount every minute or half minute. Increments of 8, 15, 17, or 25 W per minute, 10 W per half minute, or 4 W every 15 seconds have been reported.[14] We introduced the use of a continuously incrementing (ramp pattern) exercise protocol,[8,15] (Fig. 5-3) and we have used it extensively in adults and children.[16] In comparing the ramp test with 1-, 2-, and 3-minute step increments at the same overall average work rate increase, Zhang et al.[17] have shown that no significant differences were found in the $\dot{V}O_2$max, *AT*, $\dot{V}E$max, HRmax, $\Delta\dot{V}O_2/\Delta$WR, or exercise duration among the four protocols in healthy subjects. Step patterns in some measures could be seen in the 2- and 3-minute step protocols, however (see Fig. 3-3). Thus, although any of these protocols might be used, either the ramp or the 1-minute incremental test seems practical and preferable in patients.

Several investigators[18,19] have stressed the desirability of adjusting the work rate increment according to the patient's cardiorespiratory status. Tests that are too brief, that is, with the work rate increased too rapidly, may not allow a sufficient quantity of data to be accumulated. Tests that are too long, that is, with too small a work rate increase, are likely to be terminated prematurely because of boredom or "seat discomfort." We have found that tests in which the incremental part of the protocol is completed between 6 and 12 minutes' duration give the highest maximum $\dot{V}O_2$ in normal subjects, although the differences with durations outside this range are small.[20] We know of no similar study in patients with heart or lung disease; consequently, we can only assume that the findings with patients would be similar. Therefore, we attempt to select a work rate increment that will result in termination of the incremental part of the exercise test in 8 to 10 minutes.

How to Select Increment Size

We select the increment size after considering the patient's history (especially the amount and intensity of his or her daily activity), physical examination (notably obesity and evidence of cardiac or respiratory disease), and pulmonary function evaluation (particularly the FEV_1 and MVV). If we expect the patient to have a near-normal power output, we estimate the $\dot{V}O_2$ at unloaded pedalling from the patient's body weight and the maximum $\dot{V}O_2$ from the patient's age and height. We then calculate the work rate increment necessary to reach the patient's estimated maximum $\dot{V}O_2$ in 10 minutes. The steps that we use to approximate the correct increment for the cycle are: (1) $\dot{V}O_2$ unloaded in milliters per minute $= 150 + (6 \times kg)$; (2) maximum $\dot{V}O_2$ in milliters per minute $=$ (height in cm $-$ age in years) $\times$ 20 for sedentary men and $\times$ 14 for sedentary women; (3) the work rate (W) increment per minute $=$ (maximum $\dot{V}O_2$ $- \dot{V}O_2$ unloaded)/100.

For example, given an apparently healthy sedentary man 180 cm in height, 100 kg in weight, and 50 years of age, his anticipated $\dot{V}O_2$ unloaded $= 150 + 6 \times 100 = 750$ ml per minute; his anticipated maximum $\dot{V}O_2 = (180 - 50) \times 20 = 2600$ ml per minute. To obtain an incremental test duration of 10 minutes, we would calculate an increment size of $(2600 - 750)/100 = 18.5$ W per minute. Practically, we would select an increment of 20 W per minute and expect a test duration of slightly less than 10 minutes.

If we know that the patient has a MVV, FEV_1, or DL_{CO} less than 80% of that predicted, we would consider reducing the expected maximum $\dot{V}O_2$ proportionally; i.e., MVV or DL_{CO} of 50% of that

predicted reduces the expected maximum $\dot{V}O_2$ to roughly half to two thirds of normal. If the patient has resting tachycardia, symptoms suggestive of angina, or evidence of chronic heart failure, we also reduce the expected maximum $\dot{V}O_2$, the amount being judged by our pre-exercise assessment of impairment. In each case we reduce the size of the work rate increment in an attempt to keep the total incremental exercise time at about 10 minutes.

Given a choice, we would rather overestimate than underestimate the work rate increment. With too large an increment, the test will be brief and the patient will recover quickly, an advantage if retesting is necessary. With too small an increment, the patient may stop for ambiguous reasons and may feel too fatigued for retesting.

Validity of Measurements

Some investigators have expressed concern whether the maximum $\dot{V}O_2$ is as high in continuous incremental protocols as in discontinuous protocols and whether the highest $\dot{V}O_2$ reached (maximum $\dot{V}O_2$) should be identified as the $\dot{V}O_2max$. Taylor et al.[21] defined the $\dot{V}O_2max$ from a series of progressively higher constant work rate tests as that occurring when an increase in work rate resulted in an increase of $\dot{V}O_2$ of less than 150 ml per minute above the $\dot{V}O_2$ from the previous lower work rate. This criterion is appropriate for tests in fit subjects using large work rate increments, such as 2.5% grade change at a treadmill speed of 7 mph. In tests featuring a 15-W per minute increase in work rate, however, the rate of increase in $\dot{V}O_2$ is normally only 150 ml per minute. Therefore, at increments of 15 W per minute or less, it is invalid to use the criterion of Taylor et al. to determine whether the maximum $\dot{V}O_2$ is indeed the $\dot{V}O_2max$. A single study[22] reported an approximately 10% lower maximum $\dot{V}O_2$ using a continuous rather than a discontinuous graded work rate test; however, the long duration (20 to 30 minutes) of these continuous tests could have accounted for the reduction.[19] In contrast, Maksud,[23] Wyndham,[24] and McArdle[25] and their associates found no difference in maximum $\dot{V}O_2$ measured in continuous incremental tests compared with discontinuous constant work rate treadmill tests. Pollock and colleagues[26] found a plateau in $\dot{V}O_2$ in 59 to 69% of the continuous incremental treadmill tests they administered. We found a similar maximum $\dot{V}O_2$ in normal men using a ramp-pattern increase in cycle ergometer tests, whether the increase was

TABLE 5-1. *Effect of Protocol on Measurements of Pa_{O_2}, $P(A\text{-}a)_{O_2}$ and V_D/V_T During Cycling at the Same Mean $\dot{V}_{O_2}$ (0.92 $\pm$ 0.03 L/min)*

		Pa_{O_2}, mm Hg		$P(A\text{-}a)_{O_2}$, mm Hg		VD/VT	
	N	INCR.*	CONSTANT†	INCR.	CONSTANT	INCR.	CONSTANT
Normal	11	89	94	14	13	0.26	0.25
Restrictive lung disease	3	87	89	18	21	0.21	0.19
Obstructive lung disease	9	79	83	25	22	0.32	0.32
All subjects	23	85‡	89	19	17	0.27	0.28

* 1-minute incremental exercise protocol

† Constant work rate protocol; measurements made at 6 minutes.

‡ Indicates significant difference between 1 minute incremental (Incr.) and constant work rate test at $p < 0.05$ by paired t test; other measurements are not significantly different.

(Data from Furuike, A.N., Sue, D.Y., Hansen, J.E., and Wasserman, K.: Comparison of physiological dead space/tidal volume ratio and alveolar-arterial P_{O_2} difference during incremental and constant work exercise. Am. Rev. Respir. Dis., 126:579–583, 1982.)

20, 30, or 50 W per minute.[15] Thus, we believe that the $\dot{V}_{O_2}$max can be accurately measured with continuous incremental protocols of the proper duration.

Using the ramp pattern test, we also found that the *AT*, time constant for $\dot{V}_{O_2}$, work efficiency, maximum $\dot{V}_E$, and maximum HR were comparable to values found with constant work rate tests.[8,15] Because we were concerned that non-steady-state incremental exercise tests might give different values for $\dot{V}_E$, $\dot{V}_{O_2}$, $\dot{V}_{CO_2}$, $P(A\text{-}a)_{O_2}$, $P(a\text{-}ET)_{CO_2}$, and HR as compared to steady-state, we studied 23 men (11 normal, 9 with obstructive lung disease, and 3 with restrictive lung disease) during steady-state constant work rate and 1-minute incremental exercise tests (Table 5-1).[27] The steady-state exercise $P(A\text{-}a)_{O_2}$ values ranged from 1 to 43 mm Hg, and the V_D/V_T values ranged from 0.12 to 0.44. We found that $\dot{V}_{CO_2}$, $\dot{V}_E$, Pa_{O_2}, and R were slightly lower during incremental exercise than constant work rate exercise at the same $\dot{V}_{O_2}$. The $P(A\text{-}a)_{O_2}$, $P(a\text{-}ET)_{CO_2}$, Pa_{CO_2}, $\dot{V}_E/\dot{V}_{CO_2}$, and V_D/V_T values were in close agreement in both protocols for both the normal subjects and the patients, however. Thus, it is possible to make measurements of gas exchange and ventilation/perfusion matching equally well during incremental or steady-state exercise.

Special Monitoring Requirements for Rapid Incremental Tests

With rapid incremental tests, frequent and accurate measurements are needed. HR and blood pressure are not difficult to measure, but accurate measurement of $\dot{V}_E$, $\dot{V}_{CO_2}$, and $\dot{V}_{O_2}$ requires special thought and understanding of the properties of the measuring devices. The reader is referred to the Appendix, Beaver et al.,[28,29] and Sue et al.[30]

for descriptions of how to make these measurements and for an analysis of potential errors.

Cycle versus Treadmill

Whether the treadmill or the cycle ergometer is the preferable mode of exercise for exercise testing has been a subject of considerable debate (Table 5-2). The treadmill has been in common use for decades. It allows one to exercise most ambulatory patients except those who are severely dyspneic, uncoordinated, or confused or those who have significant lower extremity musculoskeletal disease. The treadmill uses an activity familiar to everyone and allows the investigator the opportunity to vary both speed and grade to change the work rate. It has several disadvantages, however.

TABLE 5-2. *Comparison of Treadmill and Cycle Ergometers for Exercise Testing*

FEATURE	TREADMILL	CYCLE
Higher maximum $\dot{V}_{O_2}$ and maximum O_2 pulse	+	
Similar maximum HR and maximum $\dot{V}_E$	+	+
Familiarity of exercise	+ +	+
Quantitation of external work	− −	+ +
Freedom from artifacts in ECG, air flow, and pressure tracing	− −	+ +
Ease of obtaining arterial blood specimens	− −	+ +
Safety (fewer musculoskeletal injuries)		+
Usefulness in supine position		+
Use of less vertical and horizontal laboratory space		+
Less noise		+
Lower cost		+
Portability	−	+
Greater experience in the United States	+	
Greater experience in Europe		+

More important advantage (+ +) or disadvantage (− −); less important advantage (+) or disadvantage (−).

The treadmill is frightening to some patients and is noisy, bulky, and expensive. Moreover, the laboratory ceiling may be too low for use at the higher treadmill grades. Repeated experience on the treadmill may lead to some increase in the efficiency of walking.[31] Probably the greatest disadvantage of the treadmill is the difficulty in quantifying work rate. Any connection between the patient and the treadmill, except that between the patient's shoes and the treadmill belt, can decrease the expected energy requirement for body movement at that grade and speed. Railings, arm boards, mouthpieces, blood pressure measuring devices, and steadying hands all have the potential to reduce the patient's actual work rate. Length of stride as speed or grade is changed, shift of center of gravity, and change from walking to jogging all can affect the patient's metabolic requirement.

Even the most athletic patients require several minutes of practice in starting and ending the treadmill exercise before beginning measurement. Although injuries are rarely reported, careful surveillance is necessary. Because patients can lose their balance on the moving belts, it is wise to have additional help immediately available on the sideboard of the treadmill, particularly for elderly patients.

The cycle ergometer allows a more accurate quantitation of external work rate and can be used when patients are in the supine or upright position. A minor disadvantage is that most individuals have a lower maximum $\dot{V}O_2$ and LAT on the cycle than on the treadmill, even though their maximum HR, maximum $\dot{V}E$, and maximum blood lactate are similar on both ergometers. In 8 studies of male subjects, the mean maximum $\dot{V}O_2$ on the cycle varied from 89 to 95% of treadmill values.[32] The cycle is less expensive, less bulky, and less noisy than the treadmill. Electromagnetically braked cycles maintain a given work rate despite appreciable fluctuations in pedalling frequency. Mechanical cycles are much less expensive but require exact pedalling frequencies for work quantitation. This may be important because some patients have difficulty cycling at a prescribed rate. None of our patients have been injured using the cycle or treadmill, but we believe that the cycle is safer for those patients who are less well coordinated. We place the patient's feet in toe clips and sometimes, if necessary, bind their shoes to the pedals with tape, so they do not slip out.

Because of less arm and torso movement on the cycle than on the treadmill, one finds less artifact in ventilatory and circulatory measurements and has greater ease in obtaining blood samples. Because the tubular post supporting our cycle seat once buckled while being used by a very obese patient, we now use a stainless steel rod to support a conventional bicycle seat (covered with sheepskin or gel) or a platform-type seat. "Seat pain" can be a problem with prolonged repeated testing, but it is uncommon with the clinical protocols described previously. In agreement with Astrand[33], we prefer the cycle to the treadmill for clinical testing because we can accurately quantify external work rate and thereby establish the patient's work rate-$\dot{V}O_2$ relationship, a critical measurement in assessing cardiovascular function.

Description and Use of Constant Work Rate Tests

DETERMINING $\dot{V}O_2$max

Historically, discontinuous constant work rate tests, each with a large increase in work rate with intervening rest periods, were used to measure $\dot{V}O_2$max.[34] When $\dot{V}O_2$ rose less than 150 ml per minute despite an increase in the work rate, Taylor et al.[21] defined $\dot{V}O_2$ as $\dot{V}O_2$max. Advantages of progressively greater constant work rate tests for determining maximum $\dot{V}O_2$ are as follows: (1) the higher intensity work rates selected can be based on the patient's cardiovascular and ventilatory responses to the lower work rate tests; (2) timed manual bag collection of mixed expired gas for measurement of $\dot{V}CO_2$ and $\dot{V}O_2$ near the end of each exercise does not require rapidly responding gas analyzers; and (3) an obligatory plateau of $\dot{V}O_2$ provides unequivocal identification of $\dot{V}O_2$max. Disadvantages are the following: (1) the repeated tests take considerable time for patient, physician, and technician; (2) these tests are tiring and exhausting and may be more likely to result in injury to the patient; and (3) although such tests are often considered "steady-state" tests, this cannot be true at work rates at or above that necessary to ensure a $\dot{V}O_2$max.

MEASURING KINETICS AND DETERMINING ANAEROBIC OR LACTIC ACIDOSIS THRESHOLD

Constant work rate tests are ideal for measuring cardiovascular, ventilatory, and gas exchange kinetics. Measurement of these variables, especially $\dot{V}O_2$, during the transition from rest to low level exercise or between two levels of exercise (see Fig. 3-4) using breath-by-breath analysis allows measurements of time constants or half-times of response.[35] Averaging the data obtained from several breath-by-breath tests may be necessary for adequate precision.[36,37] Sietsema et al.[38] used such a protocol to demonstrate striking reductions in the $\dot{V}O_2$ increase during the first 20 seconds after exercise onset in patients with cyanotic congenital heart disease. They[39] also demonstrated that, in normal subjects, the magnitude and mean response time (MRT) of $\dot{V}O_2$ correlated well with the fitness ($\dot{V}O_2max/kg$) of the individual; the lower $\dot{V}O_2max/kg$, the longer the MRT for constant work rates of 100 W or higher. Similarly, Ben-Dov et al.[40] demonstrated significantly lower increases in $\dot{V}O_2$ in the first 20 seconds of constant work rate exercise in hyperthyroidism, despite the overall higher metabolic requirement of the disease. At higher constant work rates, Koike et al.[41] demonstrated the lengthening of the $\dot{V}O_2$ time constant as carboxyhemoglobin levels were increased.

The measurement of $\dot{V}O_2$ kinetics over a 6-minute period of constant work rate can also be useful. If the *AT* is uncertain after incremental testing, a constant work rate test can be performed at a work level expected to approximate the individual's *AT*. If the work rate turns out to be above the individual's *AT*, the $\dot{V}O_2$ will not plateau by the end of the third minute, but will continue to rise.[42] The degree of rise will be greater the further the work level is above the *AT* and correlates highly with the extent of the developed lactic acidosis (see Fig. 2-37).[43,44] A repetition of the test at one or two other constant work rate levels should allow an accurate determination of the *AT*.

Several studies have shown the utility of precisely assessing the *AT* and the sensitivity of the $\Delta\dot{V}O_2(6–3)$ to disorders in O_2 transport. Casaburi et al.[45] showed the advantage of training patients with chronic obstructive pulmonary disease with constant work rates above rather than below their *AT*. Koike et al.[41] demonstrated increases in the $\Delta\dot{V}O_2(6–3)$ with reductions in hemoglobin availability, whereas Zhang et al.[46] showed the positive correlation between the $\Delta\dot{V}O_2(6–3)$ and the severity of heart failure in patients with congestive heart failure.

DETECTING EXERCISE-INDUCED BRONCHOSPASM

Although exercise-induced bronchospasm can often be demonstrated after the usual incremental testing in the afflicted individual, it may be more evident after 6 minutes of near maximal constant load exercise.[47] It is necessary to obtain good baseline measurements of FEV_1, or some other index of airway obstruction, immediately before exercise. Most investigators prefer the treadmill to the cycle ergometer for inducing post-exercise bronchospasm, although we have used both successfully. To induce post-exercise bronchospasm, it is our practice to increase the work rate to approximately 80% of the predicted maximal work rate after a 1-minute warm-up at a lower work rate. The patient inspires dry air from a bag filled with compressed air rather than room air because, according to current concepts, dry air aids in the induction of bronchospasm and reduces day-to-day variability if repeated tests are necessary.[48] After cessation of 6 minutes of heavy exercise, the mouthpiece is immediately removed. Spirometric tracings are obtained as soon as possible and at 3, 6, 10, 15, and 20 minutes after exercise.

MEASURING CAROTID BODY CONTRIBUTION TO EXERCISE VENTILATION

The effect of carotid body input to the medullary respiratory centers can be assessed by altering the PO_2 of the blood reaching the carotid bodies.[49] Normally, if the carotid bodies are contributing significantly to ventilatory drive, a rise in carotid artery PO_2 will immediately reduce the carotid body neural outflow and depress ventilation transiently. This can be detected by an immediate fall in $\dot{V}E$, V_T, and f and a rise in PET_{CO_2} approximately 6 to 10 seconds after an unobtrusive switch of inspiratory gas from room air to 100% O_2 (see Fig. 3-29). After 1 minute of 100% O_2 breathing, a switch back to room air results in a return to baseline $\dot{V}E$ and PET_{CO_2} values. Because ventilation is less variable during exercise than at rest, we prefer to perform these measurements during constant work rate exercise of moderate intensity. Steady-state levels of $\dot{V}E$ at moderate exercise are usually attained in less than 5 minutes. Thus, the effect of the change in FI_{O_2} can be more clearly detected and quantified. Maximal effect is usually seen with an increase in Pa_{O_2} to 250 mm Hg or more. If the patient has a normal arterial O_2 saturation and response, $\dot{V}E$ will decrease transiently by about 15%. If a pneumotachograph is used to determine ventilation, an adjustment must be made in calculation to account for the difference in gas viscosity between air and 100% O_2. On-line recording of breath-by-breath ventilation, V_T, f, and gas concentrations is desirable.

Treadmill Test for Detecting Myocardial Ischemia

METHOD

Bruce[1], Ellestad[3], Naughton[2], and their colleagues and other cardiologists have developed and popularized several incremental treadmill protocols for detecting ECG changes of myocardial ischemia.

The Bruce protocol (Fig. 5-4C) begins with 3-minute stages of walking at 1.7 mph at 0, 5, or 10% grade.[1] The 0 and 5% grades are omitted in more fit individuals. Thereafter, the grade is incremented 2% every 3 minutes, and the speed is incremented 0.8 mph every 3 minutes until the treadmill reaches 18% grade and 5 mph. After this, the speed is increased by 0.5 mph every 3 minutes.

Ellestad's protocol (Fig. 5-4E) uses 7 periods, each of 2 or 3 minutes' duration, at progressively increasing speeds of 1.7, 3, 4, 5, 6, 7, and 8 mph. The grade is 10% for the first 4 periods, with durations of 3, 2, 2, and 3 minutes, respectively, and 15% for the last 3 periods, each of 2 minutes' duration.[3]

Naughton's protocol (Fig. 5-4A) uses 10 exercise periods of 3 minutes' duration, each separated by rest periods of 3 minutes.[2] The grade and speed of each period are as follows: 0% and 1 mph; 0% and 1.5 mph; 0% and 2 mph; 3.5% and 2 mph; 7% and 2 mph; 5% and 3 mph; 7.5% and 3 mph; 10% and 12.5% and 3 mph; and 15% and 3 mph.

In each of the foregoing treadmill protocols, blood pressure is measured and a multiple-lead ECG is recorded at each work rate and during recovery. The patient is carefully observed, and the test is terminated at the physician's discretion (e.g., for decline in blood pressure, significant ventricular arrhythmias, progressive ST segment changes, attainment of a given HR) or by the patient's symptoms.

CRITIQUE

These treadmill tests have the advantage of extensive use for clinical testing. A survey in 1977 concluded that the complication rate for "exercise stress testing" was 3.6 myocardial infarctions, 4.8 serious arrhythmias, and 0.5 deaths per 10,000 tests.[50] In this survey, the treadmill was the ergometer used most often (71%), whereas the favorite protocol (65%) was that of Bruce. The maximum $\dot{V}O_2$ is generally 5 to 11% higher with treadmill as compared to cycle ergometer testing,[29] whereas maximum HR is similar. As usually performed, $\dot{V}E$, breathing pattern, $\dot{V}O_2$, and gas exchange are not measured during these tests, so other important cardiovascular and pulmonary system information is not available. Bruce et al. has shown a high correlation of maximum $\dot{V}O_2$ and duration of treadmill exercise in their *normal* population.[51] Nevertheless, it is invalid to consider the duration of exercise a measure of maximum $\dot{V}O_2$ in patients with cardiovascular disease. The unequal duration of increment and variability in increment size are disadvantages of these tests, although interpretation is usually not based on measurements of $\dot{V}O_2$. In addition, HR itself is a poor measure of exercise intensity in many patients with heart disease. Administration of β-adrenergic blocking drugs also modifies the HR-work rate relationship and must be taken into account when interpreting the results of exercise tests.

Rather than using the foregoing protocol for treadmill testing, we[20] and Jones[12] prefer using a constant treadmill speed and incrementing the grade by a constant amount each minute for the entire study. After 3 minutes of warm-up at zero grade and a comfortable walking speed (which may range from 1 to 4.5 mph, depending on our fitness assessment), we use a constant grade increment of 1, 2, or 3% each minute to the patient's maximum tolerance. We scale speed and grade so the test will end approximately 10 minutes after the treadmill grade incrementing begins (Fig. 5-4F). We also make measurements of $\dot{V}E$, $\dot{V}CO_2$, and $\dot{V}O_2$. Following an initial delay of about 1 minute after the incremental period begins, this protocol gives a relatively linear increase in $\dot{V}O_2$ in normal subjects. The additional measures allow us to calculate values such as maximum $\dot{V}O_2$, *AT*, R, maximum $\dot{V}E/MVV$, $\dot{V}E/\dot{V}O_2$, $\dot{V}E/\dot{V}CO_2$, and O_2 pulse, thus adding considerable insight into gas exchange, ventilatory, and cardiovascular function.

Tests Suitable for Fitness Evaluation

A variety of tests have been used to evaluate individuals or groups without attempting to ascertain whether a particular system (e.g., cardiovascular, respiratory, or musculoskeletal) or motivation of

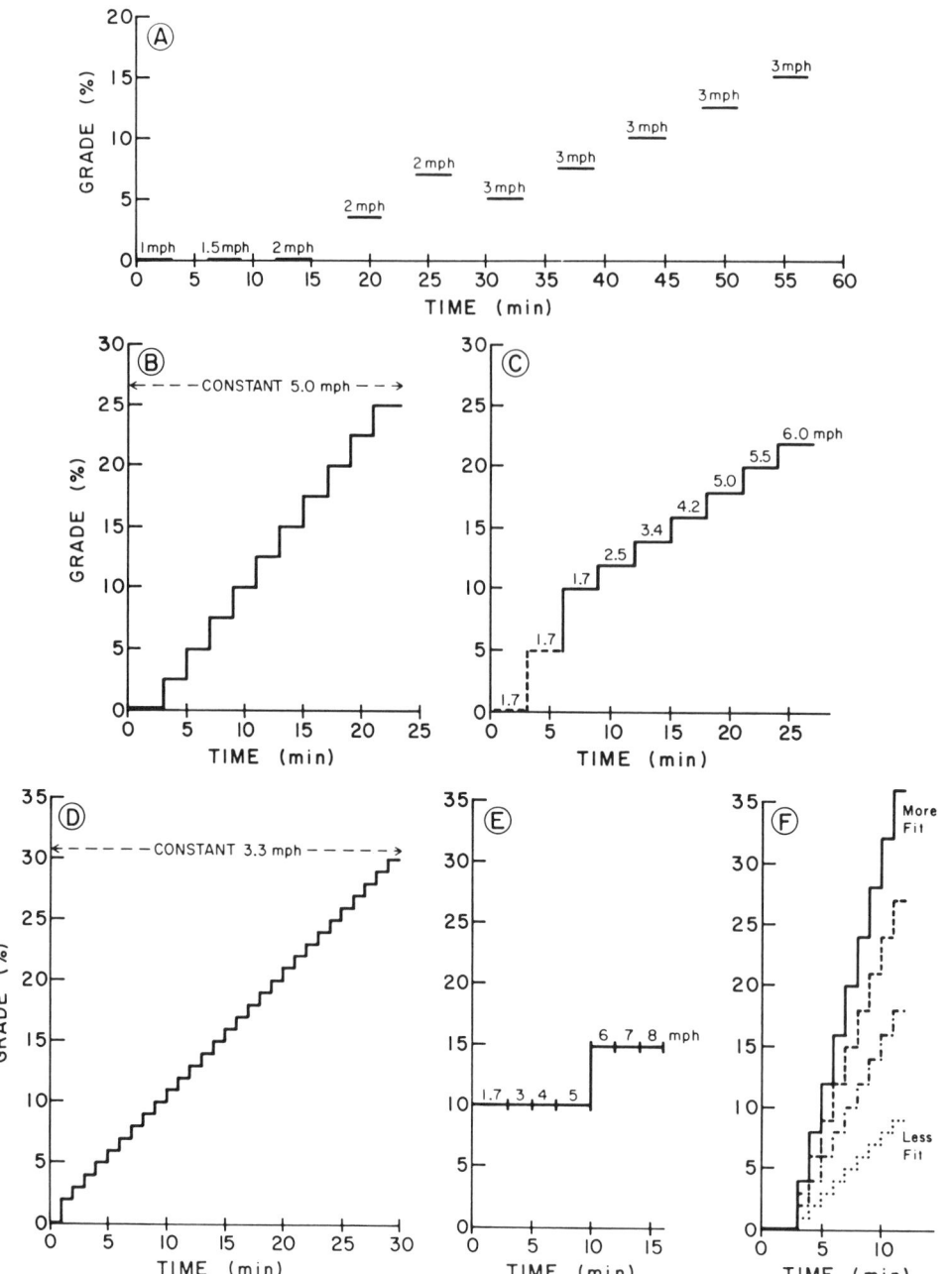

FIG. 5-4. Several treadmill protocols. A, Naughton protocol.[2] Three-minute exercise periods of increasing work rate alternate with 3-minute rest periods. The exercise periods vary in grade and speed. B, Astrand protocol.[34] The speed is constant at 5 mph. After 3 minutes at 0% grade, the grade is increased 2 1/2% every 2 minutes. C, Bruce protocol.[1] Grade and speed are changed every 3 minutes. The 0% and 5% grades are omitted in healthier subjects. D, Balke protocol.[10] After 1 minute at 0% grade and 1 minute at 2% grade, the grade is increased 1% per minute, all at a speed of 3.3 mph. E, Ellestad protocol.[3] The initial grade is 10% and the later grade is 15%, while the speed is increased every 2 or 3 minutes. F, Harbor protocol.[20] After 3 minutes of walking at a comfortable speed, the grade is increased at a constant preselected amount each minute: 1%, 2%, or 3%, so the subject reaches his or her maximum $\dot{V}_{O_2}$ in approximately 10 minutes.

the performer is limiting exercise. Such tests are likely to be used for children, young adults, military personnel, or laborers exposed to environmental stress (Fig. 5-4B and D). These tests are often considered measures of cardiovascular fitness and may allow division of the population studied into several levels of fitness. Because of

their relative simplicity, these tests can be repeated frequently with simple equipment.

HARVARD STEP TEST AND MODIFICATIONS

The original Harvard Step Test consisted of having the subject step up and down at a uniform rate of 30 step-ups per minute on a stool, bench, or platform 20 inches high for a period of 5 minutes, if possible, with measurements of pulse rate for 30 seconds after 1 minute of recovery.[52] Modifications include: (1) the addition of backpacks, which add approximately one third to the subject's weight; (2) reduction in the duration of the test to 3 minutes; (3) change in the step height to 17 inches for women; (4) measurement of HR during exercise; (5) change in the time of measurement of recovery pulse; (6) change in test scoring; and (7) use of a gradational step in which the height of the platform could be raised 2 cm every minute or 4.5 cm every 2 minutes.[52–54]

600-YARD RUN-WALK

The 600-yard run-walk requires that the subject cover a 600-yard level distance in the shortest possible time.[55] He or she may intersperse running with walking but must try to finish as quickly as possible. A properly marked track or football field is suitable. For 87 male university staff and faculty members, time for completion showed a moderately good correlation (r = 0.644) with their maximum $\dot{V}O_2$ measured by an incremental cycle ergometer test (which ranged from 25 to 50 ml/min/kg).

12-MINUTE TEST

In the 12-minute field performance test, the subjects, dressed in running attire, cover as much distance as possible by running or walking.[56] The distance covered was shown to correlate well (r = 0.897) with maximum $\dot{V}O_2$ measured during an intermittent incremental treadmill test in 115 military personnel (maximum $\dot{V}O_2$ range of 30 to 60 ml/min/kg).[56]

THREE GRADATIONAL TESTS

The inclined treadmill, cycle ergometer, and step tests used in a gradational manner for measurement of cardiorespiratory fitness all have proponents. Shephard reported the results of a study in which experienced users of each technique repeatedly evaluated their methods for 10 successive days on 24 men with maximum $\dot{V}O_2$ of 31 to 69 ml/min/kg.[57] These 24 subjects liked the treadmill most and the step tests least. When continuous incremental tests were done, maximum $\dot{V}O_2$ was highest with the step test and lowest with the cycle test, but the difference was less than 5%. The authors concluded that "central exhaustion" limited treadmill exercise, leg exhaustion limited cycle exercise, and the combination limited stepping. The authors preferred the step test for field experiments on the basis of its cheapness, simplicity, and ease of calibration. They preferred uphill treadmill running for the laboratory tests because the maximum $\dot{V}O_2$ was higher and thigh pain was less than with the cycle.

CRITIQUE

All the foregoing tests are designed for studying healthy populations. In the case of the 600-yard run-walk or 12-minute distance tests, it is impractical to measure ventilation, HR, gas exchange, or ECG changes during the test; it is also difficult with the Harvard Step Test. Thus, the ability to assess the cause of symptoms or to monitor individuals with serious cardiovascular disorders closely is limited. Although maximum $\dot{V}O_2$, maximum $\dot{V}E$, maximum HR, and maximum lactate can be measured in the three gradational tests (inclined treadmill, cycle, and increasing step height), the emphasis in all six of these tests is to compare the fitness of communities differing in habitual activities and in economic, residential, or nutritional status, or to assess fitness longitudinally. We do not recommend them for the evaluation of patients because of the difficulty in assessing relative contributions of different organ systems to alterations in work capacity and the attendant reduction in the patient's safety.

Arm Ergometry

METHOD

Arm exercise protocols are similar to those for lower extremity exercise and are usually done because of dysfunction of the lower extremities. The usual technique is to use a converted cycle ergometer with the axle placed at or below the level of the shoulders while the subject sits or stands and moves the pedals so the arms are alternately fully extended. The most common frequency is 50 rpm. Occasionally, upper extremity exercise is performed using wheelchair wheels coupled to a cycle ergometer or by rowing, paddling, or swimming. These modes may be particularly useful for paraplegics, oarsmen, or athletes. To obtain maximal cardiovascular and respiratory stress, arm cycling must be done concurrently with lower extremity exercise.

If the person performing the test is healthy and has not undergone specific upper extremity training, the maximum $\dot{V}_{O_2}$ for arm cycling will approximate 50 to 70% of that for leg cycling.[58-61] Further, the *AT* for most healthy subjects is low (in the range of 20 to 50 W). Maximum $\dot{V}_E$ is similarly reduced, whereas maximum HR is only 2 to 12% less than with leg cycle exercise. Thus, the maximum O_2 pulse is less with arm than with leg cycling.

CRITIQUE

Although arm cycling exercise has occasional uses, it does not stress the cardiovascular and respiratory systems as much as leg cycling or treadmill exercise. As such, it is a poor substitute when one assesses the cardiovascular and respiratory systems, except when lower extremity exercise is impossible.

12-Minute Walking Test

METHOD

The distance covered in 12 minutes of walking (equivalent to the original 12-minute field test described by Cooper) has been used for assessing disability in patients with chronic bronchitis.[62] Each patient is instructed to cover as much distance as possible on foot in 12 minutes, for example, walking over a marked course in a hospital corridor. The patient is told to try to keep going, but not to be concerned if he or she has to slow down or stop to rest. The aim is for the patient to feel that at the end of the test he or she could not have covered more ground in the time given. A physician or therapist accompanies the patient, acting as timekeeper and giving encouragement as necessary.

Daily repetitions of the 12-minute test in 12 hospital in-patients on 3 different days showed a significant improvement in distance on day 2 over day 1, but not on day 3 over day 2.[62] In 35 patients with lung disease, the distance correlated significantly with FVC ($r = 0.406$), but not with FEV_1 ($r = 0.283$), whereas it correlated significantly with maximum $\dot{V}_{O_2}$ ($r = 0.52$) and maximum exercise $\dot{V}_E$ ($r = 0.53$).[62]

CRITIQUE

This is a relatively simple and practical measurement of exercise tolerance in patients with respiratory disease. It depends on a variety of factors including motivation, judgment of pace, endurance, cardiovascular fitness, and neuromuscular function. Nevertheless, it may be useful in serially evaluating patients in rehabilitation programs.

Isometric Exercise

METHOD

In one isometric test, the patient's maximal force applied to a hand dynamometer is recorded. The patient then sustains one quarter to one third of this maximal force for 3 to 5 minutes while ECG and blood pressures are recorded.[63] The procedure is sometimes done in the cardiac catheterization laboratory because the patient is immobilized in the supine position by femoral vessel catheterization. Having the patient carry weights in the hands while exercising on the treadmill has also been used as a method of combining dynamic and isometric exercise.

CRITIQUE

Because sustained lifting or forceful handgrip induces angina pectoris in some patients, isometric exercise has been used in the laboratory as a method for detecting ischemic heart disease. Sustained muscle contraction causes compression of the forearm vessels with resulting muscle ischemia, pain, and hypertension. Systolic and mean blood pressure, left ventricular work, and left ventricular end-diastolic pressure rise significantly, but one sees a lesser increase in HR and $\dot{V}_{O_2}$.[64] In comparative studies, patients suspected of having coronary artery disease have less angina and less ST segment change, but a higher incidence of ventricular arrhythmia, with isometric than with dynamic exercise.[64,65] Because the muscle groups used in this test are small, this method is not satisfactory for inducing cardiorespiratory stress. Even with sustained isometric exercise of a large muscle mass, the increase in $\dot{V}_{O_2}$ is a small fraction of that for maximum dynamic exercise.[66]

Evaluating Therapy

Both incremental and constant work rate exercise tests can be useful in evaluating the response to therapy. In patients who are well enough to tolerate tests with 6 or more minutes of incremental exercise, such a protocol is often the most reasonable. Changes in maximum work rate achieved, peak $\dot{V}O_2$, *AT* (*LT* or *LAT*), and $\Delta\dot{V}O_2/\Delta WR$ can be detected with such serial tests. Peak $\dot{V}O_2$, *AT*, and $\Delta\dot{V}O_2/\Delta WR$ are likely to change significantly with changes in the degree of heart failure whether due to drug administration or other factors.[67,68]

In patients with extremely severe cardiovascular or respiratory disease, initial or serial evaluations may not allow more than a few minutes of unloaded pedalling or slow walking. In such cases, the duration of tolerable exercise or, more likely, the changes in gas exchange, ventilation, or cardiovascular responses may be useful. Sietsema et al.[38] showed that breath-by-breath $\dot{V}O_2$ measures during the transition from resting to only a few minutes of unloaded cycling can identify cardiovascular dysfunction.

In patients with moderate dysfunction, serial constant work rate tests of 6 minutes' duration, which may be easily tolerated, are useful. During such tests, changes in the time constant for $\dot{V}O_2$ at the onset of exercise can be evaluated.[38-40] For a given work rate, the $\Delta\dot{V}O_2(6-3)$ should decrease with improvement in cardiovascular fitness[43], heart failure[46], or hemoglobin availability.[41]

Summary

Numerous exercise devices, protocols, and physiologic measuring systems are available for the safe and economical evaluation of normal individuals, athletes, or patients suspected of having, or known to have, respiratory, cardiovascular, or neuromuscular disease. The specific exercise performed can be tailored to the diagnostic or therapeutic questions being asked and the facilities and technical and professional expertise available. Ordinarily, a maximum amount of information can be obtained by making ventilatory, gas exchange, ECG, blood pressure, and blood gas measurements during a cycle or treadmill test that includes: (1) sitting or standing at rest; (2) unloaded cycling or treadmill walking for 3 minutes; (3) 1-minute incremental exercise with an increment size enabling the subject to reach his or her maximally tolerated work rate in about 10 minutes; and (4) early recovery. At other times, constant work rate tests, timed walking tests, or arm ergometry may be indicated.

References

1. Bruce, R.A.: Exercise testing of patients with coronary artery disease. Ann. Clin. Res., 3:323–332, 1971.

2. Patterson, J.A., Naughton, J., Pietras, R.J., and Gumar, R.N.: Treadmill exercise in assessment of patients with cardiac disease. Am. J. Cardiol., 30:757–762, 1972.

3. Ellestad, M.H.: Stress Testing. 2nd Ed. Philadelphia, F.A. Davis, 1980.

4. American Thoracic Society: Standardization of spirometry: 1987 update. Am. Rev. Respir. Dis., 136:1285–1307, 1987.

5. Campbell, S.C.: A comparison of the maximum voluntary ventilation with forced expiratory volume in one second: an assessment of subject cooperation. J. Occup. Med., 24:531–533, 1982.

6. Seldinger, S.I.: Catheter replacement of the needle in percutaneous arteriography: a new technique. Acta Radiol., 39:368–376, 1953.

7. Huszczuk, A.: Personal communication, 1985.

8. Whipp, B.J., Davis, J.A., Torres, F., and Wasserman, K.: A test to determine parameters of aerobic function during exercise. J. Appl. Physiol., 50:217–221, 1981.

9. Balke, B.: Correlation of static and physical endurance. I. A test of physical performance based on the cardiovascular and respiratory response to gradually increased work. Project No. 21–32–004, Report No. 1. San Antonio, TX, United States Air Force School of Aviation Medicine, April 1952.

10. Balke, B., and Ware, R.W.: An experimental study of "physical fitness" of Air Force personnel. U.S. Armed Forces Med. J., 10:675–688, 1959.

11. Consolazio, C.F., Nelson, R.A., Matoush, L.O., and Hansen, J.E.: Energy metabolism at high altitude (3,475 m). J. Appl. Physiol., 21:1732–1740, 1966.

12. Jones, N.L.: Clinical Exercise Testing. 3rd Ed. Philadelphia, W.B. Saunders, 1988.

13. Spiro, S.G.: Exercise testing in clinical medicine. Br. J. Dis. Chest, 71:145–172, 1977.

14. Fairshter, R.D., Walters, J., Salvess, K., Fox, M., Minh, V.D., and Wilson, A.F.: Comparison of incremental exercise test during cycle and treadmill ergometry. Am. Rev. Respir. Dis., 125(Suppl.):254, 1982 (Abstract).

15. Davis, J.A., Whipp, B.J., Lamarra, N., Huntsman, D.J., Frank, M.H., and Wasserman, K.: Effect of ramp slope on measurement of aerobic parameters from the ramp exercise test. Med. Sci. Sports Exerc., 14:339–343, 1982.

16. Cooper, D.M., and Weiler-Ravell, D.: Gas exchange response to exercise in children. Am. Rev. Respir. Dis., 129(Suppl.):S47-S48, 1984.

17. Zhang Y.-Y., Johnson, M.C., Chow, N., and Wasserman, K.: Effect of exercise testing protocol on parameters of aerobic function. Med. Sci. Sports Exerc., 23:625–630, 1991.

18. Arstilla, M.: Pulse-conducted triangular exercise-ECG test. Acta Med. Scand., 529(Suppl.):103–109, 1972.

19. Redwood, D.R., Rosing, D.R., Goldstein, A.R., Beiser, G., and Epstein, S.E.: Importance of the design of an exercise protocol in the evaluation of patients with angina pectoris. Circulation, 43:618–628, 1971.

20. Buchfuhrer, M.J., Hansen, J.E., Robinson, T.E., Sue, D.Y., Wasserman, K., and Whipp, B.J.: Optimizing the exercise protocol for cardiopulmonary assessment. J. Appl. Physiol., 55:1558–1564, 1983.

21. Taylor, H.L., Buskirk, E., and Henschel, A.: Maximal

oxygen intake as an objective measure of cardiorespiratory performance. J. Appl. Physiol., 8:73–80, 1955.

22. Froelicher, V.F., Brammel, H., Davis, G.D., Noguera, I., Stewart, A., and Lancaster, M.D.: A comparison of three maximal treadmill exercise protocols. J. Appl. Physiol., 36:720–725, 1974.

23. Maksud, M.G., and Coutts, K.D.: Comparison of a continuous and discontinuous graded treadmill test for maximal oxygen uptake. Med. Sci. Sports Exerc., 3:63–65, 1971.

24. Wyndham, C.H., Strydom, N.B., Leary, W.P., and Williams, C.G.: Studies of the maximum capacity of men for physical effort. Arbeitsphysiologie, 22:285–295, 1966.

25. McArdle, W.D., Katch, F.I., and Pechar, G.S.: Comparison of continuous and discontinuous treadmill and bicycle tests for max $\dot{V}O_2$. Med. Sci. Sports Exerc., 5:156–160, 1972.

26. Pollock, M.L., Bohannon, R.L., Cooper, K.M., Ayres, J., Ward, A., White, S.R., and Linnerud, N.D.: A comparative analysis of four protocols for maximal treadmill stress testing. Am. Heart J., 92:39–46, 1976.

27. Furuike, A.N., Sue, D.Y., Hansen, J.E., and Wasserman, K.: Comparison of physiological dead space/tidal volume ratio and alveolar-arterial PO_2 difference during incremental and constant work exercise. Am. Rev. Respir. Dis., 126:579–583, 1982.

28. Beaver, W.L.: Water vapor corrections in oxygen consumption calculations. J. Appl. Physiol., 35:928–931, 1973.

29. Beaver, W.L., Wasserman, K., and Whipp, B.J.: On-line computer analysis and breath-by-breath graphical display of exercise function tests. J. Appl. Physiol., 34:128–132,1973.

30. Sue, D.Y., Hansen, J.E., Blais, M., and Wasserman, K.: Measurement and analysis of gas exchange during exercise using a programmable calculator. J. Appl. Physiol., 49:456–461, 1980.

31. Chester, E.H., Belman, M.J., Bahler, R.C., Baum, G.L., Schey, G., and Buch, P.: Multidisciplinary treatment of chronic pulmonary insufficiency. 3. The effect of physical training on cardiopulmonary performance in patients with chronic obstructive pulmonary disease. Chest, 72:695–702, 1977.

32. Hansen, J.E.: Exercise instruments, schemes, and protocols for evaluating the dyspneic patient. Am. Rev. Respir. Dis., 129(Suppl.):525–527, 1984.

33. Astrand, I.: Aerobic work capacity in men and women. Acta Physiol. Scand., 49(Suppl.169):l-9, 1960.

34. Astrand, P.O., and Rodahl, K.: Textbook of Work Physiology. 2nd Ed. New York, McGraw-Hill, 1977, pp. 333–365.

35. Nery, L.E., Wasserman, K., Andrews, J.D., Huntsman, D.J., Hansen, J.E., and Whipp, B.J.: Ventilatory and gas exchange kinetics during exercise in chronic airway obstruction. J. Appl. Physiol., 53:1594–1602, 1982.

36. Lamarra, N., Whipp, B.J., Blumenberg, M., and Wasserman, K.: Model-order estimation of cardiorespiratory dynamics during moderate exercise. In Modelling and Control of Breathing. Edited by B.J. Whipp and D.M. Wiberg. New York, Elsevier Science, 1983, pp. 338–345.

37. Whipp, B.J., Ward, S.A., Lamarra, N., Davis, J.A., and Wasserman, K.: Parameters of ventilatory and gas exchange dynamics during exercise. J. Appl. Physiol., 52:1506–1513, 1982.

38. Sietsema K.E., Cooper, D.M., Rosove, M.A., Perloff, J.K., Child, J.S., Canobbio, M.M., Whipp, B.J., and Wasserman, K.: Dynamics of oxygen uptake during exercise in adults with cyanotic congenital heart disease. Circulation, 73:1137–1144, 1986.

39. Sietsema K.E., Daly, J.A., and Wasserman, K.: Early dynamics of O_2 uptake and heart rate as affected by exercise work rate. J.Appl.Physiol., 67:2535–2541, 1989.

40. Ben-Dov, I., Sietsema, K.E., and Wasserman, K.: O_2 uptake in hyperthyroidism during constant work rate and incremental exercise. Eur. J. Appl. Physiol., 62:261–267, 1991.

41. Koike, A., Wasserman, K., McKenzie, D.K., Zanconato, S., and Weiler-Ravell, D.: Evidence that diffusion limitation determines oxygen uptake kinetics during exercise in humans. J. Clin. Invest., 86:1698–1706, 1990.

42. Whipp, B.J., and Wasserman, K.: Oxygen uptake kinetics for various intensities of constant load work. J. Appl. Physiol., 33:351–356, 1972.

43. Roston, W.L., Whipp, B.J., Davis, J.A., Effros, R.M., and Wasserman, K.: Oxygen uptake kinetics and lactate concentration during exercise in humans. Am. Rev. Respir. Dis., 135:1080–1084, 1987.

44. Casaburi, R., Barstow, T.J., Robinson, T., and Wasserman, K.: Influence of work rate on ventilatory and gas exchange kinetics. J. Appl. Physiol., 67:547–555, 1989.

45. Casaburi, R., Wasserman, K., Patessio, A., Ioli, F., Zanaboni, S., and Donner, C.F.: A new perspective in pulmonary rehabilitation: anaerobic threshold as a discriminant in training. Eur. J. Respir. Dis., 2:618–623, 1989.

46. Zhang, Y.-Y., Wasserman, K., Sietsema, K.E., Barstow, T.J., Mizumoto, G., and Sullivan, C.S.: O_2 uptake kinetics in response to exercise: a measure of tissue anaerobiosis in heart failure. Chest, 103:735–741, 1993.

47. Cropp, G.I.A.: The exercise bronchoprovocation test: standardization of procedures and evaluation of response. J. Allergy Clin. Immunol., 64:627–633, 1979.

48. Deal, E.C., Jr., McFadden, E.R., Jr., Ingram, R.H., Strauss, R.H., and Jaeger, J.J.: Role of respiratory heat exchange in production of exercise-induced asthma. J. Appl. Physiol., 46:467–475, 1979.

49. Wasserman, K.: Testing regulation of ventilation with exercise. Chest, 70:5173–5178, 1976.

50. Stuart, R.J., and Ellestad, M.H.: National survey of exercise stress testing facilities. Chest, 77:94–97, 1980.

51. Bruce, R.A., Kusimi, F., and Hosmer, D.: Maximal oxygen intake and nomographic assessment of functional aerobic impairment in cardiovascular disease. Am. Heart J., 85:546–562, 1973.

52. Consolazio, C.F., Johnson, R.E., and Pecora, L.I.: Physiological Measurements of Metabolic Function in Man. New York, McGraw-Hill, 1963, pp. 368–401.

53. Nagle, F.J., Balke, B., and Naughton, J.P.: Gradational step tests for assessing work capacity. J. Appl. Physiol., 21:745–748, 1965.

54. Nagle, F.J., Balke, B., Baptista, G., Alleyia, J., and Hawley, E.: Compatibility of progressive treadmill, bicycle and step tests based on oxygen uptake responses. Med. Sci. Sports Exerc., 3:149–154, 1971.

55. Fleishman, E.A.: The Structure and Measurement of Physical Fitness. Englewood Cliffs, NJ, Prentice-Hall, 1964, pp. 171–172.

56. Cooper, K.M.: A means of assessing maximal oxygen intake. JAMA, 203:201–204, 1968.

57. Shephard, R.J.: The relative merits of the step test, bicycle ergometer, and treadmill in the assessment of cardiorespiratory fitness. Arbeitsphysiologie, 23:219–230, 1966.

58. Bar-Or, O., and Zwiren, L.D.: Maximal oxygen consumption test during arm exercise-reliability and validity. J. Appl. Physiol., 38:424–426, 1975.

59. Vokac, Z., Bell, H., Bautz-Holter, E., and Rodahl, K.: Oxygen uptake/heart rate relationship in leg and arm exercise, sitting and standing. J. Appl. Physiol., 39:54–59, 1975.

60. Davis, J.A., Vodak, P., Wilmore, J.H., Vodal, J., and Kurtz, P.: Anaerobic threshold and maximal aerobic power for three modes of exercise. J. Appl. Physiol., 41:544–550, 1976.

61. Casaburi, R., Barstow, T.J., Robinson, T.E., and Wasserman, K.: Dynamic and steady-state ventilatory and gas exchange responses to arm exercise. Med. Sci. Sports Exerc., 24:1365–1374, 1992.

62. McGavin, C.R., Gupta, S.P., and McHardy, G.J.R.: Twelve minute walking test for assessing disability in chronic bronchitis. Br. Med. J., 1:822–823, 1976.

63. Helfant, R.H., DeVilla, M.A., and Meister, S.G.: Effect of sustained isometric hand grip exercise on left ventricular performance. Circulation, 44:982–993, 1971.

64. Blomquist, C.G.: Use of exercise testing for diagnostic and functional evaluation of patients with arteriosclerotic heart disease. Circulation, 44:1120–1136, 1971.

65. Haissly, J., Messin, R., Degre, S., Vandermoten, P., Demaret, B., and Denolin, H.: Comparative responses to isometric (static) and dynamic exercise tests in coronary artery disease. Am. J. Cardiol., 33:791–795, 1974.

66. Whipp, B.J., and Phillips, E.E., Jr.: Cardiopulmonary and metabolic responses to sustained isometric exercise. Arch. Phys. Med. Rehabil., 51:398–402, 1970.

67. Itoh, H., Taniguchi, K., Koike, A., and Doi, M.: Evaluation of severity of heart failure using ventilatory gas analysis. Circulation, 81(Suppl. II):II-31-II-37, 1990.

68. Winter, U.J., Wasserman, K., Treese, N., and Hopp, H.W. (Eds).: Computerized Cardiopulmonary Exercise Testing. New York, Springer Verlag, 1991.

Normal Values

INTERPRETATION OF THE results of exercise tests requires knowing the normal response. In this chapter, we compile values for important physiologic variables that we think represent the best data available for sedentary normal subjects during exercise. In some instances, several sets of normal values for the same measurement are given. When doing so, we have critiqued each set and have put forth our recommendation.

Maximum Oxygen Uptake

Recommended values for maximum $\dot{V}O_2$ are given for sedentary men and women in Table 6-1 and children of average activity levels in Table 6-2 performing cycle and, in the case of adults, treadmill exercise. Figure 6-1 gives mean predicted maximum $\dot{V}O_2$ values for sedentary men and women of normal (predicted) weight. Figure 6-2 gives mean predicted maximum $\dot{V}O_2$ values for leg cycling for children.

The selection of maximum $\dot{V}O_2$ predicted values (both mean and 95% confidence level) is a challenging problem, especially because the body sizes and activity levels of the usual clinical population differ from those of reference populations. Maximum $\dot{V}O_2$ in normal subjects during exercise varies with age, gender, body size, level of ordinary activity, and type of exercise. When comparing the maximum $\dot{V}O_2$ of an individual to the predicted maximum $\dot{V}O_2$, a predicted value generated for the same form of exercise must be used. It is preferable if the population from which the predicting equations were obtained be a large number of individuals with similar characteristics to the patient being tested.

AGE AND GENDER

Many investigators have reported that maximum $\dot{V}O_2$ is less for women than men and declines with age.[1-3] Although cross-sectional studies of change in maximum $\dot{V}O_2$ with age are easier to perform, they may be misleading because their maximum $\dot{V}O_2$ values tend to decrease more slowly than longitudinal studies in the same subject.[4] In a longitudinal study, Astrand et al.[5] measured maximum $\dot{V}O_2$ during cycling exercise in 66 well-trained, physically active men and women aged 20 to 33 years and studied them again 21 years later. The mean decrease in maximum $\dot{V}O_2$ was 22% for the 35 women and 20% for the 31 men.

Bruce et al.[6] used stepwise multiple regression analysis to identify whether gender, age, physical activity, weight, height, or smoking aided in the prediction of maximum $\dot{V}O_2$ during treadmill exercise in adults. They found that gender and age were the 2 most important factors. The maximum $\dot{V}O_2$ of women was approximately 77% of maximum $\dot{V}O_2$ of men when adjusted for body weight and activity. Astrand[7] reported 17% lower maximum $\dot{V}O_2$ for 18 women students compared to 17 male students of comparable size.

ACTIVITY LEVEL

Investigators generally agree that values obtained from athletes, physical education teachers, servicemen, or participants in organized exercise groups should not be used as reference values for a clinical population. Balke and Ware[8] found the maximum $\dot{V}O_2$ of Air Force personnel to be

---

TABLE 6-1. *Calculation of Predicted Maximum* $\dot{V}O_2$ *ml/min*[6,12]

A

Sedentary Men
Cycle factor = 50.72 − 0.372 × A
Step 1. Measure man's weight (W, kg) and height (H, cm) in light clothes without shoes and record age (A, yr)
Step 2. Calculate man's normal (predicted) W in kg as follows:
Normal (predicted) W = 0.79 × H − 60.7
Step 3A. If man's actual W equals normal W:
Predicted $\dot{V}O_2$max (ml/min) = actual W × cycle factor
Step 3B. If patient's actual W is less than normal W:
Predicted $\dot{V}O_2$max (ml/min) = [(normal W + actual W)/2] × cycle factor
Step 3C. If patient's actual W exceeds normal W:
Predicted $\dot{V}O_2$max (ml/min) = (normal W × cycle factor) + 6 × (actual W − normal W)
Step 4. If treadmill is used rather than cycle:
Multiply predicted $\dot{V}O_2$max by 1.11

B

Sedentary Women
Cycle factor = 22.78 − 0.17 × A
Step 1. Measure woman's weight (W, kg) and height (H, cm) in light clothes without shoes and record age (A, yr)
Step 2. Calculate woman's normal (predicted) W in kg as follows:
Normal (predicted) W = 0.65 × H − 42.8
Step 3A. If woman's actual W equals normal W:
Predicted $\dot{V}O_2$max (ml/min) = (actual W + 43) × cycle factor
Step 3B. If patient's actual W is less than normal W:
Predicted $\dot{V}O_2$max (ml/min) = [(normal W + actual W + 86)/2] × cycle factor
Step 3C. If patient's actual W exceeds normal W:
Predicted $\dot{V}O_2$max (ml/min) = [(normal W + 43) × cycle factor] + 6 × (actual W − normal W)
Step 4. If treadmill is used rather than cycle:
Multiply predicted $\dot{V}O_2$max by 1.11

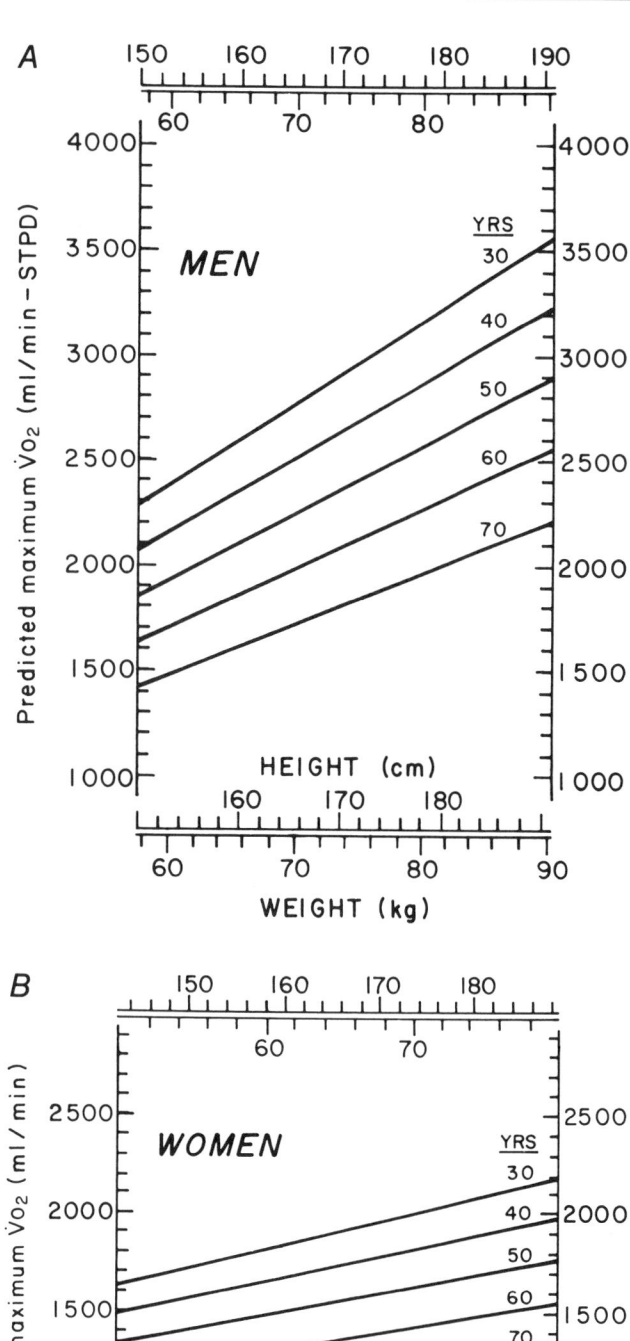

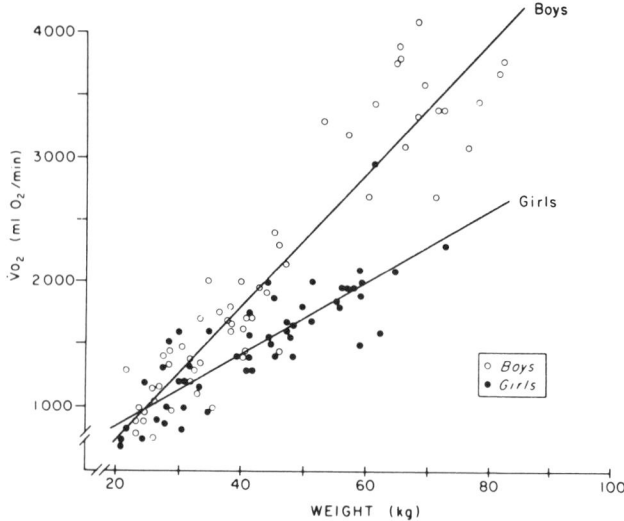

FIG. 6-2. Maximum O_2 uptake of 109 normal North American boys and girls for leg cycling. Regression equations for maximum $\dot{V}O_2$ (ml/min) as function of body weight (kg) were: for boys, $\dot{V}O_2 = 52.8 \times$ weight (kg) − 303.4, (r = 0.94); for girls, $\dot{V}O_2 = 28.5$ weight (kg) + 288.1, (r = 0.84). (From Cooper, D.M., Weiler-Ravell, D., Whipp, B.J., and Wasserman, K.: Aerobic parameters of exercise as a function of body size during growth in children. J. Appl. Physiol., 56:628–634, 1984.)

strongly related to their activity pattern. Drinkwater et al.[2] found that the maximum $\dot{V}O_2$ of extremely active women did not decline over two decades despite a gradual increase in body weight. Yet brief periods of physical training can acutely increase maximum $\dot{V}O_2$ by 15 to 25% or more.[1,9] The decline in maximum $\dot{V}O_2$ with age is more rapid in habitually inactive men, even allowing for greater weight gain in the inactive group.[4]

ADULTS OF NORMAL (PREDICTED) BODY WEIGHT

It is logical to assume that physical size would be a factor in maximum $\dot{V}O_2$ because the mass of the exercising muscles as well as the dimensions of the cardiovascular and pulmonary systems should determine the maximum quantity of O_2 that can be delivered and used. Astrand and Rodahl[10] point out that, in top male athletes, maximum $\dot{V}O_2$ expressed as (ml/min) $\times$ kg^{-1} is higher in smaller

FIG. 6-1. Mean maximum $\dot{V}O_2$ values for sedentary men (A) and women (B) of normal (predicted) weight using the cycle ergometer.[6,12,13] To use, locate the patient's height and weight on the horizontal axis. *If the patient is underweight* (i.e., the patient's actual weight is to the left of that directly above the patient's height), draw a line half-way between the marks vertically to the line that indicates the patient's age. From this intersection draw a line horizontally to the vertical axis and read off the predicted maximum $\dot{V}O_2$ in liters per

minute STPD. *If the patient is overweight* (i.e., the patient's actual weight is to the right of that directly above the patient's height), draw a line vertically from the height marker to the line that indicates the patient's age. From this intersection draw a line horizontally to the vertical axis and read off the preliminary predicted maximum $\dot{V}O_2$ in liters per minute STPD. To obtain the actual predicted maximum $\dot{V}O_2$ for the obese patient, add 6 ml/min for each kilogram the patient is overweight. Finally, if the treadmill is used, predicted cycle values should be increased 11%.

TABLE 6-2. *Predicted Maximum V̇O₂ and AT in Normal Children for Cycle Ergometry*

	BOYS ≤ 13	BOYS > 13	GIRLS ≤ 11	GIRLS > 11
Number studied	37	21	24	27
Maximum V̇O₂, ml/min/kg (mean ± SD)	42 ± 6	50 ± 8	38 ± 7	34 ± 4
lower 95% confidence limit	32	37	26	27
AT, ml/min/kg (mean ± SD)	26 ± 5	27 ± 6	23 ± 4	19 ± 3
lower 95% confidence limit	18	17	16	14

(From Cooper, D.M., and Weiler-Ravell, D.: Gas exchange response to exercise in children. Am. Rev. Respir. Dis., 129(Suppl.):S47–S48, 1984.)

than in larger athletes, even when obesity is not a factor. Expressed as (ml/min) × kg$^{-2/3}$, however, maximum V̇O₂ does not differ between smaller and larger athletes. These investigators argue against the traditional practice of using weight as a primary variable in predicting maximum V̇O₂ or fitness. Despite the variability related to activity levels, relatively good agreement among series exists for the mean predicted maximum V̇O₂ values of non-obese, sedentary populations if one uses age, gender, and height rather than age, gender, and weight. Pulmonologists are accustomed to predict most respiratory function values using height rather than weight. Jones et al.[11] found, in a population of over 1000 referrals to their laboratory, that maximum work capacity was best expressed related to gender, height, and age rather than gender, weight, and age. Davis[13] also found,

in 204 volunteers between 20 and 70 years of age, that the prediction of maximum V̇O₂ was not improved by adding weight to the values of gender, age, and height.

We have reviewed the similarities and differences in several series of men and women of relatively normal body weight.[6,12,13,15,16] Figures 6–3 and 6–4 show values of three North American and one Japanese series for sedentary men and women of normal body proportions. All four series show parallel declines, with age and similar mean values for men between 170 and 180 cm (see Fig. 6-3B and C) at all age levels. Jones' values tend to be lower at 160 cm and higher at 190 cm than the three other series. Thus, the values in these four series agree for men of average size regardless of age.

The values in the women's series show more

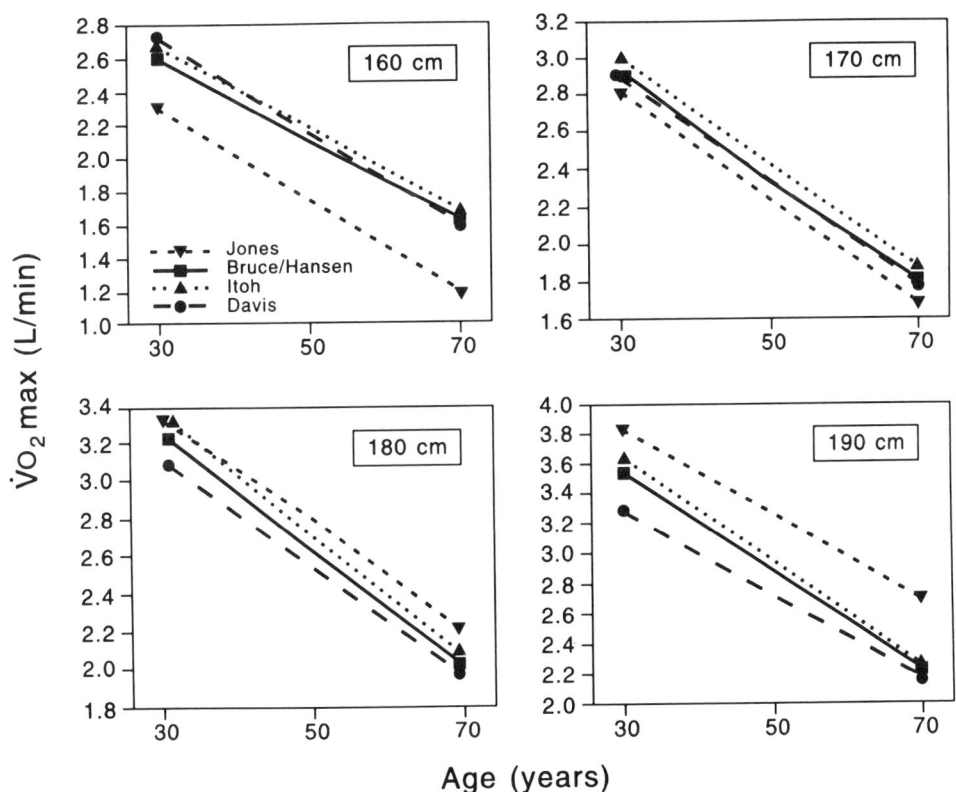

FIG. 6-3. Comparison of predicted maximum V̇O₂ for cycle ergometry of sedentary men of normal (predicted) weight calculated from four reference series for ages 30 to 70 for four different heights and weights: 160 cm and 66 kg, 170 cm and 74 kg, 180 cm and 82 kg, and 190 cm and 89 kg. Data are from Jones et al.,[15] Bruce et al. as modified by Hansen et al.,[6,12] Itoh et al.,[16] and Davis.[13]

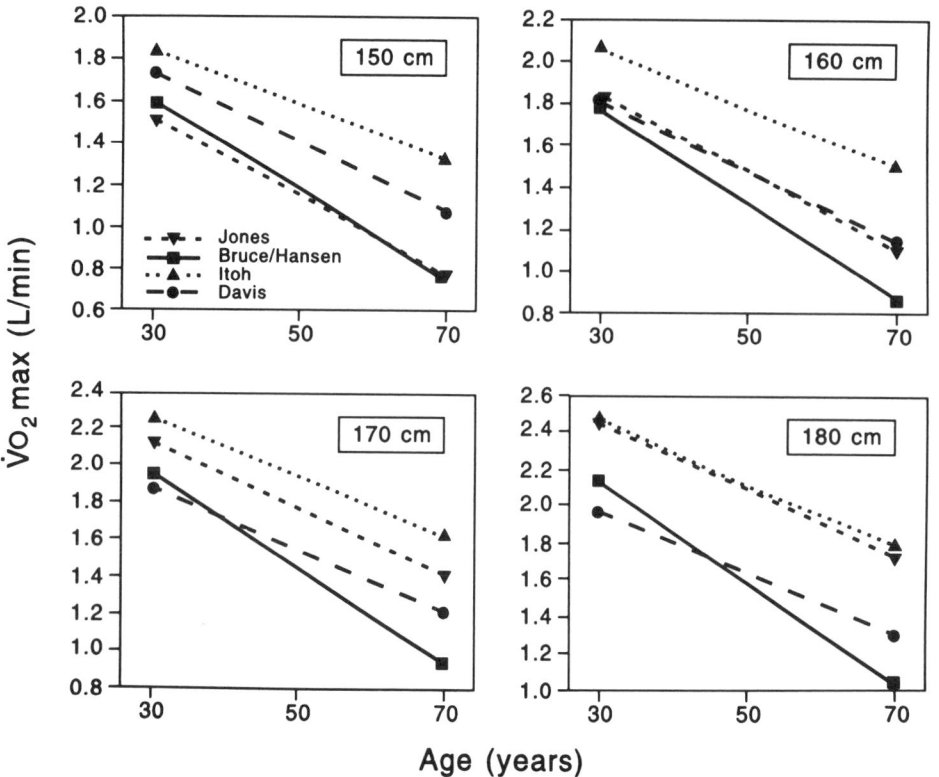

FIG. 6-4. Comparison of predicted maximum $\dot{V}O_2$ for cycle ergometry of sedentary women of normal (predicted) weight calculated from four reference series for ages 30 to 70 for four different heights and weights: 150 cm and 55 kg, 160 cm and 62 kg, 170 cm and 68 kg, and 180 cm and 74 kg. Data are from Jones et al.,[15] Bruce et al. as modified by Hansen et al.,[6,12] Itoh et al.,[16] and Davis.[13]

diversity (Fig. 6-4A to D). The values for Japanese women are invariably higher, suggesting a higher general activity level for women in that country. The closest match in the North American series is at a height of 160 cm and 30 to 50 years of age (Fig. 6-4B). Height is a more important factor in Jones' predicting equations and a less important factor in Davis' equations, with the greatest divergences at 180 cm. Bruce's values are lower in older women, but they compare reasonably well in younger women. Because we have no clear methodologic or other reasons to justify discarding any of these series, we must consider that the diversity of values reflects the differences in activity levels of women in different locales and generations. Thus, we recommend caution in using predicted values from patients that are at the extremes of height and, in the case of women, over age 60.

NUTRITIONAL STATUS

Despite the arguments of Astrand and Rodahl[10] and the obvious effect of obesity on the predicted maximum $\dot{V}O_2$ when it is expressed as (ml/min) $\times$ kg^{-1}, many exercise physiologists and clinicians continue to estimate cardiovascular function by comparing actual to predicted values based only on age, gender, and weight, even in obese indi-

viduals. We believe that this practice causes a biased interpretation by requiring too high a predicted maximum $\dot{V}O_2$ in obese individuals. We believe that sufficient evidence now exists to assert that, even though maximum $\dot{V}O_2$ values may still be expressed as (ml/min) $\times$ kg^{-1} in many publications, this practice is not optimal for the clinical evaluation of the cardiorespiratory function of patients.[11,12,13,17]

OVERWEIGHT PATIENTS

How can one best select an appropriate predicted maximum $\dot{V}O_2$ in the overweight patient? We found, in a cycle ergometer study of a population of 77 middle-aged men (mean age = 54 years, range 34 to 74 years) whom we judged to have normal cardiovascular and respiratory systems and good motivation, that when the subject was overweight,[12,17] there was better agreement with Bruce's data for maximum $\dot{V}O_2$[6] modified for cycle ergometry using normal weight (weight predicted from height) rather than actual weight. Buskirk and Taylor[18] found that maximum $\dot{V}O_2$ correlated better with a measure of fat-free body weight (r = 0.85) than total body weight (r = 0.63) in 43 healthy students and in 13 soldiers performing treadmill exercise.

Although Jones et al.[11] did not measure maximum $\dot{V}O_2$ for their 1000 normal individuals, they found that adding weight as a variable to height, age, and gender did not improve the prediction of *cycle ergometry* exercise capacity. Thus, weight alone did not appreciably influence external work capacity on the cycle. Yet we know that, in healthy individuals, maximum $\dot{V}O_2$ correlates highly with maximum external work performed. At all external work levels on the cycle, those with larger legs have higher measured $\dot{V}O_2$ than those with smaller legs. On average, we estimate that unloaded $\dot{V}O_2$ while cycling will increase approximately 6 ml/min/kg of extra body weight.[19] In addition, overweight individuals can be expected to have slightly higher maximum $\dot{V}O_2$ and anaerobic threshold (*AT*) values than others of the same age, gender, and height, because in walking the same distances they expend more energy and their muscles become more trained. Thus, body weight can change predicted maximum $\dot{V}O_2$ without affecting maximum external work capacity on the cycle ergometer.

In the first edition of this book, our prediction equation did not include an increase in predicted maximum $\dot{V}O_2$ for obesity. We now recommend increasing the predicted maximum by 6 ml/min for each kg of weight above normal (predicted) weight, whether the cycle or treadmill is used for exercise testing.

Sample calculation: Find the predicted maximum $\dot{V}O_2$ for treadmill exercise for an overweight 60-year-old sedentary man who is 180 cm tall and weighs 110 kg. Using Table 6-1A, step 2, or the horizontal axis of Figure 6-1A, we ascertain that he is overweight, his predicted weight being 81.5 kg (normal W = 0.79 × 180 − 60.7 = 142.2 − 60.7 = 81.5). Using Table 6-1A, step 3C, we find that his predicted maximum $\dot{V}O_2$ for cycle ergometry is 81.5 × (50.72 − 0.372 × 60) + 6 × (110 − 81.5) = 81.5 × 28.4 + 6 × 28.5 = 2315 + 171 = 2486 ml/min. Using step 4, the predicted maximum $\dot{V}O_2$ for treadmill ergometry is 2486 × 1.11 = 2760 ml/min. Using Figure 6-1A, by extending a line vertically from 180 cm to the 60-year line, we find that the predicted maximum $\dot{V}O_2$ for cycle ergometry is 2320 ml/min for a non-obese man. This amount, plus 6 ml/kg × 28.5 kg (for overweight), yields a predicted maximum $\dot{V}O_2$ of 2490 ml/min for cycle ergometry for this patient. This value times 1.11 yields a predicted value of 2750 ml/min for treadmill ergometry.

We realize that excess body weight may interfere with an individual's exercise capacity or with respiratory or other system functions. Thus, weight that increases the metabolic cost of moving the entire body and its parts may cause impairment in performing external work even when the measured maximum $\dot{V}O_2$ indicates normal cardiorespiratory function.

UNDERWEIGHT PATIENTS

In the first edition of this book, we decreased the predicted maximum $\dot{V}O_2$ in proportion to the actual decrease in body weight for those patients whose weight was less than normal (as if muscle were primarily reduced). Because fat as well as muscle tissue is reduced in most underweight persons, we now prefer to reduce the predicted maximum $\dot{V}O_2$ values by using the average of the actual and normal weight in the maximum $\dot{V}O_2$ and related calculations in such patients.

Sample calculation: Find the predicted maximum $\dot{V}O_2$ for a 50-year-old sedentary woman who is 160 cm tall and weighs 45 kg. Using Table 6-1B, step 2, or Figure 6-1B, we find that she is underweight and that her normal weight is 61 kg (normal W = 0.65 × 160 − 43 = 104 − 43 = 61). Using Table 6-1B, step 3B, her predicted maximum $\dot{V}O_2$ is [(45 + 61 + 86)/2] × (22.78 − 0.17 × 50) = 94 × 14.28 = 1342 ml/min. Using Figure 6-1B, by extending a line vertically from 53 kg (which is the average of her actual and normal weight) to the 50-year line, we find that the predicted maximum $\dot{V}O_2$ is 1350 ml/min.

OUR LABORATORY'S CLINICAL POPULATION

We have reviewed our experience in the last approximately 1000 clinical cardiopulmonary exercise tests performed in our laboratories. Regarding body dimensions, our clinical exercise-tested population is, on average, shorter, more obese, and more variable in weight than any of the reference populations in standard series of healthy, relatively sedentary North American older adults (Table 6-3 and Fig. 6-5). This is especially true of the women tested. For men, 70% exceeded normal (predicted) weight (see Table 6-1 equations), 45% exceeded 110% of normal weight, 26% exceeded 120% of normal weight, 6% exceeded 140% of normal weight, and 2% exceeded 160% of normal weight. For women, 70% exceeded normal weight, 56% exceeded 110% of normal weight, 42% exceeded 120% of normal weight, 25% exceeded 140% of normal weight, and 12% exceeded

TABLE 6-3. *Comparison of Physical Characteristics of Healthy Reference Populations and a Clinical Population**

		MEN		
SERIES	NUMBER	AGE	HEIGHT	WEIGHT
Bruce et al.[6]	138	48.6 + 11.1	177.5 + 6.6	78.6 + 8.6
Jones et al.[11]	732	48.0 + 12.0	174.0 + 6.5	81.8 + 12.6
Davis[13]	103	43.4 + 14.6	178.7 + 7.1	82.3 + 12.1
Harbor-UCLA†	750	54.2 + 11.7	172.8 + 7.4	83.4 + 17.1
		WOMEN		
SERIES	NUMBER	AGE	HEIGHT	WEIGHT
Bruce et al.[6]	157	41.4 + 11.2	166.0 + 6.3	62.1 + 9.8
Jones et al.[11]	339	47.0 + 13.5	162.0 + 6.2	67.3 + 12.8
Davis[13]	101	44.6 + 14.6	164.4 + 6.6	63.6 + 10.4
Harbor-UCLA†	240	49.1 + 13.5	160.5 + 8.4	71.2 + 21.6

* Values are mean ± SD.
† All groups but the Harbor-UCLA series are healthy reference populations.

160% of normal weight. These findings emphasize the importance of not using predicted maximum $\dot{V}_{O_2}$ values expressed as (ml/min) $\times$ kg^{-1} in populations of this make-up.

95% CONFIDENCE LIMITS

Because of the skew of values within each series, 95% confidence limits are likely to give a more accurate lower limit of normal than 1.65 times the standard error of the estimate (SEE) subtracted from the mean. As pointed out,[11] maximum exercise values tend to be skewed even in relatively sedentary populations because training increases

values above the mean more than inactivity decreases values below the mean. We suggest that 83% of mean predicted value is a reasonable approximation for the lower 95% confidence limit in the patient of average height, but that extremes in height, weight, or age are likely to have an even lower 95% confidence limit.

CHILDREN

Cooper and colleagues[14,20] reported maximum $\dot{V}_{O_2}$ for 109 children, aged 6 to 17 years, who performed cycle ergometry using a continuously increasing work rate protocol (see Fig. 6-2). Because

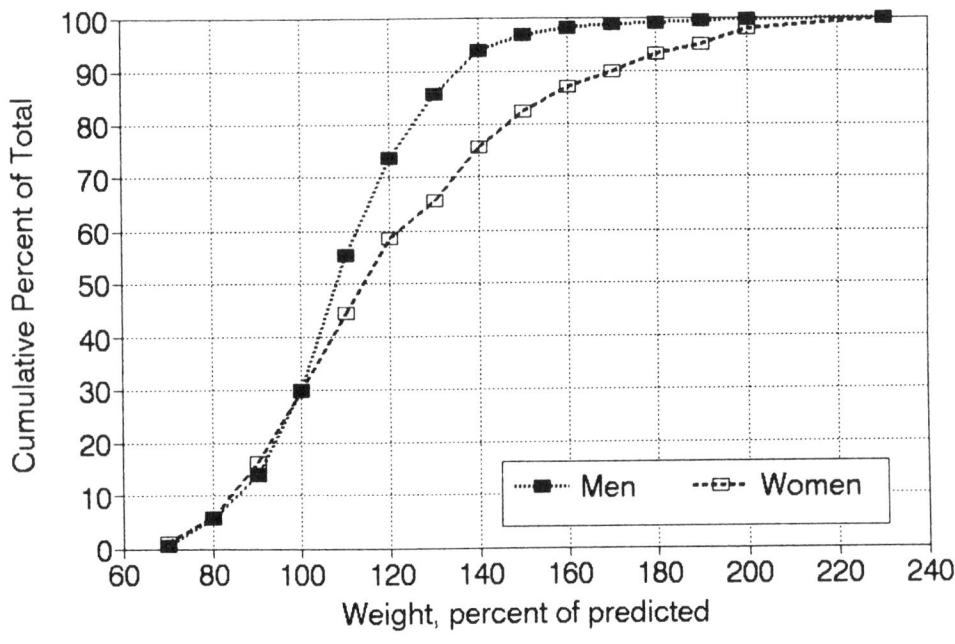

FIG. 6-5. Relationship of actual with normal (predicted) weight in approximately 1000 consecutive patients who were presented to our laboratory for diagnostic exercise testing. Normal (predicted) weight for men in kilograms = 0.79 × height in cm − 60.7;[6] for women in kilograms = 0.65 × height in cm − 42.8.[13] Our patient population can be seen to include a high proportion of overweight individuals.

the subjects were not obese, maximum $\dot{V}O_2$ correlated similarly with either weight or height. These investigators found, in addition, that their data were similar to those of Astrand[7] for the boys, but the girls studied by Astrand had a significantly higher maximum $\dot{V}O_2$ versus height relationship. Cooper et al. suggested that cultural or societal differences might account for this difference.

Exercise Mode

The type of exercise is an important determinant of maximum $\dot{V}O_2$. Maximum $\dot{V}O_2$ during arm cranking ergometer exercise is about 70% of that of leg cycling exercise[21] because of the smaller mass of muscle and lower work rate. Many studies[22–28] have shown that the maximum $\dot{V}O_2$ of leg cycling is approximately 89 to 95% of the maximal values achieved with treadmill exercise. Thus, the form of ergometry and muscle groups involved must be considered when predicting maximum $\dot{V}O_2$.

Maximum Heart Rate (HR) and Heart Rate Reserve (HRR)

The following equations can be used to estimate the maximum heart rate (HR) and the heart rate reserve (HRR) for adults and children:

Maximum heart rate (beats/min)
$$= 220 - \text{age (years)}$$

Heart rate reserve (HRR)
$$= \text{Predicted maximum HR}$$
$$- \text{observed maximum HR}$$

The maximum heart rate achieved declines with age in all studies. No consistent difference exists between men and women or among the types of exercise used, i.e., leg cycling, stepping, or inclined treadmill, walking or running.

The two most common formulae for predicting maximum HR in adults are: $220 - \text{age (years)}$ and $210 - 0.65 \times \text{age (years)}$.[29] Data from this laboratory fit the former equation slightly better. The standard deviation for each formula is 10 beats/min. As reported by Sheffield et al.[30] and Astrand and Rodahl,[10] the maximum heart rates derived from fit individuals approximate either formula reasonably well. The study of K.H. Cooper et al.[31] shows a lower maximum HR in the less fit than the more fit individual. Similarly, we found that

the maximum HR was reduced in obese men, consistent with the suggestion that a sedentary existence may reduce maximum HR even in well-motivated subjects.[12]

Scandinavian children were found to have an average maximum HR of 205 beats/min,[10] whereas North American children aged 8 to 18 had an average maximum heart rate of 187 beats/min with a lower 95% confidence limit of 160.[32]

The concept of HRR can be useful for estimating the relative stress of the cardiovascular system during exercise, but it should be used with caution. A normal HRR is zero. The mean predicted maximum HR may not be reached because of normal population variability, poor motivation, medications such as β-adrenergic blockers or because of heart, peripheral vascular, lung, endocrine, or musculoskeletal diseases.

Relationship of $\dot{V}O_2$ and Heart Rate: The Maximum Oxygen Pulse

The predicted maximum O_2 pulse is the quotient of the predicted maximum $\dot{V}O_2$ and predicted maximum HR derived from equations previously given. Adult values should be calculated from these equations.

$$\text{Predicted maximum } O_2 \text{ pulse (ml/beat)}$$
$$= \frac{\text{Predicted maximum } \dot{V}O_2 \text{ (ml/min)}}{\text{Predicted maximum HR (beats/min)}}$$

Mean values, confidence limits, and graphic data for children are given in Figure 6-6.

In a given individual, a consistent relationship exists between $\dot{V}O_2$ and HR during exercise (see Fig. 3-9). The quotient of the $\dot{V}O_2$ and HR is the O_2 pulse (see Fig. 3-10); its values are dependent on the stroke volume and the difference between the arterial and mixed venous blood O_2 content. This arterial-venous O_2 difference is, in turn, dependent on the availability of hemoglobin, blood oxygenation in the lung, and extraction of oxygen in the periphery. Examples of the normal and abnormal $\dot{V}O_2$ versus HR response and O_2 pulse response are shown in Figure 6-7. The normal relationship of $\dot{V}O_2$ with HR (patients 1 and 2) is linear over a wide range with a positive intercept on the HR axis. Although sedentary patients 1 and 2 differ considerably in their predicted maximum values (because they differ in age and gender or size), both have normal responses. An exercise re-

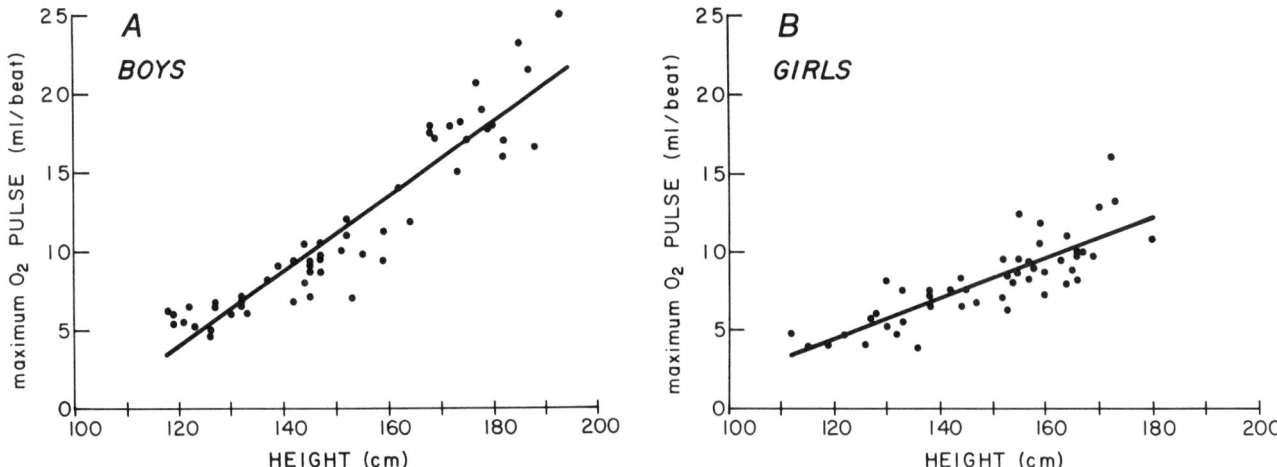

Fig. 6-6. Maximum O_2 pulse for normal North American boys (A) and girls (B). For boys, the best fit regression line is O_2 pulse (ml/beat) = 0.23 × height (cm) − 24.4. The lower 95% confidence limit is 3.8 ml/beat below the regression line. For girls, the equation is O_2 pulse (ml/beat) = 0.128 × height (cm) − 10.9 with a lower 95% confidence limit of 3.0 ml/beat below the regression line. (Modified from Cooper, D.M., Weiler-Ravell, D., Whipp, B.J., and Wasserman, K.: Growth-related changes in oxygen uptake and heart rate during progressive exercise in children. Pediatr. Res., 18:845–851, 1984.)

sponse with a higher $\dot{V}O_2$/HR than predicted indicates better than average cardiorespiratory function, whereas a response with a lower $\dot{V}O_2$/HR indicates poorer than average cardiorespiratory function (patient 3). In our clinical population, this latter response is most commonly due to low stroke volume, but it could be due to anemia or carboxyhemoglobinemia, poor blood oxygenation in the lung, right to left shunt, or (rarely) low peripheral oxygen extraction. In patient 4, the increasing slope of the HR versus $\dot{V}O_2$ relationship for the last several minutes of exercise is abnormal, indicating that the rise in $\dot{V}O_2$ is disproportionately slower than that of heart rate as work rate increases. In patient 5, the rate of rise of the HR versus $\dot{V}O_2$ plot is normal, but exercise ends at a relatively low work rate. If the cessation of incremental exercise is due to pain, musculoskeletal disease, ventilatory insufficiency, or other such factors, these factors (rather than circulatory disease) may be the cause of an abnormally low maximum O_2 pulse.

These differing responses can be seen in their entirety in Figure 6-7A, which has $\dot{V}O_2$ and HR axes and O_2 pulse isopleths. Figure 6-7B plots the O_2 pulse versus time for the same responses. Normally, the rate of increase in O_2 pulse declines gradually as the O_2 pulse approaches maximum values. (This is a necessary consequence of a linear $\dot{V}O_2$ versus HR response with a positive intercept on the HR axis.) This curvilinear response of the O_2 pulse during incremental exercise is clearly demonstrated in Figure 6-7B. Thus, both the abso-

lute values of $\dot{V}O_2$, HR, and O_2 pulse and their patterns of change are important; one or several may be abnormal in various disease states. The predicted O_2 pulse at any given work rate is strongly dependent on the individual's body size, gender, age, degree of fitness, and hemoglobin concentration. Normal values for the predicted maximum O_2 pulse on the cycle ergometer range from approximately 5 ml/beat in a 7-year-old child to 8 ml/beat in a 150 cm, 70-year-old woman to 17 ml/beat in a 190 cm, 30-year-old man. The actual O_2 pulse may be considerably higher than predicted in the cardiovascularly fit person or in the patient receiving β-adrenergic blocking drugs.

Brachial Artery Blood Pressure

The brachial artery blood pressure values of nonhypertensive men, measured directly (intra-arterially) or by cuff and sphygmomanometer during 1-minute incremental exercise, are given in Table 6-4.

Blood pressure can be measured by auscultation during exercise by skilled technicians or physicians, but assessing the fourth Korotkoff phase diastolic pressure (muffling of sound) and the fifth Korotkoff phase diastolic pressure (disappearance of sound) may be difficult because of the background noise of the ergometer. Intra-arterial pressures can be accurately and continuously measured by means of a pressure transducer attached to an indwelling catheter whenever arterial blood specimens are not being drawn, however.

A.

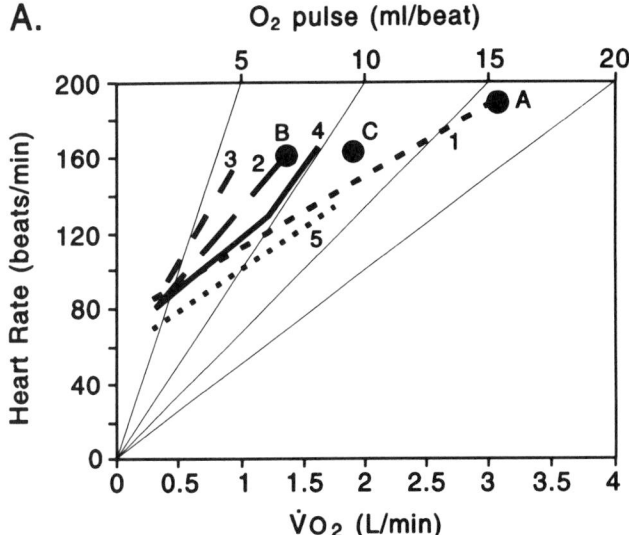

B.

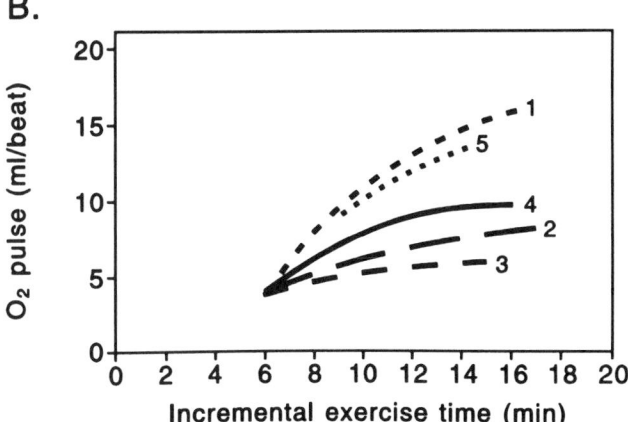

FIG. 6-7. Values of $\dot{V}_{O_2}$, heart rate, and O_2 pulse for five individuals during incremental cycle ergometer tests. For clarity, resting, unloaded pedalling, and recovery data are not shown. The upper figure has isopleths for O_2 pulse at 5, 10, 15, and 20 ml/beat. The three large solid circles are maximal exercise target values (each of which depended on each patient's age, gender, size, activity level, and exercise mode) and are labelled A for patients 1 and 5, B for patients 2 and 3, and C for patient 4. The responses for patients 1 and 2 are normal. Patient 3 had decreased cardiovascular function throughout the test and would not have reached target values even if able to exercise longer. Patient 4 manifested decreased cardiovascular function about 2 minutes before the cessation of exercise. Patient 5 stopped exercise prematurely for other than cardiovascular causes. B plots the same O_2 pulse data against time for the five patients. Patients 1 and 2 reach their target values, whereas patients 3, 4, and 5 do not. The plateau in O_2 pulse seen for patient 4 is abnormal.

The blood pressure measurements recorded in Table 6-4 are from a predominantly cigarette-smoking and sedentary normal population.[12,33] Values may be lower in non-smoking, more active individuals. Noteworthy is the striking rise in systolic (by both cuff and direct intra-arterial recording) and mean pressures, the considerable rise in intra-arterial diastolic pressures, the modest rise in fourth phase cuff diastolic pressures, and the gradual decline in fifth phase cuff diastolic pressures during incremental exercise. Although resting pressures are higher in older men, the mean maximum exercise systolic and diastolic pressures are similar in both groups. Note that the true mean arterial pressure closely approximates the diastolic pressure plus half the pulse pressure, rather than one third the pulse pressure during exercise when using a cuff.

Accurate intra-arterial blood pressure values are more difficult to obtain during treadmill ergometry because of movement artifacts. When the subject is using the cycle, the arm and transducer are stabilized by the hand on the handlebar, but tight gripping should be avoided to minimize the hypertensive effect of isometric exercise.

Anaerobic (Lactate, Lactic Acidosis) Threshold

The *AT* is expressed in units of O_2 uptake, but it can also be related to the predicted $\dot{V}_{O_2}$max. The mean values and confidence limits for the *AT* in normal children are given in Table 6-2, with the ratios of *AT*/maximum $\dot{V}_{O_2}$ in Figure 6-8. Figure 6-8 shows that the lower 95% confidence limit for the *AT*/maximum $\dot{V}_{O_2}$ is about 44%. Table 6-5 gives the mean and lower 95% confidence limit for the *AT*/maximum $\dot{V}_{O_2}$ in normal adult men and women.

The $\dot{V}_{O_2}$ at which the blood lactate level begins to rise has been used to define the *AT* in normal subjects[35,36] and noninvasively is best measured by the V-slope method.[37–39] A useful way to define abnormality is to multiply the lower 95% confidence limit of the predicted *AT*/predicted maximum $\dot{V}_{O_2}$ (Table 6-5) by the predicted maximum $\dot{V}_{O_2}$ of the subject. Thus, although the mean *AT* for men ranged between 49 and 63% of maximum $\dot{V}_{O_2}$ in several series,[40–43] the lowest value in our study of 77 middle-aged (34 to 74 years) normal sedentary men was 40% of maximum $\dot{V}_{O_2}$.[12] This lower limit of normal agrees reasonably well with the lowest value for *AT* in normal men suggested by Wasserman et al.[40] of 1 L/min of $\dot{V}_{O_2}$, approximately the cost of maintaining a moderate walking pace.

Jones et al.[15] and Davis et al.[34] have studied the effect of age on *AT*. Jones' ratios of *AT*/maximum $\dot{V}_{O_2}$ are slightly higher than Davis' ratios. Though different *AT* detection methods were used (Jones et al. used ventilatory equivalents and Davis et al.

TABLE 6-4. *Blood Pressure During 1-Minute Incremental Cycle Exercise Measured Directly from Catheter in Brachial Artery and in Opposite Arm by Cuff**

	PRIOR EXAM, AT REST	REST ON CYCLE	EXERCISE NEAR *AT*	EXERCISE NEAR MAXIMUM
	SEDENTARY, NON-HYPERTENSIVE MEN, AGES 34 TO 74			
Systolic intra-arterial		142 ± 18	182 ± 23	207 ± 27
Systolic cuff	124 ± 11	131	171	200
Diastolic intra-arterial		86 ± 10	92 ± 11	99 ± 12
Diastolic fourth phase	79 ± 7	84	86	88
Diastolic fifth phase		81	80	77
Mean intra-arterial		107	128	142
	SEDENTARY, NON-HYPERTENSIVE MEN, AGES 19 TO 24			
Systolic intra-arterial		129		203
Diastolic intra-arterial		78		106
Mean intra-arterial		96		141

* Values are mean or mean ± SD in mm Hg.
(Data are from references 12 and 33.)

used V-slope), both groups found that the absolute *AT* declines with age in both sexes, but less than the predicted maximum $\dot{V}O_2$, so the ratio of *AT*/maximum $\dot{V}O_2$ tends to increase with age. In addition to the gradual increase in the ratio with age, the ratios in women tend to be higher than those in men because of their lower $\dot{V}O_2$max.

Cooper et al.[14] tested 51 girls and 58 boys between the ages of 6 and 17 years. They were healthy and non-obese, but did not participate in vigorous sports. Mean *AT* was 58% of maximum $\dot{V}O_2$, but again, the lower limit of normal for this sample of normal children was approximately 44% of maximum $\dot{V}O_2$ (Fig. 6-8).

The mode of exercise may affect the value of *AT* in normal subjects. Davis et al.[44] studied 39 healthy college-age men. Mean $\dot{V}O_2$ at the *AT* was

46.5 ± 8.9% of maximum $\dot{V}O_2$ for arm cycling, 63.8 ± 9.0% of maximum $\dot{V}O_2$ for leg cycling, and 58.6 ± 5.8% of maximum $\dot{V}O_2$ for treadmill exercise. A substantial difference was noted between the *AT* during arm cycling and either form of leg exercise, but no significant difference existed between the *AT* obtained from cycle exercise and that obtained from treadmill exercise. Buchfuhrer et al.[45] found similar ratios of *AT*/maximum $\dot{V}O_2$ for treadmill and for cycle exercise, 50.3 ± 9.4% and 47.2 ± 11.0%, respectively. Withers et al.,[46] however, comparing highly trained cyclists and runners, found a higher *AT* for the total group on the treadmill (mean 76% of maximum $\dot{V}O_2$) than on the cycle (mean 64% of maximum $\dot{V}O_2$), with the cyclists reaching higher *AT* and *AT*/$\dot{V}O_2$max on the cycle and runners reaching higher *AT* and *AT*/$\dot{V}O_2$max on the treadmill.

Oxygen Uptake-Work Rate Relationship ($\Delta\dot{V}O_2/\Delta WR$)

The overall $\Delta\dot{V}O_2/\Delta WR$ during incremental cycle ergometer exercise of 6 to 12 minutes' duration for

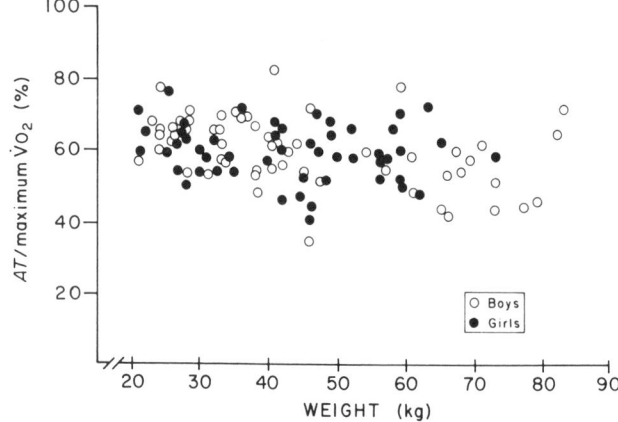

FIG. 6-8. The ratio of anaerobic threshold to maximum O_2 uptake, as a percentage, for 109 normal North American boys and girls. (From Cooper, D.M., Weiler-Ravell, D., Whipp, B.J., and Wasserman, K.: Aerobic parameters of exercise as a function of body size during growth in children. J. Appl. Physiol., 56:628–634, 1984.)

TABLE 6-5. *Mean and Lower 95% Confidence Limits for Predicted* AT/Predicted $\dot{V}O_2$ *Max in Adults, as a Percentage**

	MEN		WOMEN	
AGE (YR)	MEAN	LOWER 95% LIMIT	MEAN	LOWER 95% LIMIT
20	53	42	52	41
30	54	43	55	44
40	55	44	58	47
50	56	45	60	49
60	57	46	63	52
70	58	47	65	54

(Data from references 15 and 34.)

a population of 54 sedentary adult men was 10.3 ml/min/watt(W), with an SD of 1.0 ml/min/W and a lower limit of normal at the 95% confidence level of 8.6 ml/min/W.[47]

When a progressively increasing work rate test is initiated, a delay occurs before oxygen uptake begins to increase in a linear fashion. This delay must be considered in the calculation of the overall value of the $\Delta \dot{V}_{O_2}/\Delta WR$. This kinetic delay is equal to the time constant of $\dot{V}_{O_2}$ following a stepwise increase and is between half and three quarters of a minute. Thus, the formula used in calculation is:

$$\Delta \dot{V}_{O_2}/\Delta WR = (\text{maximum } \dot{V}_{O_2} - \text{unloaded } \dot{V}_{O_2})/[(T - 0.75) \times S]$$

where $\dot{V}_{O_2}$ is measured in milliliters per minute, T is the time of incremental exercise, and S is the slope of work rate increment in watts per minute. The overall $\Delta \dot{V}_{O_2}/\Delta WR$ during incremental cycle ergometer exercise has been found to vary modestly with the slope of work rate increase, the cardiovascular fitness of the individual, and the duration of the test.[47,48] In 10 normal young men, tests of approximately 15 minutes' duration (15-W/min increment) gave higher $\Delta \dot{V}_{O_2}/\Delta WR$ values (11.2 ± 0.15 ml/min/W) than tests of approximately 5 minutes' duration (60-W/min increment) (8.8 ± 0.15 ml/min/W). In tests of long duration, a lower fraction of the total energy cost of the work is supported from body stores of oxygen and anaerobic sources (e.g., lactate production), and a larger fraction is supported by oxygen extracted from the inspired air. The reverse allocation of energy support occurs in maximal tests of short duration. In tests of intermediate duration, however, the mean ± SD of $\Delta \dot{V}_{O_2}/\Delta WR$ found in 10 normal young men was 10.2 ± 0.16 ml/min/W,[48] and in 54 older sedentary normal men it was 10.3 ± 1.0 ml/min/ W.[47] This range is small enough so the $\Delta \dot{V}_{O_2}/\Delta WR$ is clinically useful in identifying patients with circulatory disorders.

In patients with circulatory disease (pulmonary, cardiac, or peripheral), the $\Delta \dot{V}_{O_2}/\Delta WR$ may be reduced because of either abnormally slow O_2 extraction kinetics at the muscle or the inability to raise muscle blood flow appropriately to provide oxygen rapidly enough to satisfy muscle requirements.[47,49,50] Many persons with coronary artery disease manifest a low $\Delta \dot{V}_{O_2}/\Delta WR$ relationship, primarily evident during the latter portion of their maximal exercise tests because of an inability to increase cardiac output. Many, but not all, men

with circulatory disorders have a significantly reduced $\Delta \dot{V}_{O_2}/\Delta WR$.[47] We have not analyzed data to describe the mean and range of $\Delta \dot{V}_{O_2}/\Delta WR$ for normal women or children, but we have seen that many athletes have a higher than average $\Delta \dot{V}_{O_2}/ \Delta WR$ (in the range of 11 to 12 ml/min/W).

Ventilation, Breathing Reserve, Tidal Volume, and Breathing Frequency

During sea level exercise below the AT, mean $\dot{V}_E$ (L/min, BTPS) = 24.6 × $\dot{V}_{CO_2}$ (L/min, STPD) + 3.2, with an SEE of 2.4 L/min, in normal adult men.[51]

At maximum work rates, the following values (mean ± SD) have been found for normal adult men, ages 34 to 74, for cycle ergometry using a breathing valve with a dead space of 64 ml.[12,17]

1. Maximum exercise $\dot{V}_E$/maximum voluntary ventilation (MVV),% = 72 ± 15
2. Breathing reserve = (MVV − maximum exercise $\dot{V}_E$) = 38 ± 22 L/min; lower limit of normal 11 L/min.
3. Maximum tidal volume (maximum V_T) < inspiratory capacity (IC) in all subjects
4. Maximum breathing frequency (f) < 50/min in over 95% of all subjects

Below the AT, ventilation is closely linked to metabolic requirements, with a narrow range in normal men. Whereas the $\dot{V}_E$ of a given patient is similarly linked to the metabolic demand, it is also dependent on the efficiency of ventilation, the degree of respiratory compensation for metabolic acidosis, the appropriateness of the ventilatory control mechanisms, and the mechanical capabilities of the lungs, chest wall, and respiratory muscles.

MAXIMUM EXERCISE VENTILATION

Because the maximal metabolic rate is lower when smaller muscle groups are used, maximum $\dot{V}_E$ for arm cycling is less than that for leg cycling or treadmill walk-running,[44] whereas maximum $\dot{V}_E$ is similar for the two latter forms of exercise.[3,45]

BREATHING RESERVE

The breathing reserve relates the ventilatory response during maximal exercise to the maximal ability to breathe. Because normal, untrained subjects do not ordinarily have ventilatory limitations on their ability to perform work,[19] some ability to increase ventilation further is usually present during maximal exercise. This potential increase in ventilation is generally estimated from the MVV, a test performed at rest. The MVV is highly dependent on the subject's motivation and effort. Normal values for MVV lasting 12 and 15 seconds are available.[52,53] The difference between the measured MVV and the maximum $\dot{V}_E$ during exercise is used as a measure of the ventilatory or breathing reserve. A low breathing reserve suggests that a subject's exercise capacity may be limited by his or her ventilatory capacity. The breathing reserve is usually reduced in patients with moderate to severe restrictive or obstructive lung disease (see Fig. 4-6).

Many investigators have examined the relationship between MVV and the maximum exercise $\dot{V}_E$. In general, maximum exercise $\dot{V}_E$ averages 50 to 80% of the 12- or 15-second MVV,[12] indicating a breathing reserve of 20 to 50% of the MVV.

Because the MVV is dependent on the subject's cooperation, effort, and technique of performance, the MVV is sometimes indirectly estimated from the FEV_1 or $FEV_{0.75}$. Gandevia and Hugh-Jones[54] suggested that the indirect MVV could be estimated as $FEV_1 \times 35$, whereas Cotes[55] suggested $FEV_{0.75} \times 40$ or $36.8 \times FEV_1 - 2.8$. Miller and colleagues[56] found that $FEV_1 \times 41$ or $FEV_{0.75} \times 46$ estimated MVV. Our data[12] and those of Campbell[57] indicate that $FEV_1 \times 40$ provides a good estimate of the MVV both in normal subjects and in patients with obstructive lung disease. If the direct MVV is less than the indirect MVV ($FEV_1 \times 40$), poor cooperation or understanding in the performance of the maneuver, extreme obesity, neurologic disorders, or inspiratory obstruction may be possible causes. If one is uncertain regarding a discrepancy between the direct MVV and the indirect MVV, or if the patient has variable obstruction, it may be necessary to have the patient repeat the direct MVV before performing the exercise test. We believe it preferable to use the indirect MVV ($FEV_1 \times 40$) rather than the direct MVV for calculation of the breathing reserve in patients with interstitial disease who have used inordinately high frequencies (e.g., over 100 breaths/min) in the MVV maneuver, frequencies that are unrealistic for the patient to maintain during exercise.

In 77 normal middle-aged subjects during an incremental cycle ergometer exercise test,[12] the mean measured MVV was 131 ± 23.6 L/min (range 81 to 203 L/min). The mean maximum exercise $\dot{V}_E$/MVV was $71.5 \pm 14.6\%$; only 13 subjects had a value greater than 80%. When we used $FEV_1 \times 40$ as an indirect estimate of the MVV, the mean maximum exercise $\dot{V}_E$/indirect MVV was $71.5 \pm 15.3\%$, i.e., the same percentage as for the directly measured MVV. Expressing breathing reserve as MVV − maximum exercise $\dot{V}_E$, we obtain an average of 38.1 ± 22.0 L/min using the directly measured MVV and 38.0 ± 21.5 L/min for the indirect MVV.

TIDAL VOLUME AND BREATHING FREQUENCY DURING EXERCISE

We consider that patients have ventilatory limitation if the exercise tidal volume (V_T) reaches the resting inspiratory capacity, particularly at submaximal work rates, or if the breathing frequency exceeds approximately 55 breaths/min. The maximum exercise V_T, like VC and other resting pulmonary function measurements, depends on the subject's height, age, and gender. In addition, the dead space or re-breathed volume of the breathing apparatus influences ventilation.[58–60]

Hey et al.[61] recommended that V_T be related to $\dot{V}_E$ to analyze the breathing pattern, such as is shown in Figure 3-11. At low exercise intensity, the increase in $\dot{V}_E$ is accomplished primarily by an increase in V_T. After the V_T reaches approximately 50 to 60% of the VC, further increases in $\dot{V}_E$ are accomplished primarily by increasing breathing frequency (f).[55,62] Thus, f is a curvilinear function of $\dot{V}_E$. Spiro et al.[62] found that the maximum V_T reached in normal subjects was approximately 55% of VC in normal men and 45% in normal women, whereas Cotes[63] suggested that maximum V_T is about 50% of VC for VC values between 2.0 and 5.0 L in normal men and women of European descent. Astrand[1] found that, at maximal exercise, the V_T averaged between 1.9 and 2.0 L, or 52 to 58% of the VC, whereas f at maximal exercise ranged between 34 and 46 breaths/min. Little difference in V_T/VC was noted among age groups, but f was lower in the older subjects studied.

Wasserman and Whipp[19] compared exercise V_T to IC. They found that V_T does not usually exceed approximately 70% of the IC during exercise, but it increases to a value approaching 100% in patients with restrictive lung disease, suggesting that the IC may limit the increase in V_T (see Fig. 3-11). In a series of 77 healthy middle-aged men, the mean resting V_T of 0.71 ± 0.26 L increased to 1.44 ± 0.43 L at the AT and 2.28 ± 0.43 L at maximum exercise.[12,17] Maximum f was 41.6 ± 9.6 min^{-1}.

Maximum V_T averaged $70.0 \pm 10.7\%$ of the IC and $55.0 \pm 8.7\%$ of the VC. No one had a maximum exercise V_T greater than their resting IC, and only 3 had a $f > 60$ min^{-1}.

Partitioning the duration of the ventilatory cycle (T_{TOT}) into inspiratory (T_I) and expiratory (T_E) components may also prove useful, but to date this measurement is not commonplace in clinical exercise testing, in part because most commercial exercise systems measure expiratory airflow only.

Ventilatory Equivalents for Carbon Dioxide ($\dot{V}_E/\dot{V}_{CO_2}$) and Oxygen ($\dot{V}_E/\dot{V}_{O_2}$)

The normal values (mean $\pm$ SD) during sea level exercise near the *AT* for middle-aged, normal, sedentary men are: 29.1 ± 4.3 for $\dot{V}_E/\dot{V}_{CO_2}$ and 26.5 ± 4.4 for $\dot{V}_E/\dot{V}_{O_2}$ where the $\dot{V}_E$ is expressed at BTPS with apparatus dead space ventilation subtracted, whereas $\dot{V}_{CO_2}$ and $\dot{V}_{O_2}$ are expressed as STPD.

The ratio $\dot{V}_E/\dot{V}_{CO_2}$ gives an index of the dead space ventilation, but this inference must be made with care. The following equation is a modification of the alveolar mass balance equation:

$$\frac{\dot{V}_E}{\dot{V}_{CO_2}} = \frac{k}{P_{a_{CO_2}} \times (1 - V_D/V_T)}$$

Thus, $\dot{V}_E/\dot{V}_{CO_2}$ is expected to be higher than normal when the physiologic dead space/tidal volume ratio (V_D/V_T) is high, but it also can be high when the patient hyperventilates (i.e., $P_{a_{CO_2}}$ is lower than normal) (see inset in Fig. 3-14). In an invasive exercise test, V_D/V_T can be calculated if $P_{a_{CO_2}}$ is measured. Importantly, $P_{ET_{CO_2}}$ cannot be assumed to be equal to $P_{a_{CO_2}}$ in a noninvasive test. In fact, as explained later, a low $P_{ET_{CO_2}}$ does not necessarily indicate hyperventilation because it also can be seen with a normal $P_{a_{CO_2}}$ combined with a high V_D/V_T. Situations where $P_{a_{CO_2}}$ is substantially lower than $P_{ET_{CO_2}}$ are uncommon, however. Thus, when $\dot{V}_E/\dot{V}_{CO_2}$ is high and $P_{ET_{CO_2}}$ is not low (i.e., 40 torr or above), it is likely that V_D/V_T is high.

Wasserman et al.[64] found that $\dot{V}_E/\dot{V}_{CO_2}$ declined to approximately 28 during cycle ergometer exercise in 10 healthy young men before it increased with the onset of ventilatory compensation for the exercise lactic acidosis. In steady-state exercise unaccompanied by a lactic acidosis, the $\dot{V}_E/\dot{V}_{O_2}$ is

lower than the $\dot{V}_E/\dot{V}_{CO_2}$ because the respiratory quotient is less than 1.[19] Both $\dot{V}_E/\dot{V}_{O_2}$ and $\dot{V}_E/\dot{V}_{CO_2}$ are necessarily increased at altitudes at which hyperventilation causes a decrease in $P_{a_{CO_2}}$.

Physiologic Dead Space/Tidal Volume Ratio (V_D/V_T)

Figure 6-9 shows the effect of exercise on V_D/V_T at various levels of cycle exercise in young men. We recommend the following predicted values for V_D/V_T at rest and during upright exercise after allowance for valve dead space:

1. For men under age 40: $V_D/V_T \leq 0.40$ at rest, ≤ 0.25 at *AT*, and ≤ 0.21 at maximal exercise.
2. For men over age 40: mean values $V_D/V_T = 0.30 \pm 0.08$ at rest, 0.20 ± 0.07 at *AT*, and 0.19 ± 0.07 at maximal exercise.
3. Upper 95% confidence limits for men over 40: $V_D/V_T = 0.45$ at rest, 0.33 at *AT*, and 0.29 at maximal exercise.

The physiologic dead space (V_D) is dependent on anatomic and physiologic factors, whereas the V_D/V_T is also dependent, even in normal subjects, on the pattern of breathing. At rest, the V_D/V_T may be elevated because of the rapid, shallow breathing of anxiety.

Physiologic control mechanisms usually stabilize ventilation at a slower and more efficient breathing pattern soon after the onset of exercise unless anxiety is extreme. Calculation of the V_D and V_D/V_T must be carefully performed, making an adjustment for the apparatus dead space (see Appendix D). In addition, gas exchange measurements must be synchronous with arterial blood sampling for measuring $P_{a_{CO_2}}$.

Cotes[63] suggested that V_D (ml) $= 140 + 0.07$ V_T (ml) with an SD $= 90$ ml in young men during exercise. Jones et al.[59], found the following relationship during exercise in 17 normal young men: V_D (ml) $= 138 + 0.077$ V_T (ml), with r $= 0.69$. Lifshay et al.[60] showed that men aged 50 to 81 had a significantly higher V_D than men and women aged 18 to 37. The prediction equations of Bradley et al.[65] for V_D use sex, age, height, $\dot{V}_{CO_2}$, $\dot{V}_E$, f, and temperature as factors.

All studies have shown a fall in V_D/V_T during exercise in normal subjects. Thus, whereas mean V_D/V_T at rest ranged from 0.28 to 0.35 in several studies of normal subjects, mean V_D/V_T decreased

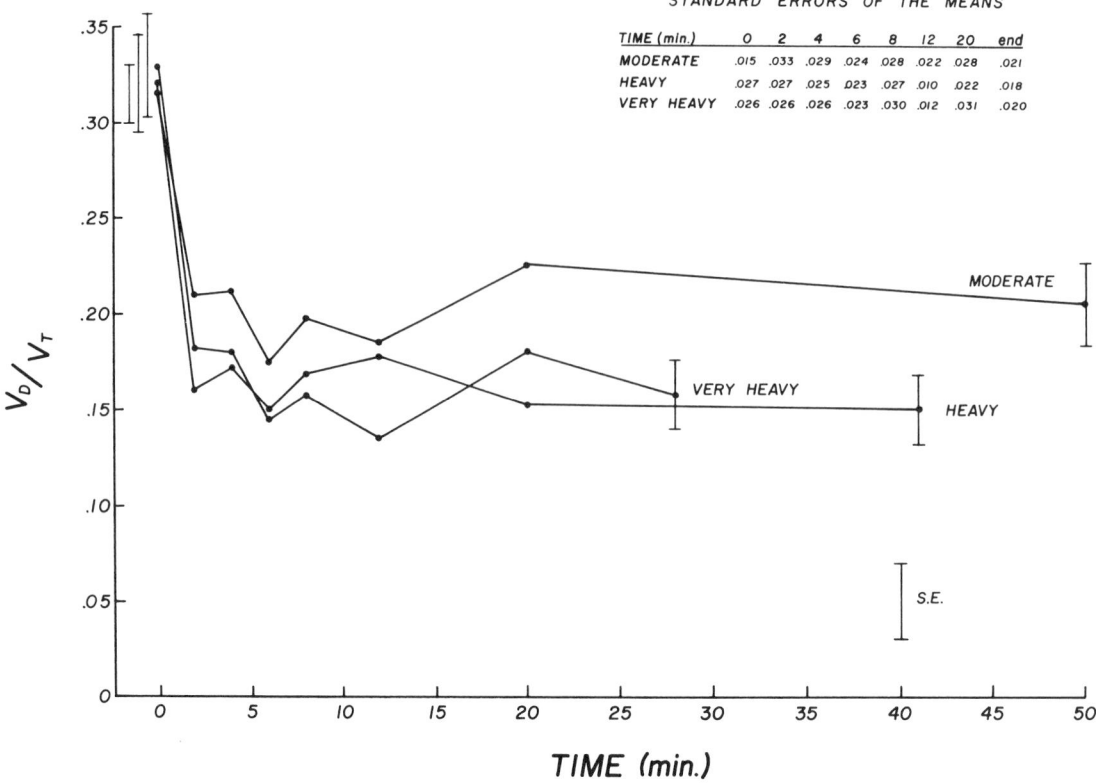

FIG. 6-9. The physiologic dead space/tidal volume ratio (VD/VT) in 10 normal young men at rest and during 3 intensities of cycle ergometer exercise as related to exercise duration. The SEM are given in the table inset. (From Wasserman, K., VanKessel, A.L., and Burton, G.G.: Interaction of physiological mechanisms during exercise. J. Appl. Physiol., 22:71–85, 1967.)

to between 0.20 and 0.25 near the *AT* and to less than 0.21 at maximal exercise.[12,59,64,66]

The practice of some manufacturers of offering a calculation of "noninvasive VD/VT" is invalid in patients and is to be condemned. This calculation substitutes $P_{ET_{CO_2}}$ for Pa_{CO_2} in the foregoing alveolar mass balance equation rearranged to allow VD/VT calculations. Because the difference between $P_{ET_{CO_2}}$ and Pa_{CO_2} is influenced by VD/VT, this calculation involves a heavy dose of circular reasoning.

Arterial and End-Tidal Carbon Dioxide (Pa_{CO_2}, $P_{ET_{CO_2}}$, and $P(a\text{-}ET)_{CO_2}$)

The normal values at sea level during upright exercise in adult men are:

1. Pa_{CO_2}: resting value = 36 to 42 mm Hg; stable during mild and moderate exercise, declining with heavy exercise.
2. $P_{ET_{CO_2}}$: resting value = 36 to 42 mm Hg; increases normally by 3 to 8 mm Hg during mild and moderate exercise (depending on breathing pattern), and decreases with heavy exercise.
3. $P(a\text{-}ET)_{CO_2}$ (mean ± SD):
   a. Exercise at the *AT* = −3 ± 3 mm Hg;
   b. At maximal exercise = −4 ± 3 mm Hg. The $P(a\text{-}ET)_{CO_2}$ is negative in more than 95% of normal men at maximal exercise.

Resting $P_{ET_{CO_2}}$ and Pa_{CO_2} values are dependent on the degree of apprehension, anxiety, and training of the subject. Many anxious subjects have a strong tendency to hyperventilate, especially while breathing through a mouthpiece and awaiting the signal to begin exercise (Fig. 6-10). Once exercise starts, however, the blood gases and pH are not discernibly different, whether performing the work while breathing through a low resistance breathing valve or breathing normally without a mouthpiece.[67] In more apprehensive individuals, the Pa_{CO_2} values rise from rest to moderate exercise as physiologic control mechanisms suppress psychogenic hyperventilation. In the relaxed individual, Pa_{CO_2} values remain relatively stable at rest and during mild and moderate exercise. Although Pa_{CO_2} values cannot be predicted accurately from Pet_{CO_2} values in an individual person, particularly in a patient with lung disease, measurement of Pet_{CO_2} is often valuable for following trends in Pa_{CO_2}. Increasing Pet_{CO_2} values, above those observed at the lowest work rate, usually mean that Pa_{CO_2} is rising.

Wasserman et al.[64] found that $P(a\text{-}et)_{CO_2}$ changed from approximately $+2.5$ mm Hg at rest to -4 mm Hg during heavy work in 10 normal men (Fig. 6-11). Jones et al.[59] found that, in 17 normal subjects at the highest work rates reached, Pet_{CO_2} was always more than 2 mm Hg higher than Pa_{CO_2}. In 5 normal men, Whipp and Wasserman[65] found $P(a\text{-}et)_{CO_2}$ was 2.8 ± 1.6 mm Hg at rest and -2.8 ± 0.6 mm Hg at a work rate of 220 W. All $P(a\text{-}et)_{CO_2}$ values were negative for work rates above 115 W. In 77 asbestos-exposed healthy men,[12] mean $P(a\text{-}et)_{CO_2}$ at rest was -0.3 ± 2.9 mm Hg and decreased to -4.1 ± 3.2 mm Hg at maximal exercise. At the peak of exercise, a $P(a\text{-}et)_{CO_2} > 0$ was rare.

Arterial, Alveolar, and End-Tidal Oxygen (Pa_{O_2}, Pa_{O_2}, Pet_{O_2}, And $P(a\text{-}a)_{O_2}$) and Arterial Oxyhemoglobin Saturation (Sa_{O_2})

The normal blood O_2 level (Pa_{O_2} and Sa_{O_2}) and alveolar-arterial P_{O_2} difference ($P(a\text{-}a)_{O_2}$) at sea level during upright exercise in adult men are:

1. Pa_{O_2}: rest = 80 mm Hg or greater; usually increasing slightly with heavy exercise.
2. Sa_{O_2}: rest = 95% or greater; no decrease with exercise.
3. Pet_{O_2}: rest = 90 mm Hg or greater; increases with heavy exercise.
4. $P(a\text{-}a)_{O_2}$:
   a. Age 20 to 39: mean $P(a\text{-}a)_{O_2} = 8$ mm Hg at rest, 11 mm Hg at *AT*, and 15 mm Hg at maximal exercise.
   b. Age 40 to 69: $P(a\text{-}a)_{O_2} = 13 \pm 7$ mm Hg at rest, 17 ± 7 mm Hg at *AT* and 19 ± 9 mm Hg at maximal exercise; upper limit of nor-

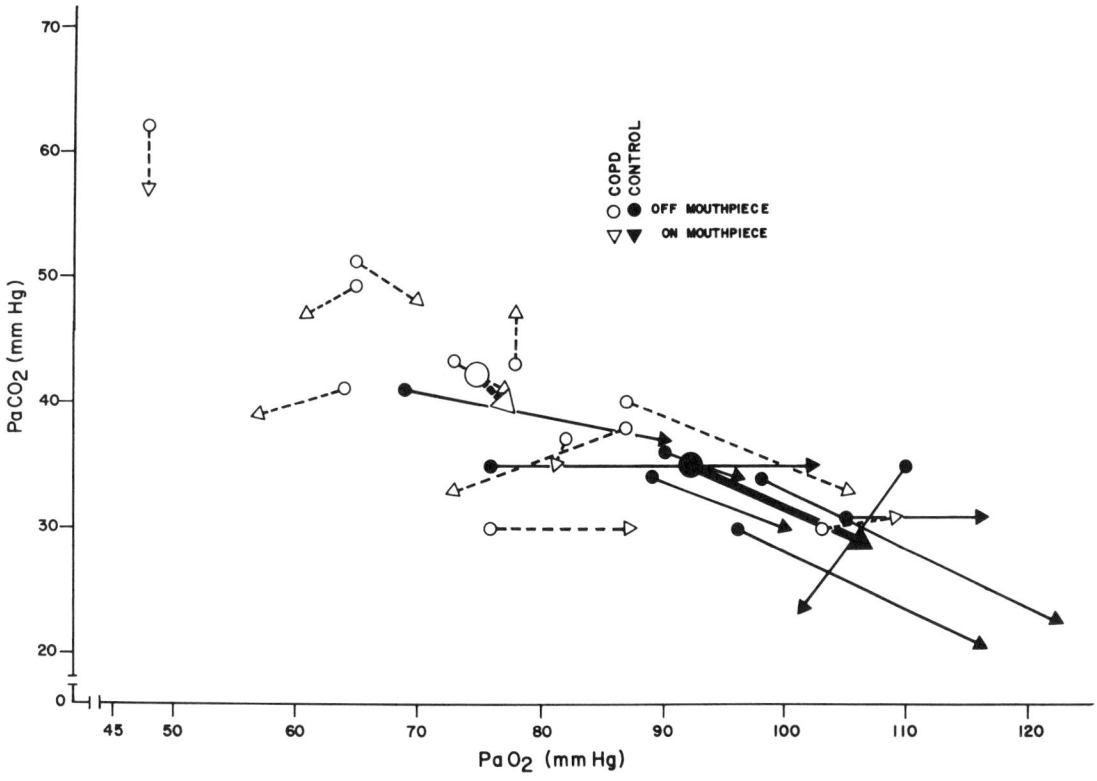

FIG. 6-10. Resting arterial partial pressures of CO_2 (Pa_{CO_2}) and O_2 (Pa_{O_2}) in normal control subjects and in patients with chronic obstructive pulmonary disease (COPD) off and acutely on the mouthpiece while awaiting cycle ergometer exercise. Small arrows show individual values and large arrows show mean values. Note the small mean decline in Pa_{CO_2} and the increase in Pa_{O_2} in the patients with COPD while breathing on the mouthpiece, whereas the controls show a larger decline in Pa_{CO_2} and a much larger rise in Pa_{O_2} with the same mouthpiece at rest (Courtesy of Dr. J.D. Andrews).

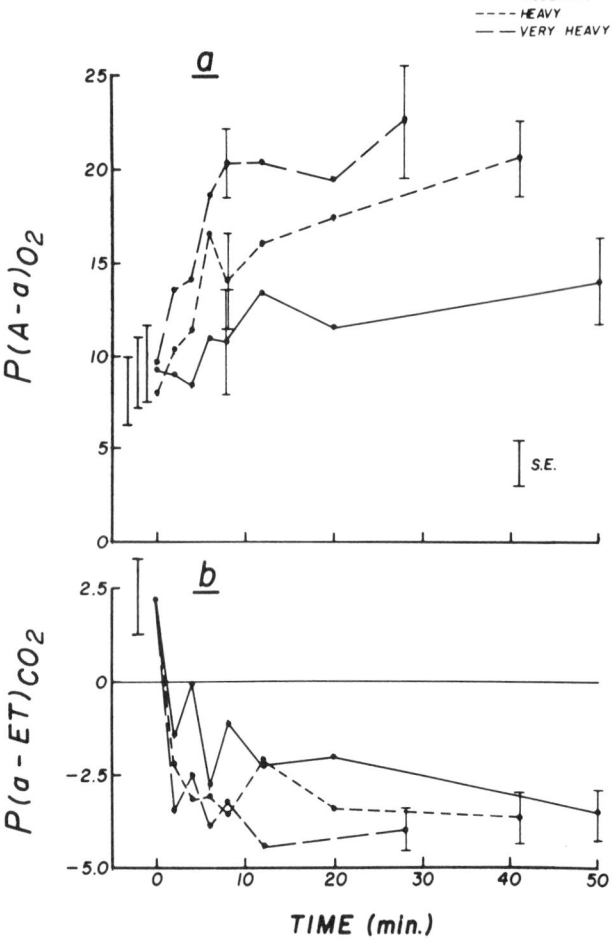

FIG. 6-11. The $P(A-a)_{O_2}$ and $P(a-ET)_{CO_2}$ in 10 normal young men at rest and during 3 intensities of cycle ergometer exercise as related to exercise duration. The mean and SEM are depicted. (From Wasserman, K., VanKessel, A.L., and Burton, G.G.: Interaction of physiological mechanisms during exercise. J. Appl. Physiol., 22:71–85, 1967.)

mal (95% confidence level) = 28 mm Hg at *AT* and 35 mm Hg at maximal exercise.

The normal resting Pa_{O_2} is dependent on age, body position, and nutritional status. Values are lower with increasing age, obesity, fasting, and in the supine position. Nevertheless, sea level values less than 80 mm Hg are not seen in normal subjects in the sitting position except in those who are obese. The PET_{O_2} and PA_{O_2} (the latter calculated from the alveolar air equation; see Appendix) are normally similar, but they may differ by 10 or more mm Hg in patients with severe maldistribution of ventilation. The PA_{O_2} and Pa_{O_2} decrease transiently soon after the start of exercise (because the rise in $\dot{V}E$ is slower than the rise in $\dot{V}O_2$, i.e., R decreases) and then increase back to approximately resting values (see Chap. 2 on O_2 uptake

kinetics, O_2 deficit, and O_2 debt). The PET_{O_2} increases 10 to 30 mm Hg above the *AT* because of metabolic acidosis-induced hyperventilation and rising R at maximal exercise.

The Sa_{O_2} normally changes less than 2% from rest to maximal exercise. In highly motivated athletes, the Sa_{O_2} has been reported to fall below resting values,[68] but this is uncommon.

Many reports show that the $P(A-a)_{O_2}$ increases during heavy exercise in normal subjects. Lilienthal et al.[69] and Asmussen and Nielsen[70] found a mean $P(A-a)_{O_2}$ of 30 mm Hg at high work rates. Jones et al.[59] found, in 17 normal active men not in physical training, a mean $P(A-a)_{O_2}$ of 12 mm Hg at rest, with an increase to approximately 20 mm Hg at work rates with a $\dot{V}O_2$ over 1.5 L/min. Whipp and Wasserman,[66] in 5 healthy young men, found a $P(A-a)_{O_2}$ of 7.4 ± 4.2 mm Hg (mean ± SD) at rest and 10.8 ± 3.6 mm Hg at heavy exercise. Cruz et al.[71] studied 4 subjects at rest and at work rates approximating 50%, 75%, and 100% of maximum $\dot{V}O_2$ at sea level and found $P(A-a)_{O_2}$ values of 11.5 ± 5.4, 11.0 ± 4.2, 16.3 ± 2.6, and 20 ± 8.8 mm Hg, respectively. Hansen et al.[72] studied 16 healthy young men, aged 18 to 24, during sea level exercise on a cycle ergometer and found that the mean $P(A-a)_{O_2}$ was 8 mm Hg while sitting at rest, 7 mm Hg during mild exercise, 11 mm Hg during moderate exercise, and 15 mm Hg during maximal exercise. Similar results were obtained by Wasserman et al.[64] in 10 healthy young men, and values are shown at rest and at 3 work intensities as related to time in Figure 6-11. We found, in 77 normal older men (ages 34 to 74 years), $P(A-a)_{O_2}$ values of 12.8 ± 7.4 mm Hg at rest and 19.0 ± 8.8 mm Hg at maximum exercise.[12] At maximum exercise, $P(A-a)_{O_2}$ was greater than 35 mm Hg in only 3 of these 77 men.

Mixed Venous Values

Mixed venous values during heavy to maximal exercise[73,74] in normal volunteers are:

1. PO_2 values as low as 15 to 20 mm Hg.
2. SO_2 values as low as 15 to 20%.
3. pH values as low as 7.00 units.
4. PCO_2 values as high as 90 mm Hg.
5. Actual bicarbonate values as high as 30 mmol/L, with standard bicarbonate values as low as 16 mmol/L.

Heavy exercise mixed venous values are unavailable for patients with diverse disease states.

TABLE 6-6. *Metabolic Acidosis at the End of and During Recovery from Maximum Incremental Cycle Ergometer Exercise in Normal Sedentary Men*

TIME	AT END OF EXERCISE		2 MINUTES INTO RECOVERY	
AGE (YEARS)	18–24	34–74	18–24	34–74
Number studied	10	77	10	77
Average exercise duration (min)	18	9	18	9
Arterial lactate increase (mmol/L*)	6.6 ± 1.4		7.6 ± 1.8	
Arterial HCO_3^- decline from rest (mmol/L*)	6.2 ± 2.3	4.0 ± 2.5	8.7 ± 2.6	8.5 ± 2.9
Arterial pH*	7.31 ± 0.04	7.37 ± 0.04	7.29 ± 0.04	7.33 ± 0.03
Gas exchange ratio (R)*		1.21 ± 0.12		1.59 ± 0.19

* Values are mean ± SD.
(Data are from references 12 and 73.)

We suspect that values even more extreme than the foregoing values for normal volunteers may be reached in some patients whose exercise is not limited by ventilatory or mechanical causes.

Historically, it has been suggested that cardiac output could be measured noninvasively during exercise with the Fick principle by estimating mixed venous CO_2 content using rebreathing techniques. This estimate of cardiac output depends on the premise that mixed venous PCO_2 values estimated by rebreathing techniques are highly correlated with mixed venous CO_2 content, even without knowing mixed venous pH or oxyhemoglobin saturation. Data obtained in our exercise laboratories indicate that the correlative relationships between serial measures of mixed venous PCO_2 and CO_2 content during incremental exercise tests are poor. These data are strong evidence that cardiac output cannot be accurately measured by CO_2 rebreathing techniques except during rest or light exercise.

Acid-Base Balance

Normally, the only acid-base disturbance that develops during exercise is metabolic acidosis. The intensity of the metabolic acidosis can be documented by arterial blood and gas exchange measurements. Normal values for younger[75] and older[12] men for incremental cycle exercise tests are given in Table 6-6.

Measurements of the acid-base status and R at the termination of an incremental exercise test are valuable in deciding whether or not the subject has made a good effort to perform maximally. Resting venous and arterial lactate values are normally less than 1 mmol/L and typically rise substantially before the termination of maximal exercise. During exercise, venous lactate values can be dependent on the site of lactate production and

the sampling site,[76] whereas arterial lactate gives a better indication of the total body lactate burden. As described in Chapter 2, the rise in blood lactate during exercise is accompanied by a nearly equimolar decline in bicarbonate and a decrease in pH. This metabolic acidosis results in hyperventilation, a decline in Pa_{CO_2}, and a further increase in $\dot{V}_{CO_2}$ so that R increases. The lactate and R reach their peak and the pH and bicarbonate reach their nadir at about 2 minutes of recovery after an incremental exercise test. The magnitude of these changes indicates the severity of exercise-induced metabolic acidosis. Small changes signify a mild degree of exercise stress secondary to low motivation or disorders that preclude the performance of exercise at a significant level above the *AT*.

Summary

Normal exercise values for maximum $\dot{V}_{O_2}$, *AT*, HR, HRR, O_2 pulse, arterial blood pressure, ventilation, ventilatory equivalents, breathing pattern, breathing reserve, arterial blood gases, $P(A-a)_{O_2}$, $P(a-ET)_{CO_2}$, V_D/V_T, mixed venous blood gases, and acid-base balance for use in assessment of patients are presented and critiqued in this chapter. In the future, new and more versatile sets of normal values will undoubtedly be compiled.

References

1. Astrand, I.: Aerobic work capacity in men and women with special reference to age. Acta Physiol. Scand., 49(Suppl. 169):1–89, 1960.
2. Drinkwater, B.L., Horvath, S.M., and Wells, C.L.: Aerobic power of females, ages 10 to 68. J. Gerontol., 30: 385–394, 1975.
3. Hermansen, L., and Saltin, B.: Oxygen uptake during maximal treadmill and bicycle exercise. J. Appl. Physiol., 26:31–37, 1969.

4. Dehn, M.M., and Bruce, R.A.: Longitudinal variations in maximal oxygen intake with age and activity. J. Appl. Physiol., 33:805–807, 1972.

5. Astrand, I., Astrand, P.O., Hallback, I., and Kilborn, A.: Reduction in maximal oxygen uptake with age. J. Appl. Physiol., 35:649–654, 1973.

6. Bruce, R.A., Kusumi, F., and Hosmer, D.: Maximal oxygen uptake and nomographic assessment of functional aerobic impairment in cardiovascular disease. Am. Heart J., 85:546–562, 1973.

7. Astrand, P.O.: Human physical fitness with special reference to sex and age. Physiol. Rev., 36:307–335, 1956.

8. Balke, I., and Ware, R.W.: An experimental study of "physical fitness" of Air Force personnel. U.S. Armed Forces Med. J., 10:675–688, 1959.

9. Davis, J.A., Frank, M.H., Whipp, B.J., and Wasserman, K.: Anaerobic threshold alterations caused by endurance training in middle-aged men. J. Appl. Physiol., 46:1039–1046, 1979.

10. Astrand, P.O., and Rodahl, K.: Textbook of Work Physiology. 3rd Ed. New York, McGraw-Hill, 1986.

11. Jones, N.L., Summers, E., and Killian, K.J.: Influence of age and stature on exercise capacity during incremental cycle ergometry in men and women. Am. Rev. Respir. Dis., 140:1373–1380, 1989.

12. Hansen, J.E., Sue, D.Y., and Wasserman, K.: Predicted values for clinical exercise testing. Am. Rev. Respir. Dis., 129(Suppl.):S49-S55, 1984.

13. Davis, J.A.: Personal communication.

14. Cooper, D.M., Weiler-Ravell, D., Whipp, B.J., and Wasserman, K.: Aerobic parameters of exercise as a function of body size during growth in children. J. Appl. Physiol., 56:628–634, 1984.

15. Jones, N.L., Makrides, L., Hitchcock, C., and McCartney, N.: Normal standards for an incremental progressive cycle ergometer test. Am. Rev. Respir. Dis., 131:700–708, 1985.

16. Itoh, H., Koike, A., Taniguchi, K., and Marumo, F.: Severity and pathophysiology of heart failure on the basis of anaerobic threshold (AT) and related parameters. Jpn. Circ. J., 53:146–154, 1989.

17. Sue, D.Y., and Hansen, J.E.: Normal values in adults during exercise testing. Clin. Chest Med., 5:89–98, 1984.

18. Buskirk, E., and Taylor, H.L.: Maximal oxygen intake and its relation to body composition, with special reference to chronic physical activity and obesity. J. Appl. Physiol., 11:72–78, 1957.

19. Wasserman, K., and Whipp, B.J.: Exercise physiology in health and disease. Am. Rev. Respir. Dis., 112:219–249, 1975.

20. Cooper, D.M., and Weiler-Ravell, D.: Gas exchange response to exercise in children. Am. Rev. Respir. Dis., 129(Suppl.):S47-S48, 1984.

21. Astrand, P.O., and Saltin, B.: Maximal oxygen uptake and heart rate in various types of muscular activity. J. Appl. Physiol., 16:977–981, 1961.

22. Wyndham, C.H., Strydom, N.B., Leary, W.P., and Williams, C.G.: Studies of the maximum capacity of men for physical effort. Arbeitsphysiologie, 22:285–295, 1966.

23. Dempsey, J.A., Reddan, W., Rankin, J., and Balke, B.: Alveolar-arterial gas exchange during muscular work in obesity. J. Appl. Physiol., 21:1807–1814, 1966.

24. Shephard, R.J., Allen, C., Benade, A.J.S., Davies, C.T.M., di Priampero, P.E., Hedman, R., Merriman, J.E., Myhre, K., and Simmons, R.: The maximum oxygen intake. Bull WHO, 38:757–764, 1968.

25. Hermansen, L., and Saltin, B.: Oxygen uptake during maximal treadmill and bicycle exercise. J. Appl. Physiol., 26:31–37, 1969.

26. Faulkner, J.A., Roberts, D.E., Elk, R.E., and Conway, J.: Cardiovascular responses to submaximum and maximum effort cyling and running. J. Appl. Physiol., 30:457–461, 1971.

27. McArdle, W.D., Katch, F.I., and Pechar, G.S.: Comparison of continuous and discontinuous treadmill and bicycle test for max $\dot{V}_{O_2}$. Med. Sci. Sports, 5:156–160, 1972.

28. Davis, J.A., and Kasch, F.W.: Aerobic and anaerobic differences between maximal running and cycling in middle-aged males. Aust. J. Sports Med., 7:81–84, 1975.

29. Jones, N.L.: Clinical Exercise Testing. 3rd Ed. Philadelphia, W.B. Saunders, 1988.

30. Sheffield, L.T., Maloof, J.A., Sawyer, J.A., and Roitman, D.: Maximal heart rate and treadmill performance of healthy women in relation to age. Circulation, 57:79–84, 1978.

31. Cooper, K.H., Purdy, J., White, S., Pollock, M., and Linnerud, A.C.: Age-fitness adjusted maximal heart rates. Med. Sci. Sports, 10:78–86, 1977.

32. Cooper, D.M., Weiler-Ravell, D., Whipp, B.J., and Wasserman, K.: Growth-related changes in oxygen uptake and heart rate during progressive exercise in children. Pediatr. Res., 18:845–851, 1984.

33. Robinson, T.R., Sue, D.Y., Huszczuk, A., Weiler-Ravell, D., and Hansen, J.E.: Intra-arterial and cuff blood pressure responses during incremental cycle ergometry. Med. Sci. Sports Exerc., 20:142–149, 1988.

34. Davis, J.A., Storer, T.W., and Caiozzo, V.J.: Prediction of normal values for lactate threshold in adult males and females. Submitted for publication.

35. Wasserman, K., and McIlroy, M.B.: Detecting the threshold of anaerobic metabolism in cardiac patients during exercise. Am. J. Cardiol., 14:844–852, 1964.

36. Wasserman, K.: The anaerobic threshold measurement to evaluate exercise performance. Am. Rev. Respir. Dis., 129(Suppl.):S35-S40, 1984.

37. Beaver, W.L., Wasserman, K., and Whipp, B.J.: A new method for detecting the anaerobic threshold by gas exchange. J. Appl. Physiol., 60:2020–2027, 1986.

38. Sue, D.Y., Wasserman, K., Morrica, R.B., and Casaburi, R.: Measurement of anaerobic threshold by V-slope method in patients with chronic obstructive lung disease and normal subjects. Chest, 94:931–938, 1988.

39. Wasserman, K., Beaver, W.L., and Whipp, B.J.: Gas exchange theory and the lactic acidosis (anaerobic) threshold. Circulation, 81(Suppl. II):II-14-II-30, 1990.

40. Wasserman, K., Whipp, B.J., Koyal, S.N., and Beaver, W.L.: Anaerobic threshold and respiratory gas exchange during exercise. J. Appl. Physiol., 35:236–243, 1973.

41. Nery, L.E., Wasserman, K., French, W., Oren, A., and Davis, J.A.: Contrasting cardiovascular and respiratory responses to exercise in mitral valve and chronic obstructive pulmonary diseases. Chest, 83:446–453, 1983.

42. Orr, G.W., Green, H.J., Hughson, R.L., and Bennett, G.W.: A computer linear regression model to determine

ventilatory anaerobic threshold. J. Appl. Physiol., 52: 1349–1352, 1982.

43. Davis, J.A., Frank, M.N., Whipp, B.J., and Wasserman, K.: Anaerobic threshold alterations caused by endurance training in middle-aged men. J. Appl. Physiol., 46: 1039–1046, 1979.

44. Davis, J.A., Vodak, P., Wilmore, J.N., Vodak, J., and Kurtz, P.: Anaerobic threshold and maximal aerobic power for three modes of exercise. J. Appl. Physiol., 41: 544–550, 1976.

45. Buchfuhrer, M.J., Hansen, J.E., Robinson, T.E., Sue, D.Y., Wasserman, K., and Whipp, B.J.: Optimizing the exercise protocol for cardiopulmonary assessment. J. Appl. Physiol., 55:1558–1564, 1983.

46. Withers, R.T., Sherman, W.M., Miller, J.M., and Costillo, D.L.: Specificity of the anaerobic threshold in endurance trained cyclists and runners. Eur. J. Appl. Physiol., 47:93–101, 1981.

47. Hansen, J.E., Sue, D.Y., Oren, A., and Wasserman, K.: Relation of oxygen uptake to work rate in normal men and men with circulatory disorders. Am. J. Cardiol., 59: 669–674, 1987.

48. Hansen, J.E., Casaburi, R., Cooper, D.M., and Wasserman, K.: Oxygen uptake as related to work rate increment during cycle ergometer exercise. Eur. J. Appl. Physiol., 57:140–145, 1988.

49. Auchincloss, J.H., Jr., Ashutosh, K., Rana, S., Peppi, D., Johnson, L.W., and Gilbert, R.: Effect of cardiac, pulmonary, and vascular disease on one-minute oxygen uptake. Chest, 70:486–93, 1976.

50. Sietsema, K.E., Cooper, D.M., Perloff, J.K., Rosove, M.H., Child, J.S., Canobbio, M.M., Whipp, B.J., and Wasserman, K.: Dynamics of oxygen uptake during exercise in adults with congenital heart disease. Circulation, 73:1137–1144, 1986.

51. Davis, J.A., Whipp, B.J., and Wasserman, K.: The relation of ventilation to metabolic rate during moderate exercise in man. Eur. J. Appl. Physiol., 44:97–108, 1980.

52. Kory, R.C., Callahan, R., Boren, N.C., and Syner, J.C.: The Veterans Administration-Army cooperative study of pulmonary function. 1. Clinical spirometry in normal men. Am. J. Med., 30:243–258, 1961.

53. Lindall, A., Medine, A., and Grismor, J.T.: A re-evaluation of normal pulmonary function measurements in the adult female. Am. Rev. Respir. Dis., 95:1061–1064, 1967.

54. Gandevia, B., and Hugh-Jones, P.: Terminology for measurements of ventilatory capacity. Thorax, 1:290–293, 1957.

55. Cotes, J.E.: Lung Function: Assessment and Application in Medicine. 3rd Ed. Oxford, Blackwell Scientific Publications, 1975, p. 104.

56. Miller, W.F., Johnson, R.L., Jr., and Wu, N.: Relationships between maximal breathing capacity and timed expiratory capacities. J. Appl. Physiol., 14:510–516, 1959.

57. Campbell, S.C.: A comparison of the maximum voluntary ventilation with forced expiratory volume in one second: an assessment of subject cooperation. J. Occup. Med., 24:531–533, 1982.

58. Bradley, P.W., and Younes, M.: Relation between respiratory valve dead space and tidal volume. J. Appl. Physiol., 49:528–532, 1980.

59. Jones, N.L., McHardy, G.J.R., Naimark, A., and Campbell, E.J.M.: Physiological dead space and alveolar-arterial gas pressure differences during exercise. Clin. Sci., 31:19–29, 1966.

60. Lifshay, A., Fast, C.W., and Glazier, J.B.: Effects of changes in respiratory pattern on physiological dead space. J. Appl. Physiol., 31:478–483, 1971.

61. Hey, E.N., Lloyd, B.B., Cunningham, D.J.C., Jukes, M.G.M., and Bolton, D.P.G.: Effects of various respiratory stimuli on the depth and frequency of breathing in man. Respir. Physiol., 1:193–205, 1966.

62. Spiro, S.C., Juniper, E., Bowman, P., and Edwards, R.H.T.: An increasing work rate test for assessing the physiological strain of submaximal exercise. Clin. Sci. Molec. Med., 46:191–206, 1974.

63. Cotes, J.E.: Lung Function: Assessment and Application in Medicine. 3rd Ed. Oxford, Blackwell Scientific Publications, 1975, p. 394.

64. Wasserman, K., VanKessel, A.L., and Burton, G.G.: Interaction of physiological mechanisms during exercise. J. Appl. Physiol., 22:71–85, 1967.

65. Bradley, C.A., Harris, E.A., Seelye, E.R., and Whitlock, R.M.L.: Gas exchange during exercise in healthy people. I. The physiological dead-space volume. Clin. Sci. Molec. Med., 51:323–333, 1976.

66. Whipp, B.J., and Wasserman, K.: Alveolar-arterial gas tension differences during graded exercise. J. Appl. Physiol., 27:361–365, 1969.

67. Ward, S.A., Wasserman, K., Davis, J.A., and Whipp, B.J.: Breathing-valve encumbrance and arterial blood gas and acid-base homeostasis during incremental exercise. Fed. Proc., 43:634, 1984 (Abstract).

68. Dempsey, J.A., Hanson, P.G., and Henderson, K.S.:. Exercise-induced arterial hypoxemia in healthy persons at sea level. J. Physiol. (Lond.), 355:161–175, 1984.

69. Lilienthal, J.L., Riley, R.L., Proemmel, D.D., and Franke, R.E.: An experimental analysis in man of the oxygen pressure gradient from alveolar air to arterial blood during rest and exercise at sea level and at altitude. Am. J. Physiol., 147:199–216, 1946.

70. Asmussen, E., and Nielsen, M.: Alveolo-arterial gas exchange at rest and during work at different O_2 tensions. Acta Physiol. Scand., 50:153–166, 1960.

71. Cruz, J.C., Hartley, L.H., and Vogel, J.A.: Effect of altitude relocations upon Aa_{DO_2} at rest and during exercise. J. Appl. Physiol., 39:469–474, 1975.

72. Hansen, J.E., Vogel, J.A., Stelter, G.P., and Consolazio, C.F.: Oxygen uptake in man during exhaustive work at sea level and high altitude. J. Appl. Physiol., 23:511–522, 1967.

73. Casaburi, R., Daly, J., Hansen, J.E., and Effros, R.M.: Abrupt changes in mixed venous blood gas compostition after the onset of exercise. J. Appl. Physiol., 67: 1106–1112, 1989.

74. Stringer, W.: Personal communication.

75. Beaver, W.L., Wasserman, K., and Whipp, B.J.: Bicarbonate buffering of lactic acid generated during exercise. J. Appl. Physiol., 60:472–478, 1986.

76. Yoshida, T., Nagata, A., Maro, M., Takeuchi, N., and Sada, Y.: The validity of anaerobic threshold determination by a Douglas bag method compared with arterial blood lactate concentration. Eur. J. Appl. Physiol., 46: 423–430, 1981.

Principles of Interpretation

CHAPTER 7

Introduction to Flow Charts

When patients complain of exercise intolerance, it is usually because they are unable to accomplish a task that they expect to complete with comparative ease and without unusual effort or undue feelings of fatigue or shortness of breath. Identifying the cause of this exercise intolerance is the major objective of integrative cardiopulmonary exercise testing.

The measurements needed for physiologic assessment are discussed in Chapter 3, and their patterns of change in response to the pathophysiology of specific diseases are described in Chapter 4. Once one has chosen the optimum exercise protocol (see Chap. 5) and has carefully selected the predicted values for the discriminating physiologic variables (see Chap. 6), the task of identifying the probable cause(s) of the exercise intolerance still remains. In this chapter, we show how the measurements made during exercise may be used in a systematic fashion to deduce pathophysiology. Although the analytic method presented here is not necessarily ideal in all instances, we have found a flow chart strategy, described in Figures 7–1 through 7–5, to be useful.

To facilitate the description of each decision based on physiologic measurements, each branchpoint is numbered on the flow charts. Furthermore, the symbol -R refers to the right branch of the numbered branchpoint and -L to the left branch of the numbered branchpoint. At the bottom of each flow chart are listed diagnoses along with additional variables that may lend support to each diagnosis.

Each branchpoint decision and the choice of which flow chart to use for data analysis should not be regarded as rigid. If the physiologic variable addressed at a particular branchpoint is not strongly in favor of one branch, or if confirmatory or supportive data are lacking, it might be helpful to consider both branches of a branchpoint. Similarly, if flow chart 3 or 4 (see Figs. 7–3 and 7–4) leads the clinician to a conclusion about pathophysiology that appears unwarranted or difficult to support, an alternative strategy may be to use flow chart 5 (see Fig. 7-5). The flow charts should be used with some degree of flexibility and always with consideration of sound physiologic principles.

Establishing the Pathophysiologic Basis of Exercise Intolerance

Maximum Exercise Capacity and Anaerobic Threshold (Flow Chart 1)

Analysis of data obtained during the exercise test begins on flow chart 1 (Fig. 7-1), which separates patients based on their measured maximum $\dot{V}O_2$ and anaerobic threshold (AT). Patients are divided into those with normal or reduced exercise capacity (normal or reduced maximum $\dot{V}O_2$) and those with reduced maximum exercise capacity into those with normal, reduced, or indeterminate AT. The analysis then proceeds to a separate flow chart (flow charts 2 to 5; see Figs. 7–2 to 7–5) for each of these groups.

Only a few conditions are associated with exercise intolerance and normal maximum $\dot{V}O_2$; these are considered in flow chart 2 (see Fig. 7-2). For those with a low maximum $\dot{V}O_2$, a normal AT suggests that O_2 flow at submaximal exercise levels is within normal limits and maximum exercise capacity is limited by one of a variety of other causes considered in flow chart 3 (see Fig. 7-3). The combination of both low maximum $\dot{V}O_2$ and AT leads to flow chart 4 (see Fig. 7-4), in which disorders that limit the capacity to transport oxygen are described. Finally, it is recognized that the AT may not always be determined; a diagnostic scheme for this circumstance is described in flow chart 5 (see Fig. 7-5).

Exercise Intolerance with Normal Maximum $\dot{V}O_2$ (Flow Chart 2)

When maximum $\dot{V}O_2$ is normal, but the patient complains of exercise intolerance, the diagnostic possibilities are described in Figure 7-2. They are: (1) a normal patient who is anxious about his or her condition and needs reassurance; (2) a person who had been fit but has recently developed a defect in the cardiovascular or respiratory system; or (3) an obese individual who, consequent to the abnormally high metabolic cost of work, has increased cardiovascular and respiratory stress during exercise and reduced ability to perform physical work. A normal maximum $\dot{V}O_2$ with a low AT is unusual, although this may be observed in a cardiac patient.

The measurements that confirm each of the diagnoses associated with a normal maximum

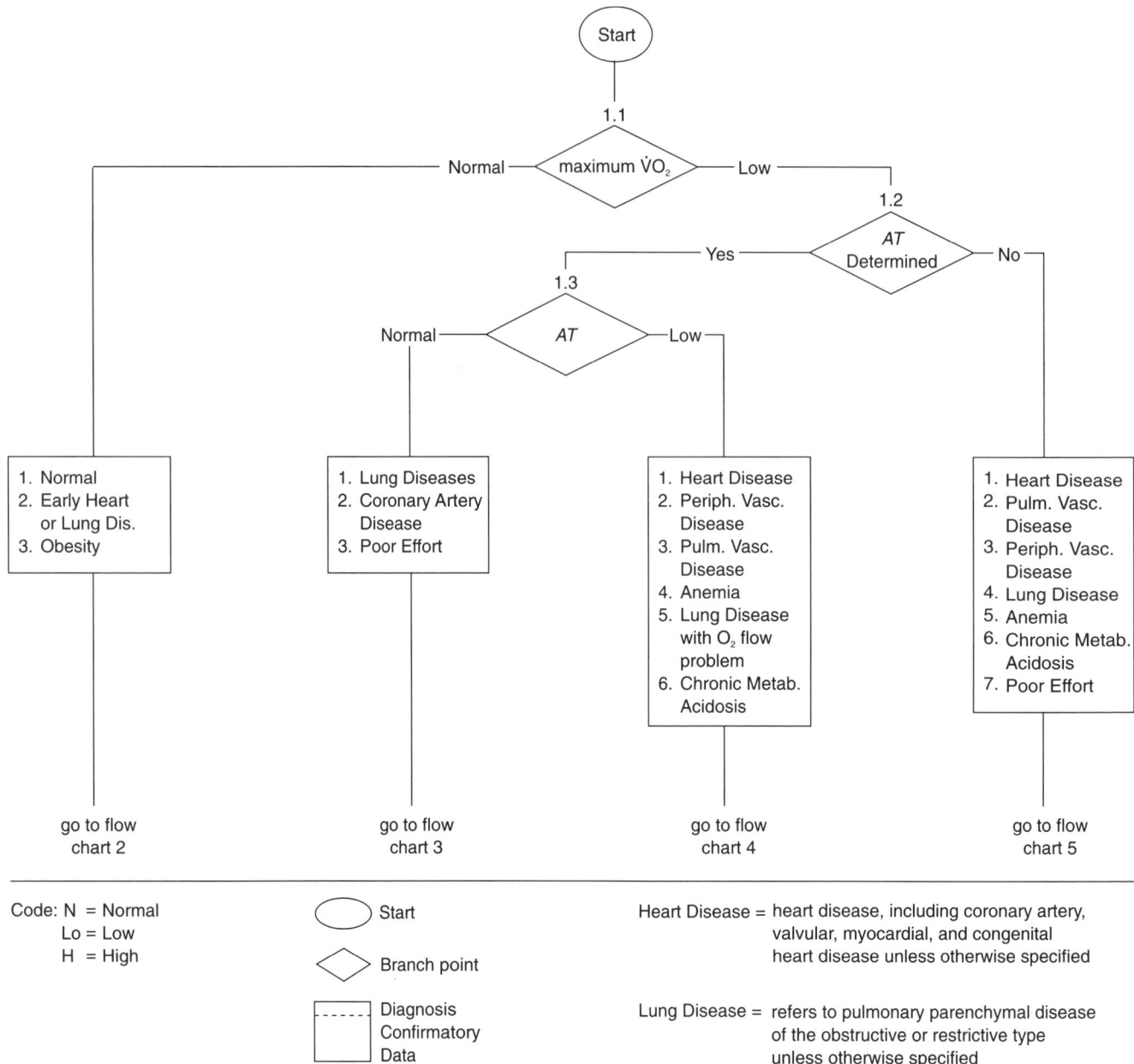

FIG. 7-1. Flow chart 1 for the differential diagnosis of the cause of exercise limitation. Analysis starts with the measurement of maximum $\dot{V}O_2$. Ellipsoids indicate starting points, diamonds indicate branchpoints, and boxes indicate diagnoses. Branchpoints are numbered to correspond to text. Measurements listed under diagnoses are used to confirm them. If the confirmatory information does not fit well, try a closely related branchpoint leading to a different diagnosis in which the confirmatory measurements fit better. The code shown at the bottom of this figure pertains to all five flow charts.

$\dot{V}O_2$ are described in the boxes in flow chart 2 (Fig. 7-2).

Normal with Anxiety State (2.1-L, 2.2-L)

People with this condition tend to be physically active and try to maintain their general state of health; otherwise, they would not be concerned. Therefore, their maximum $\dot{V}O_2$ is generally on the high side of normal, and they are not obese. If the exercise electrocardiogram, O_2 pulse, and arterial blood gases are normal at all work rates, including the maximum, the patient is probably normal. The breathing reserve is also normal, but it may be on the low side of normal if the subject has a maximum $\dot{V}O_2$ that is considerably better than the predicted normal value, i.e., the subject is in extremely good physical condition. A confirmatory measurement is a clearly normal *AT*. A patient with these findings would benefit from reassurance (see Cases 1 and 13 in Chap. 8).

Obesity (2.2-R)

Obese subjects require an increased metabolic rate ($\dot{V}O_2$ and $\dot{V}CO_2$) to perform a given physical activity compared to non-obese subjects. The increased metabolic rate results in increased cardiac output (cardiac output = $\dot{V}O_2/C(a-\bar{v})_{O_2}$) and minute ventilation ($\dot{V}E = \dot{V}CO_2/[(1 - V_D/V_T) \times (Pa_{CO_2}/P_B)]$) requirements compared to the non-obese subject

for a given level of work. When the obese individual is relatively young, the increased oxygen cost for work caused by the large body mass is tolerated generally well (see Case 15, Chap. 8). When the normal deteriorating effects of aging on maximal ventilatory capacity are combined with the extra ventilatory cost of moving the large body to perform work, however, a reduced breathing reserve results. In addition, because a higher cardiac output is needed to support the increased O_2 to perform work by the obese subject, the cardiac reserve is low. Although the *AT* expressed as a percentage of predicted maximum $\dot{V}O_2$, when ad-

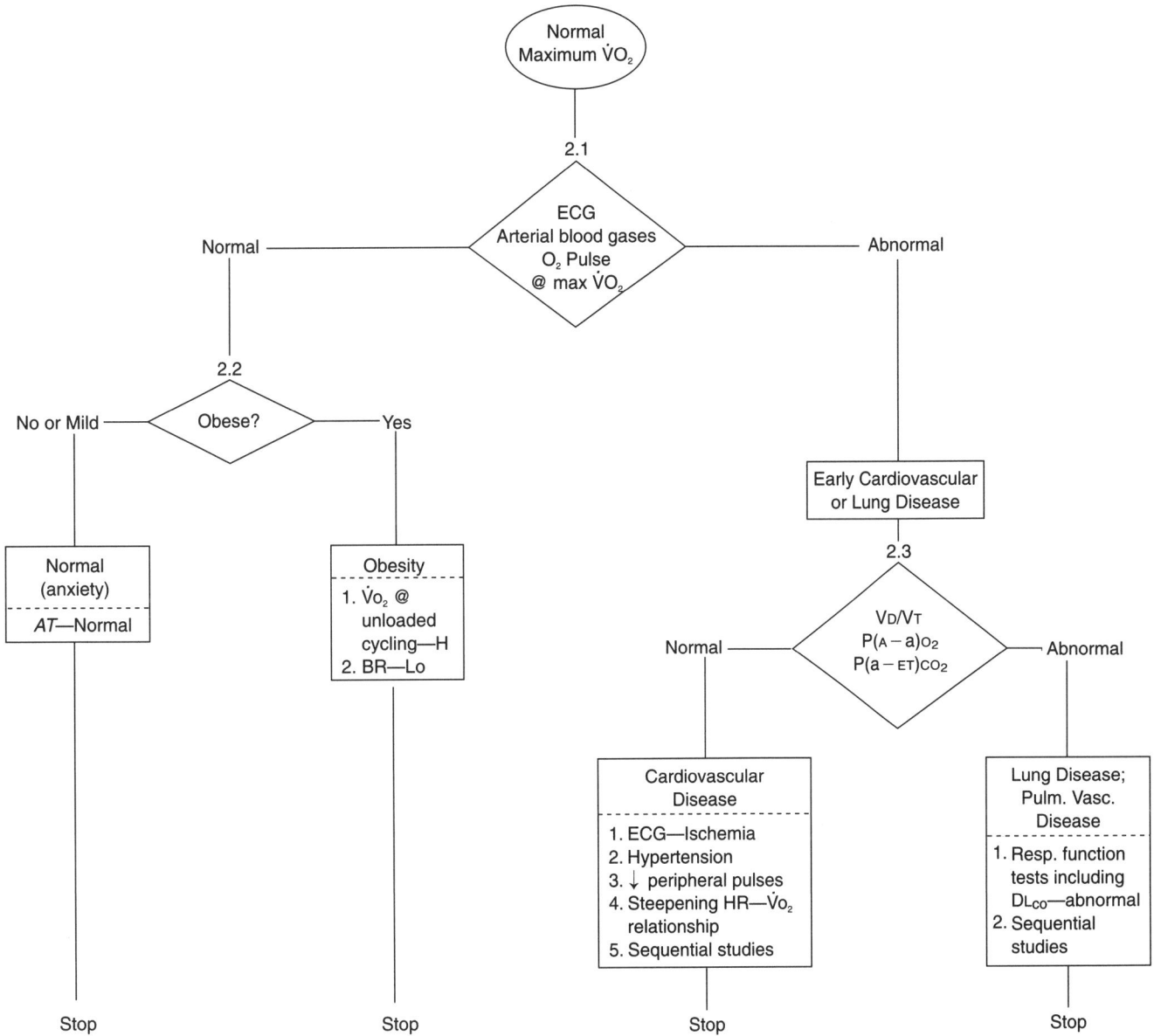

FIG. 7-2. Flow chart 2 for conditions in which maximum $\dot{V}O_2$ is normal but the patient feels limited during exercise. If the confirmatory information does not fit well, try a closely related branchpoint leading to a different diagnosis in which the confirmatory measurements fit better. Symbols and flow chart method are as described in "Introduction to Flow Charts" and Figure 7-1.

justed for height or lean body mass, is normal, the O_2 cost of walking may be too great to perform this activity without developing a metabolic acidosis. The patient's heart rate reserve is normal at maximum exercise, although the breathing reserve is usually reduced because of ventilatory restriction and increased ventilatory requirement.

Early Cardiovascular or Lung Disease (2.1-R, 2.3)

In early mild cardiovascular or lung disease, the disorder may not be severe enough to cause the maximum $\dot{V}O_2$ to be less than predicted. Specific physiologic variables may become abnormal, however, depending on the site of the defect in the metabolic-cardiovascular-ventilatory coupling. Thus, a patient may have a maximum $\dot{V}O_2$ value that falls in the normal range and yet still have a mild abnormality of the heart or lungs, perhaps only recently developed. It may be difficult to document such a developing abnormality except by sequential studies demonstrating a decline in the maximum $\dot{V}O_2$ or AT. A frequent problem of the middle-aged adult is coronary artery disease; therefore, examination of the electrocardiogram (ECG) along with gas exchange measurements that relate the increase in $\dot{V}O_2$ and $\dot{V}CO_2$ to the increase in work rate is helpful. The former provides evidence of myocardial ischemia, and the latter demonstrates whether accompanying ventricular dyskinesis is present. Moreover, the relationship between heart rate and $\dot{V}O_2$ helps to document that linearity is maintained up to the maximum value; a faster rise in heart rate than $\dot{V}O_2$ toward the end of exercise may be an indicator of heart disease. Similarly, flattening of the O_2 pulse at submaximal exercise levels also suggests the presence of heart disease. These changes, associated with evidence of myocardial ischemia on the ECG, make a strong case for the diagnosis of coronary artery disease (2.3-L) (see Case 18, Chap. 8).

Measuring arterial blood gases during incremental exercise testing is also important to determine the V_D/V_T, $P(a\text{-}ET)_{CO_2}$, and $P(A\text{-}a)_{O_2}$ in patients in this category (see Case 46, Chap. 8). Normal values generally rule out mild or developing pulmonary vascular, lung parenchymal, or airway diseases, because these measurements are usually abnormal in these pulmonary conditions (2.3-R).

Low Maximum $\dot{V}O_2$ with Normal AT (Flow Chart 3)

The breathing reserve provides a good first branchpoint for the differential diagnosis of disorders initially characterized by a low maximum $\dot{V}O_2$ and a normal AT (3.1; Fig. 7-3). Patients with a normal or high breathing reserve (3.1-R) include those making a poor effort, those who are limited by muscular and skeletal diseases, or those with coronary artery disease with or without chest pain at relatively low work rates. A low breathing reserve (3.1-L) identifies those patients with lung diseases.

Normal or High Breathing Reserve (3.1-R)

Poor Effort or Low Cardiorespiratory Stress (3.3-L). Perhaps for secondary gain, the subject may make a poor effort and may thereby have a low maximum $\dot{V}O_2$ during exercise testing. Both the breathing reserve and heart rate reserve are high, indicating that the patient has not used the full potential of either the cardiovascular or the ventilatory system. The absence of metabolic acidosis at the end of exercise is also evidence of poor effort. Additional confirmatory features include normal exercise V_D/V_T, $P(A\text{-}a)_{O_2}$, and $P(a\text{-}ET)_{CO_2}$, demonstrating that the distribution of ventilation relative to perfusion is uniform, virtually ruling out primary lung or pulmonary vascular disease (see Cases 65 to 67, Chap. 8).

Low cardiorespiratory stress is also found in conditions associated with musculoskeletal pain or weakness. Optimal cardiovascular and pulmonary evaluation is impossible when exercise is limited by arthritis or neuromuscular diseases, but this information is, of course, not without value if previously unsuspected as a cause of exercise limitation (see Cases 68 to 70, Chap. 8).

Myocardial Ischemia (3.3-R). The 12-lead ECG generally becomes abnormal when the myocardium becomes ischemic as the work rate is increased to the patient's symptom-limited maximum. The ECG abnormality may be evident only at high work rates, and the patient may or may not experience chest pain. Whereas coronary artery disease is the most frequent cause of myocardial ischemia, it may also occur in aortic valve disease or marked systemic hypertension, with or without coronary artery disease (see Cases 21 and 33, Chap. 8). The ECG may be normal in patients with posterior myocardial ischemia, but when myocardial ischemia develops, the $\dot{V}O_2$ commonly fails to increase normally as the work rate is increased (see Cases 18 and 22, Chap. 8).

Low Breathing Reserve (3.1-L)

Low breathing reserve suggests lung disease. The breathing frequency may be a useful next

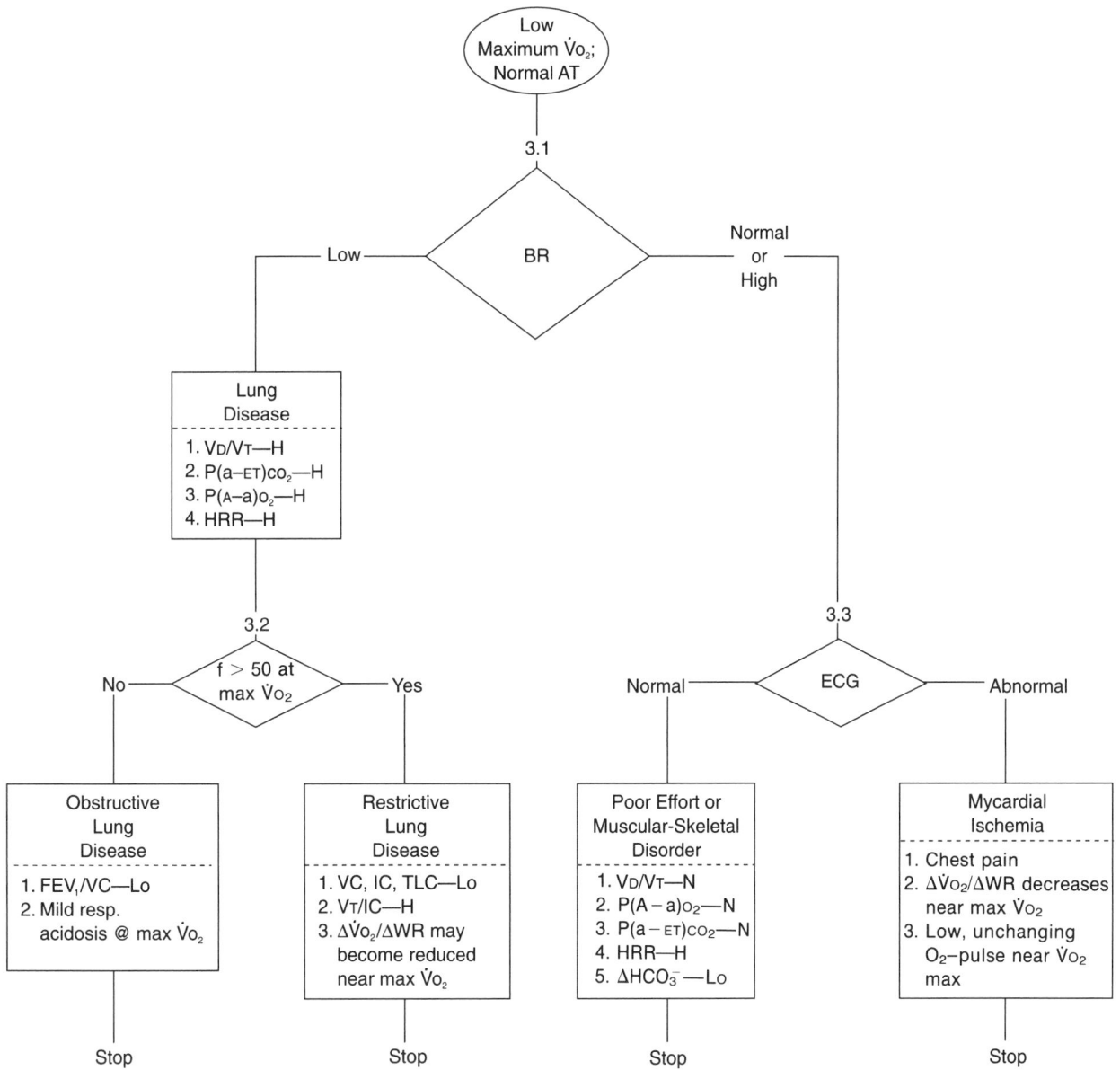

FIG. 7-3. Flow chart 3 for conditions in which maximum $\dot{V}_{O_2}$ is low but the anaerobic threshold (*AT*) is normal. If the confirmatory information does not fit well, try a closely related branchpoint leading to a different diagnosis in which the confirmatory measurements fit better. Symbols and flow chart method are as described in "Introduction to Flow Charts" and Figure 7-1.

branchpoint to distinguish obstructive from restrictive lung disease. The confirmatory data listed under each should also be noted, however. If the confirmatory data do not support the diagnosis well, the alternate branch should be tried, or a mixed disorder considered.

Obstructive Lung Diseases (3.2-L). Although the maximum $\dot{V}_{O_2}$ achieved during incremental exercise testing is low in this disorder, the *AT* is often normal. This finding suggests that the patient does not have a problem with oxygen transport to the tissues at these submaximal work rates (see Case 37, Chap. 8). Characteristically, these patients

have abnormalities in Pa_{O_2}, V_D/V_T, $P(a\text{-}ET)_{CO_2}$, and $P(A\text{-}a)_{O_2}$ during exercise consequent to ventilation-perfusion mismatching. Decreases in Pa_{O_2} commonly occur in a single step at low work rates with little further change as the work rate is increased (see Fig. 4-5). This is probably because the increased perfusion during exercise goes predominantly to normal and high $\dot{V}_A/\dot{Q}$ regions of the lungs. Except in mild obstructive disease, the breathing reserve is decreased because of the ventilatory limitation. In contrast to O_2 flow limiting disorders, however, the $\dot{V}_{O_2}$ continues to increase linearly as the work rate is increased to the patient's maximum $\dot{V}O_2$; i.e., no decrease in $\Delta\dot{V}O_2/\Delta WR$ occurs as the maximum $\dot{V}O_2$ is approached. The heart rate reserve is commonly increased because the cardiovascular capacity cannot be fully challenged as a result of the breathing limitation. Finally, expiratory flow frequently has an obstructive pattern (trapezoidal in appearance, with an early peak, as illustrated in Figure 3-28).

In patients with marked airflow obstruction, the *AT* needs to be determined by the V-slope method rather than methods that rely on the increase in ventilatory equivalent for O_2. Although CO_2 output will increase when HCO_3^- buffers lactic acid, the ventilatory response to the increased CO_2 load from buffering is often poor in these patients, and the ventilatory equivalent of O_2 does not increase measurably at the *AT* (see Cases 40 and 42, Chap. 8).

Restrictive Lung Diseases (3.2-R). Pathophysiologic responses seen in restrictive lung diseases have much in common with those of the obstructive lung diseases, but clear differences exist. The V_D/V_T and $P(a-ET)_{CO_2}$ are increased in both types of lung disorders as reflections of ventilation-perfusion mismatching. In contrast to obstructive lung diseases, however, the $P(A-a)_{O_2}$ usually increases systematically at each work rate during the incremental test. Moreoever, the V_T increases to its maximum at a relatively low work rate, and the V_T/IC ratio nears a value of one. Because V_T cannot increase normally in those with restrictive lung diseases, the ventilatory response to the increasing work rate is achieved primarily by increasing the breathing frequency, usually exceeding 50 breaths/min. Patients with restrictive lung diseases often manifest an O_2 flow problem (see Cases 49 to 53, Chap. 8). In this situation, $\dot{V}O_2$ fails to increase normally as the work rate is incremented to the patient's maximum. This may be caused both by the low arterial O_2 content and by the increased pulmonary vascular resistance (resulting from destruction of pulmonary blood vessels by the fibrosing process) that limits the cardiac output increase. Thus, these patients are classified with those with low maximum $\dot{V}O_2$ and low *AT* and will be analyzed in flow chart 4 (see Fig. 7-4).

LOW MAXIMUM $\dot{V}O_2$ WITH LOW *AT* (FLOW CHART 4)

The breathing reserve serves as a good primary branchpoint (4.1) for the differential diagnosis of disorders having a low maximum $\dot{V}O_2$ and low *AT*, as shown in flow chart 4 (Fig. 7-4, but further branching is needed to distinguish among the various conditions in this category. The V_D/V_T is a good second branchpoint (4.2) for the conditions that have a low breathing reserve; $\dot{V}E/\dot{V}CO_2$ at the *AT* is a useful second branchpoint (4.3) for the conditions with a normal or high breathing reserve.

Normal or High Breathing Reserve (4.1-R)

Normal $\dot{V}E/\dot{V}CO_2$ at **AT** *(4.3-L).* If the breathing reserve is normal or high and the $\dot{V}E/\dot{V}CO_2$ at *AT* is normal (4.3-L), then we must consider O_2 flow problems caused by nonpulmonary diseases such as heart disease, peripheral vascular disease, and anemia or hemoglobinopathy. Hematocrit (4.4) and O_2 pulse ($\dot{V}O_2/HR$) (4.6) are further branchpoints that distinguish these diagnoses.

HEART DISEASES (4.6-R). Patients with primary heart diseases (coronary artery disease, valvular heart disease, and cardiomyopathy) usually have a low maximum $\dot{V}O_2$ with a low *AT*. In these disorders, $\dot{V}O_2$ usually slows its rate of rise relative to the work rate as the maximum $\dot{V}O_2$ is approached (see Cases 16 to 28, Chap. 8). The heart rate often continues to increase as the work rate is increased despite the slower increase of $\dot{V}O_2$. This results in a steepening of the heart rate-$\dot{V}O_2$ relationship as the work rate is increased and a plateau of the O_2 pulse at subnormal values (see Fig. 3-10). In coronary artery disease, the ECG during exercise usually provides evidence of myocardial ischemia (see Table 3-3).

Patients with heart failure secondary to valvular heart diseases or cardiomyopathies may have a chronic metabolic acidosis, maintaining arterial P_{CO_2} and bicarbonate at relatively low values with a normal pH. An acute metabolic acidosis is superimposed during exercise. In rare instances, V_D/V_T may be elevated because of ventilation-perfusion mismatching. These acid-base changes and the increased V_D/V_T presumably contribute to the symptom of dyspnea.

PERIPHERAL VASCULAR DISEASE (4.6-L). In contrast to primary heart diseases, the heart rate reserve is generally high in this condition since the patient stops exercising because of claudication before the heart can be maximally stressed. Because of the failure of normal systemic vasodilatation during exercise, hypertension often develops beyond that expected with exercise. The increase in oxy-

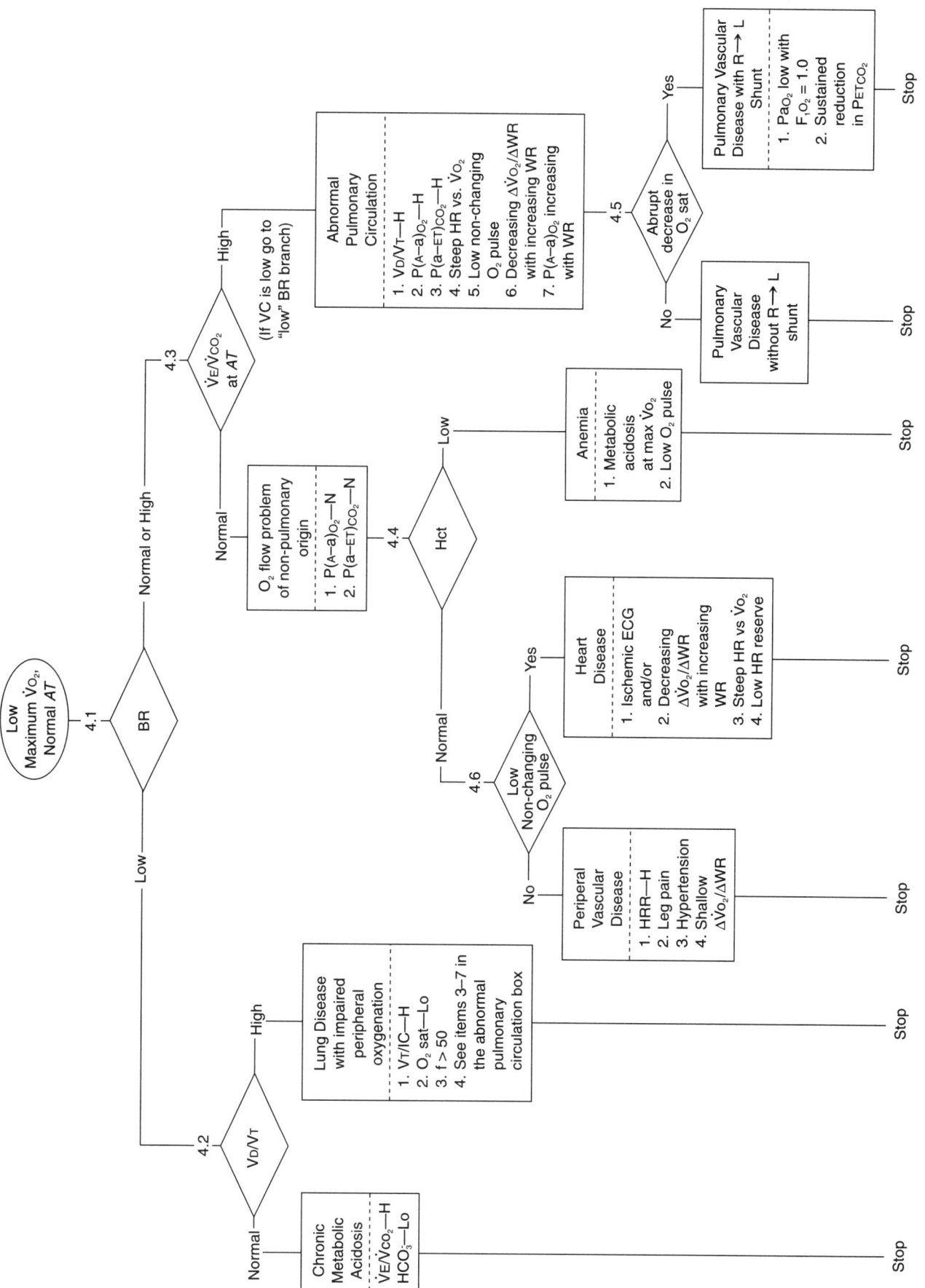

FIG. 7-4. Flow chart 4 for conditions in which maximum V̇O₂ is low and the anaerobic threshold (AT) is low. If the confirmatory information does not fit well, try a closely related branchpoint leading to a different diagnosis in which the confirmatory measurements fit better. Symbols and flow chart method are as described in "Introduction to Flow Charts" and Figure 7-1.

gen uptake relative to the increase in work rate may be diminished, resulting in a relatively shallow slope for the $\dot{V}O_2$-work rate relationship (low $\Delta\dot{V}O_2/\Delta WR$). Finally, in the absence of concomitant lung disease, measurements of VD/VT, $P(a\text{-}ET)CO_2$, and $P(A\text{-}a)O_2$, which reflect the distribution of ventilation relative to perfusion, are normal (see Cases 30 and 31, Chap. 8).

ANEMIA (4.4-R). Because of the reduced O_2 carrying capacity of the blood, lactic acidosis occurs at a relatively low work rate, causing the *AT* to be reduced. The low oxygen content of the arterial blood caused by the anemia results in decreased $C(a\text{-}\bar{v})O_2$. Thus, a high cardiac output and heart rate are required to meet the tissue O_2 requirement. The maximal O_2 pulse is reduced, reflecting the decreased $C(a\text{-}\bar{v})O_2$. The arterial blood gas tensions and the VD/VT are normal, even at maximal exercise (see Case 76, Chap. 8).

High $\dot{V}E/\dot{V}CO_2$ at **AT** *(4.3-R).* If the breathing reserve is normal or high (4.1-R) but the $\dot{V}E/\dot{V}CO_2$ at *AT* is high (4.3-R), then the most likely primary disorder is an abnormal pulmonary circulation with or without a right to left intracardiac shunt. The pattern of change in O_2 saturation (branchpoint 4.5) in response to exercise helps to distinguish these conditions.

PULMONARY VASCULAR DISEASES (4.5-L). In this category, we include those disorders that originate in the pulmonary vascular bed and cause pulmonary vascular resistance to be increased, e.g., pulmonary thromboembolic disease, primary pulmonary hypertension, and diseases that cause a pulmonary vasculitis. These disorders, when chronic, have little effect on pulmonary mechanics, but they cause abnormalities of lung gas exchange as well as limit the cardiac output increase in response to exercise.

If the pulmonary circulation, interposed between the right and left sides of the heart, does not dilate normally during exercise, the increased venous return that accompanies exercise cannot be readily transmitted to the left ventricle. When the right side of the heart cannot "feed" blood to the left side at a rate commensurate with that required for normal exercise, cardiac output cannot respond appropriately to the exercise stimulus. Because the cardiac output increase is limited, the $\dot{V}O_2$ increase relative to increase in work rate may slow at an abnormally low work rate during an incremental exercise test, resulting in a low maximal $\dot{V}O_2$. We have also noted that heart rate

increases steeply relative to $\dot{V}O_2$ and gets steeper as the maximal $\dot{V}O_2$ is approached. Thus, the O_2 pulse is reduced at maximum work and fails to increase as the work rate is increased. These findings are similar to those seen in many patients with primary heart disease.

Unlike in uncomplicated heart disease, however, these patients have high VD/VT and positive $P(a\text{-}ET)CO_2$ values. These provide evidence of poor perfusion of ventilated air spaces. Moreover, the $P(A\text{-}a)O_2$ increases abnormally as the work rate is increased, probably because of the shortened red cell transit time described in Chapter 4, as a result of the reduced capillary bed. Although these changes are similar to those seen in primary lung diseases, other measurements made during exercise distinguish these particular disorders. For instance, the breathing reserve is usually normal. In addition, rather than the mild respiratory acidosis that commonly accompanies obstructive lung diseases, metabolic acidosis develops with pulmonary vascular diseases in response to exercise.

Primary lung diseases can cause major disturbances in function of the pulmonary circulation, and the abnormal pulmonary circulation may become the dominant pathophysiologic feature limiting exercise (see Cases 41, 44, and 53, Chap. 8). In such instances, the abnormalities noted in the "abnormal pulmonary circulation" diagnostic box of flow chart 4 (Fig. 7-4) become evident during exercise testing. They cannot, however, be reliably predicted from resting measurements.

PULMONARY VASCULAR DISEASE WITH A RIGHT TO LEFT SHUNT OR CYANOTIC CONGENITAL HEART DISEASE (4.5-R). Patients with pulmonary vascular disease who open a potentially patent foramen ovale, or have congenital heart disease with a right to left shunt, may demonstrate marked reductions in arterial PO_2 during air and O_2 breathing in response to exercise (see Case 51, Chap. 8). The VD/VT, $P(a\text{-}ET)CO_2$, and $P(A\text{-}a)O_2$ values become extremely abnormal in response to exercise, depending on the degree of pulmonary hypoperfusion and the size of the shunt. These values generally increase as the work rate is increased. Patients with these disorders can be distinguished from those with other pulmonary vascular diseases by an abrupt and sustained decrease in arterial O_2 saturation and PET_{CO_2} as soon as exercise begins. $\Delta\dot{V}O_2/\Delta WR$ is reduced, and $\dot{V}CO_2$ may exceed $\dot{V}O_2$ during the first few minutes of exercise even at the lowest work rates.

Repeating the exercise test while the patient

breathes 100% O_2 is particularly helpful in distinguishing a right to left shunt from other causes of hypoxemia. If a right to left shunt exists, Pa_{O_2} falls precipitously while the patient breathes 100% O_2, and the $P(A-a)_{O_2}$ increases markedly as the venous return shunts from right to left. It can be calculated that the arterial Pa_{O_2} will decrease by approximately 100 mm Hg while the patient breathes O_2 when 3 to 5% of the venous return shunts from right to left.

Low Breathing Reserve (4.1-L)

In the category of patients with a low maximum $\dot{V}_{O_2}$ and low AT accompanied by a low breathing reserve and high V_D/V_T (4.2-R), the most likely disorder is a primary lung disease such as pulmonary fibrosis. In contrast, a low breathing reserve with a normal V_D/V_T in this category can be caused by diseases associated with chronic metabolic acidosis and hyperventilation (4.2-L). The following discussion describes further physiologic measurements that help confirm the diagnosis of each of these disorders.

Lung Disease with Impaired Peripheral Oxygenation (4.2-R). In certain patients, primarily those with severe interstitial lung disease in which the pulmonary circulation is also markedly impaired, and where there may be (not necessarily) considerable O_2 desaturation as the subject exercises, the AT and the maximum $\dot{V}_{O_2}$ are reduced. Moreover, the slope of the $\dot{V}_{O_2}$-work rate relationship may be reduced as the work rate is increased. Other abnormalities in pulmonary gas exchange characteristic of restrictive lung disease are present as described in the earlier section of this chapter on restrictive lung diseases (see Cases 51 and 53, Chap. 8).

Chronic Metabolic Acidosis (4.2-L). Patients with chronic heart failure, diabetes mellitus, renal failure, and those taking medications causing a metabolic acidosis (e.g., acetazolamide) may have a chronic metabolic acidosis. Because Pa_{CO_2} is reduced in these conditions (low Pa_{CO_2} set-point), exercise alveolar and minute ventilation are elevated; i.e., a higher than normal alveolar ventilation is needed to clear the increased metabolic CO_2 generated during exercise (see Fig. 2-31). This reduces the breathing reserve and causes the ventilatory equivalents for CO_2 and O_2 to be increased. Because of the high ventilation requirement, these patients may experience exertional dyspnea before reaching their predicted maximum $\dot{V}_{O_2}$, particularly if they have lung or heart disease, anemia, or obesity. The AT may be reduced because of their underlying disease process. The chronic metabolic acidosis is easily identified from arterial blood gas and pH measurements.

LOW MAXIMUM $\dot{V}_{O_2}$ WITH AT NOT DETERMINED (FLOW CHART 5)

The AT may not be measured during a test, or it may be too difficult to determine reliably. The latter usually results because of an irregular breathing pattern or because the AT occurs at such a low work rate that the dynamics of gas exchange at the start of exercise blur the changes in gas exchange at the AT. If it is particularly important to know the patient's AT, it can be ascertained by doing several constant work rate tests and measuring the increase in $\dot{V}_{O_2}$ from 3 to 6 minutes (see Fig. 3-23) or by measuring lactate in the arterial blood.

An alternative strategy to using the AT as the second major branchpoint (1.2) in the decision-making process shown in flow chart 1 is described in flow chart 5 (Fig. 7-5). Using flow chart 5 in patients with a low maximum $\dot{V}_{O_2}$, we next consider tests that detect mismatching of ventilation to perfusion. This allows us to distinguish disorders associated with inefficiency of lung gas exchange from disorders with normal lung function and pulmonary circulation but limited ability to increase O_2 flow to the tissues. Thus, branchpoint 5.1 requires simultaneous arterial blood gas and pulmonary gas exchange information. As shown in flow chart 5 (Fig. 7-5), if V_D/V_T, $P(a-ET)_{CO_2}$, and $P(A-a)_{O_2}$ values are normal (5.1-L), we examine the heart rate reserve (HRR) (5.2); if V_D/V_T, $P(a-ET)_{CO_2}$, and $P(A-a)_{O_2}$ values are abnormal (5.1-R), we examine the breathing reserve (5.3) in the decision-making process. The possible diagnoses at each of these branchpoints separate into two major groups, depending on whether the heart rate reserve is normal or high or the breathing reserve is normal or low. The next level of branching allows specific diagnoses to be made.

Whereas the first step in flow chart 5 (5.1) depends on knowledge of arterial P_{CO_2} and P_{O_2}, it may not be feasible to collect arterial blood under some circumstances. An alternative is to approximate Pa_{CO_2} from venous blood drawn from a superficial vein of a warmed hand or from capillary blood from a finger or ear lobe and, from these

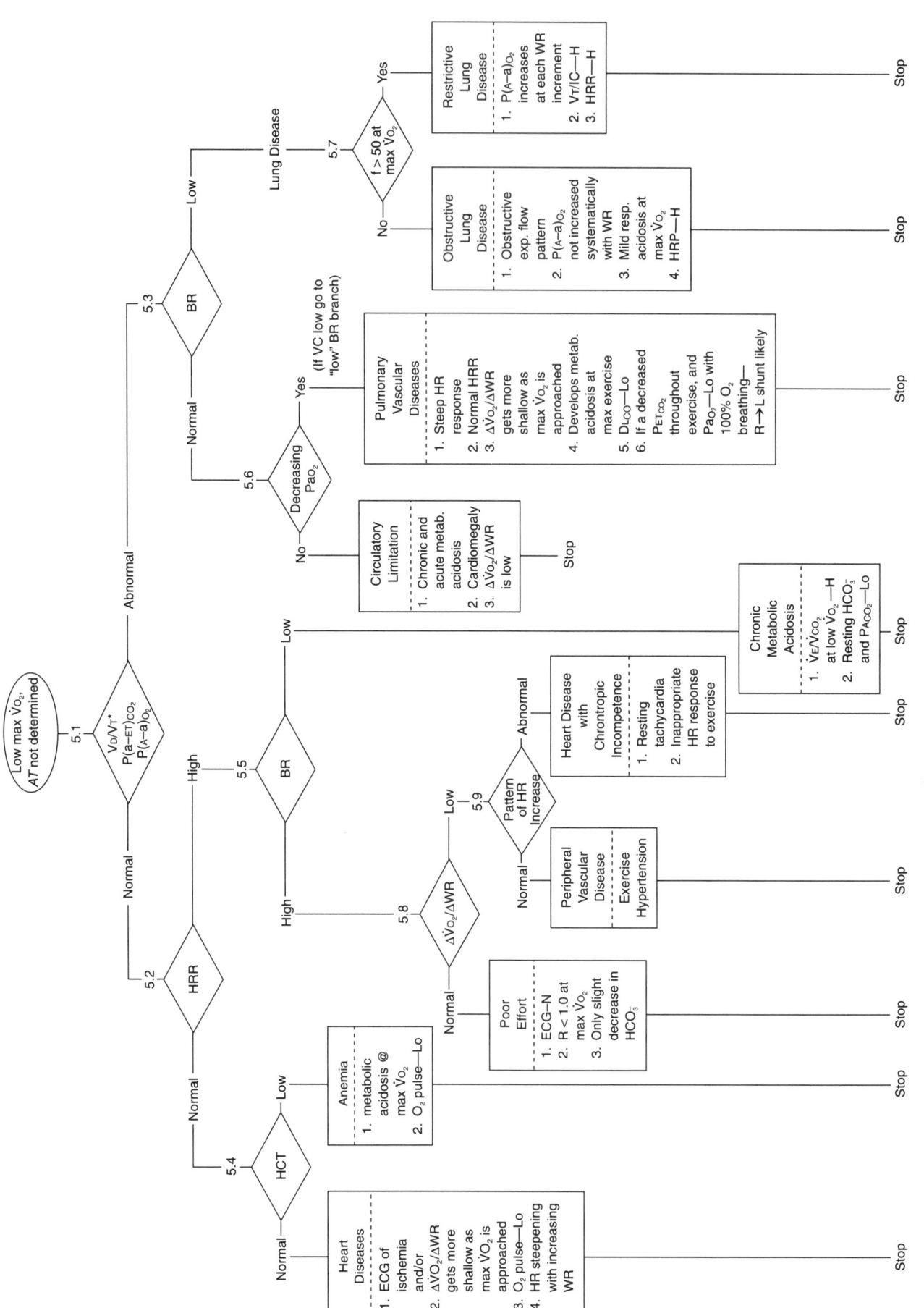

Fig. 7-5. Flow chart 5 for conditions in which maximum $\dot{V}O_2$ is low but the anaerobic threshold (AT) has not been measured or cannot be reliably determined. If the confirmatory information does not fit well, try a closely related branchpoint leading to a different diagnosis in which the confirmatory measurements fit better. Symbols and flow chart method are as described in "Introduction to Flow Charts" and Figure 7-1.

measurements, to estimate V_D/V_T and $P(a\text{-}ET)_{CO_2}$.* Normal values would direct the analysis to the left (5.1-L), and abnormal values would direct the analysis to the right (5.1-R).

Normal Distribution of Ventilation-perfusion (5.1-L)

Heart disease, anemia, poor effort, peripheral vascular disease, and chronic metabolic acidosis are all associated with a low maximum $\dot{V}_{O_2}$, but they have normal indices of gas exchange efficiency (uniform $\dot{V}_A/\dot{Q}$). The HRR allows this group to be further subdivided into those with a normal HRR (5.2-L) (heart disease and anemia) and a high HRR (5.2-R) (poor effort, peripheral vascular disease, and chronic metabolic acidosis).

The two disorders with a low maximum $\dot{V}_{O_2}$, uniform $\dot{V}_A/\dot{Q}$, and normal HRR (5.2-L) are heart diseases (ischemic, valvular, cardiomyopathic, or non-cyanotic congenital) and anemia. They can be distinguished on the basis of the hematocrit (5.4), and the diagnosis can be confirmed by examining the measurements listed in the diagnostic boxes for these categories.

Poor effort, peripheral vascular disease, or chronic metabolic acidosis can cause a low maximum $\dot{V}_{O_2}$, uniform $\dot{V}_A/\dot{Q}$, and high HRR (5.2-R). A chronic metabolic acidosis is often associated with a low breathing reserve (5.5-R), especially when accompanied by a cardiorespiratory disorder. A poor effort can be confirmed by other measurements, including a high breathing reserve (5.5-L), failure to develop a significant metabolic acidosis at end-exercise, an R < 1.0 at the maximum $\dot{V}_{O_2}$, and a normal ECG.

The low $\Delta\dot{V}_{O_2}/\Delta WR$ value (5.8-R) also distinguishes peripheral vascular disease and patients with primary heart disease accompanied by pacemaker incompetency from those subjects making a poor effort. The measurements listed in the respective diagnostic boxes confirm these diagnoses.

Non-uniform Distribution of Ventilation to Perfusion (5.1-R)

Chronic heart failure, pulmonary vascular diseases, and obstructive and restrictive lung dis-

eases are all associated with a low maximum $\dot{V}_{O_2}$ and abnormal indices of gas exchange efficiency (non-uniform $\dot{V}_A/\dot{Q}$). The breathing reserve (5.3) allows this group to be further subdivided into those with a normal breathing reserve (heart failure and pulmonary vascular diseases) and those with a low breathing reserve (obstructive and restrictive lung diseases).

The two disorders with a low maximum $\dot{V}_{O_2}$ and a non-uniform $\dot{V}_A/\dot{Q}$, but a normal breathing reserve (5.3-L), can usually be distinguished by the Pa_{O_2} or arterial O_2 saturation (5.6) measurement. The patient with pulmonary vascular disease without a right to left shunt generally has a mildly reduced Pa_{O_2} or arterial O_2 saturation at rest that decreases progressively as the work rate increases (5.6-R). If the pulmonary vascular disease is accompanied by a right to left shunt, such as in cyanotic congenital heart disease or the opening of an unsealed foramen ovale, then the decrement in O_2 saturation at the start of exercise will be marked. Item 6 in the diagnostic box for pulmonary vascular diseases describes simple measurements that can support the development of a right to left shunt during exercise (Fig. 7-5).

The patient with chronic heart failure will have a normal or only a slightly reduced O_2 saturation at rest that remains largely unaffected by exercise (5.6-L). The box identifying this diagnosis lists confirmatory measurements.

The two lung disorders with a low maximum $\dot{V}_{O_2}$ and a non-uniform $\dot{V}_A/\dot{Q}$, but with a low breathing reserve (5.3-R), can generally be distinguished by the breathing frequency and supported by the measurements listed in the respective diagnostic boxes for obstructive and restrictive lung disease. A breathing frequency > 50 at the patient's maximum $\dot{V}_{O_2}$ is commonly associated with restrictive lung disease (5.7-R), whereas a breathing frequency < 50 at the maximum $\dot{V}_{O_2}$ is characteristic of the patient with obstructive lung disease (5.7-L). The distinction is more simply made with standard pulmonary function measurements, however.

Interpretation of Constant Work Rate Tests

Whereas the foregoing analyses use measurements obtained from incremental exercise tests, certain information can best be obtained from constant work rate tests. For example, it is possible to evaluate the role of the carotid bodies in the

---

* A noninvasive, although less satisfactory, alternative is to examine $\dot{V}_E/\dot{V}_{CO_2}$ and $\dot{V}_E/\dot{V}_{O_2}$ values at moderate work rates. If these values are normal, $\dot{V}_A/\dot{Q}$ disturbances are unlikely, but normal values may be obtained when hypoventilation offsets the increase that would be caused by an elevated V_D/V_T. If the $\dot{V}_E/\dot{V}_{CO_2}$ and $\dot{V}_E/\dot{V}_{O_2}$ are elevated, $\dot{V}_A/\dot{Q}$ disturbances are likely, but alveolar hyperventilation must be excluded as the cause. For this, an estimate of arterial P_{CO_2} from capillary blood is helpful.

exercise hyperpnea by surreptitiously switching the inspired gas from air to 100% oxygen during steady-state exercise (see Fig. 3-29). One notes a decrease in ventilation within two breaths or so as arterial blood with a high P_{O_2} reaches the carotid bodies. The maximum decrement in ventilation can be measured by monitoring ventilation on a breath-by-breath basis. The proportional decrease in ventilation is the minimum contribution of the carotid bodies to ventilatory drive. The consequent increase in Pa_{CO_2}, as the ventilation falls, leads to chemoreceptor stimulation and offsets some of the carotid body inhibition induced by hyperoxia.

Constant work exercise of moderately severe intensity can also be used to identify exercise-induced bronchospasm (see Chap. 5) by comparing indices of airflow obstruction during the first 20 minutes of recovery with those before exercise. Normally, the FEV_1 is unchanged or increased after exercise, but reductions in FEV_1 of 10% or greater accompany exercise-induced asthma.

Constant work rate tests can also be used to determine the magnitude of the cardiac output increase at the start of exercise (Phase I). After the first 15 seconds of exercise, the time constant (time to reach 63% of steady-state) for $\dot{V}_{O_2}$ kinetics (Phase II) can be used to estimate the effectiveness of cardiovascular transport of O_2 to the metabolically active muscles. If O_2 transport is adequate to meet the O_2 requirement, the time constant for $\dot{V}_{O_2}$ will be about 30 seconds, and $\dot{V}_{O_2}$ will be in a steady-state by 3 minutes. If the work is above the AT, however, the $\dot{V}_{O_2}$ kinetics will be slowed, with $\dot{V}_{O_2}$ not reaching a steady-state by 3 minutes, and $\dot{V}_{CO_2}$ will exceed $\dot{V}_{O_2}$ (see Fig. 1-2). The difference between the 6- and the 3-minute $\dot{V}_{O_2}$ is quantitatively related to the increase in lactate. This is associated with an increase in $\dot{V}_{CO_2}$ caused by the CO_2 released from HCO_3^- as it buffers newly formed lactic acid (see Chap. 3). Thus, constant work rate tests are valuable in assessing cardiovascular and metabolic function.

Summary

To determine the likely pathophysiologic causes of exercise limitation, we have found that a logical approach can be expressed in a series of five flow charts (see Figs. 7–1 to 7–5). Physiologic measurements relating heart rate, ventilation, and gas exchange to work rate are used in the decision-making process. The first flow chart (see Fig. 7-1) separates four major categories of patients: (1) those with a normal maximum $\dot{V}_{O_2}$; (2) those with a reduced maximum $\dot{V}_{O_2}$ but with a normal AT; (3) those with a reduced maximum $\dot{V}_{O_2}$ but with a reduced AT; and (4) those with a reduced maximum $\dot{V}_{O_2}$ but with the AT not determined. Flow charts 2 to 5 analyze these four categories further (see Figs. 7–2 to 7–5), usually allowing a specific organ-related physiologic diagnosis to be made. The flow charts are designed only as guides to an orderly decision-making process, however. The final judgment must be made by the examiner.

Case Presentations

W E SELECTED THE cases presented in this section because they are either representative of specific pathophysiology or they teach a unique lesson. They were not selected because they show data from especially cooperative subjects or are pretty records. In fact, these studies were done on typical patients evaluated in our clinical exercise laboratory and therefore include records that range between the best and the worst with respect to appearance. The primary goal of this chapter is to offer a systematic approach to interpretation of exercise performance. We demonstrate how measurements can be used as decision-making branchpoints for reaching an appropriate diagnosis and apply these measurements to a spectrum of abnormalities.

The data given in these case presentations are restricted to information needed to interpret the exercise test. Generally, two sets of resting blood gas data are included in Table 3 of each report. The first is obtained with the subject sitting on the ergometer but before breathing on the mouthpiece (i.e., *without* accompanying respiratory gas exchange data), and the second is obtained with the subject on the ergometer while breathing on the mouthpiece prior to exercise (i.e., *with* accompanying gas exchange data). Both sets of data are reported for comparison.

The graphic data given in Figures A and B display data points every 30 seconds, calculated as the average of whole breath-by-breath measurements over the preceding 15- to 20-second period. On panels 1, 2, 3, 6, 8, and 9 of these figures, after a period of rest and unloaded pedalling (0 W), the work rate is increased in equal increments each minute; various variables are plotted on the vertical axes. The increments begin at the left vertical dashed line, and the termination of exercise is indicated by the right vertical dashed line. Two minutes of recovery data are also plotted. In panel 3, work rate is scaled to be $\frac{1}{10}$ of that of $\dot{V}_{O_2}$. Thus, when the $\dot{V}_{O_2}$ increase exactly parallels the work rate increase, $\Delta\dot{V}_{O_2}/\Delta$ work rate = 10 ml/W. Interrelated ventilatory and cardiovascular variables are plotted on panels 4, 5, and 7 during rest and exercise, but not recovery. In panel 5, the mean predicted maximum $\dot{V}O_2$ and maximum HR for a sedentary person of the same sex, age, and body size are marked with an "X." Moreover, plotted on panel 5 is $\dot{V}CO_2$ as a function of $\dot{V}O_2$. The dashed diagonal line through this plot has a slope of 1. Thus, when $\dot{V}CO_2$ versus $\dot{V}O_2$ increases more steeply than this line, the $\dot{V}O_2$ is above the subject's anaerobic threshold, and the break-point is the anaerobic threshold. The summary data shown in Table 2 are taken from Table 3 (and Table 4, if provided) and Figure A (and Figure B, if provided).

The predicted values given for each case are the mean values taken from Chapter 6. As with any predicted values there are normal ranges. To the best of our knowledge, our interpretations take the range of normal values into account.

Seventy-nine cases are presented for interpretation. Practical considerations limited our ability to provide more examples, and of course, there are many disorders of exercise performance that we have not studied directly. Because each category of disease can have perturbations that are instructive to review, however, we find it desirable sometimes to present more than one case of each type of disorder. Moreover, patients frequently have more than one abnormality. Thus, we thought it important to present some of these complex cases and to provide our rationale for our conclusions regarding the dominant pathophysiology.

Of the 79 cases, the first 15 are of men and women whom we concluded were normal. They were selected to show the effect of age, gender, form of ergometry used for testing, effect of O_2 breathing, effect of β-adrenergic blockade, effect of obesity, and effect of cigarette smoking on the test results.

Cases 16 to 29 are examples of coronary artery disease, valvular heart disease, cardiomyopathies, and congenital heart disease. Other examples of heart diseases are provided in the "complex" case category described later.

Cases 30 to 35 are examples of peripheral vascular diseases. Again, some examples are included in the "complex" case category because these disorders are commonly associated with primary heart disease.

Cases 36 to 45 include several types and severity of diseases primarily associated with airflow obstruction. Other examples of obstructive airway disease can be found in the "complex" category.

Cases 46 to 58 are examples of pulmonary fibrosis or respiratory restriction of various causes and that identified as idiopathic. Two cases show results before and after treatment.

Cases 59 to 64 are examples of chronic pulmonary vascular diseases of several types. One of the major roles of exercise testing is diagnosis and the noninvasive evaluation of the effect of therapy in these disorders. Other examples of pulmonary vascular diseases are presented in the group of patients with lung diseases.

Cases 65 to 67 are examples of subjects who were classified as having made a poor effort during exercise testing. It was concluded that they did not have evidence of organic disease reducing exercise tolerance.

Examples of disorders of the respiratory "pump" are presented in cases 68 to 70. These disorders can be found in many forms, and the three cases presented are representative.

The last and perhaps the most challenging and interesting group of patients, cases 71 to 79, are those with multiple abnormalities (complex cases). We have analyzed these cases with the intent of diagnosing the limiting disorder or disorders.

In a few instances, the conclusions we reached in the case analysis will not be easily obtained from the logical sequence suggested by the flow charts. Nevertheless, we started each analysis by using the flow charts. The supporting data listed under each diagnosis in the flow chart should always be considered to confirm the diagnosis derived from the flow chart analysis.

We recommend, therefore, that students of these cases ought not to be too rigid in the use of the flow charts. For instance, we point out that a measurement (branchpoint) that distinguishes obstructive from restrictive lung disease is the breathing frequency at the maximum work rate performed. Generally this value is greater than 50 per minute in patients with restrictive lung disease and less than 50 per minute in patients with obstructive lung disease. Although this distinction usually exists, exceptions will almost inevitably occur.

Whereas this section is intended to be on atlas of types of disorders reducing exercise tolerance, it is necessarily incomplete because of the variety of conditions that can interfere with the coupling of external to cellular respiration. Nevertheless, we hope that the principles taught by these cases and the preparatory chapters will provide the reader with the necessary physiologic background to interpret the many pathophysiologic conditions not described.

CASE 1 *Normal man*

CLINICAL FINDINGS

This 55-year-old executive was referred for exercise testing because of his complaint of decreased exercise tolerance. He complained of weakness, fatigue, and some dyspnea after jogging 1 block, but he could walk 3 miles on the level without difficulty. He had become symptomatic following recovery from an ankle injury 2 years earlier and felt unable to satisfactorily improve his exercise tolerance. He denied chest pain, syncope, palpitations, coughing, or wheezing. He had smoked half a pack of cigarettes per day for 10 years but had reduced his smoking to 3 to 4 cigarettes per week. He took no medications. Physical examination, chest roentgenograms, and resting ECG were normal.

EXERCISE FINDINGS

The patient performed exercise on a cycle ergometer. He pedalled at 60 rpm without added load for 3 minutes. The work rate was then increased 20 W per minute to his symptom-limited maximum. Arterial blood was sampled every second minute, and intra-arterial blood pressure was recorded from a percutaneously placed brachial artery catheter. The patient stopped exercise because of thigh fatigue. Twelve-lead ECG recordings remained normal during exercise.

TABLE 1-1. *Selected Respiratory Function Data*

MEASUREMENT	PREDICTED	MEASURED
Age, yr		55
Sex		Male
Height, cm		182
Weight, kg	83	80
Hematocrit, %		41
VC, L	4.75	6.06
IC, L	3.17	4.16
TLC, L	7.08	8.24
FEV_1, L	3.76	4.52
FEV_1/VC, %	79	75
MVV, L/min	151	200
$D_{L_{CO}}$, ml/mm Hg/min	28.8	28.3

TABLE 1-2. *Selected Exercise Data*

MEASUREMENT	PREDICTED	MEASURED
Maximum $\dot{V}_{O_2}$, L/min	2.47	2.53
Maximum HR, beats/min	165	176
Maximum O_2 pulse, ml/beat	15.0	14.5
$\Delta\dot{V}_{O_2}/\Delta$WR, ml/min/W	10.3	9.8
AT, L/min	> 1.07	1.2
Blood pressure, mm Hg (rest, max)		144/81,225/87
Maximum $\dot{V}_E$, L/min		107
Exercise breathing reserve, L/min	> 15	93
Pa_{O_2}, mm Hg (rest, max ex)		98,110
$P(A-a)_{O_2}$, mm Hg (rest, max ex)		5,15
$P(a-ET)_{CO_2}$, mm Hg (rest, max ex)		0,−5
V_D/V_T (rest, heavy ex)		0.26,0.15
HCO_3^-, mEq/L (rest, 2-min recov)		25,12

Fɪɢ. 1-A.

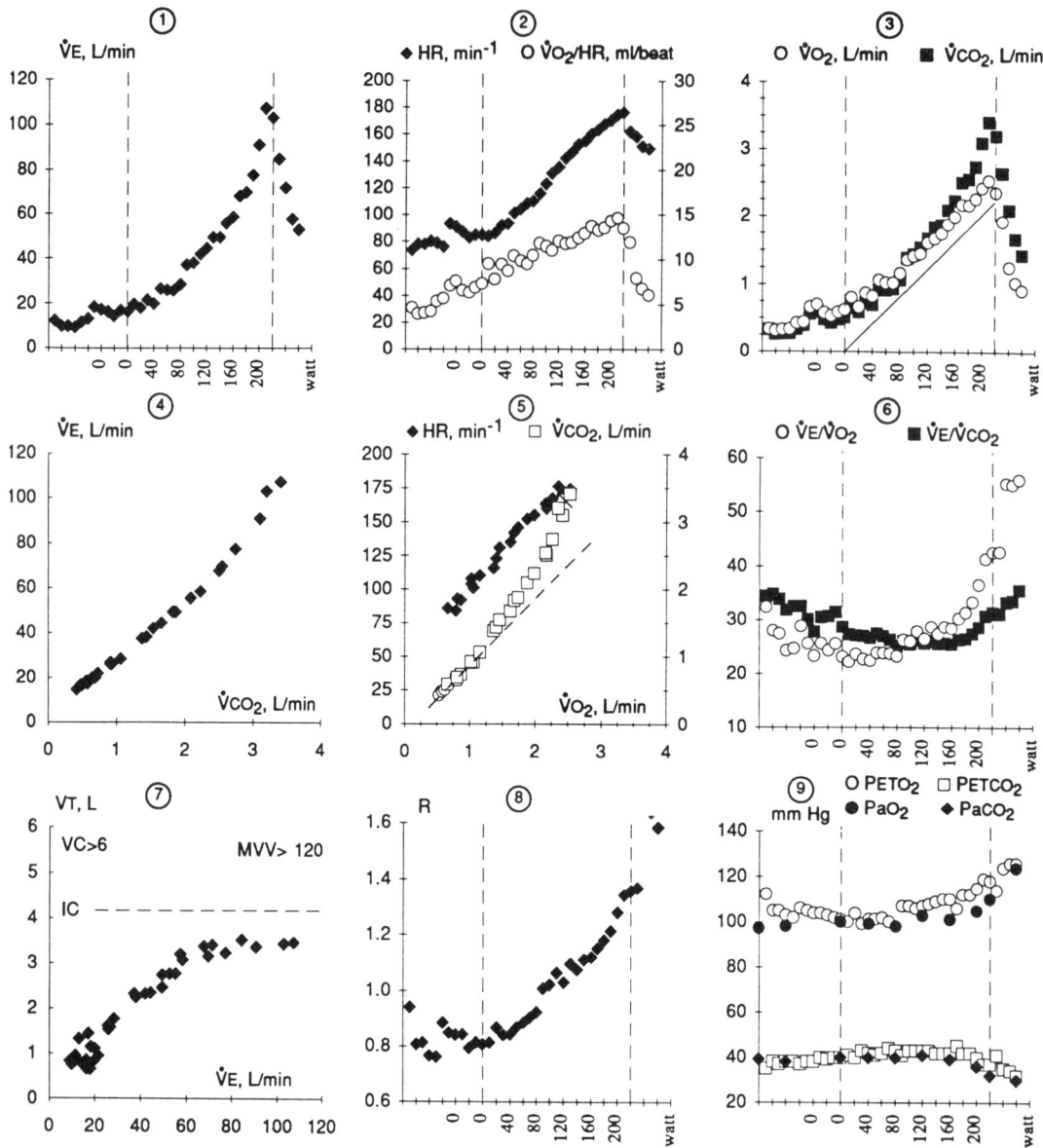

1. Vertical dashed lines in panels 1 to 3 and 6, 8, and 9 indicate the beginning and the end of increasing work period.

2. Unloaded cycling is performed for 3 minutes before the left vertical dashed line.

3. In panel 3, the diagonal line shows the increase of $\dot{V}O_2$ at a slope of 10 ml/min/W.

4. In panel 5, the diagonal dashed line has a slope of 1; the "x" in the upper right is the predicted maximum heart rate and $\dot{V}O_2$ for the subject.

TABLE 1-3.

Time min	Work rate watts	BP mm Hg	HR min⁻¹	f min⁻¹	$\dot{V}E$ L/min BTPS	$\dot{V}CO_2$ L/min STPD	$\dot{V}O_2$ L/min STPD	$\dfrac{\dot{V}O_2}{HR}$ ml/beat	R	pH	HCO₃ meq/L	PO2, mm Hg			PCO2, mm Hg			$\dfrac{\dot{V}E}{\dot{V}CO_2}$	$\dfrac{\dot{V}E}{\dot{V}O_2}$
												ET	a	(A-a)	ET	a	(a-ET)		
	Rest	153/87								7.42	25	97			39				
	Rest		74	14	12.2	0.32	0.34	4.6	0.94			112			35			34	32
	Rest		78	13	9.8	0.25	0.31	4.0	0.81			105			38			35	28
	Rest		78	13	9.9	0.26	0.32	4.1	0.81			105			37			34	27
	Rest	144/81	80	11	9.2	0.26	0.34	4.3	0.76	7.42	24	103	98	5	38	38	0	32	24	0.26
	Rest		79	12	11.4	0.32	0.42	5.3	0.76			102			38			32	25
	Rest		76	10	13.2	0.38	0.43	5.7	0.88			106			37			33	29
	Unloaded		93	16	18.2	0.56	0.66	7.1	0.85			105			38			30	26
	Unloaded		91	12	17.1	0.58	0.69	7.6	0.84			104			38			28	23
	Unloaded		87	19	16.2	0.48	0.57	6.6	0.84			104			40			30	26
	Unloaded		83	19	14.5	0.42	0.53	6.4	0.79			103			39			31	24
	Unloaded		85	22	16.9	0.48	0.59	6.9	0.81			102			40			31	25
	Unloaded	171/87	85	25	16.4	0.50	0.62	7.3	0.81	7.41	25	101	100	2	40	40	0	29	23	0.21
0.5	20		84	24	19.7	0.65	0.80	9.5	0.81			100			41			27	22
1.0	20		86	28	18.1	0.58	0.67	7.8	0.87			104			40			27	23
1.5	40		92	23	21.6	0.73	0.87	9.5	0.84			99			43			27	23
2.0	40	183/84	93	18	19.9	0.69	0.82	8.8	0.84	7.40	24	101	99	5	42	40	-2	27	22	0.18
2.5	60		101	17	26.7	0.92	1.06	10.5	0.87			101			41			27	24
3.0	60		104	17	26.0	0.91	1.03	9.9	0.88			102			42			27	24
3.5	80		108	16	25.8	0.93	1.03	9.5	0.90			100			44			26	24
4.0	80	195/81	110	16	28.4	1.07	1.16	10.5	0.92	7.38	23	103	98	9	43	40	-3	25	23	0.14
4.5	100		116	16	37.3	1.38	1.37	11.8	1.01			107			41			26	26
5.0	100		123	17	38.1	1.44	1.41	11.5	1.02			107			43			25	26
5.5	120		131	18	42.0	1.54	1.45	11.1	1.06			106			43			26	28
6.0	120	207/87	135	19	44.5	1.67	1.62	12.0	1.03	7.37	23	107	103	7	43	41	-2	26	26	0.17
6.5	140		142	18	49.4	1.83	1.67	11.8	1.10			108			43			26	29
7.0	140		146	20	49.4	1.87	1.74	11.9	1.07			109			42			26	27
7.5	160		152	20	55.5	2.09	1.88	12.4	1.11			110			42			26	29
8.0	160	213/90	155	19	58.3	2.23	1.99	12.8	1.12	7.35	21	110	101	13	42	39	-3	25	28	0.13
8.5	180		160	20	67.7	2.51	2.18	13.6	1.15			106			45			26	30
9.0	180		163	22	69.5	2.55	2.16	13.3	1.18			112			42			27	31
9.5	200		167	24	77.3	2.74	2.26	13.5	1.21			112			42			27	33
10.0	200	225/87	170	27	90.7	3.10	2.42	14.2	1.28	7.31	18	115	105	15	40	36	-4	29	37	0.16
10.5	220		174	31	107.2	3.40	2.53	14.5	1.34			119			37			31	41
11.0	220	216/90	176	30	102.9	3.20	2.36	13.4	1.36	7.30	15	118	110	15	37	32	-5	31	43	0.14
	Recovery		162	24	84.3	2.64	1.93	11.9	1.37			114			41			31	43
	Recovery		158	21	71.5	2.10	1.26	8.0	1.67			124			35			33	55
	Recovery		151	18	57.6	1.67	1.02	6.8	1.64			126			34			34	55
	Recovery	165/75	149	19	52.7	1.44	0.91	6.1	1.58	7.22	12	126	124	5	32	30	-2	35	56	0.18

Interpretation

COMMENTS

The results of the respiratory function studies are within normal limits (Table 1-1).

ANALYSIS

In flow chart 1, the maximum $\dot{V}O_2$ and anaerobic threshold are normal (Table 1-2). See flow chart 2: The ECG and arterial blood gases (Table 1-3) are normal throughout exercise; the O_2-pulse at the maximum work rate is normal.

CONCLUSION

This is a normal man, with high level of anxiety regarding his physical status.

CASE 2   *Normal athlete*

CLINICAL FINDINGS

This 31-year-old physiologist was a frequent marathon runner. He had no known health problems and trained several times weekly.

EXERCISE FINDINGS

The subject performed exercise on a cycle ergometer. He pedalled without added load at 60 rpm for 2 minutes. The work rate was then increased 30 W every minute to his symptom-limited maximum. There were no arrhythmias, and the ECG remained normal.

TABLE 2-1. *Selected Respiratory Function Data*

MEASUREMENT	PREDICTED	MEASURED
Age, yr		31
Sex		Male
Height, cm		182
Weight, kg	83	81
Hematocrit, %		43
VC, L	5.48	6.27
IC, L	3.65	3.56
FEV$_1$, L	4.43	4.51
FEV$_1$/VC, %	81	72
MVV, L/min	182	185

TABLE 2-2. *Selected Exercise Data*

MEASUREMENT	PREDICTED	MEASURED
Maximum $\dot{V}O_2$, L/min	3.22	4.95
Maximum HR, beats/min	189	175
Maximum O_2 pulse, ml/beat	17.0	28.3
$\Delta\dot{V}O_2/\Delta WR$, ml/min/W	10.3	11.5
AT, L/min	> 1.32	2.5
Maximum $\dot{V}E$, L/min		186
Exercise breathing reserve, L/min	> 15	−1

Fig. 2-A.

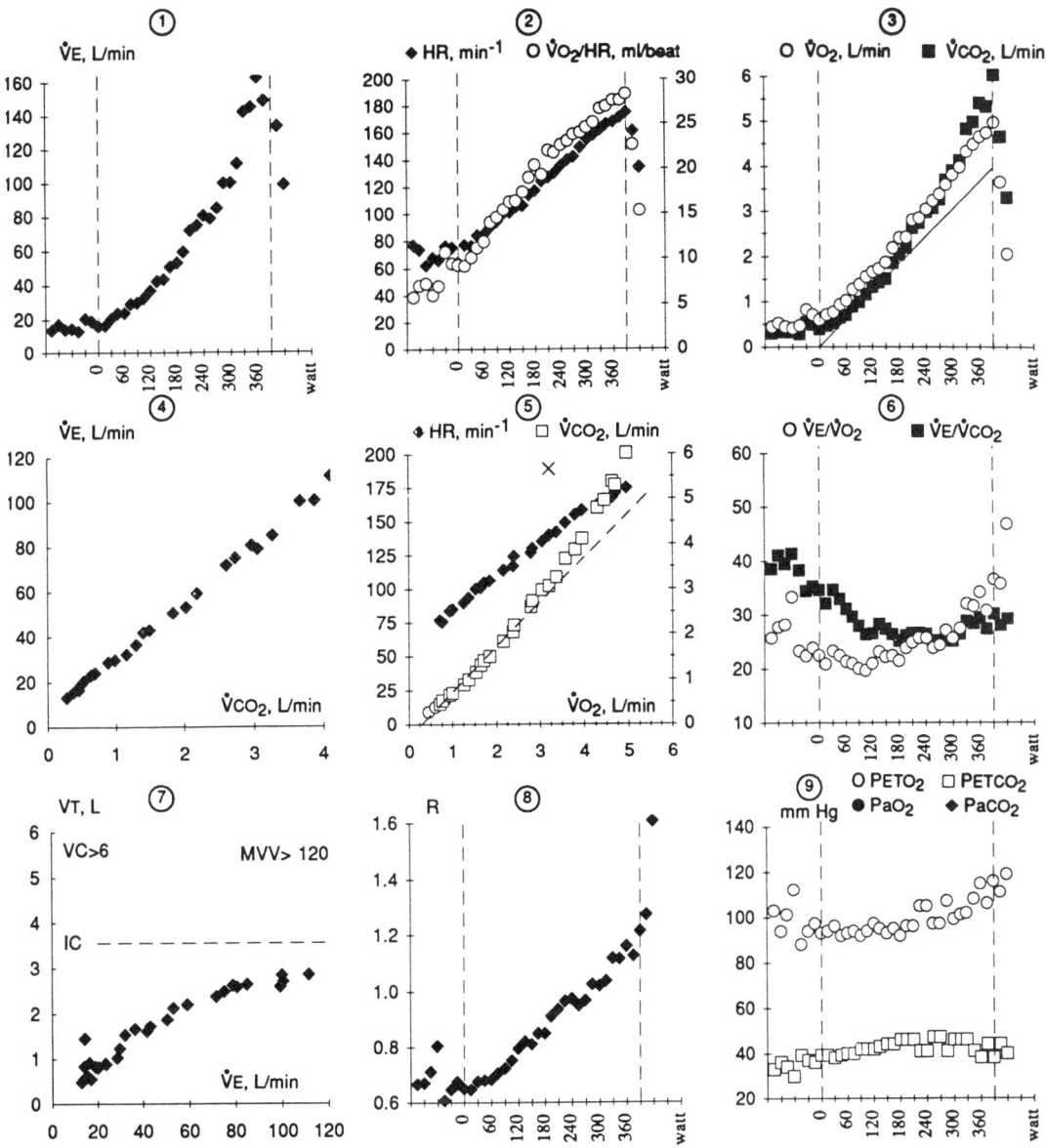

1. Vertical dashed lines in panels 1 to 3 and 6, 8, and 9 indicate the beginning and the end of increasing work period.

2. Unloaded cycling is performed for 3 minutes before the left vertical dashed line.

3. In panel 3, the diagonal line shows the increase of $\dot{V}_{O_2}$ at a slope of 10 ml/min/W.

4. In panel 5, the diagonal dashed line has a slope of 1; the "x" in the upper right is the predicted maximum heart rate and $\dot{V}_{O_2}$ for the subject.

TABLE 2-3.

Time min	Work rate watts	BP mm Hg	HR min⁻¹	f min⁻¹	$\dot{V}E$ L/min BTPS	$\dot{V}CO_2$ L/min STPD	$\dot{V}O_2$ L/min STPD	$\dfrac{\dot{V}O_2}{HR}$ ml/beat	R	pH	HCO₃ meq/L	PO2, mm Hg ET	a	(A-a)	PCO2, mm Hg ET	a	(a-ET)	$\dfrac{\dot{V}E}{\dot{V}CO_2}$	$\dfrac{\dot{V}E}{\dot{V}O_2}$	$\dfrac{VD}{VT}$
	Rest		77	25	13.7	0.30	0.45	5.8	0.67			103			33			39	26	
	Rest		74	31	17.0	0.35	0.52	7.0	0.67			94			36			41	28	
	Rest		62	17	14.1	0.32	0.45	7.3	0.71			101			34			40	28	
	Rest		68	10	14.5	0.33	0.41	6.0	0.80			112			30			41	33	
	Unloaded		66	27	13.0	0.28	0.46	7.0	0.61			88			39			38	23	
	Unloaded		76	25	20.4	0.53	0.82	10.8	0.65			94			37			34	22	
	Unloaded		75	23	18.9	0.48	0.71	9.5	0.68			97			36			35	24	
	Unloaded		64	26	15.7	0.39	0.60	9.4	0.65			93			39			35	22	
0.5	30		77	18	16.3	0.46	0.71	9.2	0.65			94			39			32	21	
1.0	30		76	25	20.1	0.52	0.77	10.1	0.68			96			38			35	23	
1.5	60		84	26	23.3	0.64	0.94	11.2	0.68			92			39			33	22	
2.0	60		85	27	23.8	0.69	1.01	11.9	0.68			93			40			31	21	
2.5	90		90	28	28.7	0.89	1.26	14.0	0.71			94			40			30	21	
3.0	90		94	24	29.6	0.99	1.37	14.6	0.72			92			42			28	20	
3.5	120		100	21	32.2	1.16	1.54	15.4	0.75			94			42			26	20	
4.0	120		101	22	36.5	1.31	1.65	16.3	0.79			97			42			26	21	
4.5	150		105	26	41.9	1.41	1.72	16.4	0.82			95			43			28	23	
5.0	150		106	25	43.1	1.50	1.85	17.5	0.81			93			44			27	22	
5.5	180		114	27	50.6	1.84	2.17	19.0	0.85			95			44			26	22	
6.0	180		117	25	53.2	2.03	2.39	20.4	0.85			92			46			25	21	
6.5	210		124	27	59.3	2.19	2.40	19.4	0.91			96			46			26	24	
7.0	210		127	30	71.7	2.61	2.79	22.0	0.94			96			46			26	25	
7.5	240		130	30	75.0	2.73	2.83	21.8	0.96			105			41			27	26	
8.0	240		135	31	80.6	2.97	3.05	22.6	0.97			105			41			26	26	
8.5	270		140	30	78.9	3.06	3.22	23.0	0.95			97			47			25	24	
9.0	270		142	32	85.0	3.27	3.38	23.8	0.97			97			47			25	24	
9.5	300		149	35	100.0	3.67	3.58	24.0	1.03			107			41			26	27	
10.0	300		155	37	100.4	3.88	3.80	24.5	1.02			99			46			25	26	
10.5	330		158	39	111.6	4.11	3.96	25.1	1.04			101			46			26	27	
11.0	330		162	48	142.4	4.81	4.31	26.6	1.12			102			46			29	32	
11.5	360		166	48	144.8	4.97	4.46	26.9	1.11			108			41			28	32	
12.0	360		168	53	162.6	5.38	4.64	27.6	1.16			115			38			29	34	
12.5	390		171	50	149.1	5.31	4.71	27.5	1.13			106			44			27	31	
13.0	390		175	63	186.0	6.01	4.95	28.3	1.21			116			38			30	36	
	Recovery		161	46	133.7	4.63	3.64	22.6	1.27			111			44			28	36	
	Recovery		134	38	99.1	3.29	2.05	15.3	1.60			119			40			29	47	

Interpretation

COMMENTS

This case is presented to illustrate results of a normal, athletic subject.

ANALYSIS

In flow chart 1, the maximum $\dot{V}O_2$ and the anaerobic threshold are considerably above the predicted values (Table 2-2). The predicted values are, of course, those for a sedentary population. The results of this study demonstrate how much better an athlete can perform than the average member of the sedentary group. The exceptionally high O_2 pulse at maximum work rate reflects the large stroke volume and $C(a-\bar{v})O_2$ that this subject must have. Assuming that the mixed venous O_2 saturation were as low as 20%, the O_2 pulse of 28.3 ml/beat would indicate that the subject's stroke volume must be approximately 175 ml. The normal ventilatory equivalent for O_2 and CO_2 at the anaerobic threshold (panel 6, Fig. 2-A) reflects the ventilation-perfusion matching of a normal subject. The maximum exercise ventilation is approximately equal to his MVV. Thus, his breathing reserve is approximately zero, a common finding in exceptionally fit people.

CONCLUSION

This is an exceptionally fit, normal subject.

CASE 3 *Normal man: Air and oxygen breathing*

CLINICAL FINDINGS

The patient was a 59-year-old retired shipyard worker with a history of asbestos exposure and a 2 pack year history of cigarette smoking. He had stopped working 4 years previously. He was asymptomatic at the time of this examination. Physical and laboratory examinations were normal; chest roentgenograms revealed focal pleural plaques with calcification.

EXERCISE FINDINGS

After we obtained informed consent, the patient participated in a blind-crossover exercise study on a cycle ergometer, receiving one of two humidified gas mixtures (compressed air or 100% oxygen) just prior to and during each study. He pedalled at 60 rpm without added load for 3 minutes. The work rate was then increased 15 W per minute to his symptom-limited maximum. Arterial blood was sampled every second minute, and intra-arterial blood pressure was recorded from a percutaneously placed brachial artery catheter. He rested 1 hour between the two studies and exercised to his maximum tolerance on each occasion. On both occasions he stopped exercise because of general fatigue. Resting and exercise ECG readings were normal.

TABLE 3-1. *Selected Respiratory Function Data*

MEASUREMENT	PREDICTED	MEASURED
Age, yr		59
Sex		Male
Height, cm		155
Weight, kg	62	53
Hematocrit, %		46
VC, L	2.90	3.19
IC, L	1.94	2.12
TLC, L	4.51	4.62
FEV_1, L	2.26	2.49
FEV_1/VC, %	78	78
MVV, L/min	112	118
DL_{CO}, ml/mm Hg/min	19.9	20.7

TABLE 3-2. *Selected Exercise Data*

MEASUREMENT	PREDICTED	AIR	O_2
Maximum $\dot{V}CO_2$, L/min		2.03	1.93
Maximum $\dot{V}O_2$, L/min	1.65	1.57	
Maximum HR, beats/min	161	192	188
Maximum O_2 pulse, ml/beat	10.2	8.2	
$\Delta\dot{V}O_2/\Delta WR$, ml/min/W	10.3	9.7	
AT, L/min	> 0.73	0.8	
Blood pressure, mm Hg (rest, max)		100/56,213/88	100/63,231/94
Maximum $\dot{V}E$, L/min		89	72
Exercise breathing reserve, L/min	> 15	29	46
Pa_{O_2}, mm Hg (rest, max ex)		102,101	585,586
$P(A-a)_{O_2}$, mm Hg (rest, max ex)		24,25	103,93
$P(a-ET)_{CO_2}$, mm Hg (rest, max ex)		-4,-4	1,-2
VD/VT (rest, heavy ex)		0.19,0.27	0.37,0.26
HCO_3^-, mEq/L (rest, 2-min recov)		23,12	19,14

FIG. 3-A. *Air breathing.*

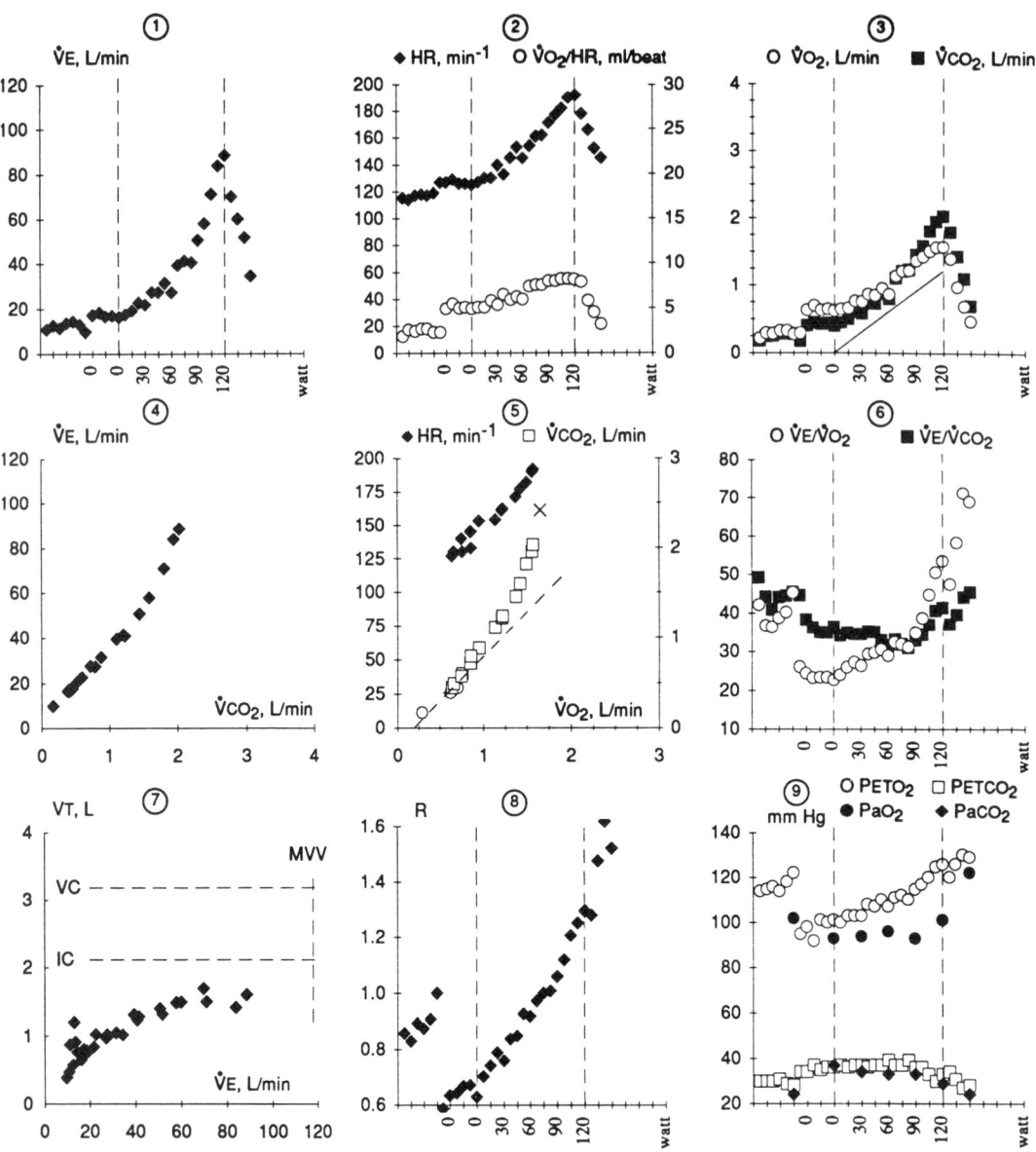

1. Vertical dashed lines in panels 1 to 3 and 6, 8, and 9 indicate the beginning and the end of increasing work period.

2. Unloaded cycling is performed for 3 minutes before the left vertical dashed line.

3. In panel 3, the diagonal line shows the increase of $\dot{V}O_2$ at a slope of 10 ml/min/W.

4. In panel 5, the diagonal dashed line has a slope of 1; the "x" in the upper right is the predicted maximum heart rate and $\dot{V}O_2$ for the subject.

FIG. 3-B. *Oxygen breathing.*

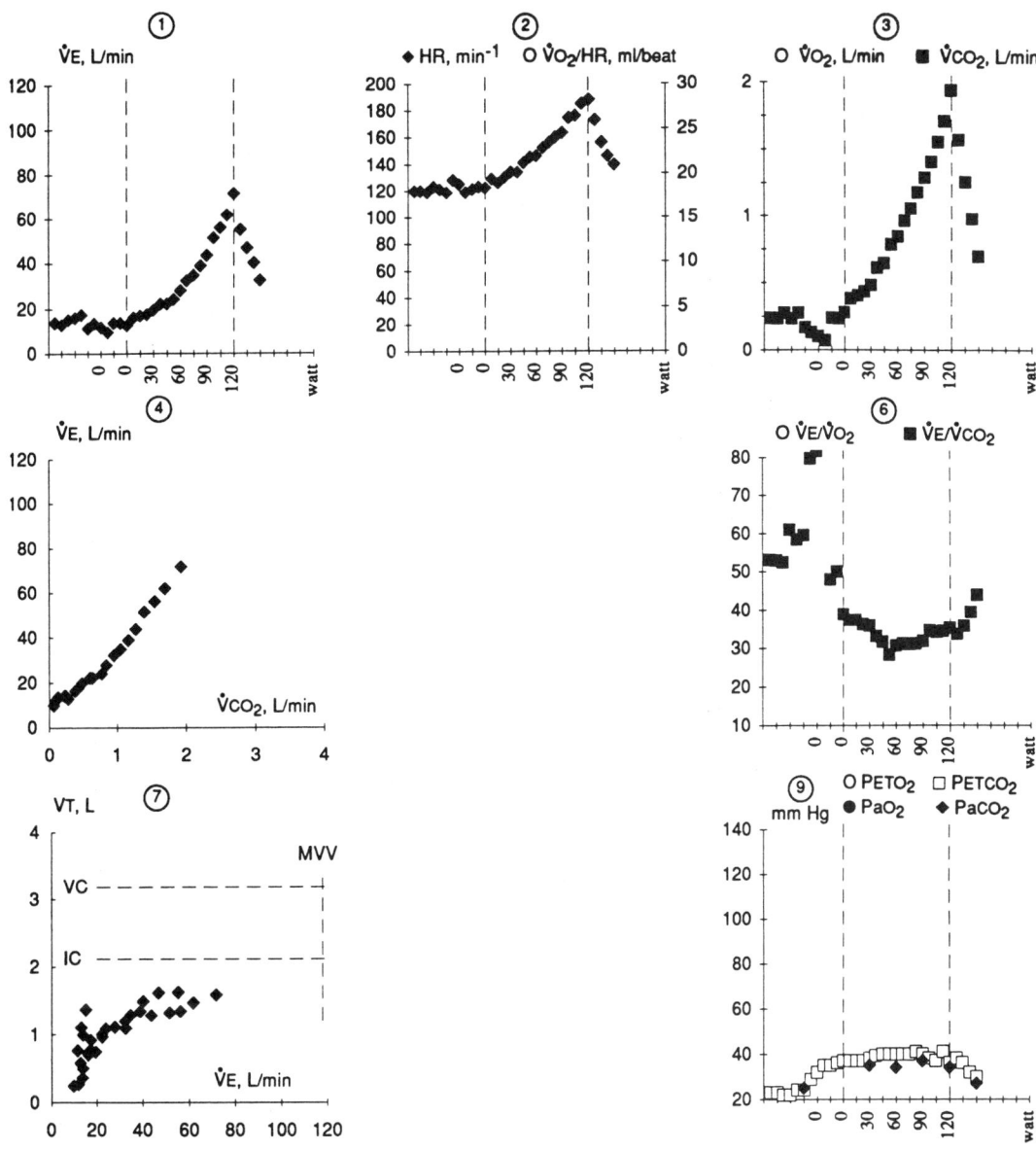

1. Vertical dashed lines in panels 1 to 3 and 6 and 9 indicate the beginning and the end of increasing work period.
2. Unloaded cycling is performed for 3 minutes before the left vertical dashed line.

TABLE 3-3. *Air breathing.*

Time min	Work rate watts	BP mm Hg	HR min⁻¹	f min⁻¹	V̇E L/min BTPS	V̇CO2 L/min STPD	V̇O2 L/min STPD	V̇O2/HR ml/beat	R	pH	HCO3 meq/L	PO2, mm Hg ET	a	(A-a)	PCO2, mm Hg ET	a	(a-ET)	V̇E/V̇CO2	V̇E/V̇O2	VD/VT
	Rest		115	23	10.8	0.18	0.21	1.8	0.86			114			30			49	42	
	Rest		114	22	12.5	0.24	0.29	2.5	0.83			115			30			44	37	
	Rest		117	13	11.3	0.25	0.28	2.4	0.89			116			30			41	36	
	Rest		118	15	13.6	0.28	0.32	2.7	0.88			114			31			44	39	
	Rest		117	19	14.5	0.29	0.32	2.7	0.91			118			29			44	40	
	Rest	100/56	119	11	13.2	0.27	0.27	2.3	1.00	7.48	18	122	102	24	28	24	-4	45	45	0.19
	Unloaded		127	25	9.7	0.17	0.29	2.3	0.59			95			34			45	26	
	Unloaded		127	21	17.1	0.40	0.63	5.0	0.63			98			34			38	24	
	Unloaded		129	23	18.2	0.45	0.70	5.4	0.64			92			37			36	23	
	Unloaded		126	23	16.7	0.42	0.63	5.0	0.67			101			35			35	23	
	Unloaded		126	24	17.0	0.43	0.64	5.1	0.67			100			36			35	23	
	Unloaded	150/75	125	25	16.3	0.39	0.62	5.0	0.63	7.41	23	101	93	3	36	37	1	36	23	0.31
0.5	15		127	23	17.3	0.45	0.64	5.0	0.70			100			37			34	24	
1.0	15		130	25	19.2	0.49	0.66	5.1	0.74			103			36			35	26	
1.5	30		130	22	22.6	0.60	0.76	5.8	0.79			103			37			35	27	
2.0	30	163/75	140	26	21.9	0.57	0.75	5.4	0.76	7.40	21	103	94	14	37	34	-3	35	26	0.24
2.5	45		133	27	27.6	0.72	0.86	6.5	0.84			108			36			35	29	
3.0	45		145	28	27.6	0.72	0.85	5.9	0.85			107			37			35	30	
3.5	60		153	30	31.5	0.88	0.95	6.2	0.93			110			37			33	30	
4.0	60	194/81	145	28	27.2	0.79	0.86	5.9	0.92	7.40	20	107	96	19	39	33	-6	31	29	0.15
4.5	75		154	30	39.4	1.11	1.14	7.4	0.97			111			37			33	32	
5.0	75		161	32	41.4	1.21	1.21	7.5	1.00			112			37			32	32	
5.5	90		162	33	40.8	1.23	1.22	7.5	1.01			110			39			31	31	
6.0	90	194/75	171	36	50.8	1.45	1.37	8.0	1.06	7.39	20	115	93	25	36	33	-3	33	35	0.19
6.5	105		177	39	58.0	1.59	1.42	8.0	1.12			117			36			34	39	
7.0	105		182	47	71.0	1.81	1.50	8.2	1.21			120			33			37	45	
7.5	120		190	59	83.9	1.95	1.56	8.2	1.25			125			30			40	51	
8.0	120	213/88	192	55	88.6	2.03	1.57	8.2	1.29	7.37	16	126	101	25	33	29	-4	41	53	0.27
	Recovery		178	41	69.9	1.79	1.40	7.9	1.28			120			34			37	47	
	Recovery		166	40	60.0	1.43	0.97	5.8	1.47			126			31			40	58	
	Recovery		152	39	51.8	1.10	0.68	4.5	1.62			130			27			44	71	
	Recovery	169/63	145	34	34.6	0.70	0.46	3.2	1.52	7.33	12	129	122	11	28	24	-4	45	69	0.19

Interpretation

COMMENTS

Resting respiratory function is normal (Table 3-1). The exercise test was repeated with the patient breathing O_2, as part of an experimental study. At rest, the patient acutely hyperventilated while breathing with the mouthpiece; this ceased as soon as the exercise started. The associated relative hypoventilation noted in the transition from rest to unloaded cycling (panel 9, Fig. 3-A) caused a simultaneous marked decrease in R (panel 8, Fig. 3-A). This does not affect the final interpretation but does caution the examiner on the use of the resting bicarbonate values.

ANALYSIS

In flow chart 1, the maximum $\dot{V}O_2$ is normal (Table 3-2 and panel 3 of Fig. 3-A). See flow chart 2. The

TABLE 3-4. *Oxygen breathing.*

Time min	Work rate watts	BP mm Hg	HR min⁻¹	f min⁻¹	V̇E L/min BTPS	V̇CO2 L/min STPD	V̇O2 L/min STPD	V̇O2/HR ml/beat	R	pH	HCO3 meq/L	PO2, mm Hg ET	a	(A-a)	PCO2, mm Hg ET	a	(a-ET)	V̇E/V̇CO2	V̇E/V̇O2	VD/VT
	Rest		120	14	13.9	0.24									23			53		
	Rest		120	12	13.2	0.23									23			53		
	Rest		119	11	15.1	0.27									22			52		
	Rest		123	22	15.9	0.23									22			61		
	Rest		121	19	17.4	0.27									24			58		
	Rest	100/63	119	15	11.4	0.17				7.49	19		585	103	24	25	1	60		0.37
	Unloaded		128	38	13.6	0.13									29			80		
	Unloaded		125	44	11.9	0.10									32			82		
	Unloaded		119	41	9.8	0.07									35			90		
	Unloaded		121	28	13.9	0.24									35			48		
	Unloaded		123	28	13.9	0.23									36			50		
	Unloaded	163/81	122	22	12.7	0.28									37			39		
0.5	15		129	23	16.1	0.38									37			37		
1.0	15		126	22	16.8	0.40									37			37		
1.5	30		130	23	17.5	0.43									37			36		
2.0	30	181/88	134	26	19.4	0.48				7.40	21		591	87	38	35	-3	36		0.28
2.5	45		134	23	22.2	0.61									39			33		
3.0	45		141	22	22.1	0.64									40			32		
3.5	60		145	22	23.9	0.78									40			28		
4.0	60	206/88	146	25	27.9	0.84				7.38	20		576	103	40	34	-6	31		0.16
4.5	75		152	27	32.3	0.96									40			31		
5.0	75		156	27	34.8	1.05									40			31		
5.5	90		160	29	39.0	1.17									41			31		
6.0	90	225/91	163	34	43.7	1.28				7.37	21		581	95	40	37	-3	32		0.25
6.5	105		174	39	51.6	1.40									38			34		
7.0	105		176	42	56.3	1.55									37			34		
7.5	120		185	42	62.0	1.70									41			34		
8.0	120	231/94	188	45	71.7	1.93				7.35	18		586	93	36	34	-2	35		0.26
	Recovery		173	34	55.3	1.56									38			34		
	Recovery		156	29	46.9	1.25									36			36		
	Recovery		146	27	40.3	0.97									32			39		
	Recovery	219/75	140	30	32.7	0.69				7.33	14		584	102	30	27	-3	44		0.25

ECG, arterial blood gases, and O_2 pulse at maximum $\dot{V}O_2$ are normal (branchpoint 2.1). The subject is not obese (branchpoint 2.2). Thus, the cardiorespiratory response to exercise is normal, consistent with this patient's history and clinical findings.

The major difference between the air and O_2 breathing studies is a significantly reduced exercise ventilation in the latter when performing at the same work rate (Table 3-3 and 3-4 and panel 1 of Fig. 3-A and 3-B). Consistent with this is the higher Pa_{CO_2} at maximum exercise during the O_2 breathing study. Arterial oxygen tension was normal (585 mm Hg) at rest and remained unchanged throughout exercise during the oxygen breathing study, demonstrating the absence of a significant right to left shunt.

CONCLUSION

This is a normal subject.

CASE 4 *Normal woman: Air and oxygen breathing*

CLINICAL FINDINGS

This 45-year-old housewife was referred for evaluation of dyspnea. She had recently begun to increase her activity and felt that she was shorter of breath than she should be. Physical and laboratory examinations revealed no abnormalities.

EXERCISE FINDINGS

The patient performed exercise on a cycle ergometer. She pedalled at 60 rpm without added load for 3 minutes. The work rate was then increased 10 W per minute to her symptom-limited maximum. Arterial blood was sampled every second minute, and intra-arterial blood pressure was recorded from a percutaneously placed brachial artery catheter. A second incremental exercise test was performed with O_2 breathing, 1½ hours after recovery from the first, with work rate increments of 20 W per minute. She stopped exercise in each case complaining of general fatigue and shortness of breath. Resting and exercise ECGs were normal.

TABLE 4-1. *Selected Respiratory Function Data*

MEASUREMENT	PREDICTED	MEASURED
Age, yr		45
Sex		Female
Height, cm		165
Weight, kg	64	61
Hematocrit, %		40
VC, L	3.30	3.21
IC, L	2.20	1.99
FEV_1, L	2.68	2.71
FEV_1/VC, %	81	84
MVV, L/min	112	117
$D_{L_{CO}}$, ml/mm Hg/min	24.1	21.1

TABLE 4-2. *Selected Exercise Data*

MEASUREMENT	PREDICTED	ROOM AIR	O_2
Maximum work rate, W		130	160
Maximum $\dot{V}O_2$, L/min	1.60	1.71	
Maximum HR, beats/min	175	160	155
Maximum O_2 pulse, ml/beat	9.1	10.7	
$\Delta\dot{V}O_2/\Delta WR$, ml/min/W	10.3	11.9	
AT, L/min	> 0.78	0.9	
Blood pressure, mm Hg (rest, max)		138/81,194/81	106/75,181/88
Maximum $\dot{V}E$, L/min		70	54
Exercise breathing reserve, L/min	> 15	47	63
Pa_{O_2}, mm Hg (rest, max ex)		105,108	643,552
$P(A-a)_{O_2}$, mm Hg (rest, max ex)		5,16	33,117
$P(a-ET)_{CO_2}$, mm Hg (rest, max ex)		−1,−6	4,−3
V_D/V_T (rest, heavy ex)		0.21,0.11	0.34,0.18
HCO_3^-, mEq/L (rest, 2-min recov)		25,13	25, unknown

Fɪɢ. 4-A. *Air breathing.*

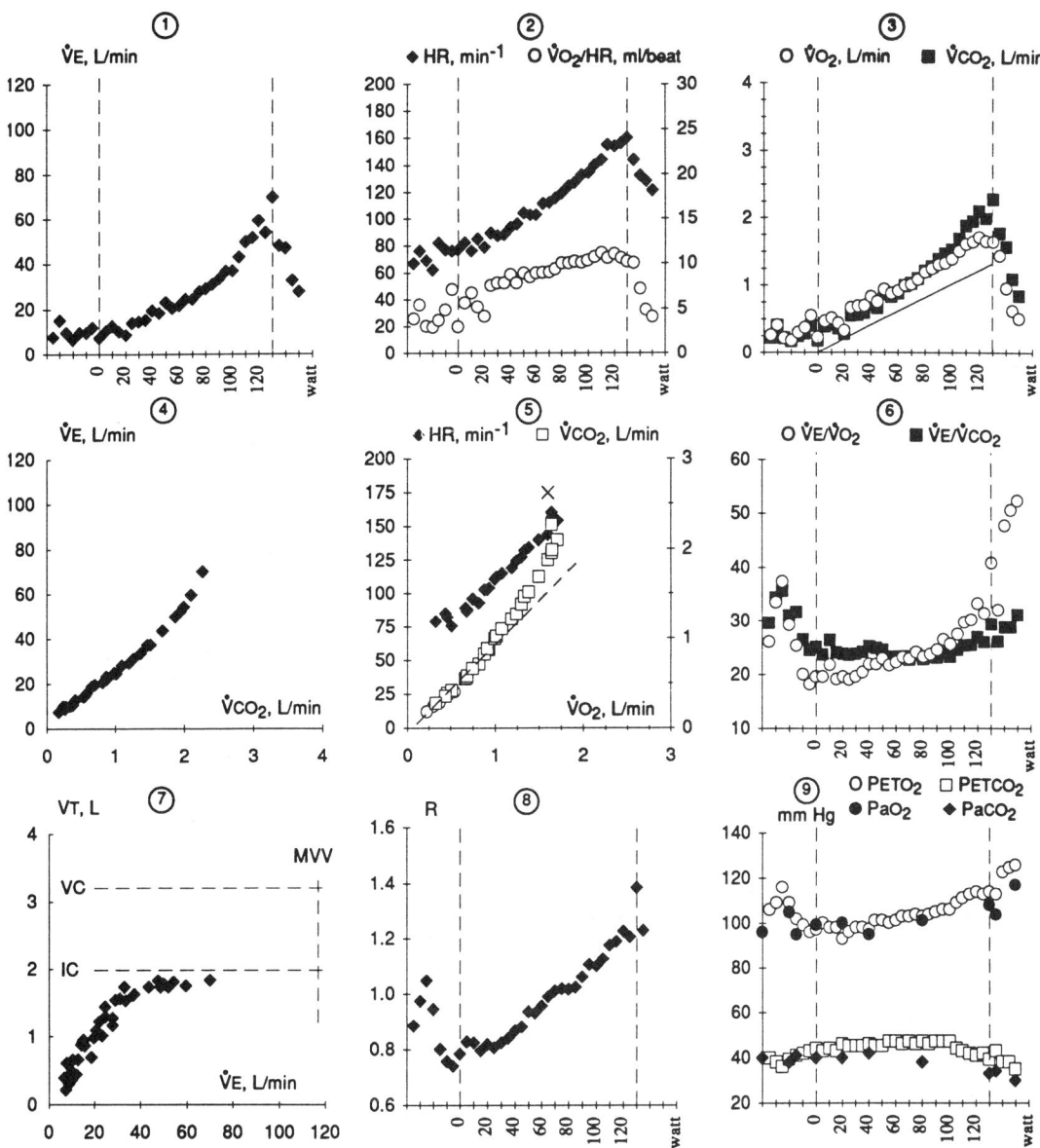

1. Vertical dashed lines in panels 1 to 3 and 6, 8, and 9 indicate the beginning and the end of increasing work period.

2. Unloaded cycling is performed for 3 minutes before the left vertical dashed line.

3. In panel 3, the diagonal line shows the increase of $\dot{V}O_2$ at a slope of 10 ml/min/W.

4. In panel 5, the diagonal dashed line has a slope of 1; the "x" in the upper right is the predicted maximum heart rate and $\dot{V}O_2$ for the subject.

Fig. 4-B. *Oxygen breathing.*

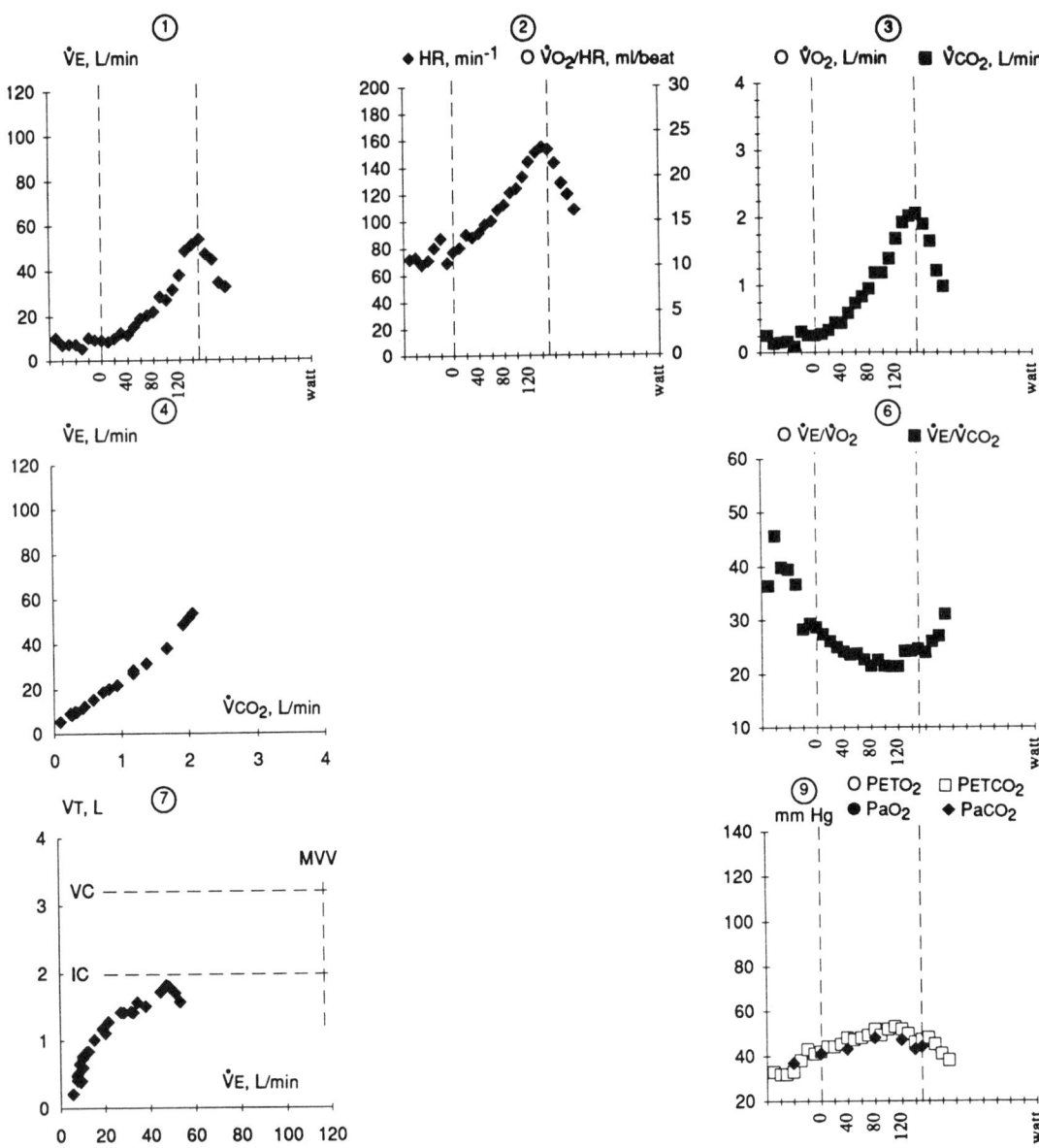

1. Vertical dashed lines in panels 1 to 3 and 6 and 9 indicate the beginning and the end of increasing work period.
2. Unloaded cycling is performed for 3 minutes before the left vertical dashed line.

TABLE 4-3. *Air breathing.*

Time min	Work rate watts	BP mm Hg	HR min^{-1}	f min^{-1}	$\dot{V}_E$ L/min BTPS	$\dot{V}_{CO_2}$ L/min STPD	$\dot{V}_{O_2}$ L/min STPD	$\frac{\dot{V}_{O_2}}{HR}$ ml/beat	R	pH	HCO$_3$ meq/L	PO2, mm Hg ET	a	(A-a)	PCO2, mm Hg ET	a	(a-ET)	$\frac{\dot{V}_E}{\dot{V}_{CO_2}}$	$\frac{\dot{V}_E}{\dot{V}_{O_2}}$	$\frac{V_D}{V_T}$
	Rest	138/81								7.42	25		96			40				
	Rest		67	13	7.9	0.23	0.26	3.9	0.88			106			40			30	26	
	Rest		76	16	15.1	0.40	0.41	5.4	0.98			109			38			34	34	
	Rest		69	22	9.7	0.22	0.21	3.0	1.05			116			36			36	37	
	Rest	138/75	62	17	6.7	0.17	0.18	2.9	0.94	7.43	25	109	105	5	39	38	-1	31	29	0.21
	Unloaded	138/81	82	27	9.9	0.24	0.30	3.7	0.80	7.41	26	102	95	6	41	41	0	32	25	0.26
	Unloaded		77	28	9.8	0.28	0.37	4.8	0.76			99			42			27	20	
	Unloaded		76	27	12.1	0.40	0.54	7.1	0.74			96			43			25	18	
	Unloaded	144/75	77	34	7.4	0.18	0.23	3.0	0.78	7.41	25	97	99	2	44	40	-4	25	20	0.08
0.5	10		82	16	10.4	0.38	0.46	5.6	0.83			100			43			24	20	
1.0	10		76	19	12.7	0.42	0.51	6.7	0.82			98			44			26	22	
1.5	20		85	21	10.2	0.35	0.44	5.2	0.80			98			43			24	19	
2.0	20	144/75	79	29	8.9	0.27	0.33	4.2	0.82	7.41	25	93	100	3	46	40	-6	24	20	0.07
2.5	30		89	16	14.1	0.54	0.67	7.5	0.81			96			45			24	19	
3.0	30		87	16	14.7	0.56	0.68	7.8	0.82			98			45			24	20	
3.5	40		88	18	15.6	0.58	0.69	7.8	0.84			98			45			24	20	
4.0	40	144/75	93	20	19.6	0.71	0.82	8.8	0.87	7.39	25	97	95	8	46	42	-4	25	22	0.17
4.5	50		96	27	18.7	0.66	0.75	7.8	0.88			101			45			25	22	
5.0	50		104	23	23.3	0.87	0.93	8.9	0.94			101			45			25	23	
5.5	60		103	19	20.7	0.82	0.88	8.5	0.93			100			47			23	22	
6.0	60	156/75	103	18	22.0	0.88	0.92	8.9	0.96			101			47			23	22	
6.5	70		111	19	24.7	0.99	1.00	9.0	0.99			103			46			23	23	
7.0	70		112	17	24.6	1.02	1.01	9.0	1.01			103			47			23	23	
7.5	80		115	24	28.0	1.10	1.08	9.4	1.02			104			46			24	24	
8.0	80	163/75	119	19	29.3	1.21	1.19	10.0	1.02	7.37	22	103	101	11	47	38	-9	23	23	0.01
8.5	90		124	20	31.2	1.27	1.24	10.0	1.02			104			46			23	24	
9.0	90		127	22	33.7	1.38	1.30	10.2	1.06			105			47			23	24	
9.5	100		132	23	37.1	1.47	1.33	10.1	1.11			106			47			24	26	
10.0	100	175/81	134	23	37.4	1.52	1.38	10.3	1.10			106			47			23	26	
10.5	110		140	25	43.5	1.69	1.50	10.7	1.13			109			44			24	28	
11.0	110		144	28	50.0	1.88	1.60	11.1	1.18			111			43			25	30	
11.5	120		155	30	52.1	1.95	1.64	10.6	1.19			113			42			25	30	
12.0	120		154	34	59.6	2.10	1.71	11.1	1.23			114			41			27	33	
12.5	130		156	30	54.3	1.99	1.65	10.6	1.21			113			42			26	31	
13.0	130	194/81	160	38	70.0	2.27	1.64	10.3	1.38	7.31	16	114	108	16	39	33	-6	29	41	0.11
	Recovery	156/69	144	28	48.6	1.77	1.44	10.0	1.23	7.28	16	113	104	17	43	34	-9	26	32	0.03
	Recovery		132	26	47.5	1.57	0.95	7.2	1.65			123			38			29	48	
	Recovery		128	19	33.0	1.09	0.62	4.8	1.76			125			38			29	51	
	Recovery	131/63	121	22	28.0	0.84	0.50	4.1	1.68	7.26	13	126	117	13	35	30	-5	31	52	0.07

TABLE 4-4. *Oxygen breathing.*

Time min	Work rate watts	BP mm Hg	HR min⁻¹	f min⁻¹	$\dot{V}_E$ L/min BTPS	$\dot{V}CO_2$ L/min STPD	$\dot{V}O_2$ L/min STPD	$\dfrac{\dot{V}O_2}{HR}$ ml/beat	R	pH	HCO₃ meq/L	PO2, mm Hg ET	a	(A-a)	PCO2, mm Hg ET	a	(a-ET)	$\dfrac{\dot{V}_E}{\dot{V}CO_2}$	$\dfrac{\dot{V}_E}{\dot{V}O_2}$	$\dfrac{VD}{VT}$
	Rest		72	14	10.3	0.25									33			36		
	Rest		73	15	7.2	0.13									32			46		
	Rest		68	18	7.5	0.15									32			40		
	Rest	106/75	71	15	7.6	0.16				7.44	25	643	33		33	37	4	40		0.34
	Unloaded		80	27	5.6	0.09									38			37		
	Unloaded		87	17	10.2	0.31									43			28		
	Unloaded		69	23	9.3	0.25									41			29		
	Unloaded	113/69	77	24	9.2	0.25				7.39	24	605	67		42	41	-1	29		0.21
0.5	20		80	13	8.5	0.27									44			27		
1.0	20		90	13	10.0	0.34									44			26		
1.5	40		88	15	12.5	0.45									45			25		
2.0	40	125/69	91	14	11.6	0.43				7.39	26	595	75		48	43	-5	24		0.15
2.5	60		97	15	15.2	0.59									47			24		
3.0	60		100	16	18.8	0.73									48			24		
3.5	80		108	18	20.1	0.82									49			23		
4.0	80	144/75	112	17	21.7	0.94				7.34	25	601	64		52	48	-4	22		0.15
4.5	100		121	20	28.3	1.18									49			23		
5.0	100		124	19	27.1	1.18									52			22		
5.5	120		133	22	31.5	1.38									53			21		
6.0	120	169/81	144	25	38.0	1.68				7.29	22	587	79		52	47	-5	21		0.13
6.5	140		151	27	48.7	1.92									50			24		
7.0	140	175/81	155	30	51.4	2.01				7.30	21	564	106		46	43	-3	24		0.17
7.5	160	181/88	153	34	53.6	2.06				7.28	20	552	117		47	44	-3	25		0.19
	Recovery		143	26	47.4	1.89									48			24		
	Recovery		128	26	44.8	1.64									45			26		
	Recovery		120	22	34.6	1.21									41			27		
	Recovery		108	23	32.5	0.98									38			31		

Interpretation

COMMENTS

Resting respiratory function (Table 4-1) and ECG are normal.

ANALYSIS

In flow chart 1, the maximum $\dot{V}O_2$ and anaerobic threshold are normal (Table 4-2). See flow chart 2 for further analysis. There are no ECG abnormalities, and arterial blood gas values and VD/VT are normal throughout exercise (Table 4-3) (branchpoint 2.1). The patient is not obese (Table 4-1) (branchpoint 2.2). Thus, this patient has no limitation to exercise for her age and has no physiologic evidence of cardiovascular or pulmonary disease.

Pa_{O_2} is also normal during 100% O_2 breathing (Table 4-4), ruling out a significant right to left shunt.

Of special note is that the patient was able to exercise to a higher work rate with a slightly lower heart rate during O_2 breathing instead of air breathing. Moreover, respiratory compensation for the metabolic acidosis (decrease in Pa_{CO_2}) was less evident during the O_2 breathing study.

CONCLUSION

Our final assessment is that this patient was actually normal and her symptoms were the result of anxiety regarding her performance at sports.

CASE 5 *Normal woman*

CLINICAL FINDINGS

This non-smoking occupational therapist was referred for evaluation of dyspnea. She described the sensation as the inability to take a deep breath. She also noted nervousness, dizziness, and shortness of breath while eating. She was usually active in sports, but also noted shortness of breath in these activities. Physical examination was normal except for resting tachycardia and a $\frac{2}{6}$ systolic ejection murmur. Echocardiogram revealed a mitral valve prolapse. There were no dysrhythmias on 24 hour Holter monitoring. Chest roentgenograms, ECG, and respiratory function tests were normal, except for some reduction in expiratory flow rates attributable to reduced effort.

EXERCISE FINDINGS

The patient performed exercise on a cycle ergometer. She pedalled at 60 rpm without added load for 3 minutes. The work rate was then increased 15 W per minute to her symptom-limited maximum. Arterial blood was sampled every second minute, and intra-arterial blood pressure was recorded from a percutaneously placed brachial artery catheter. She stopped pedalling at 150 W complaining of fatigue and a feeling of palpitations. She felt somewhat short of breath. There were no abnormal ST changes or arrhythmia. No wheezing or diminution of FEV_1 occurred in the post-exercise period.

TABLE 5-1. *Selected Respiratory Function Data*

MEASUREMENT	PREDICTED	MEASURED
Age, yr		24
Sex		Female
Height, cm		159
Weight, kg	61	51
Hematocrit, %		40
VC, L	3.60	3.50
IC, L	2.40	2.11
TLC, L	4.91	4.71
FEV_1, L	3.01	2.55
FEV_1/VC, %	84	73
MVV, L/min	115	118
D_{LCO}, ml/mm Hg/min	26.5	29.8

TABLE 5-2. *Selected Exercise Data*

MEASUREMENT	PREDICTED	MEASURED
Maximum $\dot{V}_{O_2}$, L/min	1.84	1.62
Maximum HR, beats/min	196	198
Maximum O_2 pulse, ml/beat	9.4	8.2
$\Delta\dot{V}_{O_2}/\Delta WR$, ml/min/W	10.3	9.1
AT, L/min	> 0.83	1.0
Blood pressure, mm Hg (rest, max)		135/84,177/87
Maximum $\dot{V}_E$, L/min		64
Exercise breathing reserve, L/min	> 15	54
Pa_{O_2}, mm Hg (rest, max ex)		95,100
$P(A-a)_{O_2}$, mm Hg (rest, max ex)		14,17
$P(a-ET)_{CO_2}$, mm Hg (rest, max ex)		−1,−3
V_D/V_T (rest, heavy ex)		0.20,0.16
HCO_3^-, mEq/L (rest, 2-min recov)		25,15

FIG. 5-A.

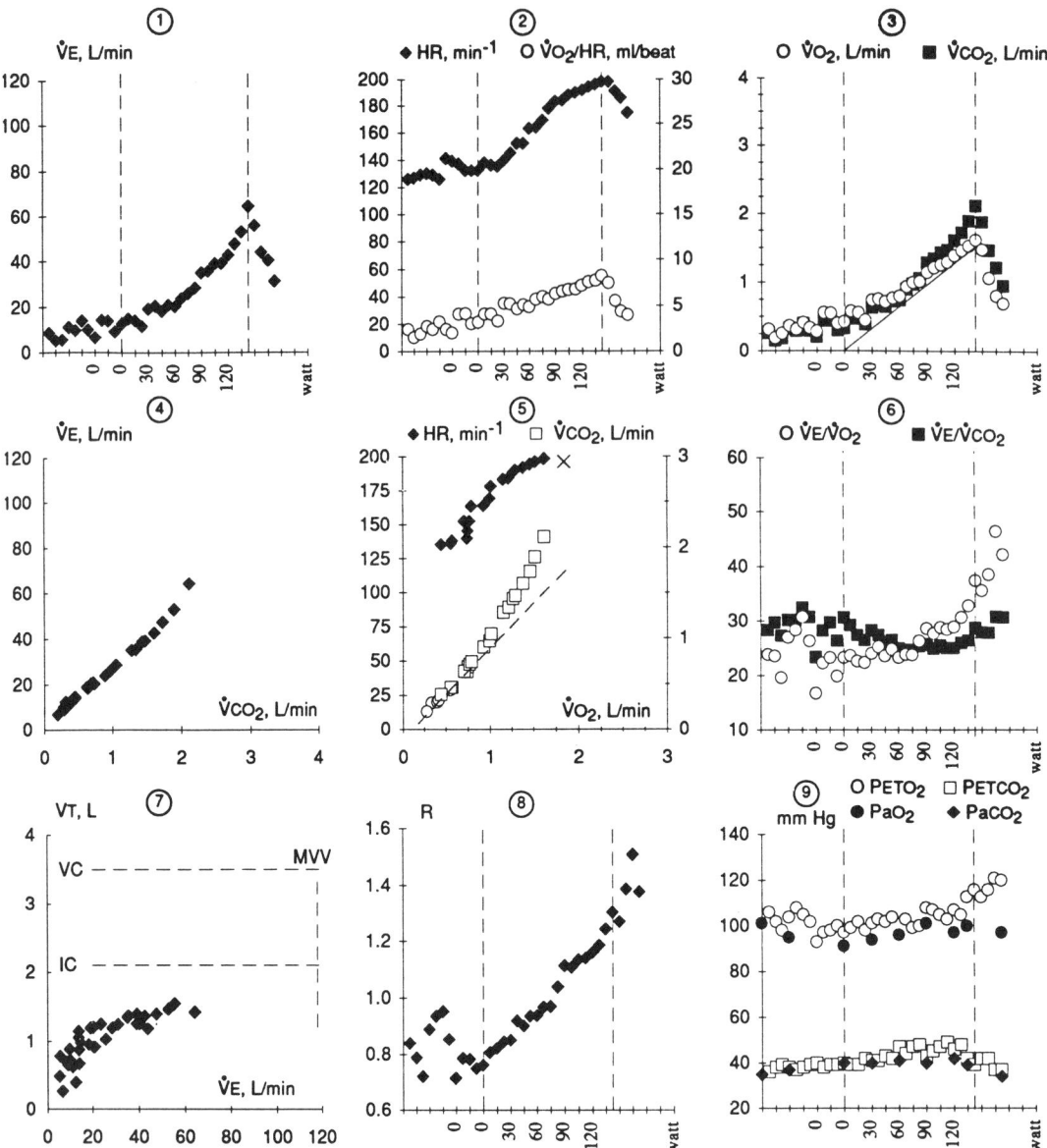

1. Vertical dashed lines in panels 1 to 3 and 6, 8, and 9 indicate the beginning and the end of increasing work period.

2. Unloaded cycling is performed for 3 minutes before the left vertical dashed line.

3. In panel 3, the diagonal line shows the increase of $\dot{V}O_2$ at a slope of 10 ml/min/W.

4. In panel 5, the diagonal dashed line has a slope of 1; the "x" in the upper right is the predicted maximum heart rate and $\dot{V}O_2$ for the subject.

TABLE 5-3.

Time min	Work rate watts	BP mm Hg	HR min⁻¹	f min⁻¹	V̇E L/min BTPS	V̇CO₂ L/min STPD	V̇O₂ L/min STPD	V̇O₂/HR ml/beat	R	pH	HCO₃ meq/L	PO₂, mm Hg ET	a	(A-a)	PCO₂, mm Hg ET	a	(a-ET)	V̇E/V̇CO₂	V̇E/V̇O₂	VD/VT
	Rest	135/84								7.47	25		101			35				
	Rest		126	12	8.4	0.26	0.31	2.5	0.84			106			36			28	24	
	Rest		127	11	5.4	0.15	0.19	1.5	0.79			102			38			30	24	
	Rest		129	7	5.5	0.18	0.25	1.9	0.72			98			39			27	20	
	Rest	144/84	130	18	11.2	0.32	0.36	2.8	0.89	7.44	25	104	95	14	38	37	-1	30	27	0.20
	Rest		129	11	9.7	0.29	0.31	2.4	0.94			108			37			30	28	
	Rest		126	13	13.7	0.39	0.41	3.3	0.95			105			38			32	31	
	Unloaded		141	14	10.1	0.29	0.34	2.4	0.85			102			39			31	26	
	Unloaded		139	25	6.8	0.20	0.28	2.0	0.71			93			40			23	17	
	Unloaded		137	21	14.2	0.44	0.56	4.1	0.79			97			38			28	22	
	Unloaded		132	12	13.8	0.43	0.55	4.2	0.78			98			39			30	23	
	Unloaded		132	14	9.1	0.30	0.40	3.0	0.75			100			39			26	20	
	Unloaded	141/81	132	32	12.5	0.32	0.42	3.2	0.76	7.42	25	97	91	9	40	40	0	31	23	0.23
0.5	15		138	15	14.7	0.46	0.57	4.1	0.81			99			39			29	24	
1.0	15		136	16	14.0	0.46	0.56	4.1	0.82			102			39			27	23	
1.5	30		135	17	11.5	0.38	0.45	3.3	0.84			98			42			26	22	
2.0	30	150/84	140	16	19.1	0.63	0.74	5.3	0.85	7.42	25	101	94	10	41	40	-1	28	24	0.22
2.5	45		145	17	20.4	0.69	0.75	5.2	0.92			103			41			27	25	
3.0	45		152	19	18.3	0.64	0.71	4.7	0.90			102			43			26	24	
3.5	60		152	23	21.0	0.72	0.77	5.1	0.94			104			42			26	25	
4.0	60	159/84	163	22	20.3	0.74	0.79	4.8	0.94	7.40	25	96	96	11	47	41	-6	25	23	0.14
4.5	75		164	19	23.8	0.90	0.93	5.7	0.97			103			44			25	24	
5.0	75		169	25	25.9	0.97	1.00	5.9	0.97			99			47			25	24	
5.5	90		178	24	28.6	1.05	1.01	5.7	1.04			100			48			25	26	
6.0	90	171/81	183	26	35.1	1.28	1.15	6.3	1.11	7.38	23	108	101	12	43	40	-3	26	29	0.15
6.5	105		184	26	35.6	1.34	1.21	6.6	1.11			107			45			25	28	
7.0	105		188	31	39.0	1.43	1.26	6.7	1.13			105			47			25	29	
7.5	120		190	28	39.1	1.47	1.29	6.8	1.14			103			49			25	28	
8.0	120	174/87	192	31	42.6	1.60	1.38	7.2	1.16	7.32	21	107	97	16	46	42	-4	25	29	0.17
8.5	135		194	34	47.6	1.73	1.46	7.5	1.18			105			48			26	31	
9.0	135	177/87	196	36	52.8	1.89	1.52	7.8	1.24	7.31	19	113	100	17	42	39	-3	26	33	0.15
9.5	150		198	45	64.2	2.11	1.62	8.2	1.30			116			39			29	37	
	Recovery		198	36	55.6	1.88	1.48	7.5	1.27			113			42			28	36	
	Recovery		191	37	43.9	1.47	1.06	5.5	1.39			116			42			28	38	
	Recovery		186	32	40.3	1.22	0.81	4.4	1.51			121			37			31	46	
	Recovery	153/78	175	25	31.2	0.95	0.69	3.9	1.38	7.27	15	120	97	26	37	34	-3	31	42	0.16

Interpretation

COMMENTS

This young woman, who experienced occasions of dyspnea, has normal lung volumes and flow rates indicating the absence of restrictive or obstructive lung disease (Table 5-1). In addition, her diffusing capacity is normal. Her resting ECG is also normal.

ANALYSIS

In flow chart 1, the maximum V̇O₂ and anaerobic threshold are normal (Table 5-2). See flow chart 2: Her ECG and O₂ pulse at maximum exercise are normal and her arterial blood gases remain normal through exercise (branchpoint 2.1). This patient is not obese (branchpoint 2.2). This leads to the diagnosis of a normal subject with anxiety; however, she has a marked tachycardia at rest and an appropriate heart rate response to exercise. Hyperthyroidism was ruled out and the tachycardia was not a persistent observation (Holter monitoring), as might be found with vasoregulatory asthenia.

CONCLUSION

This is a normal young woman with anxiety; however, the sensation of palpitations was not related to a cardiac arrhythmia. The patient deserves follow-up for endocrine disorders or other conditions that might account for her symptoms.

CASE 6 *Normal man*

CLINICAL FINDINGS

This 37-year-old shipyard machinist was evaluated because of complaints of dyspnea. He stated that he had been unable to play a full game of baseball for the last 6 years and that he gets out of breath and has to stop after climbing 3 to 4 flights on shipboard. He never smoked. He denied cough, chest pain, edema, or other symptoms. Physical, roentgenographic, and laboratory examinations were normal.

EXERCISE FINDINGS

The patient performed exercise on a cycle ergometer. He pedalled at 60 rpm without added load for 3 minutes. The work rate was then increased 25 W per minute to his symptom-limited maximum. Arterial blood was sampled every second minute, and intra-arterial blood pressure was recorded from a percutaneously placed brachial artery catheter. He stopped exercise because of general fatigue. Resting and exercise ECGs were normal.

TABLE 6-1. *Selected Respiratory Function Data*

MEASUREMENT	PREDICTED	MEASURED
Age, yr		37
Sex		Male
Height, cm		157
Weight, kg	63	67
Hematocrit, %		45
VC, L	3.30	4.38
IC, L	2.20	2.80
TLC, L	4.52	5.30
FEV_1, L	2.66	3.52
FEV_1/VC, %	81	80
MVV, L/min	127	124
DL_{CO}, ml/mm Hg/min	22.4	29.8

TABLE 6-2. *Selected Exercise Data*

MEASUREMENT	PREDICTED	MEASURED
Maximum $\dot{V}_{O_2}$, L/min	2.36	2.23
Maximum HR, beats/min	183	188
Maximum O_2 pulse, ml/beat	12.9	11.9
$\Delta\dot{V}_{O_2}/\Delta$WR, ml/min/W	10.3	10.4
AT, L/min	> 0.99	1.1
Blood pressure, mm Hg (rest, max)		125/75,188/94
Maximum $\dot{V}_E$, L/min		90
Exercise breathing reserve, L/min	> 15	34
Pa_{O_2}, mm Hg (rest, max ex)		84,114
$P(A-a)_{O_2}$, mm Hg (rest, max ex)		7,2
$P(a-ET)_{CO_2}$, mm Hg (rest, max ex)		0, −4
V_D/V_T (rest, heavy ex)		0.31,0.16
HCO_3^-, mEq/L (rest, 2-min recov)		24,16

Fig. 6-A.

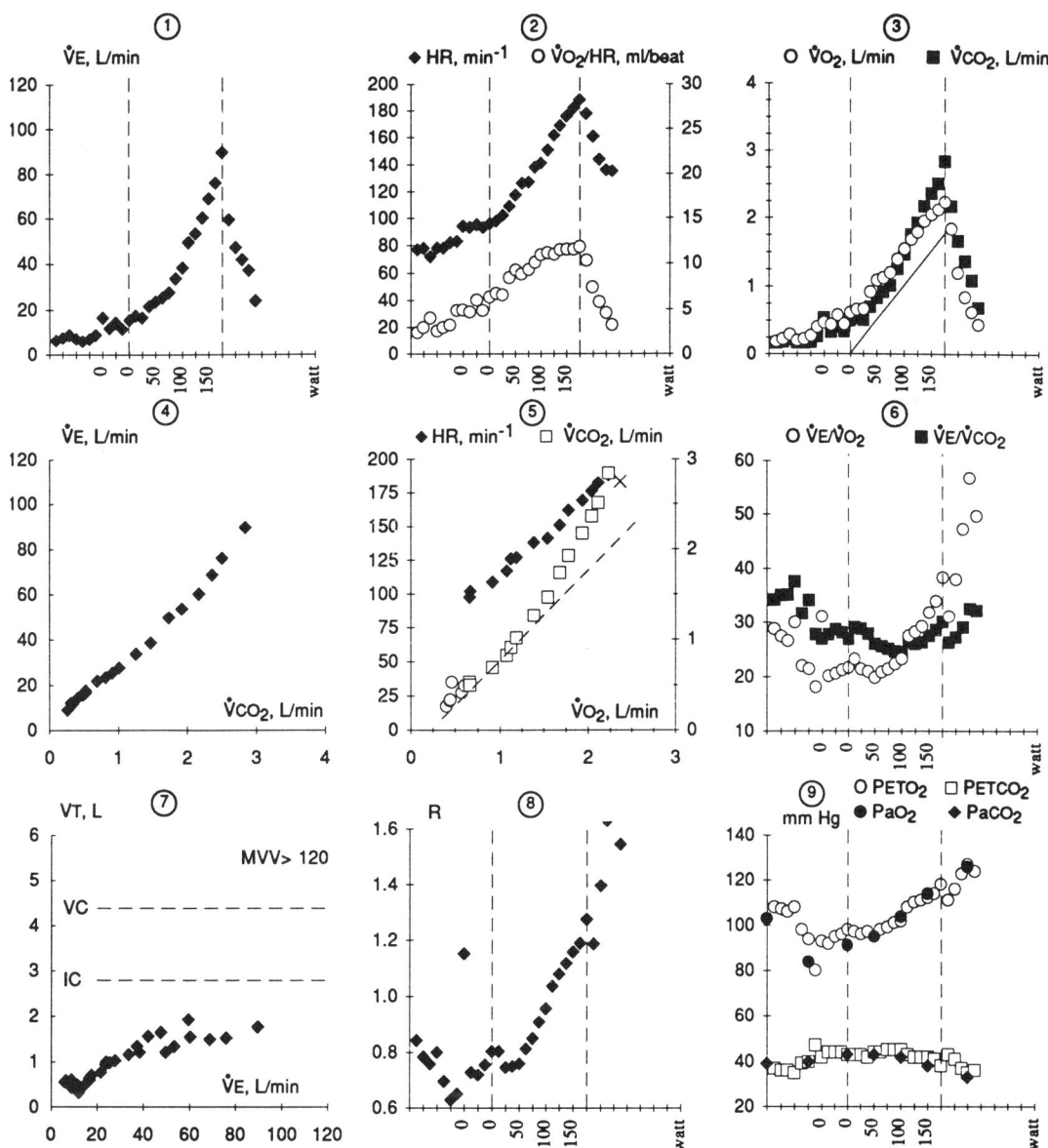

1. Vertical dashed lines in panels 1 to 3 and 6, 8, and 9 indicate the beginning and the end of increasing work period.

2. Unloaded cycling is performed for 3 minutes before the left vertical dashed line.

3. In panel 3, the diagonal line shows the increase of $\dot{V}O_2$ at a slope of 10 ml/min/W.

4. In panel 5, the diagonal dashed line has a slope of 1; the "x" in the upper right is the predicted maximum heart rate and $\dot{V}O_2$ for the subject.

TABLE 6-3.

Time min	Work rate watts	BP mm Hg	HR min⁻¹	f min⁻¹	$\dot{V}E$ L/min BTPS	$\dot{V}CO_2$ L/min STPD	$\dot{V}O_2$ L/min STPD	$\dfrac{\dot{V}O_2}{HR}$ ml/beat	R	pH	HCO₃ meq/L	PO2, mm Hg ET	a	(A-a)	PCO2, mm Hg ET	a	(a-ET)	$\dfrac{\dot{V}E}{\dot{V}CO2}$	$\dfrac{\dot{V}E}{\dot{V}O2}$	$\dfrac{VD}{VT}$
	Rest	125/75								7.41	24	103			39					
	Rest		77	11	6.4	0.16	0.19	2.5	0.84			108			37			34	29	
	Rest		78	14	7.5	0.18	0.23	2.9	0.78			107			36			35	27	
	Rest		72	15	9.0	0.22	0.29	4.0	0.76			106			36			35	27	
	Rest		78	13	7.1	0.16	0.20	2.6	0.80			108			35			37	30	
	Rest		78	11	6.0	0.16	0.23	2.9	0.70			98			39			32	22	
	Rest	125/81	82	13	6.9	0.17	0.27	3.3	0.63	7.39	24	94	84	7	40	40	0	34	21	0.31
	Unloaded		83	21	9.0	0.26	0.40	4.8	0.65			80			47			28	18	
	Unloaded		94	28	16.7	0.53	0.46	4.9	1.15			93			42			27	31	
	Unloaded		93	38	12.1	0.32	0.44	4.7	0.73			92			44			28	20	
	Unloaded		95	31	14.4	0.41	0.57	6.0	0.72			95			44			29	21	
	Unloaded		93	23	11.5	0.34	0.45	4.8	0.76			96			44			28	21	
	Unloaded	144/81	96	28	15.6	0.49	0.61	6.4	0.80	7.37	24	98	91	8	43	43	0	27	22	0.22
0.5	25		98	25	17.5	0.53	0.66	6.7	0.80			97			43			29	23	
1.0	25		102	26	16.6	0.50	0.67	6.6	0.75			96			43			29	21	
1.5	50		109	28	21.6	0.69	0.92	8.4	0.75			97			42			28	21	
2.0	50	150/81	117	25	23.5	0.82	1.08	9.2	0.76	7.38	25	95	95	1	44	43	-1	26	20	0.21
2.5	75		126	26	25.5	0.91	1.12	8.9	0.81			98			44			26	21	
3.0	75		127	27	27.7	1.01	1.19	9.4	0.85			99			45			25	21	
3.5	100		138	29	33.6	1.26	1.39	10.1	0.91			101			45			25	22	
4.0	100	181/94	141	32	38.6	1.47	1.54	10.9	0.95	7.37	24	102	104	2	45	42	-3	24	23	0.15
4.5	125		151	41	49.7	1.74	1.68	11.1	1.04			108			43			27	28	
5.0	125		162	40	53.5	1.92	1.78	11.0	1.08			110			42			26	28	
5.5	150		169	39	60.2	2.17	1.94	11.5	1.12			111			42			26	29	
6.0	150	188/94	176	46	68.8	2.36	2.04	11.6	1.16	7.37	22	112	114	2	42	38	-4	27	32	0.16
6.5	175		182	50	76.0	2.51	2.11	11.6	1.19			114			41			29	34	
7.0	175		188	51	89.7	2.84	2.23	11.9	1.27			118			38			30	38	
	Recovery		178	31	59.6	2.17	1.83	10.3	1.19			111			43			26	31	
	Recovery		161	29	47.5	1.66	1.19	7.4	1.39			116			41			27	38	
	Recovery		144	27	42.0	1.37	0.84	5.8	1.63			123			37			29	47	
	Recovery	181/100	136	28	37.5	1.08	0.62	4.6	1.74	7.30	16	127	126	2	35	33	-2	33	57	0.18
	Recovery		135	24	23.9	0.68	0.44	3.3	1.55			124			36			32	50	

Interpretation

COMMENTS

The results of this patient's resting respiratory function studies are normal (Table 6-1). The resting ECG is normal.

ANALYSIS

In flow chart 1, maximum $\dot{V}O_2$ and the anaerobic threshold are within normal limits (Table 6-2). See flow chart 2: ECG, O_2 pulse at maximum $\dot{V}O_2$, and arterial blood gases are normal (branchpoint 2.1). The patient is not obese (branchpoint 2.2).

CONCLUSION

This is a normal 37-year-old man. Symptoms probably relate to anxiety and lack of fitness.

CASE 7 Normal man

CLINICAL FINDINGS

This 74-year-old retired shipyard worker was referred for evaluation and exercise testing because work-up at another institution had resulted in a diagnosis of "emphysema" despite no evidence of airway obstruction. The patient had a mild, nonproductive cough, had smoked approximately 35 cigarette pack years, and continued to smoke. He had no other circulatory or respiratory symptoms, except for shortness of breath from climbing 2 flights of stairs but not from walking for 1 mile on the level. Physical examination was normal. Exercise testing was performed to help resolve the difference between clinical impressions.

EXERCISE FINDINGS

The patient performed exercise on a cycle ergometer. He pedalled at 60 rpm without added load for 3 minutes. The work rate was then increased 15 W per minute to his symptom-limited maximum. Arterial blood was sampled every second minute, and intra-arterial blood pressure was recorded from a percutaneously placed brachial artery catheter. The patient stopped exercise because of shortness of breath. Resting and exercise ECGs were normal.

TABLE 7-1. *Selected Respiratory Function Data*

MEASUREMENT	PREDICTED	MEASURED
Age, yr		74
Sex		Male
Height, cm		169
Weight, kg	73	82
Hematocrit, %		44
VC, L	3.37	4.88
IC, L	2.25	4.12
TLC, L	5.60	6.05
FEV_1, L	2.58	3.96
FEV_1/VC, %	77	81
MVV, L/min	110	107
D_{LCO}, ml/mm Hg/min	21.6	24.8

TABLE 7-2. *Selected Exercise Data*

MEASUREMENT	PREDICTED	MEASURED
Maximum $\dot{V}O_2$, L/min	1.74	1.95
Maximum HR, beats/min	146	132
Maximum O_2 pulse, ml/beat	11.9	14.8
$\Delta\dot{V}O_2/\Delta WR$, ml/min/W	10.3	10.6
AT, L/min	> 0.78	1.4
Blood pressure, mm Hg (rest, max)		150/84,177/79
Maximum $\dot{V}E$, L/min		68
Exercise breathing reserve, L/min	> 15	39
PaO_2, mm Hg (rest, max ex)		97,101
$P(A-a)O_2$, mm Hg (rest, max ex)		20,16
$P(a-ET)CO_2$, mm Hg (rest, max ex)		3,0
VD/VT (rest, heavy ex)		0.35,0.22
HCO_3^-, mEq/L (rest, 2-min recov)		20,15

Fig. 7-A.

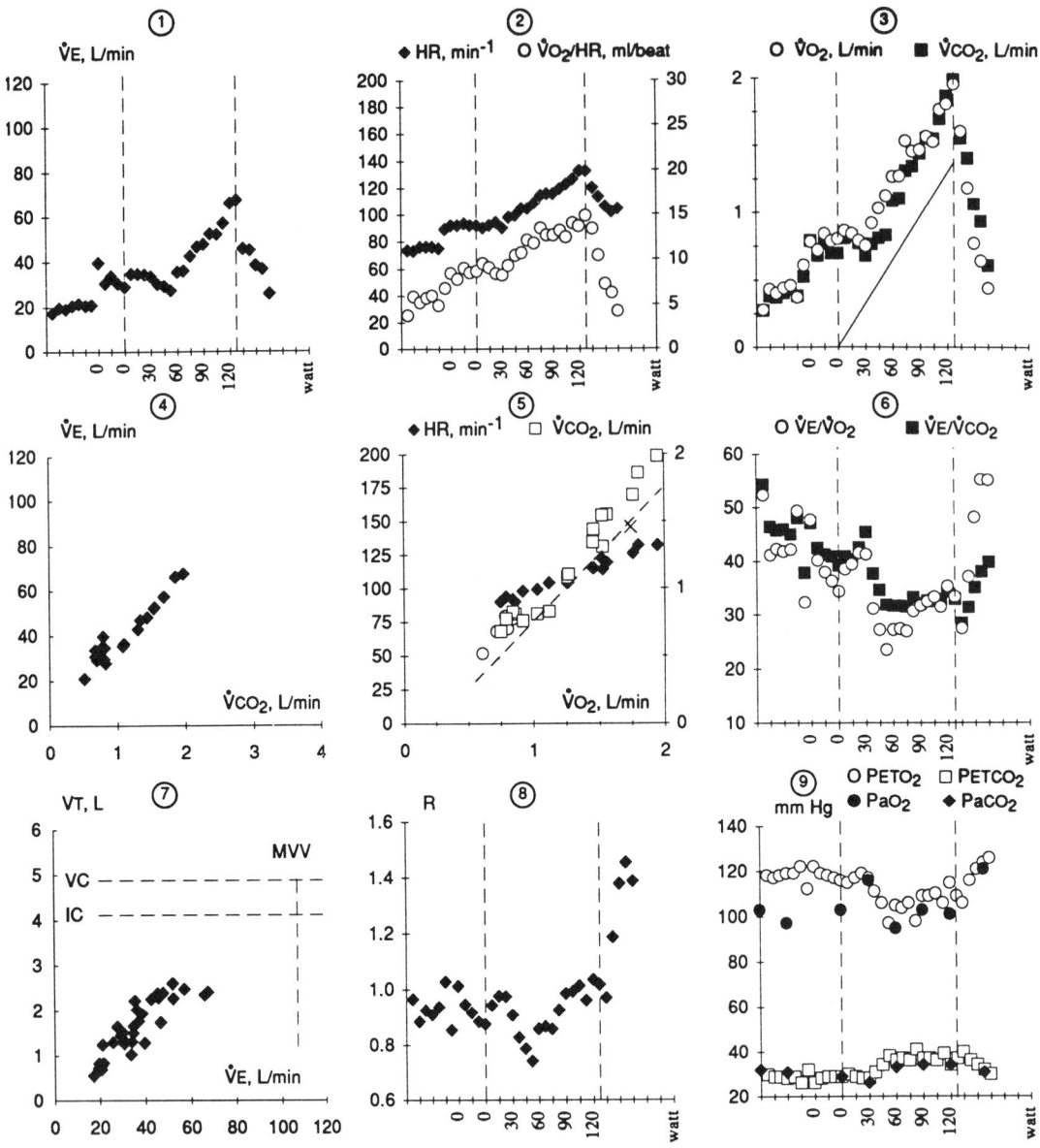

1. Vertical dashed lines in panels 1 to 3 and 6, 8, and 9 indicate the beginning and the end of increasing work period.

2. Unloaded cycling is performed for 3 minutes before the left vertical dashed line.

3. In panel 3, the diagonal line shows the increase of $\dot{V}O_2$ at a slope of 10 ml/min/W.

4. In panel 5, the diagonal dashed line has a slope of 1; the "x" in the upper right is the predicted maximum heart rate and $\dot{V}O_2$ for the subject.

TABLE 7-3.

Time min	Work rate watts	BP mm Hg	HR min⁻¹	f min⁻¹	$\dot{V}E$ L/min BTPS	$\dot{V}CO_2$ L/min STPD	$\dot{V}O_2$ L/min STPD	$\dfrac{\dot{V}O_2}{HR}$ ml/beat	R	pH	HCO₃ meq/L	PO2 ET	PO2 a	PO2 (A-a)	PCO2 ET	PCO2 a	PCO2 (a-ET)	$\dfrac{\dot{V}E}{\dot{V}CO_2}$	$\dfrac{\dot{V}E}{\dot{V}O_2}$	VD/VT
	Rest	150/82								7.41	20		103			32				
	Rest		74	31	17.3	0.27	0.28	3.8	0.96			118			30			54	52	
	Rest		73	24	19.7	0.38	0.43	5.9	0.88			117			29			46	41	
	Rest		76	27	19.2	0.37	0.40	5.3	0.93			118			29			46	42	
	Rest	147/84	76	27	20.7	0.40	0.44	5.8	0.91	7.42	20	119	97	20	28	31	3	46	42	0.35
	Rest		76	26	21.6	0.43	0.46	6.1	0.93			119			29			45	42	
	Rest		75	30	20.8	0.38	0.37	4.9	1.03			122			26			48	49	
	Unloaded		89	17	21.1	0.52	0.61	6.9	0.85			112			32			38	32	
	Unloaded		92	31	39.8	0.79	0.78	8.5	1.01			122			26			47	48	
	Unloaded		92	23	30.8	0.68	0.72	7.8	0.94			119			28			42	40	
	Unloaded		93	26	34.0	0.77	0.84	9.0	0.92			118			29			41	38	
	Unloaded		92	24	30.7	0.70	0.79	8.6	0.89			117			29			41	36	
	Unloaded	162/84	92	20	29.1	0.70	0.80	8.7	0.88	7.42	18	116	103	15	29	29	0	39	34	0.23
0.5	15		90	21	34.9	0.81	0.86	9.6	0.94			115			30			41	39	
1.0	15		92	21	34.8	0.82	0.84	9.1	0.98			117			29			40	39	
1.5	30		94	23	34.7	0.77	0.79	8.4	0.97			119			28			43	41	
2.0	30	159/81	90	33	33.7	0.68	0.75	8.3	0.91	7.44	17	117	116	6	28	26	-2	45	41	0.25
2.5	45		98	20	30.3	0.76	0.92	9.4	0.83			111			31			38	31	
3.0	45		99	20	29.7	0.81	1.03	10.4	0.79			106			34			35	27	
3.5	60		104	17	27.8	0.83	1.12	10.8	0.74			97			38			32	24	
4.0	60	168/84	104	16	35.6	1.08	1.26	12.1	0.86	7.37	19	105	95	18	36	33	-3	32	27	0.17
4.5	75		108	18	36.4	1.10	1.27	11.8	0.87			104			37			32	27	
5.0	75		114	19	42.8	1.31	1.53	13.4	0.86			106			36			31	27	
5.5	90		115	27	46.8	1.34	1.45	12.6	0.92			98			41			33	31	
6.0	90	186/90	115	20	47.9	1.44	1.46	12.7	0.99	7.36	19	109	103	13	37	34	-3	32	32	0.20
6.5	105		119	23	52.5	1.55	1.56	13.1	0.99			109			37			33	32	
7.0	105		122	20	52.2	1.54	1.52	12.5	1.01			110			36			33	33	
7.5	120		126	23	57.2	1.69	1.76	14.0	0.96			106			39			33	31	
8.0	120	177/79	132	28	66.1	1.86	1.80	13.6	1.03	7.33	18	115	101	16	34	34	0	34	35	0.25
8.5	135		132	28	67.5	1.98	1.95	14.8	1.02			109			37			33	33	
	Recovery		120	20	45.8	1.55	1.60	13.3	0.97			106			40			28	28	
	Recovery		113	19	45.4	1.40	1.18	10.4	1.19			116			36			31	37	
	Recovery		106	20	38.8	1.06	0.77	7.3	1.38			121			34			35	48	
	Recovery	168/78	102	21	37.1	0.93	0.64	6.3	1.45	7.31	15	124	121	6	32	31	-1	38	55	0.25
	Recovery		104	20	25.9	0.61	0.44	4.2	1.39			126			30			40	55	

Interpretation

COMMENTS

This patient's resting respiratory function is normal (Table 7-1). The resting ECG is normal.

ANALYSIS

In flow chart 1, the maximum $\dot{V}O_2$ is normal. The anaerobic threshold is normal (Table 7-2). See flow chart 2: The ECG, O_2 pulse, arterial blood gases, and VD/VT are normal (branchpoint 2.1). The patient is not obese (branchpoint 2.2).

CONCLUSION

This is a normal cardiovascular and respiratory response to exercise. The patient has no evidence of abnormalities consistent with the diagnosis of "emphysema" given to the patient in a previous examination.

CASE 8 *Normal, with ventilatory chemoreflex insensitivity*

CLINICAL FINDINGS

This 67-year-old retired man had worked for 30 years in the shipyards. He had never smoked. Three months previously, he was found to have hypertension for which he was treated with triamterene and hydrochlorothiazide. He noted shortness of breath after climbing 2 flights of stairs and frequent mild substernal pressure not related to exertion, meals, body position, or stress. Physical, roentgenographic, laboratory, and ECG examinations were normal.

EXERCISE FINDINGS

The patient performed exercise on a cycle ergometer. He pedalled at 60 rpm without added load for 3 minutes. The work rate was then increased 20 W per minute to his symptom-limited maximum. Arterial blood was sampled every second minute, and intra-arterial blood pressure was recorded from a percutaneously placed brachial artery catheter. He stopped exercise with shortness of breath, but without chest pain or pressure. ECG pattern remained normal.

TABLE 8-1. *Selected Respiratory Function Data*

MEASUREMENT	PREDICTED	MEASURED
Age, yr		67
Sex		Male
Height, cm		173
Weight, kg	76	80
Hematocrit, %		48
VC, L	3.82	3.86
IC, L	2.55	2.42
TLC, L	6.06	6.04
FEV_1, L	2.97	3.07
FEV_1/VC, %	78	80
MVV, L/min	124	121
DL_{CO}, ml/mm Hg/min	26.3	32.3

TABLE 8-2. *Selected Exercise Data*

MEASUREMENT	PREDICTED	MEASURED
Maximum $\dot{V}_{O_2}$, L/min	1.98	1.94
Maximum HR, beats/min	153	142
Maximum O_2 pulse, ml/beat	13.0	13.7
$\Delta\dot{V}_{O_2}/\Delta WR$, ml/min/W	10.3	9.9
AT, L/min	> 0.89	1.5
Blood pressure, mm Hg (rest, max)		176/92,215/92
Maximum $\dot{V}_E$, L/min		56
Exercise breathing reserve, L/min	> 15	65
Pa_{O_2}, mm Hg (rest, max ex)		96,81
$P(A-a)_{O_2}$, mm Hg (rest, max ex)		8,22
$P(a-ET)_{CO_2}$, mm Hg (rest, max ex)		1,−6
V_D/V_T (rest, heavy ex)		0.39,0.26
HCO_3^-, mEq/L (rest, 2-min recov)		27,22

F IG. 8-A.

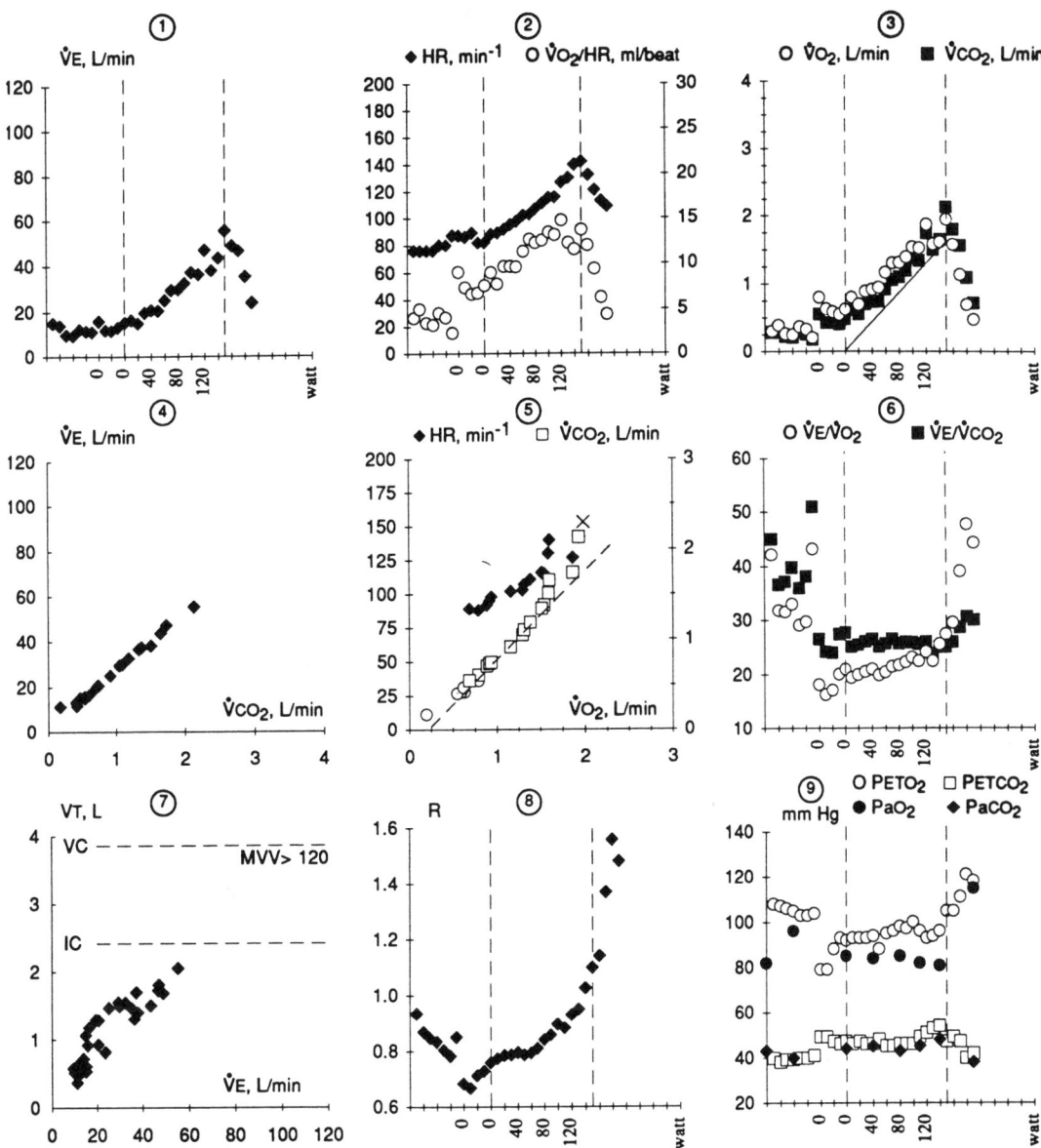

1. Vertical dashed lines in panels 1 to 3 and 6, 8, and 9 indicate the beginning and the end of increasing work period.

2. Unloaded cycling is performed for 3 minutes before the left vertical dashed line.

3. In panel 3, the diagonal line shows the increase of $\dot{V}O_2$ at a slope of 10 ml/min/W.

4. In panel 5, the diagonal dashed line has a slope of 1; the "x" in the upper right is the predicted maximum heart rate and $\dot{V}O_2$ for the subject.

TABLE 8-3.

Time min	Work rate watts	BP mm Hg	HR min⁻¹	f min⁻¹	V̇E L/min BTPS	V̇CO₂ L/min STPD	V̇O₂ L/min STPD	V̇O₂/HR ml/beat	R	pH	HCO₃ meq/L	PO₂ ET	PO₂ a	PO₂ (A-a)	PCO₂ ET	PCO₂ a	PCO₂ (a-ET)	V̇E/V̇CO₂	V̇E/V̇O₂	VD/VT
	Rest	176/92								7.41	27	82			40	43				
	Rest		76	28	15.0	0.28	0.30	3.9	0.93			108			40			45	42	
	Rest		76	19	13.7	0.33	0.38	5.0	0.87			107			38			37	32	
	Rest		76	19	9.8	0.22	0.26	3.4	0.85			106			39			37	31	
	Rest	164/92	76	16	9.3	0.20	0.24	3.2	0.83	7.43	26	105	96	8	39	40	1	40	33	0.39
	Rest		80	22	12.3	0.29	0.36	4.5	0.81			103			40			36	29	
	Rest		80	22	11.4	0.25	0.32	4.0	0.78			103			40			38	30	
	Unloaded		87	30	11.2	0.17	0.20	2.3	0.85			104			41			51	43	
	Unloaded		87	17	15.7	0.54	0.79	9.1	0.68			79			49			26	18	
	Unloaded		86	19	11.8	0.42	0.63	7.3	0.67			79			49			24	16	
	Unloaded		89	18	11.6	0.42	0.59	6.6	0.71			88			47			24	17	
	Unloaded		82	25	13.1	0.40	0.55	6.7	0.73			93			46			27	20	
	Unloaded	185/92	82	25	15.1	0.47	0.62	7.6	0.76	7.40	27	92	85	10	47	44	-3	28	21	0.25
0.5	20		88	14	16.5	0.61	0.79	9.0	0.77			93			46			25	19	
1.0	20		89	14	14.9	0.54	0.69	7.8	0.78			93			47			25	20	
1.5	40		92	15	19.5	0.70	0.89	9.7	0.79			93			46			26	20	
2.0	40	194/89	95	16	20.7	0.73	0.92	9.7	0.79	7.40	27	94	84	12	46	45	-1	26	21	0.26
2.5	60		98	22	20.5	0.74	0.94	9.6	0.79			88			48			25	20	
3.0	60		102	17	25.1	0.92	1.16	11.4	0.79			95			45			26	20	
3.5	80		103	19	29.5	1.05	1.30	12.6	0.81			96			45			27	21	
4.0	80	203/89	107	20	30.0	1.10	1.31	12.2	0.84	7.40	26	98	85	16	46	43	-3	26	22	0.21
4.5	100		111	21	32.6	1.19	1.39	12.5	0.86			97			46			26	22	
5.0	100		115	22	37.4	1.38	1.54	13.4	0.90			100			46			26	23	
5.5	120	209/89	116	28	36.6	1.34	1.52	13.1	0.88	7.38	26	96	82	18	49	45	-4	26	23	0.23
6.0	120		127	26	47.2	1.74	1.87	14.7	0.93			93			51			26	24	
6.5	140		130	27	38.1	1.51	1.59	12.2	0.95			94			53			24	23	
7.0	140	215/92	140	29	43.6	1.65	1.61	11.5	1.02	7.35	26	96	81	22	54	48	-6	25	26	0.26
7.5	160		142	27	55.5	2.13	1.94	13.7	1.10			105			47			25	27	
	Recovery		132	29	49.0	1.80	1.58	12.0	1.14			105			49			26	29	
	Recovery		121	27	46.8	1.56	1.14	9.4	1.37			111			47			29	39	
	Recovery		113	24	35.4	1.09	0.70	6.2	1.56			121			40			31	48	
	Recovery	209/92	109	29	23.7	0.71	0.48	4.4	1.48	7.37	22	118	115	7	42	38	-4	30	44	0.22

Interpretation

COMMENTS

Results of the resting respiratory function studies are normal (Table 8-1). The resting ECG is normal.

ANALYSIS

In flow chart 1, the maximum V̇O₂ and anaerobic threshold are normal (Table 8-2). See flow chart 2: The exercise ECG, arterial blood gases, VD/VT, and O₂ pulse at maximum V̇O₂ are normal (branchpoint 2.1). The patient is not obese (branchpoint 2.2). While the arterial CO₂ tension is normal at rest, the increase in ventilation lagged the increase in CO₂ production, causing arterial PCO₂ to rise gradually during exercise (panel 9, Fig. 8-A and Table 8-3). This is occasionally seen when the ventilatory chemoreflex is relatively insensitive to the exercise metabolic acidosis. Because the CO₂ stores are increasing in the body as a consequence of the rising PaCO₂, CO₂ output does not rise as steeply as it otherwise might, particularly above the anaerobic threshold. Thus, V̇E/V̇CO₂ at the termination of work is not increased over that at the AT (panel 6, Fig. 8-A) and there is no steepening in the V̇E-work rate relationship (panels 1 and 4, Fig. 8-A).

CONCLUSION

This is normal cardiovascular and respiratory function in a patient likely to have a ventilatory chemoreflex that is relatively insensitive to pH decrease.

CASE 9 *Exceptionally fit man with mild lung disease*

CLINICAL FINDINGS

This 59-year-old worker had no complaints or history of heart or lung disease. He had sustained a gunshot wound to the right chest at age 24 that was not surgically treated. He had been exposed to asbestos 20 years previously and had smoked 1 package of cigarettes daily for 12 years until 20 years ago. He cycled approximately 50 miles a week. Physical, roentgenographic, and ECG examinations were normal except for evidence of focal, old granulomatous disease and an old rib fracture.

EXERCISE FINDINGS

The patient performed exercise on a cycle ergometer. He pedalled at 60 rpm without added load for 3 minutes. The work rate was then increased 20 W per minute to his symptom-limited maximum. Arterial blood was sampled every second minute, and intra-arterial blood pressure was recorded from a percutaneously placed brachial artery catheter. He stopped exercise because of general exhaustion. Exercise ECGs were normal.

TABLE 9-1. *Selected Respiratory Function Data*

MEASUREMENT	PREDICTED	MEASURED
Age, yr		59
Sex		Male
Height, cm		175
Weight, kg	78	
Hematocrit, %		46
VC, L	4.21	4.34
IC, L	2.79	3.57
TLC, L	6.36	5.86
FEV_1, L	3.58	3.57
FEV_1/VC, %	80	82
MVV, L/min	137	152
D_{LCO}, ml/mm Hg/min	28.2	29.5

TABLE 9-2. *Selected Exercise Data*

MEASUREMENT	PREDICTED	MEASURED
Maximum $\dot{V}_{O_2}$, L/min	2.32	3.40
Maximum HR, beats/min	161	195
Maximum O_2 pulse, ml/beat	14.4	17.4
$\Delta\dot{V}_{O_2}/\Delta WR$, ml/min/W	10.3	12.7
AT, L/min	> 1.02	1.4
Blood pressure, mm Hg (rest, max)		125/75,200/88
Maximum $\dot{V}_E$, L/min		174
Exercise breathing reserve, L/min	> 15	− 22
Pa_{O_2}, mm Hg (rest, max ex)		120,71
$P(A-a)_{O_2}$, mm Hg (rest, max ex)		5,49
$P(a-ET)_{CO_2}$, mm Hg (rest, max ex)		−4, −13
V_D/V_T (rest, heavy ex)		0.17,0.02
HCO_3^-, mEq/L (rest, 2-min recov)		25,10

TABLE 9-3.

Time min	Work rate watts	BP mm Hg	HR min^{-1}	f min^{-1}	$\dot{V}E$ L/min BTPS	$\dot{V}CO_2$ L/min STPD	$\dot{V}O_2$ L/min STPD	$\dfrac{\dot{V}O_2}{HR}$ ml/beat	R	pH	HCO$_3$ meq/L	PO2, mm Hg ET	a	(A-a)	PCO2, mm Hg ET	a	(a-ET)	$\dfrac{\dot{V}E}{\dot{V}CO_2}$	$\dfrac{\dot{V}E}{\dot{V}O_2}$	VD VT
	Rest	125/75								7.45	25		75			36				
	Rest		77	11	20.9	0.48	0.36	4.7	1.33			123			30			42	55	
	Rest		77	17	17.3	0.36	0.28	3.6	1.29			124			29			44	57	
	Rest		79	11	16.2	0.39	0.34	4.3	1.15			122			29			39	45	
	Rest	119/75	84	8	14.6	0.36	0.33	3.9	1.09	7.52	22	118	120	5	31	27	-4	39	42	0.17
	Unloaded		96	7	16.4	0.54	0.67	7.0	0.81			97			39			29	24	
	Unloaded		84	12	21.9	0.65	0.74	8.8	0.88			106			36			32	28	
	Unloaded		81	13	23.9	0.68	0.72	8.9	0.94			110			35			34	32	
	Unloaded		81	17	26.2	0.68	0.70	8.6	0.97			111			34			36	35	
	Unloaded		82	10	23.0	0.66	0.71	8.7	0.93			108			35			34	31	
	Unloaded	156/81	82	16	23.3	0.65	0.69	8.4	0.94	7.47	22	110	103	14	35	31	-4	34	32	0.17
0.5	20		79	15	24.7	0.73	0.82	10.4	0.89			107			35			32	29	
1.0	20		84	18	23.3	0.70	0.78	9.3	0.90			99			39			31	28	
1.5	40		82	8	18.9	0.66	0.88	10.7	0.75			91			41			28	21	
2.0	40	163/81	89	8	24.0	0.87	1.11	12.5	0.78	7.43	24	92	77	28	42	37	-5	27	21	0.13
2.5	60		91	13	23.5	0.89	1.15	12.6	0.77			89			44			25	19	
3.0	60		99	16	24.2	0.90	1.18	11.9	0.76			84			47			25	19	
3.5	80		98	21	35.2	1.28	1.53	15.6	0.84			78			50			26	22	
4.0	80	175/81	107	14	36.1	1.38	1.54	14.4	0.90	7.41	24	95	85	24	45	38	-7	25	23	0.10
4.5	100		107	15	41.1	1.55	1.63	15.2	0.95			96			47			26	24	
5.0	100		113	16	43.4	1.72	1.82	16.1	0.95			97			47			24	23	
5.5	120		117	22	52.0	1.93	1.95	16.7	0.99			99			45			26	26	
6.0	120		123	20	56.5	2.08	2.07	16.8	1.00	7.37	21	99	86	27	46	37	-9	26	26	0.11
6.5	140		119	20	60.0	2.20	2.17	18.2	1.01			100			46			27	27	
7.0	140		128	21	61.2	2.33	2.26	17.7	1.03			101			46			26	26	
7.5	160		131	25	72.5	2.61	2.44	18.6	1.07			105			44			27	29	
8.0	160	200/88	147	21	69.8	2.65	2.50	17.0	1.06	7.35	18	102	75	43	46	34	-12	26	27	0.01
8.5	180		148	27	82.1	3.03	2.74	18.5	1.11			106			44			26	29	
9.0	180		161	26	82.2	3.11	2.79	17.3	1.11			104			46			26	29	
9.5	200		166	26	85.0	3.24	2.85	17.2	1.14			104			47			26	29	
10.0	200		167	30	90.6	3.40	2.90	17.4	1.17	7.29	16	106	71	49	47	34	-13	26	30	0.02
10.5	220		176	31	105.5	3.74	3.06	17.4	1.22			109			44			28	34	
11.0	220		189	34	117.3	4.01	3.13	16.6	1.28			112			42			29	37	
11.5	240		195	55	174.5	4.75	3.40	17.4	1.40			122			34			36	50	
	Recovery	200/88	180	35	121.1	3.52	2.68	14.9	1.31	7.26	13	118	83	43	36	29	-7	34	44	0.11
	Recovery		171	33	113.3	3.15	1.99	11.6	1.58			118			38			35	56	
	Recovery		159	26	89.2	2.42	1.35	8.5	1.79			125			36			36	64	
	Recovery	163/75	147	28	83.7	2.01	1.09	7.4	1.84	7.20	10	128	113	20	32	26	-6	40	75	0.17
	Recovery		145	27	67.1	1.50	0.90	6.2	1.67			128			31			43	72	
	Recovery																			

Interpretation

COMMENTS

The results of this patient's respiratory function studies are within normal limits (Table 9-1). The resting ECG is normal. The respiratory alkalosis at rest, while breathing on the mouthpiece, is acute, developing in anticipation of exercise. It disappears after exercise started. When starting to breathe on the mouthpiece, the patient hyperventilates to a pH of 7.52, Pa$_{CO_2}$ of 27 mm Hg and Pa$_{O_2}$ of 120. The extraordinarily large increase in Pa$_{O_2}$ when starting to breathe on the mouthpiece at rest is probably due to: (1) hypoxemia off the mouthpiece due to microatelectasis associated with obesity (a common problem in overweight subjects); and (2) the large increase in Pa$_{O_2}$, which accompanies acute hyperventilation, and a high R.

ANALYSIS

In flow chart 1, this patient's maximum $\dot{V}O_2$ and anaerobic threshold are above predicted (Table

Fig. 9-A.

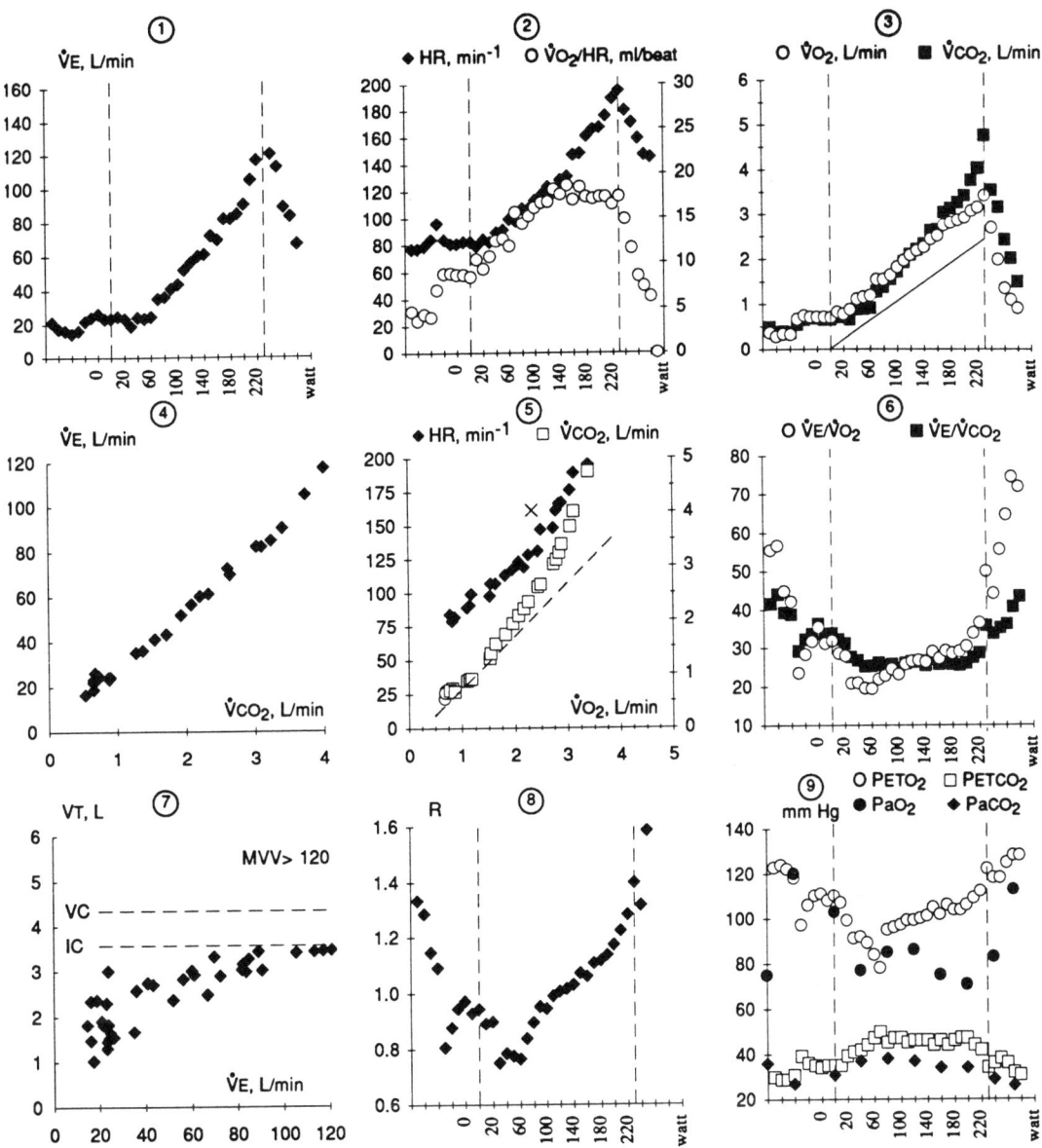

1. Vertical dashed lines in panels 1 to 3 and 6, 8, and 9 indicate the beginning and the end of increasing work period.

2. Unloaded cycling is performed for 3 minutes before the left vertical dashed line.

3. In panel 3, the diagonal line shows the increase of $\dot{V}O_2$ at a slope of 10 ml/min/W.

4. In panel 5, the diagonal dashed line has a slope of 1; the "x" in the upper right is the predicted maximum heart rate and $\dot{V}O_2$ for the subject.

9-2). Because he cycled regularly to maintain his fitness, he performed exceedingly well. See flow chart 2: The ECG and O_2 pulse (high because of fitness) at maximal exercise are normal, but the blood gases are abnormal (branchpoint 2.1). V_D/V_T and $P(a-ET)_{CO_2}$ are normal, but $P(A-a)_{O_2}$ at maximum exercise is increased and suggests the presence of mild lung disease (branchpoint 2.3).

CONCLUSION

This exceptionally fit man of 59 years has features of mild lung disease.

CASE 10 *Normal: Cycle and treadmill*

CLINICAL FINDINGS

This 37-year-old hospital employee was asymptomatic and volunteered for an exercise study. He did not exercise regularly or smoke. Physical examination, chest roentgenograms and resting ECG were normal.

EXERCISE FINDINGS

On 2 separate days, 1 month apart, the subject exercised to maximum tolerance using an incremental protocol, first on the cycle and second on the treadmill. He stopped on both occasions because of calf fatigue. There was no arrhythmia or abnormality in the ECG.

TABLE 10-1. *Selected Respiratory Function Data*

MEASUREMENT	PREDICTED	MEASURED
Age, yr		37
Sex		Male
Height, cm		161
Weight, kg	66	53
Hematocrit, %		45
VC, L	3.56	3.21
IC, L	2.37	2.51
TLC, L	4.90	5.01
FEV_1, L	2.87	2.64
FEV_1/VC, %	81	82
MVV, L/min	132	107
D_{LCO}, ml/mm Hg/min	23.1	22.3

TABLE 10-2. *Selected Exercise Data*

MEASUREMENT	PREDICTED cycle	PREDICTED treadmill	MEASURED cycle	MEASURED treadmill
Maximum $\dot{V}O_2$, L/min	2.21	2.45	1.87	2.07
Maximum HR, beats/min	183	183	173	183
Maximum O_2 pulse, ml/beat	12.1	13.4	10.8	11.3
$\Delta\dot{V}O_2/\Delta WR$, ml/min/W	10.3		8.4	
AT, L/min	> 0.93	> 1.03	1.1	1.15
Maximum $\dot{V}E$, L/min			76	85
Exercise breathing reserve, L/min	> 15	> 15	31	22

TABLE 10-3. *Cycle ergometry.*

Time min	Work rate watts	BP mm Hg	HR min⁻¹	f min⁻¹	$\dot{V}E$ L/min BTPS	$\dot{V}CO_2$ L/min STPD	$\dot{V}O_2$ L/min STPD	$\frac{\dot{V}O_2}{HR}$ ml/beat	R	pH	HCO_3 meq/L	PO2, mm Hg ET	PO2, mm Hg a	PO2, mm Hg (A-a)	PCO2, mm Hg ET	PCO2, mm Hg a	PCO2, mm Hg (a-ET)	$\frac{\dot{V}E}{\dot{V}CO_2}$	$\frac{\dot{V}E}{\dot{V}O_2}$	$\frac{VD}{VT}$
	Rest		79	15	9.5	0.28	0.33	4.2	0.85			99			44			29	25	
	Rest		95	14	11.1	0.36	0.42	4.4	0.86			97			45			28	24	
	Rest		78	13	7.8	0.23	0.26	3.3	0.88			101			44			29	26	
	Rest		74	14	7.3	0.19	0.21	2.8	0.90			102			43			32	29	
	Unloaded		109	18	17.3	0.58	0.55	5.0	1.05			105			44			27	29	
	Unloaded		97	8	11.1	0.44	0.52	5.4	0.85			96			46			24	20	
	Unloaded		103	17	14.3	0.53	0.63	6.1	0.84			92			48			24	20	
	Unloaded		104	16	15.1	0.56	0.65	6.3	0.86			94			47			25	21	
	Unloaded		108	16	17.7	0.67	0.71	6.6	0.94			97			47			24	23	
	Unloaded		97	16	14.8	0.55	0.55	5.7	1.00			103			46			24	24	
0.5	25		107	16	16.4	0.61	0.60	5.6	1.02			104			46			25	25	
1.0	25		108	18	16.2	0.57	0.57	5.3	1.00			103			45			26	26	
1.5	50		113	18	15.8	0.58	0.64	5.7	0.91			96			47			25	22	
2.0	50		110	17	17.1	0.67	0.74	6.7	0.91			94			50			23	21	
2.5	75		122	19	22.0	0.86	0.89	7.3	0.97			99			48			24	23	
3.0	75		129	17	19.8	0.85	0.90	7.0	0.94			93			52			22	20	
3.5	100		132	21	26.4	1.07	1.04	7.9	1.03			99			50			23	24	
4.0	100		133	17	22.9	1.07	1.12	8.4	0.96			89			57			20	19	
4.5	125		143	21	31.1	1.40	1.29	9.0	1.09			97			55			21	23	
5.0	125		147	22	35.1	1.64	1.50	10.2	1.09			95			56			20	22	
5.5	150		155	26	41.4	1.82	1.52	9.8	1.20			102			53			22	26	
6.0	150		159	27	44.4	1.94	1.58	9.9	1.23			103			53			22	27	
6.5	175		168	31	53.2	2.24	1.71	10.2	1.31			107			52			23	30	
7.0	175		173	44	75.8	2.79	1.87	10.8	1.49			114			46			26	39	
	Recovery		167	34	60.1	2.31	1.67	10.0	1.38			109			50			25	34	
	Recovery		158	30	49.5	1.88	1.29	8.2	1.46			112			49			25	36	
	Recovery		146	31	48.8	1.68	0.98	6.7	1.71			118			44			27	47	
	Recovery		140	27	40.1	1.30	0.73	5.2	1.78			121			42			29	52	

FIG. 10-A. *Cycle ergometry.*

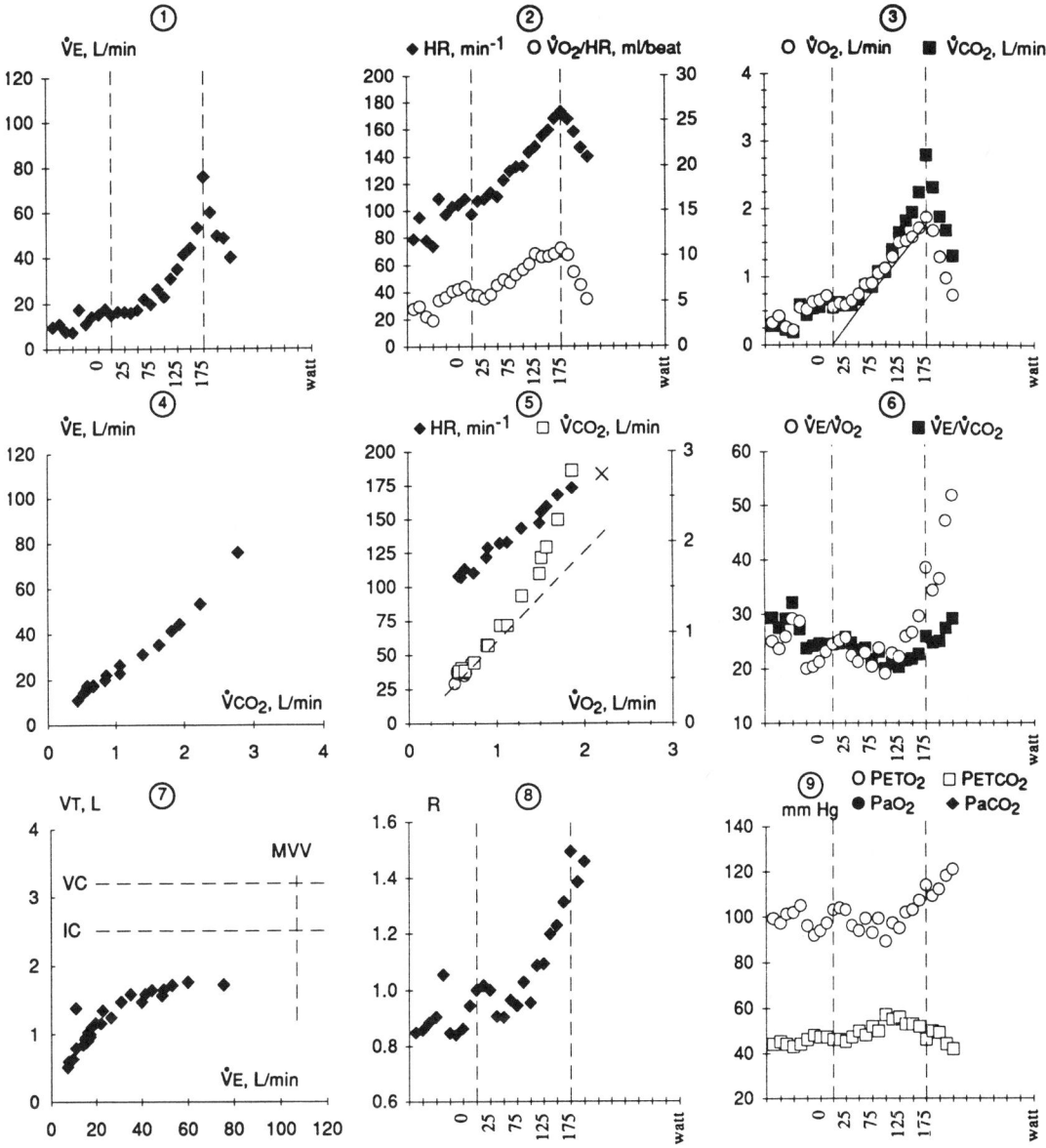

1. Vertical dashed lines in panels 1 to 3 and 6, 8, and 9 indicate the beginning and the end of increasing work period.
2. Unloaded cycling is performed for 3 minutes before the left vertical dashed line.
3. In panel 3, the diagonal line shows the increase of $\dot{V}O_2$ at a slope of 10 ml/min/W.
4. In panel 5, the diagonal dashed line has a slope of 1; the "x" in the upper right is the predicted maximum heart rate and $\dot{V}O_2$ for the subject.

FIG. 10-B. *Treadmill ergometry.*

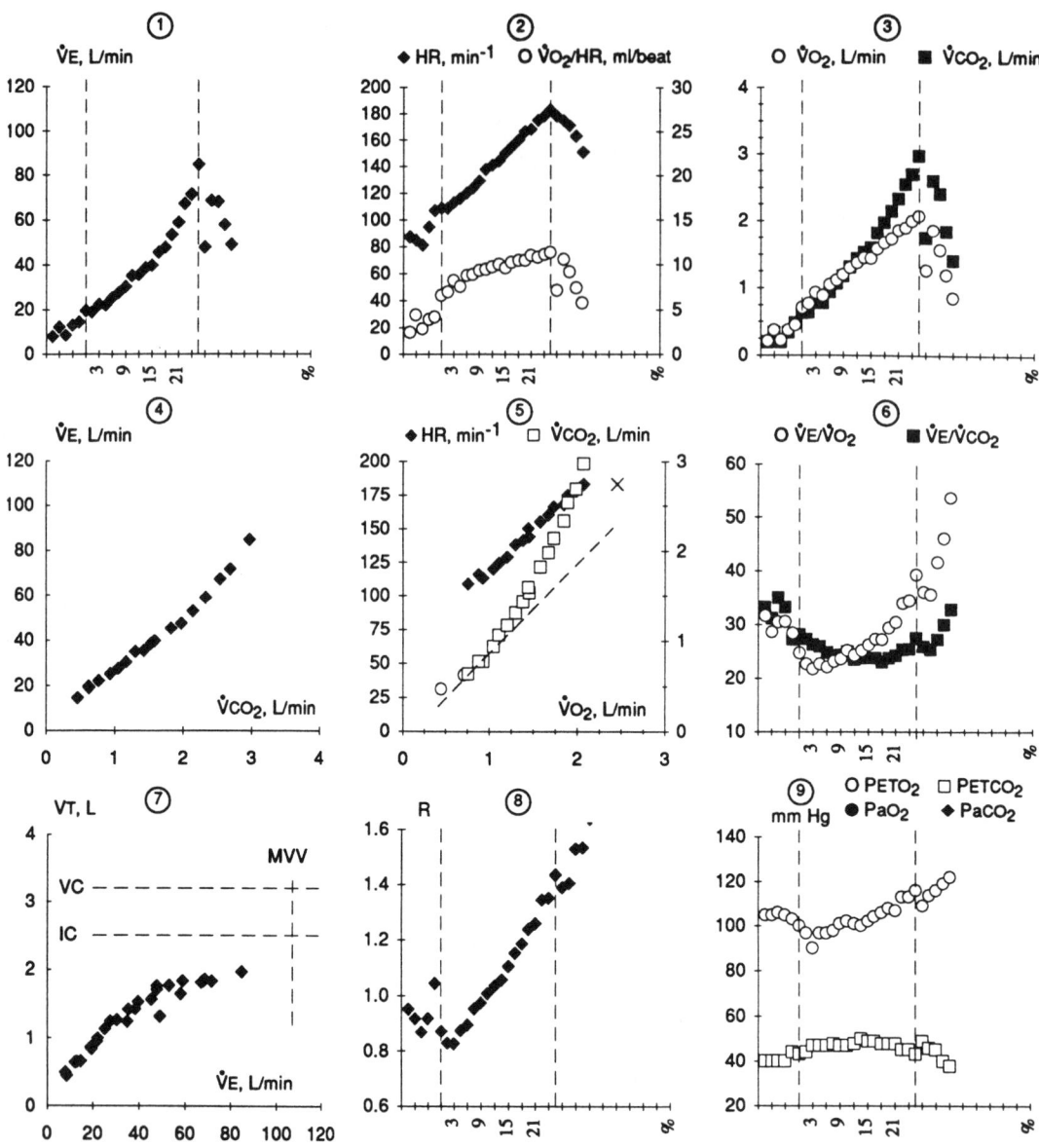

1. Vertical dashed lines in panels 1 to 3 and 6, 8, and 9 indicate the beginning and the end of increasing work period.

2. Zero grade walking is performed for 1 minute before the left vertical dashed line.

3. In panel 5, the diagonal dashed line has a slope of 1; the "x" in the upper right is the predicted maximum heart rate and $\dot{V}O_2$ for the subject.

TABLE 10-4. *Treadmill ergometry.*

Time min	Treadmill grade, %	BP mm Hg	HR min⁻¹	f min⁻¹	V̇E L/min BTPS	V̇CO₂ L/min STPD	V̇O₂ L/min STPD	V̇O₂/HR ml/beat	R	pH	HCO₃ meq/L	PO2 ET	a	(A-a)	PCO2 ET	a	(a-ET)	V̇E/V̇CO₂	V̇E/V̇O₂	VD/VT
	Rest		87	16	8.0	0.20	0.21	2.4	0.95			105			40			33	32	
	Rest		85	19	12.2	0.34	0.37	4.4	0.92			105			40			31	29	
	Rest		81	19	8.6	0.20	0.23	2.8	0.87			106			40			35	30	
	Rest		95	20	13.0	0.34	0.37	3.9	0.92			105			40			33	31	
	0		107	22	14.6	0.47	0.45	4.2	1.04			103			44			27	28	
	0		109	23	19.4	0.62	0.71	6.5	0.87			100			43			28	25	
0.5	3		109	22	19.1	0.63	0.76	7.0	0.83			97			44			27	23	
1.0	3		113	22	22.1	0.77	0.93	8.2	0.83			90			47			26	22	
1.5	6		116	23	21.9	0.77	0.88	7.6	0.88			97			47			26	23	
2.0	6		120	22	25.1	0.94	1.05	8.8	0.90			97			47			25	22	
2.5	9		124	22	27.5	1.06	1.11	9.0	0.95			98			48			24	23	
3.0	9		129	24	30.4	1.17	1.20	9.3	0.98			101			47			24	24	
3.5	12		138	28	35.0	1.31	1.30	9.4	1.01			102			47			25	25	
4.0	12		141	25	35.6	1.43	1.38	9.8	1.04			101			48			23	24	
4.5	15		144	27	38.6	1.53	1.45	10.1	1.06			100			50			24	25	
5.0	15		150	26	39.8	1.59	1.44	9.6	1.10			102			49			24	26	
5.5	18		155	29	45.6	1.82	1.58	10.2	1.15			104			49			24	27	
6.0	18		160	27	47.8	1.98	1.67	10.4	1.19			106			48			23	27	
6.5	21		166	30	53.3	2.14	1.73	10.4	1.24			108			48			24	29	
7.0	21		168	32	59.0	2.33	1.85	11.0	1.26			107			48			24	30	
7.5	24		175	37	67.3	2.54	1.89	10.8	1.34			113			45			25	34	
8.0	24		178	39	71.7	2.69	1.99	11.2	1.35			113			45			25	34	
8.5	27		183	43	84.9	2.97	2.07	11.3	1.43			116			43			27	39	
	Recovery		178	28	47.8	1.75	1.26	7.1	1.39			109			49			26	36	
	Recovery		175	37	68.8	2.60	1.85	10.6	1.41			114			46			25	35	
	Recovery		171	37	68.3	2.40	1.57	9.2	1.53			116			45			27	42	
	Recovery		163	35	58.1	1.84	1.20	7.4	1.53			119			40			30	46	
	Recovery		151	37	49.2	1.41	0.86	5.7	1.64			122			38			33	54	

Interpretation

COMMENTS

The results of this subject's resting respiratory function studies are normal (Table 10-1). The resting ECG is normal. This study is presented to contrast the results when the same subject performed on the cycle and on the treadmill.

ANALYSIS

In flow chart 1, the maximum V̇O₂ and the anaerobic threshold are normal for both cycle and treadmill exercise (Table 10-2). The ECG and O₂ pulse are normal at maximum work rate (branchpoint 2.1). See flow chart 2: The subject is not obese (branchpoint 2.2). The maximum V̇O₂ is about 10% higher on the treadmill than on the cycle.

CONCLUSION

This subject shows normal exercise performance.

CASE 11 *Normal: Pre- and post-β-adrenergic blockade*

CLINICAL FINDINGS

This 23-year-old asthmatic student voluntarily participated in a double-blind study evaluating the effect of a β-adrenergic blocker, pindolol, on exercise-induced asthma. He had had hay fever and asthma since childhood but was otherwise in excellent health. He was taking no medications. Physical examination, chest roentgenograms, ECG, and hemogram were normal. He became familiar with the procedures 1 week prior to the following studies.

EXERCISE FINDINGS

Two similar cycle exercise studies were performed a week apart. After baseline spirometry, 0.4 mg of pindolol or placebo was given over a 20-minute period through a venous catheter. After repeat spirometry, the subject pedalled without added resistance at 60 rpm for 3 minutes and at 60 W for an additional 3 minutes. Thereafter, the work rate was increased 20 W every minute. On each occasion the subject stopped because of fatigue. ECG pattern remained normal. Repeat spirometry in duplicate or triplicate, performed 2, 7, 12, 17, 22, and 27 minutes after exercise, did not reveal exercise-induced bronchospasm.

TABLE 11-1. *Selected Respiratory Function Data*

MEASUREMENT	PREDICTED	MEASURED
Age, yr		23
Sex		Male
Height, cm		170
Weight, kg	68	64
Hematocrit, %		45
VC, L	4.79	4.86
IC, L	3.21	3.40
TLC, L	6.46	6.72
FEV$_1$, L	4.04	3.58
FEV$_1$/VC, %	84	74
MVV, L/min	175	142
D$_{LCO}$, ml/mm Hg/min	33.2	32.5

TABLE 11-2. *Selected Exercise Data*

MEASUREMENT	PREDICTED	PLACEBO	PINDOLOL
Maximum $\dot{V}O_2$, L/min	2.90	2.57	2.39
Maximum HR, beats/min	197	189	156
Maximum O$_2$ pulse, ml/beat	14.7	13.6	15.3
$\Delta\dot{V}O_2/\Delta$WR, ml/min/W	10.3	10.5	9.7
AT, L/min	> 1.16	1.5	1.4
Maximum $\dot{V}E$, L/min		94	85
Exercise breathing reserve, L/min	> 15	48	57

Fig. 11-A. *Pre-β-adrenergic blockade.*

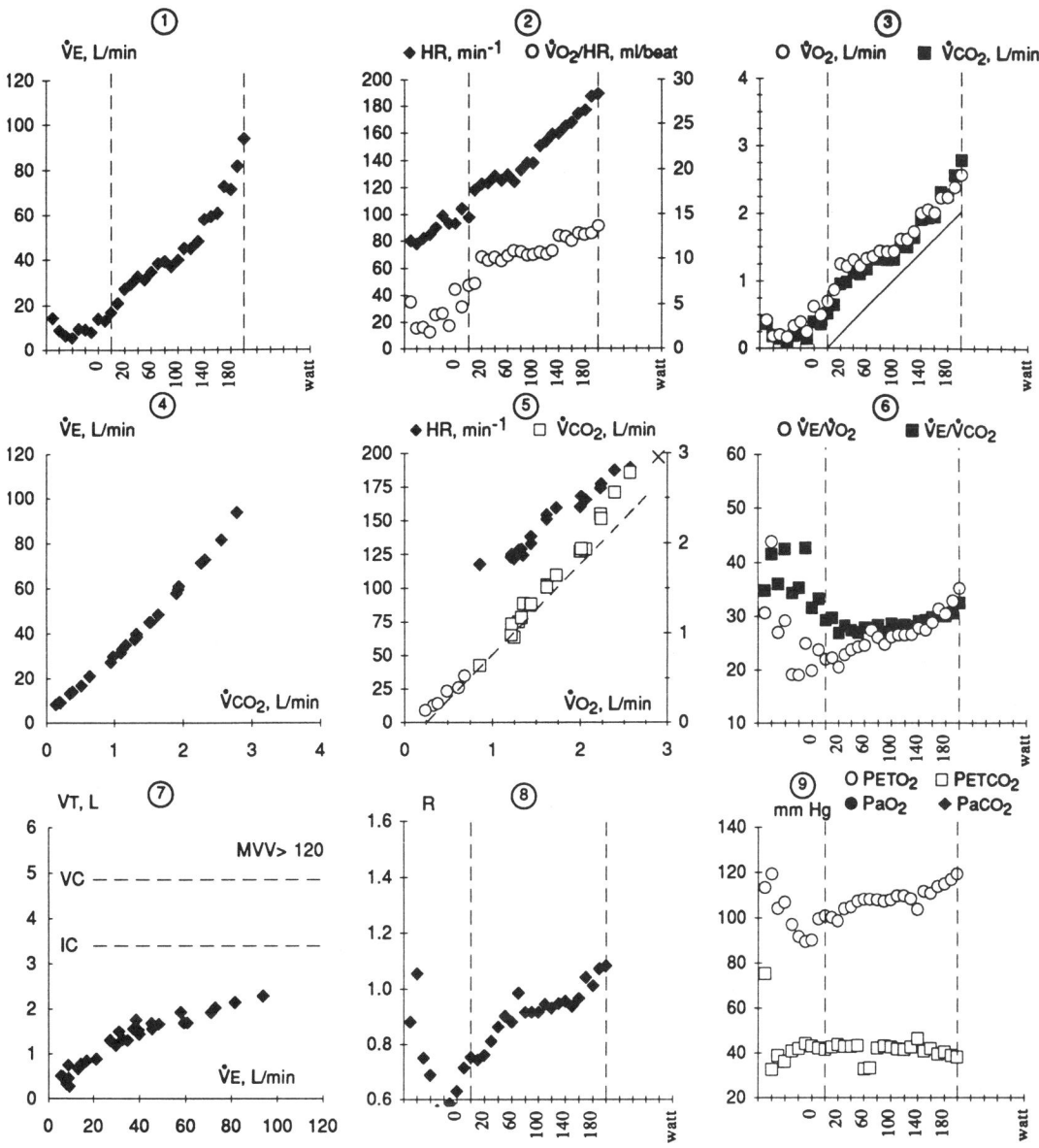

1. Vertical dashed lines in panels 1 to 3 and 6, 8, and 9 indicate the beginning and the end of increasing work period.

2. Unloaded cycling is performed for 3 minutes before the left vertical dashed line.

3. In panel 3, the diagonal line shows the increase of $\dot{V}O_2$ at a slope of 10 ml/min/W.

4. In panel 5, the diagonal dashed line has a slope of 1; the "x" in the upper right is the predicted maximum heart rate and $\dot{V}O_2$ for the subject.

FIG. 11-B. *Post-β-adrenergic blockade.*

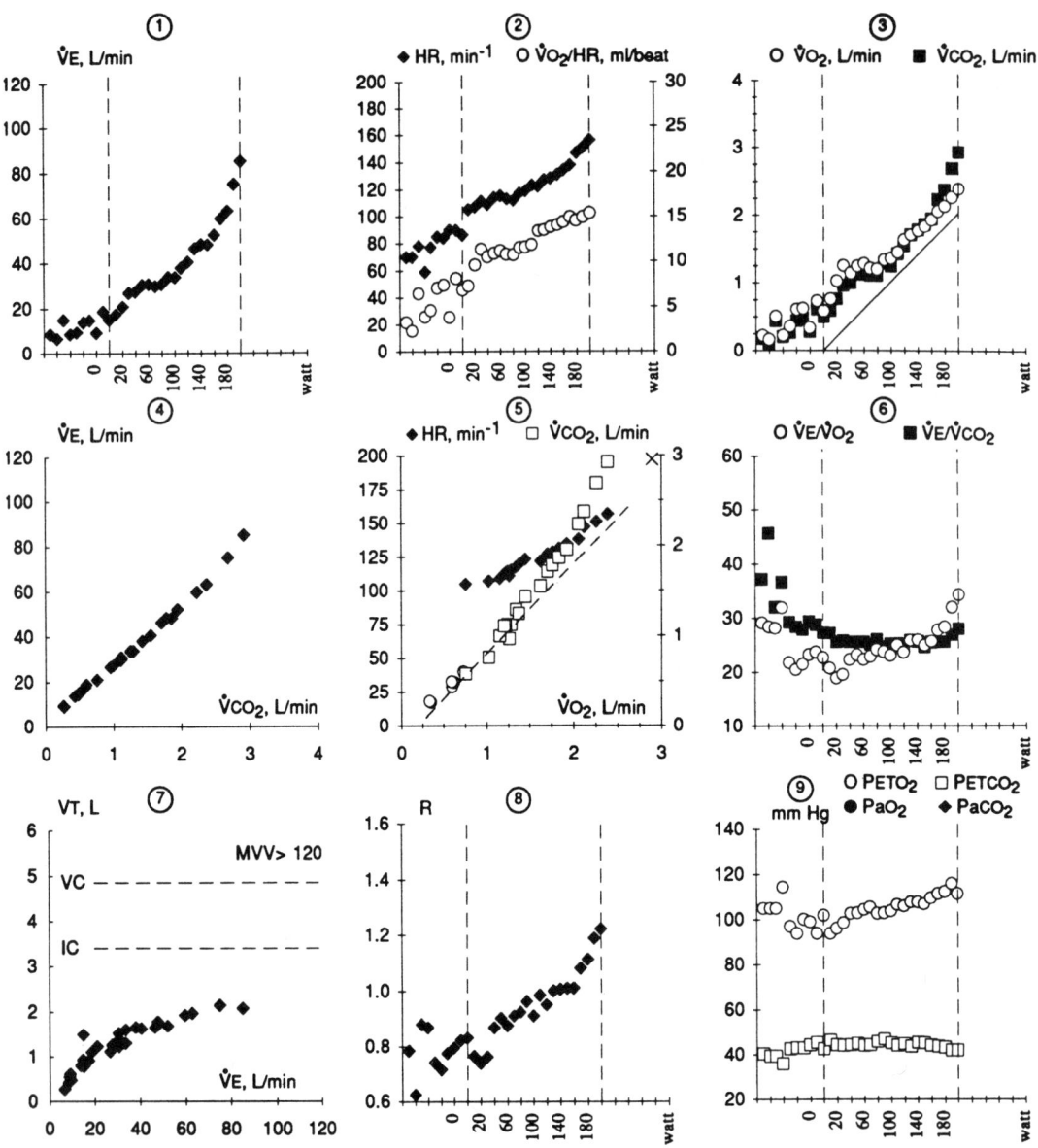

1. Vertical dashed lines in panels 1 to 3 and 6, 8, and 9 indicate the beginning and the end of increasing work period.

2. Unloaded cycling is performed for 3 minutes before the left vertical dashed line.

3. In panel 3, the diagonal line shows the increase of $\dot{V}O_2$ at a slope of 10 ml/min/W.

4. In panel 5, the diagonal dashed line has a slope of 1; the "x" in the upper right is the predicted maximum heart rate and $\dot{V}O_2$ for the subject.

TABLE 11-3. *Pre-β-adrenergic blockade.*

Time min	Work rate watts	BP mm Hg	HR min⁻¹	f min⁻¹	$\dot{V}E$ L/min BTPS	$\dot{V}CO_2$ L/min STPD	$\dot{V}O_2$ L/min STPD	$\frac{\dot{V}O_2}{HR}$ ml/beat	R	pH	HCO₃ meq/L	PO2 ET	a	(A-a)	PCO2 ET	a	(a-ET)	$\frac{\dot{V}E}{\dot{V}CO_2}$	$\frac{\dot{V}E}{\dot{V}O_2}$	VD/VT
	Rest		80	19	14.5	0.37	0.42	5.3	0.88			113			75			35	31	
	Rest		78	12	8.9	0.19	0.18	2.3	1.06			119			32			41	44	
	Rest		82	13	6.5	0.15	0.20	2.4	0.75			104			39			36	27	
	Rest		85	11	5.6	0.11	0.16	1.9	0.69			107			36			42	29	
	Unloaded		90	34	9.4	0.19	0.34	3.8	0.56			97			41			34	19	
	Unloaded		99	20	9.1	0.21	0.39	3.9	0.54			92			42			35	19	
	Unloaded		93	25	8.1	0.14	0.24	2.6	0.58			90			44			43	25	
	Unloaded		93	20	14.0	0.39	0.62	6.7	0.63			90			43			32	20	
	Unloaded		104	20	13.3	0.35	0.49	4.7	0.71			99			42			33	24	
	Unloaded		98	20	16.9	0.52	0.69	7.0	0.75			101			41			29	22	
0.5	20		118	24	21.1	0.64	0.86	7.3	0.74			100			42			30	22	
1.0	20		122	21	27.3	0.95	1.25	10.2	0.76			99			44			27	20	
1.5	40		123	25	29.8	0.98	1.21	9.8	0.81			104			43			28	23	
2.0	40		128	25	32.9	1.12	1.30	10.2	0.86			105			43			27	24	
2.5	60		125	21	31.4	1.10	1.22	9.8	0.90			107			43			27	24	
3.0	60		129	27	34.9	1.17	1.33	10.3	0.88			108			33			28	25	
3.5	80		124	22	38.7	1.33	1.35	10.9	0.99			108			33			28	27	
4.0	80		133	26	39.7	1.32	1.44	10.8	0.92			108			42			28	26	
4.5	100		138	24	37.5	1.31	1.43	10.4	0.92			107			43			27	25	
5.0	100		138	28	40.1	1.32	1.44	10.4	0.92			108			42			29	26	
5.5	120		151	27	45.3	1.53	1.62	10.7	0.94			110			42			28	27	
6.0	120		154	29	45.4	1.51	1.62	10.5	0.93			110			41			28	27	
6.5	140		159	29	48.5	1.64	1.73	10.9	0.95			108			42			28	27	
7.0	140		160	30	58.0	1.91	2.00	12.5	0.96			104			46			29	28	
7.5	160		165	35	59.4	1.93	2.06	12.5	0.94			112			41			29	27	
8.0	160		168	36	61.0	1.94	2.01	12.0	0.97			111			42			30	29	
8.5	180		174	36	72.9	2.32	2.23	12.8	1.04			114			39			30	31	
9.0	180		177	37	71.3	2.27	2.24	12.7	1.01			115			40			30	30	
9.5	200		187	38	81.7	2.56	2.39	12.8	1.07			117			39			31	33	
10.0	200		189	41	93.8	2.78	2.57	13.6	1.08			119			38			32	35	

Interpretation

COMMENTS

This study is presented to demonstrate the effect of β-adrenergic blockade on exercise. The lowest work rate after unloaded cycling is 60 W, followed by 1-minute increments of 20 W. This uneven increase in the work rate increment causes the upward distortion in the $\dot{V}O_2$-work rate slope (panel 3, Fig. 11-A and B). Results of respiratory function testing are normal at the time of study (Table 11-1).

ANALYSIS

In flow chart 1, the maximum aerobic capacity and AT are within normal limits on both pre- and post-β-adrenergic blockade exercise tests (Table 11-2). See flow chart 2: The ECG and O_2 pulse at maximum work rate are normal (branchpoint 2.1). The large reduction in maximum HR, with slight reduction in maximum $\dot{V}O_2$ and increase in maximum O_2 pulse, is typical of the effect of β-adrenergic blockade. The chronotropic effect of the β-blockade increases the time for ventricular filling and results in a larger O_2 pulse at the same work rate.

CONCLUSION

This study is normal with demonstration of heart rate slowing and the slight decrease in maximum $\dot{V}O_2$ following β-adrenergic blockade.

TABLE 11-4. *Post-β-adrenergic blockade.*

Time min	Work rate watts	BP mm Hg	HR min^{-1}	f min^{-1}	$\dot{V}E$ L/min BTPS	$\dot{V}CO_2$ L/min STPD	$\dot{V}O_2$ L/min STPD	$\dfrac{\dot{V}O_2}{HR}$ ml/beat	R	pH	HCO$_3$ meq/L	PO2, mm Hg ET	a	(A-a)	PCO2, mm Hg ET	a	(a-ET)	$\dfrac{\dot{V}E}{\dot{V}CO_2}$	$\dfrac{\dot{V}E}{\dot{V}O_2}$	$\dfrac{VD}{VT}$
	Rest		70	20	8.4	0.18	0.23	3.3	0.78			105			40			37	29	
	Rest		70	24	6.6	0.10	0.16	2.3	0.63			105			39			46	29	
	Rest		78	10	14.9	0.44	0.50	6.4	0.88			105			39			32	28	
	Rest		59	16	8.7	0.20	0.23	3.9	0.87			114			36			37	32	
	Unloaded		77	20	9.3	0.26	0.35	4.5	0.74			97			42			29	22	
	Unloaded		85	17	13.7	0.43	0.60	7.1	0.72			94			43			29	20	
	Unloaded		84	16	14.7	0.48	0.62	7.4	0.77			100			43			28	22	
	Unloaded		90	15	9.2	0.27	0.34	3.8	0.79			99			44			29	23	
	Unloaded		90	17	18.7	0.60	0.73	8.1	0.82			94			46			29	24	
	Unloaded		86	19	15.0	0.49	0.59	6.9	0.83			102			42			27	23	
0.5	20		105	19	17.4	0.58	0.76	7.2	0.76			94			47			27	21	
1.0	20		107	17	20.9	0.76	1.03	9.6	0.74			96			44			26	19	
1.5	40		111	24	26.8	0.96	1.26	11.4	0.76			99			44			26	20	
2.0	40		109	22	27.5	1.00	1.15	10.6	0.87			103			45			26	22	
2.5	60		114	20	30.4	1.12	1.24	10.9	0.90			103			45			26	23	
3.0	60		115	25	30.7	1.12	1.28	11.1	0.88			104			44			26	22	
3.5	80		113	23	29.9	1.11	1.22	10.8	0.91			106			44			25	23	
4.0	80		112	22	30.7	1.11	1.20	10.7	0.93			103			46			26	24	
4.5	100		117	21	33.6	1.29	1.34	11.5	0.96			103			47			25	24	
5.0	100		119	26	33.7	1.25	1.37	11.5	0.91			104			45			25	23	
5.5	120		123	23	38.0	1.43	1.45	11.8	0.99			107			44			25	25	
6.0	120		122	25	40.6	1.55	1.63	13.4	0.95			106			45			25	24	
6.5	140		127	28	46.5	1.71	1.71	13.5	1.00			108			44			26	26	
7.0	140		128	28	48.2	1.78	1.77	13.8	1.01			108			46			26	26	
7.5	160		131	27	48.1	1.86	1.84	14.0	1.01			107			45			25	25	
8.0	160		134	31	52.2	1.95	1.93	14.4	1.01			110			44			25	26	
8.5	180		138	31	59.8	2.23	2.06	14.9	1.08			111			44			26	28	
9.0	180		147	32	63.1	2.37	2.13	14.5	1.11			112			43			25	28	
9.5	200		151	35	75.1	2.69	2.26	15.0	1.19			116			42			27	32	
10.0	200		156	41	85.2	2.92	2.39	15.3	1.22			111			42			28	34	

CASE 12 *Normal: Immediate effects of cigarette smoking*

CLINICAL FINDINGS

This 27-year-old subject was one of several men who volunteered for a study to investigate the effect of recent cigarette smoking on cardiovascular and respiratory function during exercise. The subject was apparently in excellent general health, but had smoked cigarettes for 10 years. Physical examination, chest roentgenogram, and ECG were normal.

EXERCISE FINDINGS

Two similar exercise studies were performed 6 days apart on a cycle ergometer. In the 5 hours before the first study the subject smoked 15 medium tar cigarettes. In the second study, the subject was under observation for 5 hours without smoking. He breathed oxygen for the first 3 of those 5 hours to reduce the carboxyhemoglobin in his blood. On both occasions he pedalled without added load at 60 rpm for 3 minutes. The work rate was then increased 25 W every minute to his symptom-limited maximum. On both occasions the subject stopped exercise because of fatigue. ECG remained normal. Carboxyhemoglobin levels were 6.1% at the start of the first study and 1.5% at the start of the second study.

TABLE 12-1. *Selected Respiratory Function Data*

MEASUREMENT	PREDICTED	WITH PRIOR SMOKING	WITHOUT PRIOR SMOKING
Age, yr		27	
Sex		Male	
Height, cm		168	
Weight, kg	69	83	
Hematocrit, %		47	47
VC, L	4.65	4.18	4.20
IC, L	3.10	3.43	3.43
TLC, L	6.19	6.26	6.68
FEV$_1$, L	3.79	3.57	3.55
FEV$_1$/VC, %	81	85	85
MVV, L/min	168	149	163
D$_{LCO}$, ml/mm Hg/min	31.2	34.7	37.4

TABLE 12-2. *Selected Exercise Data*

MEASUREMENT	PREDICTED	WITH PRIOR SMOKING	WITHOUT PRIOR SMOKING
Maximum V̇$_{O_2}$, L/min	2.99	2.55	2.73
Maximum HR, beats/min	193	178	182
Maximum O$_2$ pulse, ml/beat	15.5	14.3	15.0
ΔV̇$_{O_2}$/ΔWR, ml/min/W	10.3	9.0	9.9
AT, L/min	> 1.23	1.1	1.25
Blood pressure, mm Hg (rest, max)		138/84,183/110	132/84,186/105
Maximum V̇$_E$, L/min		110	121
Exercise breathing reserve, L/min	> 15	39	42
Pa$_{O_2}$, mm Hg (rest, max ex)		102,103	109,106
P(A−a)$_{O_2}$, mm Hg (rest, max ex)		5,19	−1,16
P(a−ET)$_{CO_2}$, mm Hg (rest, max ex)		−1,−3	−2,−3
V$_D$/V$_T$ (rest, heavy ex)		0.37,0.18	0.27,0.20
HCO$_3^-$, mEq/L (rest, 2-min recov)		25,14	26,15

FIG. 12-A. *With prior smoking.*

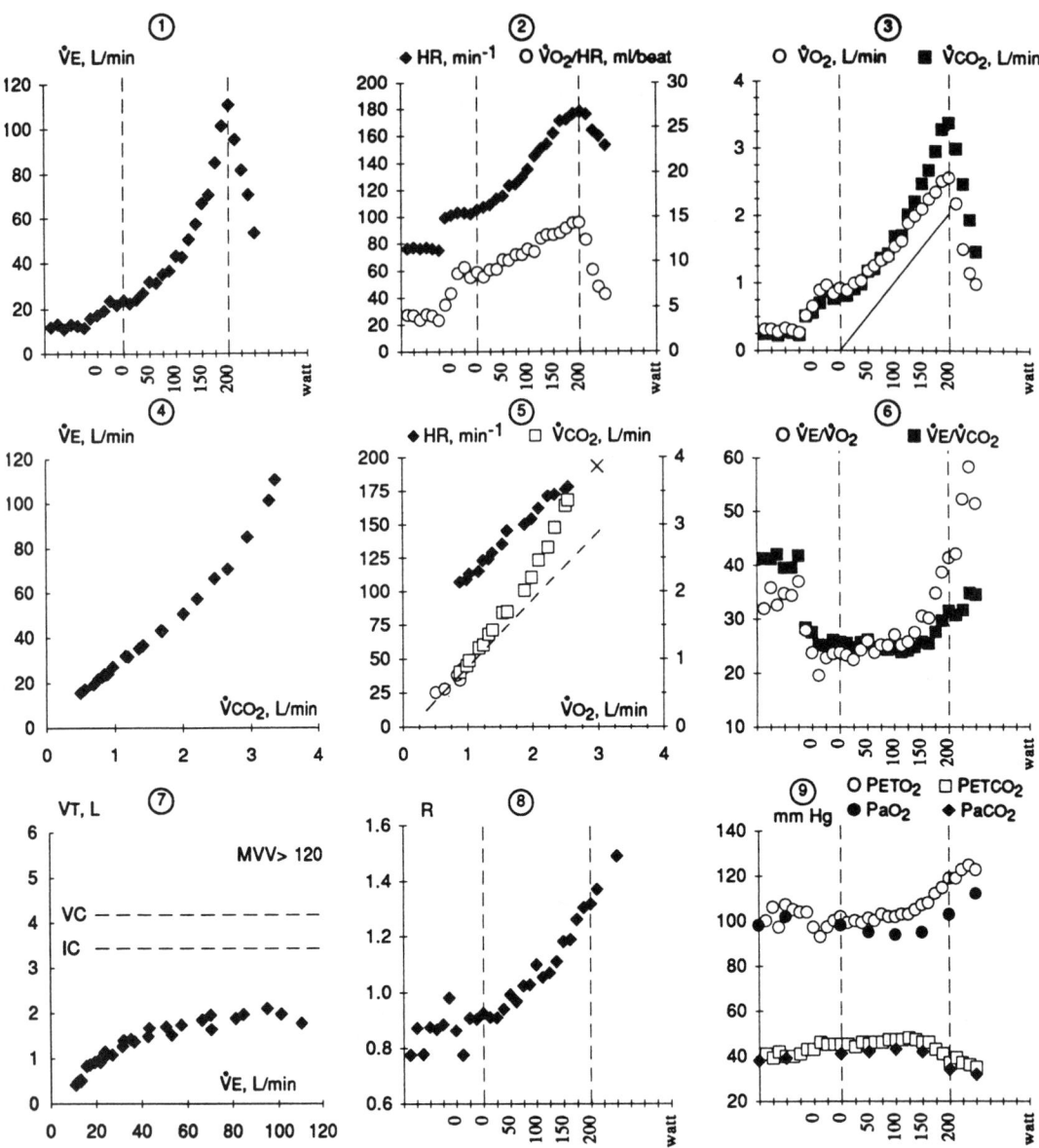

1. Vertical dashed lines in panels 1 to 3 and 6, 8, and 9 indicate the beginning and the end of increasing work period.
2. Unloaded cycling is performed for 3 minutes before the left vertical dashed line.
3. In panel 3, the diagonal line shows the increase of $\dot{V}O_2$ at a slope of 10 ml/min/W.
4. In panel 5, the diagonal dashed line has a slope of 1; the "x" in the upper right is the predicted maximum heart rate and $\dot{V}O_2$ for the subject.

FIG. 12-B. *Without prior smoking.*

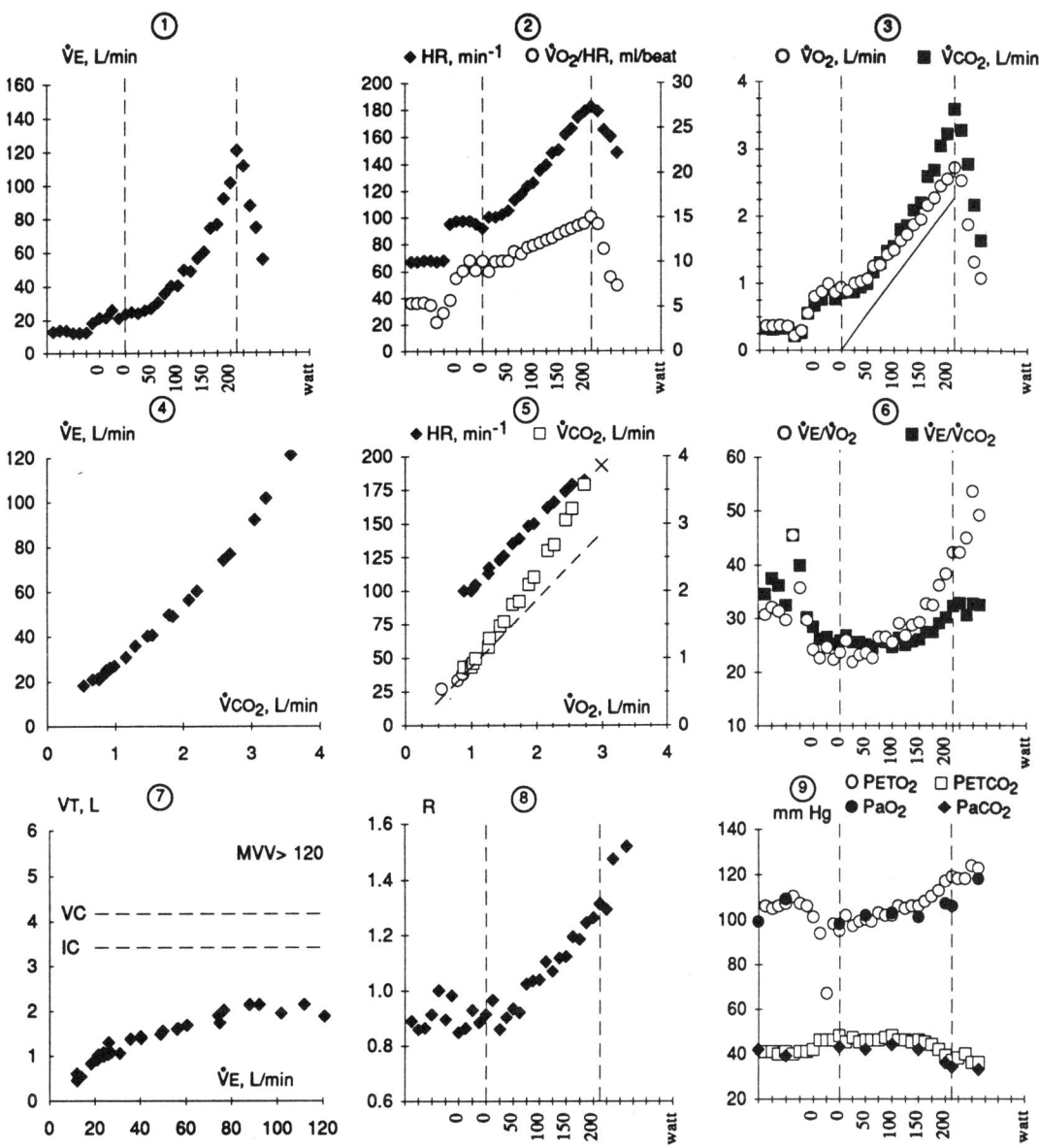

1. Vertical dashed lines in panels 1 to 3 and 6, 8, and 9 indicate the beginning and the end of increasing work period.

2. Unloaded cycling is performed for 3 minutes before the left vertical dashed line.

3. In panel 3, the diagonal line shows the increase of $\dot{V}_{O_2}$ at a slope of 10 ml/min/W.

4. In panel 5, the diagonal dashed line has a slope of 1; the "x" in the upper right is the predicted maximum heart rate and $\dot{V}_{O_2}$ for the subject.

TABLE 12-3. *With prior smoking.*

Time min	Work rate watts	BP mm Hg	HR min⁻¹	f min⁻¹	V̇E L/min BTPS	V̇CO2 L/min STPD	V̇O2 L/min STPD	V̇O2/HR ml/beat	R	pH	HCO3 meq/L	PO2 ET	PO2 a	PO2 (A-a)	PCO2 ET	PCO2 a	PCO2 (a-ET)	V̇E/V̇CO2	V̇E/V̇O2	VD/VT
	Rest	138/84								7.42	24		98			38				
	Rest		76	26	12.1	0.24	0.31	4.1	0.77			100			41			41	32	
	Rest		77	27	13.4	0.27	0.31	4.0	0.87			106			39			41	36	
	Rest		76	27	11.1	0.21	0.27	3.6	0.78			97			42			42	33	
	Rest	138/84	77	25	13.2	0.28	0.32	4.2	0.88	7.42	25	107	102	5	40	39	-1	40	35	0.37
	Rest		76	25	12.4	0.26	0.30	3.9	0.87			105			40			40	34	
	Rest		75	25	11.7	0.23	0.26	3.5	0.88			104			41			42	37	
	Unloaded		99	19	15.8	0.50	0.51	5.2	0.98			104			43			28	28	
	Unloaded		101	20	17.1	0.56	0.65	6.4	0.86			97			43			28	24	
	Unloaded		103	21	19.2	0.69	0.89	8.6	0.78			93			46			25	20	
	Unloaded		103	21	23.6	0.87	0.96	9.3	0.91			97			45			25	23	
	Unloaded		102	24	21.8	0.76	0.84	8.2	0.90			100			45			26	24	
	Unloaded	156/96	105	23	23.8	0.85	0.92	8.8	0.92	7.39	24	102	98	8	45	41	-4	26	24	0.17
0.5	25		107	22	22.5	0.81	0.89	8.3	0.91			99			45			25	23	
1.0	25		109	21	24.0	0.90	0.99	9.1	0.91			100			44			25	22	
1.5	50		113	25	27.0	0.97	1.03	9.1	0.94			99			46			26	24	
2.0	50	165/93	115	23	32.1	1.16	1.17	10.2	0.99	7.38	24	101	95	13	45	42	-3	26	26	0.20
2.5	75		123	25	31.6	1.20	1.24	10.1	0.97			100			46			25	24	
3.0	75		124	25	35.4	1.36	1.33	10.7	1.02			103			46			24	25	
3.5	100		129	27	36.8	1.42	1.38	10.7	1.03			102			47			24	25	
4.0	100	177/96	135	26	43.4	1.68	1.53	11.3	1.10	7.36	24	102	94	16	47	43	-4	25	27	0.17
4.5	125		145	29	43.0	1.70	1.61	11.1	1.06			103			47			24	25	
5.0	125		150	30	50.8	2.01	1.88	12.5	1.07			103			48			24	26	
5.5	150		154	33	57.5	2.21	1.99	12.9	1.11			105			47			25	27	
6.0	150	177/99	162	36	66.6	2.47	2.09	12.9	1.18	7.33	22	107	95	18	46	42	-4	26	30	0.19
6.5	175		171	36	70.4	2.66	2.24	13.1	1.19			108			46			25	30	
7.0	175		172	43	84.8	2.95	2.34	13.6	1.26			112			43			28	35	
7.5	200		176	51	101.2	3.27	2.51	14.3	1.30			115			41			30	39	
8.0	200		178	62	110.6	3.36	2.55	14.3	1.32	7.32	17	119	103	19	37	34	-3	31	41	0.18
	Recovery		176	45	95.2	2.99	2.18	12.4	1.37			119			39			31	42	
	Recovery		164	43	81.4	2.46	1.49	9.1	1.65			123			37			32	52	
	Recovery		160	43	70.6	1.93	1.15	7.2	1.68			125			36			35	58	
	Recovery	165/84	153	35	53.3	1.46	0.98	6.4	1.49	7.27	14	123	112	14	35	32	-3	34	51	0.21

Interpretation

COMMENTS

This study is presented because it illustrates small but significant effects of short-term cigarette smoking on the maximum $\dot{V}O_2$ and the anaerobic threshold. It also illustrates the reproducibility of the cardiac and gas exchange responses to exercise performed on different days, and the effects of obesity.

Results of resting respiratory function studies are normal (Table 12-1). The resting ECG is normal.

ANALYSIS

In flow chart 1, the maximum $\dot{V}O_2$ is borderline with prior smoking but clearly normal without prior smoking (Table 12-2). The anaerobic threshold is reduced after smoking but is normal without prior smoking (Table 12-2). See flow chart 2: The subject is 20% overweight (branchpoint 2.2). It should be noted that this obese subject's $\dot{V}O_2$ dur-

TABLE 12-4. *Without prior smoking.*

Time min	Work rate watts	BP mm Hg	HR min⁻¹	f min⁻¹	$\dot{V}_E$ L/min BTPS	$\dot{V}_{CO_2}$ L/min STPD	$\dot{V}_{O_2}$ L/min STPD	$\dfrac{\dot{V}_{O_2}}{HR}$ ml/beat	R	pH	HCO₃ meq/L	PO₂, mm Hg ET	a	(A-a)	PCO₂, mm Hg ET	a	(a-ET)	$\dfrac{\dot{V}_E}{\dot{V}_{CO_2}}$	$\dfrac{\dot{V}_E}{\dot{V}_{O_2}}$	$\dfrac{V_D}{V_T}$
	Rest	129/84								7.40	26	99			42					
	Rest		67	24	13.1	0.32	0.36	5.4	0.89			106			41			35	31	
	Rest		67	26	13.8	0.31	0.36	5.4	0.86			105			41			37	32	
	Rest		68	26	13.8	0.32	0.37	5.4	0.86			106			40			36	31	
	Rest	132/84	68	20	12.1	0.32	0.35	5.1	0.91	7.43	25	107	109	-1	41	39	-2	33	30	0.27
	Rest		67	27	12.3	0.22	0.22	3.3	1.00			110			40			45	45	
	Rest		68	25	12.5	0.26	0.29	4.3	0.90			107			41			40	36	
	Unloaded		95	22	18.2	0.54	0.55	5.8	0.98			106			41			30	30	
	Unloaded		97	23	21.0	0.67	0.79	8.1	0.85			101			42			28	24	
	Unloaded		97	21	21.4	0.75	0.87	9.0	0.86			94			46			26	23	
	Unloaded		97	20	26.0	0.92	0.99	10.2	0.93			67			46			26	25	
	Unloaded		95	21	21.0	0.76	0.86	9.1	0.88			98			46			25	22	
	Unloaded	141/87	92	22	23.8	0.85	0.93	10.1	0.91	7.39	26	95	98	6	48	43	-5	26	24	0.20
0.5	25		100	24	25.0	0.86	0.89	8.9	0.97			102			45			27	26	
1.0	25		100	24	24.0	0.86	1.00	10.0	0.86			97			47			26	22	
1.5	50		102	25	25.9	0.93	1.03	10.1	0.90			99			45			26	23	
2.0	50	153/90	105	25	27.0	0.99	1.06	10.1	0.93	7.39	25	100	102	4	46	42	-4	25	23	0.17
2.5	75		113	29	30.9	1.16	1.26	11.2	0.92			99			46			25	23	
3.0	75		117	26	35.8	1.30	1.27	10.9	1.02			103			46			26	26	
3.5	100		123	28	40.3	1.48	1.43	11.6	1.03			102			47			26	27	
4.0	100	168/93	126	29	40.6	1.55	1.49	11.8	1.04	7.37	25	102	103	4	48	44	-4	25	26	0.19
4.5	125		135	32	50.0	1.80	1.63	12.1	1.10			106			46			26	29	
5.0	125		139	33	49.0	1.85	1.73	12.4	1.07			105			46			25	27	
5.5	150		148	35	56.6	2.09	1.87	12.6	1.12			106			45			26	29	
6.0	150	177/99	150	36	60.4	2.20	1.96	13.1	1.12	7.36	23	106	101	11	46	42	-4	26	29	0.20
6.5	175		162	39	74.3	2.59	2.17	13.4	1.19			108			45			27	33	
7.0	175		166	38	76.8	2.69	2.27	13.7	1.19			110			44			27	32	
7.5	200		174	43	92.2	3.05	2.45	14.1	1.24			113			42			29	36	
8.0	200	186/105	179	52	101.8	3.22	2.55	14.2	1.26	7.35	20	117	107	13	39	36	-3	30	38	0.20
8.5	225		182	64	121.0	3.58	2.73	15.0	1.31	7.32	17	119	106	16	37	34	-3	32	42	0.20
	Recovery		179	52	111.9	3.28	2.54	14.2	1.29			118			38			33	42	
	Recovery		165	41	88.0	2.77	1.88	11.4	1.47			118			40			31	45	
	Recovery		160	43	74.9	2.18	1.33	8.3	1.64			124			36			33	54	
	Recovery	162/90	148	35	56.1	1.64	1.08	7.3	1.52	7.26	15	123	118	8	36	33	-3	32	49	0.18

ing unloaded cycling is approximately 0.95 L/min. (Table 12-3 and panel 3 of Fig. 12-A and B).

Indices other than maximum $\dot{V}_{O_2}$ and *AT* that might reflect the effect of the increased carboxyhemoglobin during exercise are the O_2 pulse and $\Delta\dot{V}_{O_2}/\Delta WR$. These are both reduced following cigarette smoking (Table 12-2). Although the indices of ventilation-perfusion matching are normal at maximum exercise in this and most normal subjects, they tend to become abnormal immediately after smoking.[1]

CONCLUSION

Cigarette smoking and obesity have affected exercise performance in an otherwise normal subject.

Reference

1. Hirsch, G.L., Sue, D.Y., Wasserman, K., Robinson, T.E., and Hansen, J.E.: Immediate effects of cigarette smoking on cardiorespiratory responses to exercise. J. Appl. Physiol., *58*:1975–1981, 1985.

CASE 13 *Normal, Suspected of Cardiomyopathy: Air and 15% Oxygen Breathing*

CLINICAL FINDINGS

This 65-year-old male self-employed cameraman referred himself for cardiopulmonary exercise testing to evaluate dyspnea that had occurred while he was hiking with a group of young men at an altitude of 10,000 ft (3 km). He had been an avid hiker but had noted a decreased ability to hike at high altitudes in the last 3 to 4 years. He was referred by his private physician to a cardiologist, who gave him an extensive cardiologic workup, including treadmill exercise tests (without metabolic measurements), gated cardiac wall motion studies, echocardiogram, and a coronary angiogram. The results of these were negative. He was told that he probably had heart failure secondary to a cardiomyopathy and was prescribed an ACE inhibitor. The patient believed that the drug did not help him but caused untoward side effects.

EXERCISE FINDINGS

The patient performed exercise on a cycle ergometer while he breathed room air and a second time breathing 15% O_2 (equivalent to 8000-ft altitude). On both occasions, he pedalled at 60 rpm without an added load for 3 minutes. The work rate was then increased 20 W per minute to tolerance. Arterial blood was sampled every second minute, and intra-arterial pressure was recorded from a percutaneously placed brachial artery catheter. The patient stopped exercise because of fatigue and shortness of breath on both occasions. No ECG abnormalities were noted at rest or during exercise.

TABLE 13-1. *Selected Respiratory Function Data*

MEASUREMENT	PREDICTED	MEASURED
Age, yr		65
Sex		Male
Height, cm		183
Weight, kg	83	83
Hematocrit, %		44
VC, L	4.60	4.70
IC, L	3.06	3.70
FEV$_1$, L	3.45	3.47
FEV$_1$/VC, %	75	74
MVV, L/min	142	129
D$_{LCO}$, ml/mm Hg/min	28.0	28.6

TABLE 13-2. *Selected Exercise Data*

MEASUREMENT	PREDICTED (ROOM AIR)	MEASURED AIR	MEASURED 15% O_2
Maximum $\dot{V}_{O_2}$, L/min	2.21	2.69	2.19
Maximum HR, beats/min	155	175	172
Maximum O_2 pulse, ml/beat	14.3	15.9	12.9
$\Delta\dot{V}_{O_2}/\Delta$WR, ml/min/W	10.3	10.3	7.8
AT, L/min	> 0.99	1.9	1.2
Blood pressure, mm Hg (rest, max ex)		132/72,210/90	114/66,198/96
Maximum $\dot{V}_E$, L/min		115	108
Exercise breathing reserves, L/min	> 15	14	21
Pa$_{O_2}$, mm Hg (rest, max ex)		113,106	77,52
P(A−a)$_{O_2}$ mm Hg (rest, max ex)		−1,16	0,27
P(a−ET)$_{CO_2}$, mm Hg (rest, max ex)		1,−3	2,0
V$_D$/V$_T$ (rest, max ex)		0.25,0.21	0.36,0.19
HCO$_3^-$, mEq/L (rest, 2-min recovery)		21,15	21,17

Fig. 13-A. *Room air.*

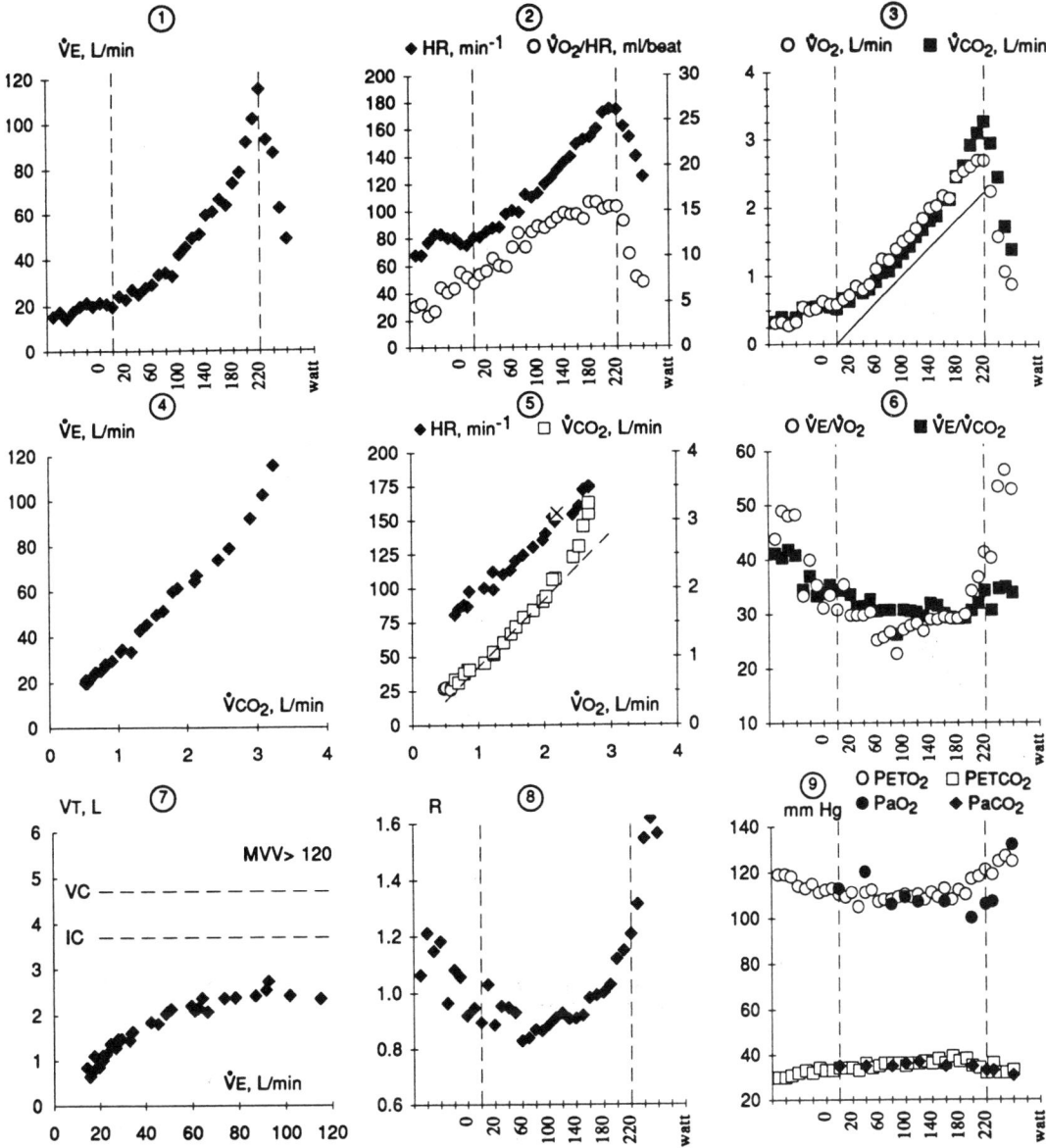

1. Vertical dashed lines in panels 1 to 3 and 6, 8, and 9 indicate the beginning and the end of increasing work period.
2. Unloaded cycling is performed for 3 minutes before the left vertical dashed line.
3. In panel 3, the diagonal line shows the increase of $\dot{V}O_2$ at a slope of 10 ml/min/W.
4. In panel 5, the diagonal dashed line has a slope of 1; the "x" in the upper right is the predicted maximum heart rate and $\dot{V}O_2$ for the subject.

Fig. 13-B. *15% oxygen.*

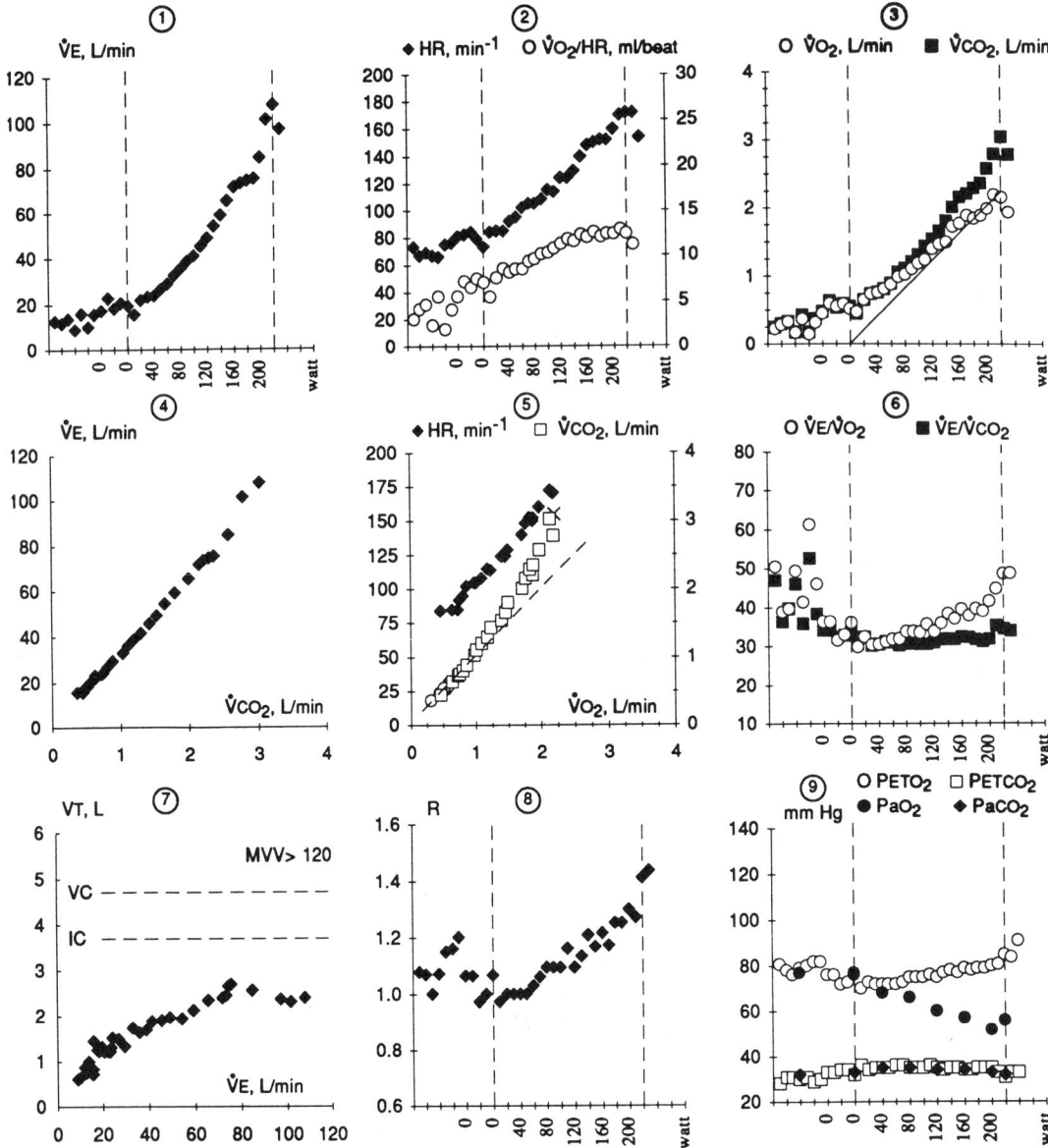

1. Vertical dashed lines in panels 1 to 3 and 6, 8, and 9 indicate the beginning and the end of increasing work period.

2. Unloaded cycling is performed for 3 minutes before the left vertical dashed line.

3. In panel 3, the diagonal line shows the increase of $\dot{V}O_2$ at a slope of 10 ml/min/W.

4. In panel 5, the diagonal dashed line has a slope of 1; the "x" in the upper right is the predicted maximum heart rate and $\dot{V}O_2$ for the subject.

TABLE 13-3. *Room air.*

Time min	Work rate watts	BP mm Hg	HR min^{-1}	f min^{-1}	$\dot{V}_E$ L/min BTPS	$\dot{V}_{CO_2}$ L/min STPD	$\dot{V}_{O_2}$ L/min STPD	$\frac{\dot{V}_{O_2}}{HR}$ ml/beat	R	pH	HCO$_3$ meq/L	PO2, mm Hg ET	a	(A-a)	PCO2, mm Hg ET	a	(a-ET)	$\frac{\dot{V}_E}{\dot{V}_{CO_2}}$	$\frac{\dot{V}_E}{\dot{V}_{O_2}}$	$\frac{V_D}{V_T}$
	Rest		68	24	15.6	0.33	0.31	4.6	1.06			119			30			41	44	
	Rest		68	16	17.5	0.40	0.33	4.9	1.21			119			30			40	49	
	Rest		77	17	14.4	0.31	0.27	3.5	1.15			118			31			42	48	
	Rest		83	22	17.8	0.39	0.33	4.0	1.18			114			32			41	48	
	Unloaded		83	19	19.9	0.53	0.55	6.6	0.96			113			33			35	33	
	Unloaded		80	21	21.3	0.53	0.49	6.1	1.08			115			32			37	40	
	Unloaded		80	19	19.9	0.55	0.52	6.5	1.06			111			34			33	35	
	Unloaded		76	19	21.2	0.58	0.63	8.3	0.92			112			33			34	31	
	Unloaded		75	19	21.0	0.55	0.58	7.7	0.95			113			33			35	33	
	Unloaded	135/72	81	23	19.8	0.52	0.58	7.2	0.90	7.40	21	110	113	-1	34	35	1	34	31	0.25
0.5	20		81	18	24.5	0.67	0.65	8.0	1.03			109			34			34	35	
1.0	20		85	20	22.8	0.63	0.71	8.4	0.89			111			34			33	30	
1.5	40		87	21	27.1	0.81	0.85	9.8	0.95			105			33			31	30	
2.0	40	144/75	88	19	25.1	0.75	0.79	9.0	0.95	7.40	21	111	120	-6	36	35	-1	31	30	0.20
2.5	60		98	19	28.0	0.81	0.87	8.9	0.93			112			34			33	30	
3.0	60		100	20	29.4	0.91	1.10	11.0	0.83			107			35			30	25	
3.5	80		99	21	33.7	1.04	1.24	12.5	0.84			108			36			31	26	
4.0	80	144/75	112	21	34.5	1.07	1.23	11.0	0.87	7.40	21	108	106	5	36	35	-1	31	27	0.18
4.5	100		110	23	33.3	1.20	1.39	12.6	0.86			109			36			26	23	
5.0	100	162/84	113	23	42.6	1.33	1.50	13.3	0.89	7.40	22	110	109	1	35	36	1	31	27	0.21
5.5	120		120	25	45.6	1.43	1.57	13.1	0.91			109			36			30	28	
6.0	120	168/84	124	24	49.6	1.57	1.69	13.6	0.93	7.40	23	110	107	4	36	37	1	30	28	0.22
6.5	140		130	24	51.2	1.67	1.84	14.2	0.91			108			37			29	27	
7.0	140		135	27	59.8	1.81	1.99	14.7	0.91			111			36			32	29	
7.5	160		140	29	61.2	1.87	2.03	14.5	0.92			109			38			31	29	
8.0	160	174/84	149	32	66.7	2.14	2.18	14.6	0.98	7.40	21	113	107	7	36	35	-1	30	29	0.17
8.5	180		152	27	64.3	2.12	2.14	14.1	0.99			108			39			29	29	
9.0	180		154	31	73.7	2.45	2.45	15.9	1.00			112			37			29	29	
9.5	200		160	33	78.7	2.61	2.54	15.9	1.03			110			38			29	30	
10.0	200	207/84	172	36	91.8	2.91	2.60	15.1	1.12	7.40	21	117	100	18	35	35	0	30	34	0.19
10.5	220		175	42	102.1	3.09	2.69	15.4	1.15			118			34			32	37	
11.0	220	210/90	174	49	115.3	3.25	2.69	15.5	1.21	7.40	20	121	106	15	32	33	1	34	41	0.23
	Recovery		162	34	92.9	2.94	2.24	13.8	1.31	7.30	16	119	107	16	36	33	-3	31	40	0.14
	Recovery		154	36	87.3	2.44	1.58	10.3	1.54			125			32			35	53	
	Recovery		140	29	62.8	1.73	1.07	7.6	1.62			127			32			35	56	
	Recovery		125	24	49.1	1.39	0.89	7.1	1.56	7.30	15	125	132	-4	33	31	-2	34	53	0.17

Interpretation

COMMENTS

Resting respiratory function studies were normal.

ANALYSIS

In flow chart 1, maximum $\dot{V}_{O_2}$ and the anaerobic threshold are both normal, well above predicted values for sedentary men. Proceeding to flow chart 2 through branchpoints 2.1 and 2.2, it is apparent that the patient is an exceptionally fit man. The low breathing reserve is compatible with good motivation. While the patient was breathing 15% O_2, maximum $\dot{V}_{O_2}$ and the anaerobic threshold decreased modestly and exercise tolerance decreased somewhat; these are normal findings.

CONCLUSION

This is a fit 65-year-old man with excellent cardiovascular function who has no evidence to support the diagnosis of cardiomyopathy. His symptoms are most likely due to the decrease in cardiovascular function associated with aging while he tries to continue his physical feats of earlier years.

PRINCIPLES OF EXERCISE TESTING AND INTERPRETATION

TABLE 13-4. *15% oxygen.*

Time min	Work rate watts	BP mm Hg	HR min⁻¹	f min⁻¹	V̇E L/min BTPS	V̇CO₂ L/min STPD	V̇O₂ L/min STPD	V̇O₂/HR ml/beat	R	pH	HCO₃ meq/L	PO₂, mm Hg ET	a	(A-a)	PCO₂, mm Hg ET	a	(a-ET)	V̇E/V̇CO₂	V̇E/V̇O₂	VD/VT
	Rest		73	17	12.7	0.24	0.22	3.0	1.08			81			28			47	51	
	Rest		67	14	12.1	0.30	0.28	4.2	1.07			78			31			36	39	
	Rest		69	14	13.9	0.32	0.32	4.6	1.00			76			31			40	40	
	Rest	114/66	67	15	9.1	0.17	0.16	2.4	1.07	7.44	21	79	77	0	30	32	2	46	49	0.36
	Rest		66	11	16.0	0.42	0.37	5.5	1.15			80			31			36	41	
	Rest		75	16	10.3	0.17	0.15	2.0	1.16			82			29			53	61	
	Unloaded		76	19	15.8	0.37	0.31	4.0	1.20			82			30			38	46	
	Unloaded		81	14	17.5	0.48	0.45	5.6	1.07			76			33			34	36	
	Unloaded		82	19	23.1	0.63	0.59	7.2	1.07			76			33			34	36	
	Unloaded		84	15	18.4	0.53	0.54	6.5	0.97			72			34			32	31	
	Unloaded		79	17	20.8	0.59	0.59	7.5	1.00			73			34			33	33	
	Unloaded	132/36	73	15	19.8	0.55	0.51	7.1	1.07	7.39	20	77	76	0	32	33	1	34	36	0.21
0.5	20		84	22	15.7	0.45	0.46	5.5	0.97			70			36			31	30	
1.0	20		85	18	22.2	0.64	0.64	7.5	1.00			73			34			32	32	
1.5	40		85	18	23.6	0.73	0.73	8.6	1.00			72			35			30	30	
2.0	40	114/60	92	16	24.2	0.75	0.75	8.1	1.00	7.41	22	72	68	4	35	35	0	30	30	0.18
2.5	60		95	18	26.8	0.81	0.81	8.5	1.00			72			35			31	31	
3.0	60		102	22	29.4	0.89	0.86	8.5	1.03			72			36			31	32	
3.5	80		105	19	33.0	1.04	0.98	9.3	1.06			73			36			30	32	
4.0	80	144/66	105	22	36.0	1.11	1.01	9.7	1.10	7.42	22	75	66	9	35	35	0	31	34	0.19
4.5	100		108	23	38.9	1.20	1.10	10.1	1.10			75			35			31	34	
5.0	100		115	22	41.5	1.30	1.19	10.3	1.10			75			35			30	33	
5.5	120		114	24	45.7	1.43	1.23	10.8	1.16			76			36			31	36	
6.0	120	144/66	124	25	49.2	1.53	1.40	11.3	1.10	7.42	22	75	60	15	35	34	-1	31	34	0.17
6.5	140		124	28	54.5	1.65	1.45	11.7	1.14			77			34			32	36	
7.0	140		129	28	59.4	1.80	1.49	11.5	1.21			78			35			32	38	
7.5	160		140	28	65.7	2.00	1.71	12.2	1.17			77			35			32	37	
8.0	160	174/73	148	30	72.0	2.15	1.77	11.9	1.22	7.41	21	79	57	21	34	34	0	32	39	0.21
8.5	180		150	30	73.6	2.21	1.88	12.5	1.17			78			34			32	38	
9.0	180		152	28	74.6	2.29	1.83	12.0	1.25			79			35			32	39	
9.5	200		152	28	75.6	2.36	1.88	12.4	1.25			79			35			31	39	
10.0	200	195/84	160	33	84.8	2.57	1.98	12.4	1.30	7.38	19	80	52	28	35	33	-2	32	41	0.17
10.5	220		170	44	101.6	2.78	2.19	12.9	1.27			81			33			35	45	
11.0	220	198/96	172	45	107.9	3.03	2.15	12.5	1.41	7.33	17	85	56	27	31	32	1	34	49	0.21
	Recovery		172	41	97.3	2.77	1.93	11.2	1.44			84			33			34	49	
	Recovery		154									91			33					

CASE 14 *Obesity*

CLINICAL FINDINGS

This 53-year-old former mechanic had retired because of medical disability 3 years previously with symptoms of vertigo, nausea, and ataxia and a diagnosis of vestibular neuronitis. He had no other complaints except for some shortness of breath when bicycling uphill. He had 30 pack years of cigarette smoking and claimed to be smoking one-half pack per day. Hypertension, diagnosed 14 years ago, was being treated with methyldopa. Chest roentgenograms were normal except for symmetric pleural thickening considered to represent extrapleural fat.

EXERCISE FINDINGS

The patient performed exercise on a cycle ergometer. He pedalled at 60 rpm without added load for 3 minutes. The work rate was then increased 15 W per minute to his symptom-limited maximum. Arterial blood was sampled every second minute, and intra-arterial blood pressure was recorded from a percutaneously placed brachial artery catheter. Resting and exercise ECGs were normal. Resting carboxyhemoglobin was 7.4%. The patient stopped exercise complaining of leg fatigue.

TABLE 14-1. *Selected Respiratory Function Data*

MEASUREMENT	PREDICTED	MEASURED
Age, yr		53
Sex		Male
Height, cm		171
Weight, kg	74	104
Hematocrit, %		51
VC, L	4.15	4.00
IC, L	2.77	3.64
TLC, L	6.15	5.69
FEV_1, L	3.28	3.25
FEV_1/VC, %	79	81
MVV, L/min	140	126
DL_{CO}, ml/mm Hg/min	28.8	29.8

TABLE 14-2. *Selected Exercise Data*

MEASUREMENT	PREDICTED	MEASURED
Maximum $\dot{V}O_2$, L/min	2.48	2.45
Maximum HR, beats/min	167	168
Maximum O_2 pulse, ml/beat	14.9	15.6
$\Delta\dot{V}O_2/\Delta WR$, ml/min/W	10.3	10.4
AT, L/min	> 1.07	1.45
Blood pressure, mm Hg (rest, max)		
Maximum $\dot{V}E$, L/min		116
Exercise breathing reserve, L/min	> 15	10
Pa_{O_2}, mm Hg (rest, max ex)		81,85
$P(A-a)_{O_2}$, mm Hg (rest, max ex)		26,37
$P(a-ET)_{CO_2}$, mm Hg (rest, max ex)		1,−7
VD/VT (rest, heavy ex)		0.31,0.23
HCO_3^-, mEq/L (rest, 2-min recov)		24,14

FIG. 14-A.

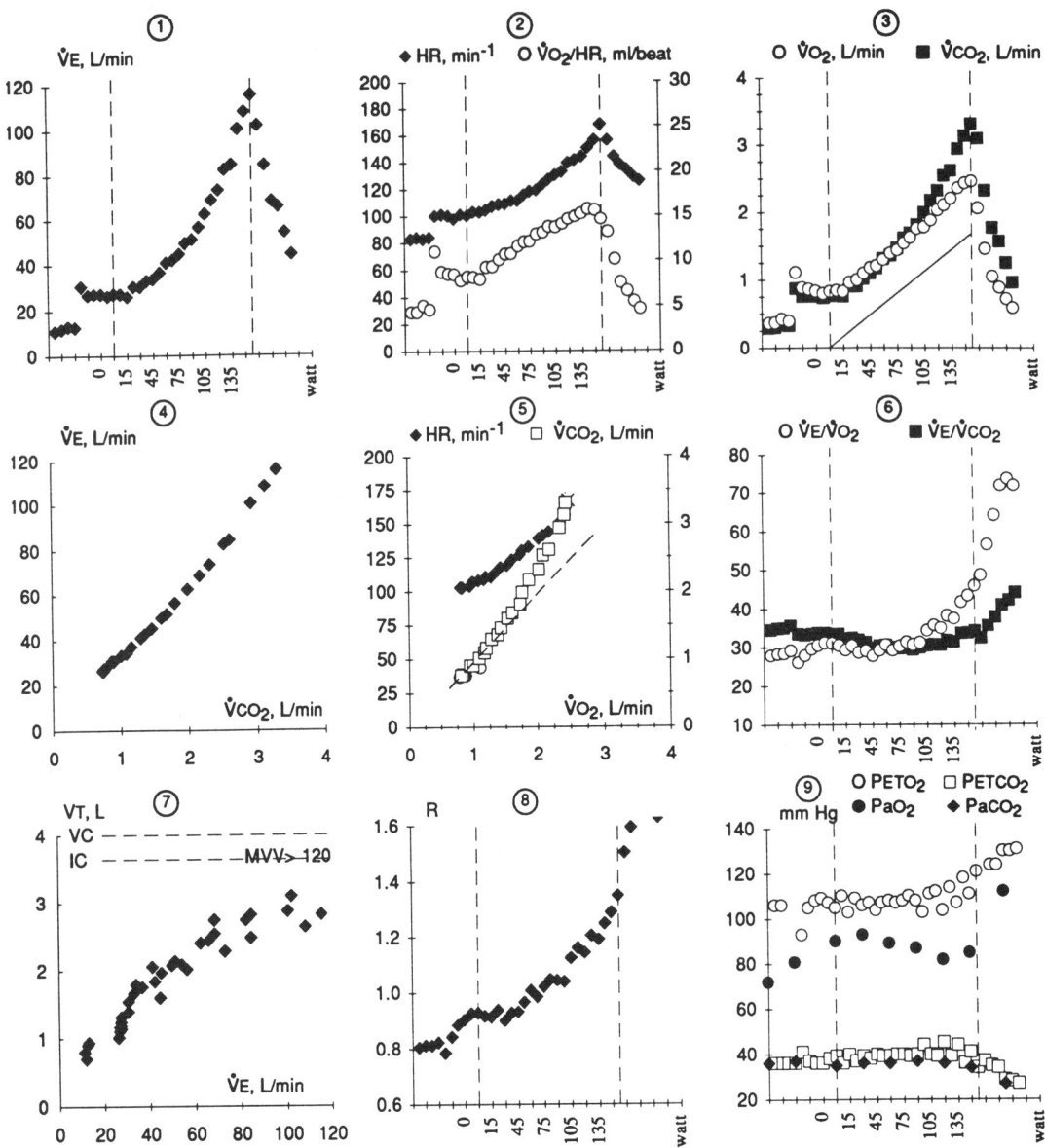

1. Vertical dashed lines in panels 1 to 3 and 6, 8, and 9 indicate the beginning and the end of increasing work period.

2. Unloaded cycling is performed for 3 minutes before the left vertical dashed line.

3. In panel 3, the diagonal line shows the increase of $\dot{V}O_2$ at a slope of 10 ml/min/W.

4. In panel 5, the diagonal dashed line has a slope of 1; the "x" in the upper right is the predicted maximum heart rate and $\dot{V}O_2$ for the subject.

TABLE 14-3.

Time min	Work rate watts	BP mm Hg	HR min⁻¹	f min⁻¹	$\dot{V}E$ L/min BTPS	$\dot{V}CO_2$ L/min STPD	$\dot{V}O_2$ L/min STPD	$\frac{\dot{V}O_2}{HR}$ ml/beat	R	pH	HCO₃ meq/L	PO2, mm Hg ET	a	(A-a)	PCO2, mm Hg ET	a	(a-ET)	$\frac{\dot{V}E}{\dot{V}CO_2}$	$\frac{\dot{V}E}{\dot{V}O_2}$	$\frac{VD}{VT}$
	Rest									7.44	24		72			36				
	Rest		83	14	11.2	0.29	0.36	4.3	0.81			106			36			35	28	
	Rest		84	17	11.9	0.30	0.37	4.4	0.81			106			36			35	28	
	Rest		83	14	13.1	0.34	0.42	5.1	0.81			167			36			35	28	
	Rest		84	14	12.6	0.32	0.39	4.6	0.82	7.43	24	168	81	26	36	37	1	36	29	0.31
	Unloaded		100	20	30.8	0.87	1.11	11.1	0.78			93			41			33	26	
	Unloaded		101	23	26.9	0.75	0.89	8.8	0.84			105			37			33	28	
	Unloaded		100	22	27.3	0.76	0.86	8.6	0.88			108			36			33	30	
	Unloaded		98	23	27.3	0.75	0.83	8.5	0.90			109			36			34	31	
	Unloaded		101	24	26.6	0.73	0.79	7.8	0.92			107			38			34	31	
	Unloaded		100	24	27.4	0.76	0.82	8.2	0.93	7.43	23	105	90	23	39	35	-4	33	31	0.24
0.5	15		103	21	27.5	0.77	0.84	8.2	0.92			110			36			33	31	
1.0	15		103	26	26.3	0.75	0.82	8.0	0.91			103			40			32	29	
1.5	30		104	20	30.8	0.90	0.96	9.2	0.94			109			37			32	30	
2.0	30		107	22	30.6	0.90	1.00	9.3	0.90	7.43	23	106	93	18	39	36	-3	32	29	0.23
2.5	45		108	20	33.3	1.01	1.09	10.1	0.93			107			38			31	29	
3.0	45		109	19	34.0	1.09	1.17	10.7	0.93			104			40			30	28	
3.5	60		111	21	36.9	1.16	1.20	10.8	0.97			107			39			30	29	
4.0	60		111	20	41.2	1.30	1.29	11.6	1.01	7.42	23	108	89	25	39	36	-3	30	31	0.20
4.5	75		115	23	42.4	1.36	1.38	12.0	0.99			107			40			30	29	
5.0	75		118	23	45.2	1.46	1.43	12.1	1.02			108			40			30	30	
5.5	90		119	24	49.9	1.60	1.53	12.9	1.05			110			39			30	31	
6.0	90		123	24	51.4	1.68	1.61	13.1	1.04	7.39	22	108	87	27	40	37	-3	29	31	0.20
6.5	105		127	28	56.6	1.81	1.74	13.7	1.04			103			44			30	31	
7.0	105		130	26	62.6	1.99	1.77	13.6	1.12			111			40			30	34	
7.5	120		133	27	68.8	2.17	1.87	14.1	1.16			112			39			31	36	
8.0	120		139	32	73.3	2.32	2.03	14.6	1.14	7.38	21	104	82	36	45	36	-9	30	35	0.20
8.5	135		141	30	82.4	2.53	2.10	14.9	1.20			114			39			32	38	
9.0	135		144	34	84.5	2.61	2.19	15.2	1.19			107			44			31	37	
9.5	150		150	35	100.8	2.93	2.35	15.7	1.25			118			36			33	42	
10.0	150		156	41	108.4	3.13	2.43	15.6	1.29	7.37	19	111	85	37	41	34	-7	34	43	0.23
10.5	165		168	41	115.8	3.30	2.45	14.6	1.35			121			34			34	46	
	Recovery		156	33	102.3	3.08	2.05	13.1	1.50			1			37			32	49	
	Recovery		144	30	84.5	2.31	1.45	10.1	1.59			124			35			35	57	
	Recovery		138	25	68.7	1.76	1.04	7.5	1.69			124			34			38	64	
	Recovery		134	27	66.1	1.56	0.89	6.6	1.75	7.32	14	130	112	20	29	27	-2	41	72	0.21
	Recovery		129	26	54.4	1.24	0.71	5.5	1.75			130			28			42	74	
	Recovery		126	28	44.7	0.96	0.59	4.7	1.63			131			27			44	72	

Interpretation

COMMENTS

Results of this patient's resting respiratory function studies are normal except for a low ERV/IC ratio consistent with obesity (Table 14-1). The resting ECG is normal. The patient is 30 kg overweight (Table 14-1); his resting carboxyhemoglobin of 7.4% suggests recent cigarette smoking.

ANALYSIS

In flow chart 1, maximum $\dot{V}O_2$ and anaerobic threshold are within normal limits (Table 14-2).

See flow chart 2: The ECG, arterial blood gases, and O_2 pulse at maximum $\dot{V}O_2$ are normal (branchpoint 2.1). The patient is 30 kg overweight (branchpoint 2.2). Supporting the diagnosis of obesity as the cause of this patient's shortness of breath is his high oxygen cost for unloaded cycling ($\dot{V}O_2 = 0.9$ L/min.), and low breathing reserve at the maximum work rate (Table 14-2).

CONCLUSION

Obesity has contributed to dyspnea in an otherwise normal, cigarette-smoking patient.

CASE 15 *Extreme Obesity*

CLINICAL FINDINGS

This 45-year-old man was referred for an exercise study to evaluate his capacity for work as a security guard. Because of his obesity, his employer believed that he was unable to perform his duties, which could include running up stairs and chasing after thieves. The evaluee denied any exercise limitation and is not taking any medications. He does not smoke or drink alcoholic beverages. Resting ECG was normal.

EXERCISE FINDINGS

The patient performed exercise on a treadmill because this was believed to best simulate the tasks he might be called on to perform. He walked on the level at 3 miles per hour (4.8 km per hour) for 3 minutes, after which the grade was increased 2° per minute to tolerance. Heart rate and rhythm were continuously monitored. Blood pressure was measured by sphygmomanometry and oxygen saturation by ear oximetry. Multiple-lead ECGs were taken during rest, exercise, and recovery. The patient appeared to give an excellent effort and stopped exercise because of fatigue; he denied chest pain or dyspnea during or after the study. No ectopy or abnormal ECG changes occurred during or after exercise.

TABLE 15-1. *Selected Respiratory Function Data*

MEASUREMENT	PREDICTED	MEASURED
Age, yr		45
Sex		Male
Height, cm		168
Weight, kg	72	157
Hematocrit, %		47
VC, L	4.11	3.67
IC, L	2.74	3.63
FEV$_1$, L	3.31	3.19
FEV$_1$/VC, %	81	87
MVV, L/min	132	140

TABLE 15-2. *Selected Exercise Data*

MEASUREMENT	PREDICTED	MEASURED
Maximum $\dot{V}O_2$, L/min	3.28	4.14
Maximum HR, beats/min	175	191
Maximum O$_2$ pulse, ml/beat	18.7	21.8
AT, L/min	> 1.39	3.25
Blood pressure, mm Hg (rest, max)		160/90,225/100
Maximum $\dot{V}E$, L/min		128
Exercise breathing reserve, L/min	> 15	12

Fig. 15-A.

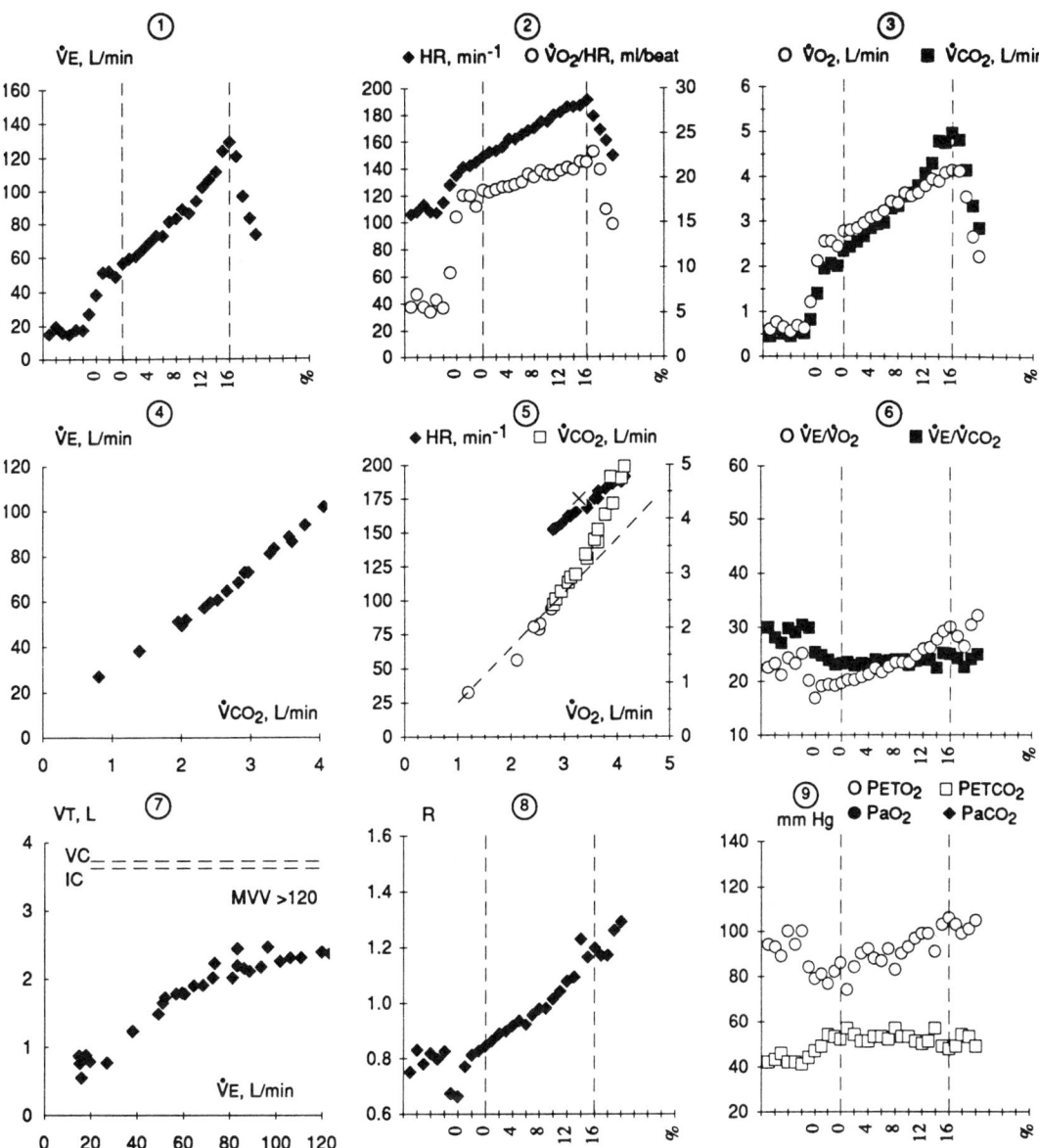

1. Vertical dashed lines in panels 1 to 3 and 6, 8, and 9 indicate the beginning and the end of increasing work period.

2. Zero grade walking is performed for 3 minutes before the left vertical dashed line.

3. In panel 5, the diagonal dashed line has a slope of 1; the "x" in the upper right is the predicted maximum heart rate and $\dot{V}O_2$ for the subject.

TABLE 15-3.

Time min	Treadmill grade, %	BP mm Hg	HR min^{-1}	f min^{-1}	$\dot{V}_E$ L/min BTPS	$\dot{V}CO_2$ L/min STPD	$\dot{V}O_2$ L/min STPD	$\frac{\dot{V}O_2}{HR}$ ml/beat	R	pH	HCO$_3$ meq/L	PO2, mm Hg ET	a	(A-a)	PCO2, mm Hg ET	a	(a-ET)	$\frac{\dot{V}_E}{\dot{V}CO_2}$	$\frac{\dot{V}_E}{\dot{V}O_2}$	$\frac{V_D}{V_T}$
	Rest	160/90																		
	Rest		106	20	15.2	0.45	0.60	5.7	0.75			94			42			30	23	
	Rest		108	25	19.8	0.63	0.76	7.0	0.83			93			43			28	23	
	Rest		113	29	16.0	0.50	0.64	5.7	0.78			89			46			27	21	
	Rest	150/100	108	17	14.8	0.45	0.55	5.1	0.82			100			42			30	24	
	Rest		107	20	17.7	0.55	0.69	6.4	0.80			94			42			29	23	
	Rest		115	20	17.5	0.52	0.63	5.5	0.83			100			41			30	25	
0.5	0		128	35	27.1	0.81	1.20	9.4	0.68			84			44			30	20	
1.0	0		135	31	38.1	1.40	2.11	15.6	0.66			79			47			25	17	
1.5	0		141	31	51.1	1.96	2.54	18.0	0.77			81			49			25	19	
2.0	0		142	30	52.0	2.07	2.55	18.0	0.81			77			54			24	19	
2.5	0		145	33	49.2	2.01	2.43	16.8	0.83			82			53			23	19	
3.0	0	210/100	149	32	57.0	2.34	2.77	18.6	0.84			86			52			23	20	
3.5	2		152	33	59.5	2.42	2.80	18.4	0.86			74			57			23	20	
4.0	2		153	34	60.6	2.53	2.85	18.6	0.89			84			54			23	20	
4.5	4		156	34	64.6	2.66	2.96	19.0	0.90			90			51			23	21	
5.0	4	210/90	162	36	68.6	2.83	3.08	19.0	0.92			92			51			23	21	
5.5	6		162	36	72.7	2.92	3.12	19.3	0.94			88			53			24	22	
6.0	6		165	36	72.8	2.97	3.22	19.5	0.92			87			53			23	22	
6.5	8		168	40	81.1	3.28	3.43	20.4	0.96			92			52			24	23	
7.0	8	210/90	170	38	83.4	3.34	3.41	20.1	0.98			83			57			24	24	
7.5	10		175	42	88.7	3.56	3.63	20.7	0.98			90			53			24	23	
8.0	10		175	40	86.3	3.61	3.56	20.3	1.01			93			53			23	23	
8.5	12		180	43	93.6	3.79	3.64	20.2	1.04			97			51			24	25	
9.0	12	220/90	182	45	101.8	4.07	3.78	20.8	1.08			99			50			24	26	
9.5	14		186	46	106.3	4.28	3.92	21.1	1.09			99			51			24	26	
10.0	14		186	48	111.0	4.77	3.88	20.9	1.23			91			57			22	28	
10.5	16		187	52	123.5	4.75	4.08	21.8	1.16			103			49			25	29	
11.0	16	225/100	191	53	128.4	4.96	4.14	21.7	1.20			106			48			25	30	
	Recovery		179	50	120.1	4.80	4.10	22.9	1.17			103			49			24	28	
	Recovery	200/80	169	39	96.4	4.13	3.53	20.9	1.17			99			54			23	26	
	Recovery		161	34	83.2	3.34	2.65	16.5	1.26			101			53			24	30	
	Recovery	180/80	150	33	73.6	2.85	2.21	14.7	1.29			105			49			25	32	

Interpretation

COMMENTS

Resting lung studies are typical of extreme obesity.

ANALYSIS

In flow chart 1, maximum $\dot{V}O_2$ and the anaerobic threshold are high normal as predicted from height. Through branchpoints 1.1 in this flow chart and branchpoints 2.1 and 2.2 in flow chart 2, the diagnosis of obesity is confirmed. The breathing reserve is low at maximal exercise. The metabolic cost ($\dot{V}O_2$) of walking at zero grade at 3 miles per hour is seen to be 2.5 L/min, which is much higher than would be seen in an individual of normal weight. The anaerobic threshold is reached at a grade of 6 to 8%, and $\dot{V}O_2$max is reached at a 16% grade. These are roughly the tasks that would correspond to the anaerobic threshold and $\dot{V}O_2$max in a subject of normal weight (albeit at a much lower $\dot{V}O_2$ cost).

CONCLUSION

Except for systolic hypertension, no evidence of cardiopulmonary disease was found. There is a fit thin person hiding in this obese man! Despite his fitness, obesity has added a significant burden to his ability to move to sustain an exercise task as well as a normal weight person of equal fitness.

CASE 16 *Coronary artery disease*

CLINICAL FINDINGS

This 58-year-old man had been exposed to asbestos, sandblasting, and 35 pack years of cigarettes. On questioning, he admitted to a grinding chest pain, originating in the midback and radiating around the left chest into the substernal area. The pain, brought on when walking on cold days and relieved in a few minutes by rest, had not previously been treated or diagnosed. He denied shortness of breath. A physical examination revealed no evidence of peripheral vascular disease, heart murmurs, or abnormal heart sounds. The resting 12-lead ECG was within normal limits.

EXERCISE FINDINGS

The patient performed exercise on a cycle ergometer. He pedalled at 60 rpm without added load for 3 minutes. The work rate was then increased 20 W per minute to his symptom-limited maximum. Arterial blood was sampled every second minute, and intra-arterial blood pressure was recorded from a percutaneously placed brachial artery catheter. The patient stopped exercise because of interscapular pain and right anterior chest pain. The ECG showed a 2-mm ST segment depression in leads 2, 3, AVF, and V3 through V6 during exercise but returned to normal after 9 minutes of recovery. The chest pain resolved within 1 minute of cessation of exercise.

TABLE 16-1. *Selected Respiratory Function Data*

MEASUREMENT	PREDICTED	MEASURED
Age, yr		58
Sex		Male
Height, cm		173
Weight, kg	76	82
Hematocrit, %		41
VC, L	4.09	4.04
IC, L	2.73	3.39
TLC, L	6.20	5.93
FEV$_1$, L	3.21	3.43
FEV$_1$/VC, %	79	85
MVV, L/min	135	155
D$_{LCO}$, ml/mm Hg/min	25.5	25.9

TABLE 16-2. *Selected Exercise Data*

MEASUREMENT	PREDICTED	MEASURED
Maximum V̇$_{O_2}$, L/min	2.25	1.47
Maximum HR, beats/min	162	146
Maximum O$_2$ pulse, ml/beat	13.9	10.3
ΔV̇$_{O_2}$/ΔWR, ml/min/W	10.3	7.2
AT, L/min	> 0.99	1.0
Blood pressure, mm Hg (rest, max)		174/81,222/99
Maximum V̇$_E$, L/min		75
Exercise breathing reserve, L/min	> 15	80
Pa$_{O_2}$, mm Hg (rest, max ex)		87,115
P(A−a)$_{O_2}$, mm Hg (rest, max ex)		18,10
P(a−ET)$_{CO_2}$, mm Hg (rest, max ex)		−3,−6
V$_D$/V$_T$ (rest, heavy ex)		0.21,0.12
HCO$_3^-$, mEq/L (rest, 2-min recov)		22,16

Fɪɢ. 16-A.

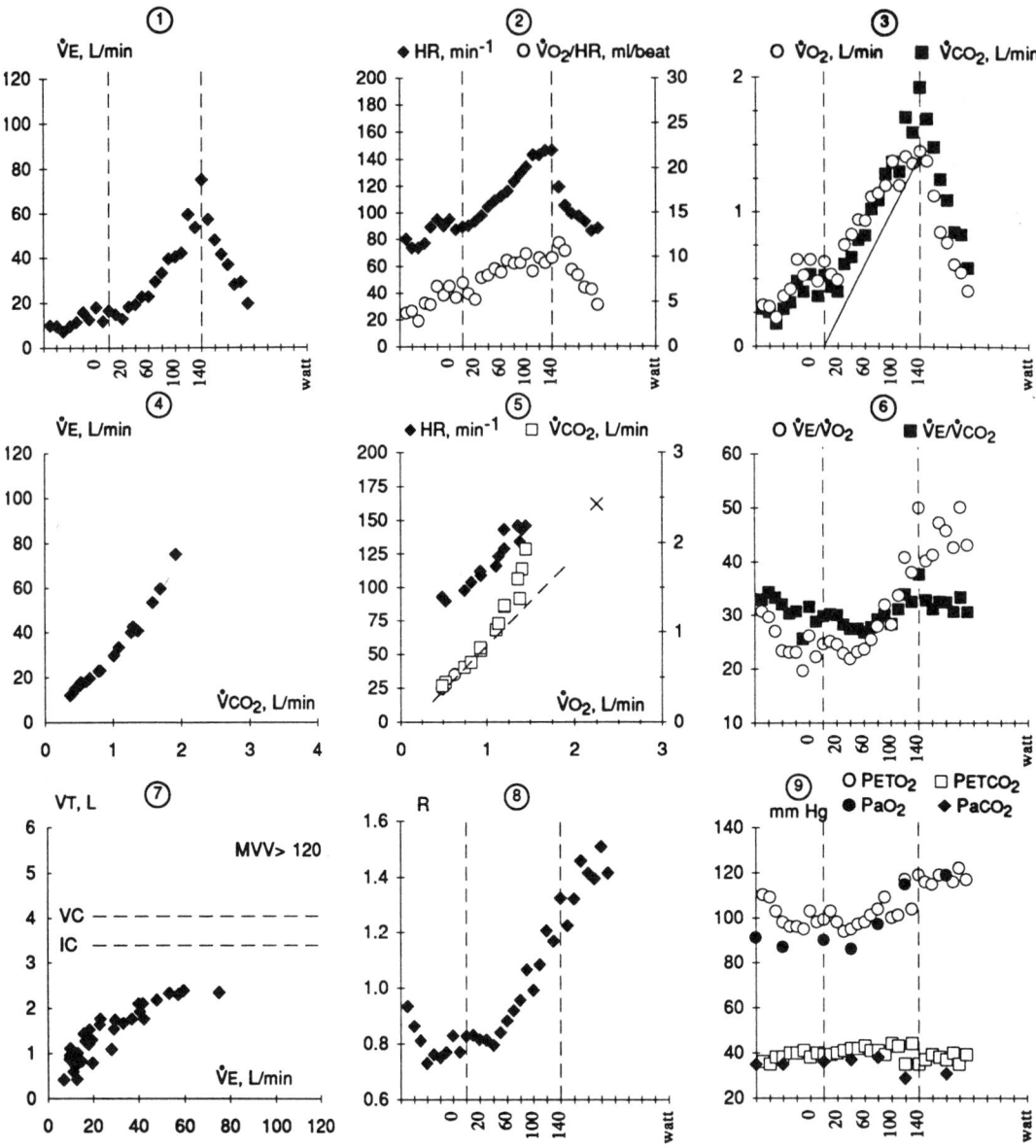

1. Vertical dashed lines in panels 1 to 3 and 6, 8, and 9 indicate the beginning and the end of increasing work period.

2. Unloaded cycling is performed for 2 minutes before the left vertical dashed line.

3. In panel 3, the diagonal line shows the increase of $\dot{V}O_2$ at a slope of 10 ml/min/W.

4. In panel 5, the diagonal dashed line has a slope of 1; the "x" in the upper right is the predicted maximum heart rate and $\dot{V}O_2$ for the subject.

TABLE 16-3.

Time min	Work rate watts	BP mm Hg	HR min⁻¹	f min⁻¹	V̇E L/min BTPS	V̇CO2 L/min STPD	V̇O2 L/min STPD	V̇O2/HR ml/beat	R	pH	HCO3 meq/L	PO2, mm Hg ET	a	(A-a)	PCO2, mm Hg ET	a	(a-ET)	V̇E/V̇CO2	V̇E/V̇O2	VD/VT
	Rest									7.42	22		91			35				
	Rest		80	9	10.0	0.28	0.30	3.8	0.93			110			36			33	31	
	Rest		74	11	9.5	0.25	0.29	3.9	0.86			109			35			34	30	
	Rest		74	17	7.1	0.17	0.21	2.8	0.81			103			38			33	27	
	Rest		77	10	9.5	0.27	0.37	4.8	0.73	7.41	22	98	87	18	38	35	-3	32	23	0.21
	Rest		89	19	11.3	0.32	0.42	4.7	0.76			96			40			30	23	
	Rest		95	11	15.7	0.48	0.64	6.7	0.75			96			40			31	23	
	Unloaded		90	30	12.8	0.40	0.52	5.8	0.77			95			41			26	20	
	Unloaded		95	15	18.0	0.53	0.64	6.7	0.83			103			38			32	26	
	Unloaded		87	17	12.1	0.37	0.48	5.5	0.77			98			40			29	22	
	Unloaded	174/81	89	13	16.6	0.52	0.63	7.1	0.83	7.41	22	99	90	18	39	36	-3	30	25	0.18
0.5	20		90	18	14.8	0.44	0.53	5.9	0.83			103			39			30	25	
1.0	20		93	13	13.1	0.40	0.49	5.3	0.82			98			40			30	24	
1.5	40		98	12	18.2	0.61	0.75	7.7	0.81			94			41			28	23	
2.0	40	192/84	104	15	19.4	0.66	0.83	8.0	0.80	7.40	23	95	86	19	42	37	-5	27	22	0.14
2.5	60		109	14	22.9	0.79	0.94	8.6	0.84			97			42			27	23	
3.0	60		112	13	23.0	0.82	0.93	8.3	0.88			98			43			27	24	
3.5	80		116	17	29.6	1.02	1.11	9.6	0.92			101			41			28	25	
4.0	80	204/90	123	20	33.4	1.09	1.14	9.3	0.96	7.39	23	104	97	14	41	38	-3	29	28	0.21
4.5	100		129	19	39.9	1.28	1.20	9.3	1.07			109			39			30	32	
5.0	100		134	21	40.5	1.37	1.38	10.3	0.99			100			44			28	28	
5.5	120		143	24	42.4	1.30	1.20	8.4	1.08			101			43			31	34	
6.0	120	222/99	143	25	59.6	1.70	1.41	9.9	1.21	7.42	18	117	115	10	35	29	-6	34	41	0.12
6.5	140		146	23	53.6	1.59	1.36	9.3	1.17			104			44			32	38	
7.0	140		146	32	75.1	1.92	1.45	9.9	1.32			119			35			38	50	
	Recovery		119	25	57.4	1.69	1.38	11.6	1.22			116			37			33	40	
	Recovery		105	22	48.0	1.48	1.12	10.7	1.32			115			39			31	41	
	Recovery		99	20	41.9	1.24	0.85	8.6	1.46			119			38			32	47	
	Recovery	210/72	97	21	37.0	1.09	0.77	7.9	1.42	7.34	16	119	119	7	37	31	-6	32	46	0.13
	Recovery		93	26	28.2	0.85	0.61	6.6	1.39			116			40			31	43	
	Recovery		86	19	29.2	0.83	0.55	6.4	1.51			122			35			33	50	
	Recovery		88	25	19.8	0.58	0.41	4.7	1.41			117			39			30	43	

Interpretation

COMMENTS

Resting respiratory function is normal (Table 16-1).

ANALYSIS

In flow chart 1, the maximum $\dot{V}O_2$ is reduced, whereas the anaerobic threshold is normal (Table 16-2), which directs us through branchpoints 1.1, 1.2, and 1.3 to flow chart 3. The breathing reserve (branchpoint 3.1) is high while the ECG (branchpoint 3.3) is abnormal, directing us to "myocardial ischemia." The patient's chest pain and low $\Delta\dot{V}O_2/\Delta WR$ are confirmatory; even more significant are the plateau in $\dot{V}O_2$ and O_2 pulse concurrently with the onset of abnormal ST segment changes. The rise in O_2 pulse after heavy exercise ceased is evidence for recovery of stroke volume from ischemia-induced left ventricular dysfunction. None of these abnormalities would have been evident if exercise had been terminated at a pulse rate below 140 beats per minute.

CONCLUSION

Myocardial ischemia is secondary to coronary artery disease.

CASE 17 *Coronary artery disease*

CLINICAL FINDINGS

This 61-year-old retired shipyard worker complained of breathing difficulties that he could not quantify or describe well. He denied shortness of breath but stated that he stopped using stairs because of a "peculiar feeling in his chest." He also complained of a stabbing substernal and right flank pain not associated with exertion or stress and neck pain, associated with movement of the head attributed to degenerative cervical spine arthritis. He had never smoked cigarettes. Examination revealed psoriasis and normal blood pressure, heart sounds, and peripheral pulses. He had bilateral pleural plaques on chest roentgenograms. He also had ECG findings suggestive of left ventricular hypertrophy.

EXERCISE FINDINGS

The patient performed exercise on a cycle ergometer. He pedalled at 60 rpm without added load for 3 minutes. The work rate was then increased 20 W per minute to his symptom-limited maximum. Arterial blood was sampled every second minute, and intra-arterial blood pressure was recorded from a percutaneously placed brachial artery catheter. The patient stopped exercise because of shortness of breath and tired thighs. He denied chest pain. The ECG developed slight ST segment depression in leads 2, 3, AVF, V5, and V6 at 120 W of exercise (HR 150) that gradually became more prominent with a maximum ST depression of 5 mm at the cessation of exercise (180 W). A rare, unifocal, premature ventricular contraction was noted. The ECG returned to baseline after 14 minutes of recovery.

TABLE 17-1. *Selected Respiratory Function Data*

MEASUREMENT	PREDICTED	MEASURED
Age, yr		61
Sex		Male
Height, cm		176
Weight, kg	78	70
Hematocrit, %		39
VC, L	4.23	3.95
IC, L	2.82	2.60
TLC, L	6.47	6.01
FEV_1, L	3.32	3.25
FEV_1/VC, %	78	82
MVV, L/min	137	121
$D_{L_{CO}}$, ml/mm Hg/min	25.5	33.3

TABLE 17-2. *Selected Exercise Data*

MEASUREMENT	PREDICTED	MEASURED
Maximum $\dot{V}_{O_2}$, L/min	2.08	1.90
Maximum HR, beats/min	159	180
Maximum O_2 pulse, ml/beat	13.1	10.6
$\Delta\dot{V}_{O_2}/\Delta WR$, ml/min/W	10.3	8.8
AT, L/min	> 0.91	1.1
Blood pressure, mm Hg (rest, max)		144/75,246/108
Maximum $\dot{V}_E$, L/min		86
Exercise breathing reserve, L/min	> 15	35
Pa_{O_2}, mm Hg (rest, max ex)		87,103
$P(A-a)_{O_2}$, mm Hg (rest, max ex)		5,15
$P(a-ET)_{CO_2}$, mm Hg (rest, max ex)		2,−1
V_D/V_T (rest, heavy ex)		0.48,0.24
HCO_3^-, mEq/L (rest, 2-min recov)		26,20

Fig. 17-A.

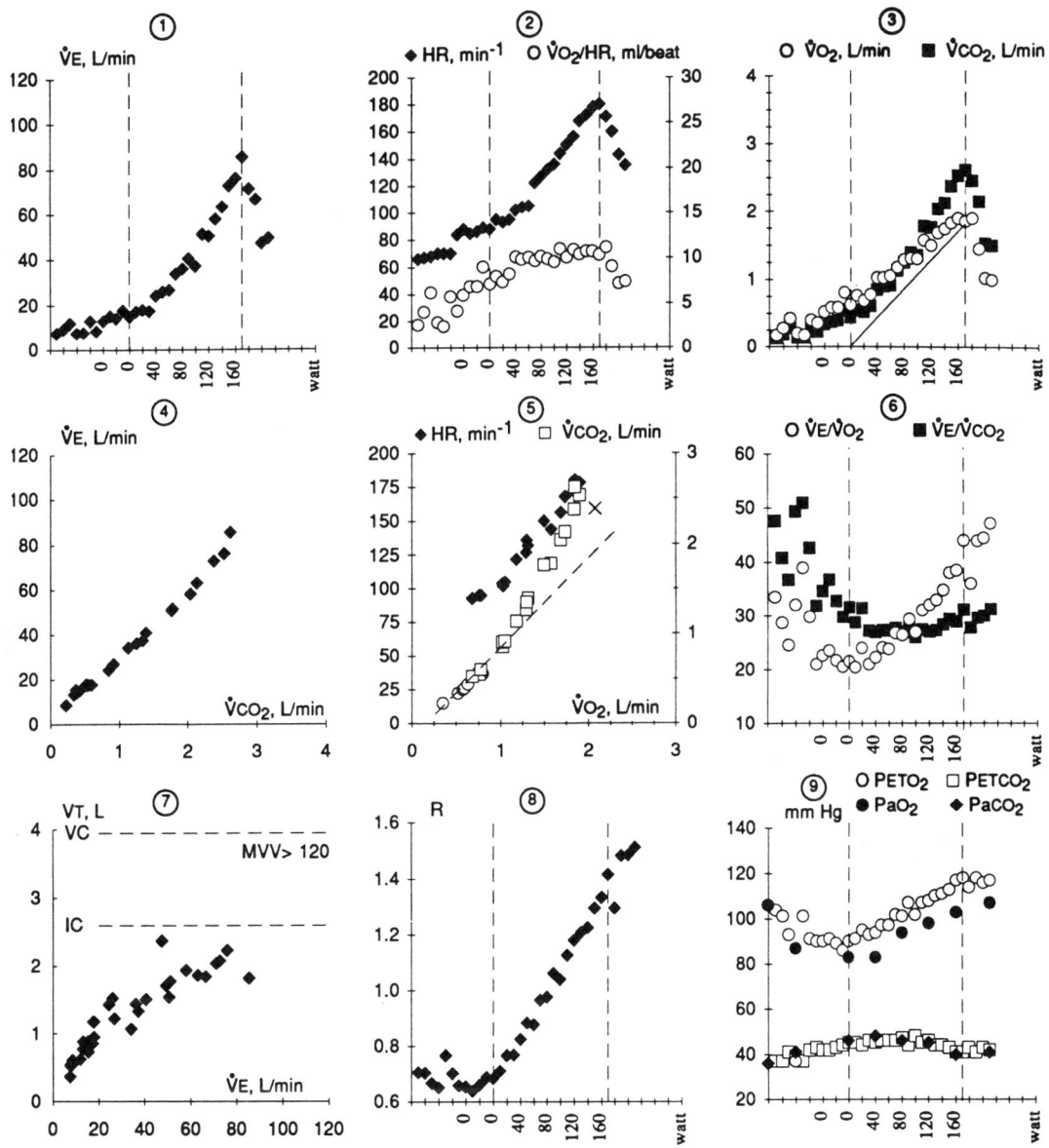

1. Vertical dashed lines in panels 1 to 3 and 6, 8, and 9 indicate the beginning and the end of increasing work period.

2. Unloaded cycling is performed for 3 minutes before the left vertical dashed line.

3. In panel 3, the diagonal line shows the increase of $\dot{V}O_2$ at a slope of 10 ml/min/W.

4. In panel 5, the diagonal dashed line has a slope of 1; the "x" in the upper right is the predicted maximum heart rate and $\dot{V}O_2$ for the subject.

TABLE 17-3.

Time min	Work rate watts	BP mm Hg	HR min^{-1}	f min^{-1}	$\dot{V}E$ L/min BTPS	$\dot{V}CO_2$ L/min STPD	$\dot{V}O_2$ L/min STPD	$\frac{\dot{V}O_2}{HR}$ ml/beat	R	pH	HCO$_3$ meq/L	PO2, mm Hg ET	a	(A-a)	PCO2, mm Hg ET	a	(a-ET)	$\frac{\dot{V}E}{\dot{V}CO_2}$	$\frac{\dot{V}E}{\dot{V}O_2}$	VD VT
	Rest	144/75								7.48	26		106			36				
	Rest		66	20	7.4	0.12	0.17	2.6	0.71			104			37			48	34	
	Rest		67	16	9.1	0.19	0.27	4.0	0.70			101			37			41	29	
	Rest		68	19	11.9	0.28	0.42	6.2	0.67			93			41			37	24	
	Rest	150/75	70	14	7.6	0.13	0.20	2.9	0.65	7.44	27	37	87	5	39	41	2	49	32	0.48
	Rest		70	15	7.9	0.13	0.17	2.4	0.76			101			37			51	39	
	Rest		70	15	13.2	0.28	0.40	5.7	0.70			91			42			43	30	
	Unloaded		84	14	8.5	0.23	0.35	4.2	0.66			90			43			32	21	
	Unloaded		88	17	13.2	0.34	0.52	5.9	0.65			90			42			35	23	
	Unloaded		85	21	15.4	0.37	0.58	6.8	0.64			91			42			37	23	
	Unloaded		86	17	14.2	0.39	0.59	6.9	0.66			89			43			33	22	
	Unloaded		89	15	17.7	0.55	0.80	9.0	0.69			86			44			30	21	
	Unloaded	171/78	88	17	15.0	0.43	0.63	7.2	0.68	7.41	29	90	83	4	45	46	1	32	22	0.37
0.5	20		95	20	17.2	0.54	0.76	8.0	0.71			91			45			29	20	
1.0	20		93	19	17.9	0.52	0.68	7.3	0.76			95			44			31	24	
1.5	40		95	15	17.6	0.60	0.78	8.2	0.77			93			46			27	21	
2.0	40	192/78	102	17	24.3	0.85	1.03	10.1	0.83	7.40	29	94	83	11	45	48	3	27	22	0.31
2.5	60		104	17	26.0	0.90	1.02	9.8	0.88			97			46			27	24	
3.0	60		105	22	26.9	0.92	1.05	10.0	0.88			97			46			27	24	
3.5	80		122	32	34.2	1.14	1.18	9.7	0.97			102			46			28	27	
4.0	80	216/87	127	25	36.1	1.26	1.29	10.2	0.98	7.40	28	101	94	9	47	46	-1	27	26	0.29
4.5	100		132	27	40.8	1.39	1.31	9.9	1.06			107			44			28	29	
5.0	100		136	28	37.4	1.35	1.30	9.6	1.04			102			48			26	27	
5.5	120		144	29	51.4	1.78	1.58	11.0	1.13			107			45			27	31	
6.0	120	231/96	150	33	50.8	1.77	1.50	10.0	1.18	7.39	27	108	98	12	46	45	-1	27	32	0.28
6.5	140		156	30	58.1	2.04	1.69	10.8	1.21			110			44			27	33	
7.0	140		168	34	63.3	2.13	1.74	10.4	1.22			111			44			28	35	
7.5	160		172	35	72.8	2.38	1.84	10.7	1.29			113			43			29	38	
8.0	160	234/99	178	34	76.0	2.53	1.90	10.7	1.33	7.39	24	117	103	15	41	40	-1	29	38	0.24
8.5	180	246/108	180	47	85.5	2.62	1.85	10.3	1.42			118			41			31	44	
	Recovery		171	35	71.3	2.46	1.90	11.1	1.29			114			43			28	36	
	Recovery		160	36	66.6	2.15	1.45	9.1	1.48			118			41			30	44	
	Recovery		143	20	47.5	1.53	1.03	7.2	1.49			116			43			30	44	
	Recovery	192/78	135	29	49.6	1.51	1.00	7.4	1.51	7.30	20	117	107	13	42	41	-1	31	47	0.31

Interpretation

COMMENTS

Resting respiratory function (Table 17-1) and ECG are normal.

ANALYSIS

In flow chart 1, the maximum $\dot{V}O_2$ and anaerobic threshold are normal (Table 17-2), which directs us through branchpoint 1.1 to flow chart 2. The ECG is abnormal and the O_2 pulse is reduced, reaching a plateau for the last 5 minutes of incremental exercise (panel 2, Fig. 17-A) (branchpoint 2.1). The indices of ventilation-perfusion matching are normal (branchpoint 2.3). The low O_2 pulse, steep heart rate-$\dot{V}O_2$ relationship and borderline low $\Delta\dot{V}O_2/\Delta WR$ indicate that the ST segment changes are functionally significant, i.e., consistent with coronary artery disease.

CONCLUSION

Myocardial ischemia is secondary to coronary artery disease, despite the absence of chest pain or reduced maximum oxygen uptake.

CASE 18 *Small vessel coronary artery disease*

CLINICAL FINDINGS

This 47-year-old asymptomatic man was referred for cardiopulmonary exercise testing because of a strong family history of coronary artery disease and the finding of coronary artery calcification on an ultrafast CT cardiac scan. Physical examination, chest roentgenograms, and resting ECGs were normal.

EXERCISE FINDINGS

The patient performed exercise on a cycle ergometer. He pedalled at 60 rpm without an added load for 3 minutes. The work rate was then increased 25 W per minute to tolerance. Heart rate and rhythm were continuously monitored; 12-lead ECGs were obtained during rest, exercise, and recovery. Blood pressure was measured with a sphygmomanometer and oxygen saturation with an ear oximeter. The patient appeared to give an excellent effort and stopped exercise because of leg fatigue. He denied chest pain during or after the study. The ECGs showed progressive down-sloping ST segment depression in leads II, III, AVF, and V3 to V6 after 150 W of exercise and reached approximately 3 mm in leads II and V4 at the cessation of exercise. These changes resolved by 5 minutes of recovery. No ectopy was present.

TABLE 18-1. *Selected Respiratory Function Data*

MEASUREMENT	PREDICTED	MEASURED
Age, yr		47
Sex		Male
Height, cm		175
Weight, kg	78	64
Hematocrit, %		42
VC, L	4.78	5.04
IC, L	3.19	3.70
FEV$_1$, L	3.91	4.03
FEV$_1$/VC, %	81	80
MVV, L/min	153	180

TABLE 18-2. *Selected Exercise Data*

MEASUREMENT	PREDICTED	MEASURED
Maximum $\dot{V}O_2$, L/min	2.35	1.88
Maximum HR, beats/min	173	181
Maximum O$_2$ pulse, ml/beat	13.6	10.4
$\Delta \dot{V}O_2/\Delta$WR, ml/min/W	10.3	6.4
AT, L/min	> 1.01	1.3
Blood pressure, mm Hg (rest, max)		125/82,160/90
Maximum $\dot{V}E$, L/min		78
Exercise breathing reserve, L/min	> 15	102
O$_2$ saturation, oximeter (rest, max)		99,95

FIG. 18-A.

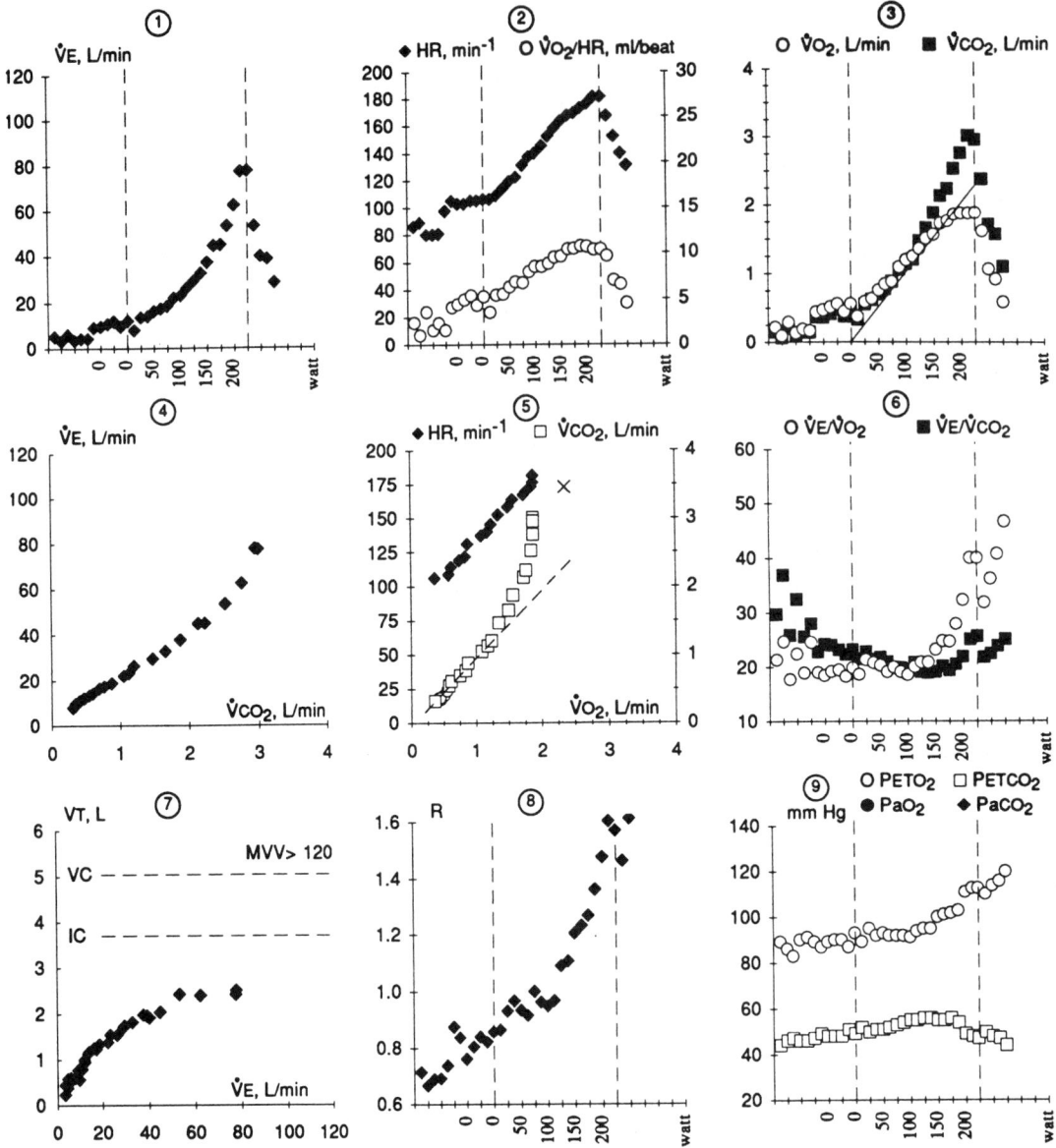

1. Vertical dashed lines in panels 1 to 3 and 6, 8, and 9 indicate the beginning and the end of increasing work period.

2. Unloaded cycling is performed for 3 minutes before the left vertical dashed line.

3. In panel 3, the diagonal line shows the increase of $\dot{V}O_2$ at a slope of 10 ml/min/W.

4. In panel 5, the diagonal dashed line has a slope of 1; the "x" in the upper right is the predicted maximum heart rate and $\dot{V}O_2$ for the subject.

TABLE 18-3.

Time min	Work rate watts	BP mm Hg	HR min⁻¹	f min⁻¹	$\dot{V}E$ L/min BTPS	$\dot{V}CO_2$ L/min STPD	$\dot{V}O_2$ L/min STPD	$\dfrac{\dot{V}O_2}{HR}$ ml/beat	R	pH	HCO₃ meq/L	PO2, mm Hg ET	a	(A-a)	PCO2, mm Hg ET	a	(a-ET)	$\dfrac{\dot{V}E}{\dot{V}CO_2}$	$\dfrac{\dot{V}E}{\dot{V}O_2}$	VD VT
	Rest	125/82																		
	Rest		86	11	5.4	0.15	0.21	2.4	0.71			89			44			30	21	
	Rest		89	14	3.4	0.06	0.09	1.0	0.67			86			46			37	25	
	Rest		80	10	6.0	0.20	0.29	3.6	0.69			83			47			26	18	
	Rest	110/60	80	8	3.6	0.09	0.13	1.6	0.69			90			46			32	22	
	Rest		81	12	4.6	0.14	0.19	2.3	0.74			91			46			26	19	
	Rest		98	8	4.6	0.14	0.16	1.6	0.88			89			47			28	25	
	Unloaded		105	12	9.2	0.36	0.43	4.1	0.84			87			49			23	19	
	Unloaded		103	12	9.5	0.35	0.46	4.5	0.76			89			48			24	18	
	Unloaded		103	14	11.0	0.41	0.51	5.0	0.80			90			48			24	19	
	Unloaded		105	12	11.9	0.47	0.56	5.3	0.84			90			48			23	19	
	Unloaded		105	17	9.7	0.37	0.45	4.3	0.82			87			51			22	18	
	Unloaded	120/82	106	13	12.2	0.48	0.56	5.3	0.86			93			49			23	20	
0.5	25		106	13	8.0	0.32	0.37	3.5	0.86			89			52			22	19	
1.0	25		109	12	13.6	0.55	0.59	5.4	0.93			95			50			23	21	
1.5	50		114	12	14.1	0.61	0.63	5.5	0.97			92			51			21	21	
2.0	50	130/90	119	13	16.3	0.70	0.75	6.3	0.93			93			51			22	20	
2.5	75		122	14	17.3	0.77	0.84	6.9	0.92			92			52			21	19	
3.0	75		131	14	18.7	0.88	0.88	6.7	1.00			92			53			20	20	
3.5	100		137	16	22.2	1.05	1.09	8.0	0.96			92			54			20	19	
4.0	100	130/90	140	15	23.3	1.13	1.19	8.5	0.95			91			55			19	19	
4.5	125		145	17	26.3	1.20	1.24	8.6	0.97			94			55			21	20	
5.0	125		152	17	29.5	1.47	1.35	8.9	1.09			95			56			19	21	
5.5	150		158	18	32.8	1.66	1.50	9.5	1.11			95			56			19	21	
6.0	150	145/90	163	19	37.7	1.88	1.56	9.6	1.21			100			55			19	23	
6.5	175		167	22	44.8	2.13	1.73	10.4	1.23			101			55			20	25	
7.0	175		169	22	45.1	2.23	1.76	10.4	1.27			102			56			19	25	
7.5	200		173	22	53.4	2.52	1.85	10.7	1.36			103			54			20	28	
8.0	200	160/90	176	26	62.5	2.76	1.87	10.6	1.48			111			49			22	32	
8.5	225		181	32	77.5	3.00	1.87	10.3	1.60			113			48			25	40	
9.0	225		181	31	77.8	2.95	1.88	10.4	1.57			113			47			25	40	
	Recovery		167	22	53.4	2.37	1.62	9.7	1.46			110			50			22	32	
	Recovery		152	21	40.2	1.71	1.06	7.0	1.61			114			48			22	36	
	Recovery		140	20	39.1	1.57	0.92	6.6	1.71			116			47			24	41	
	Recovery	160/75	131	17	28.9	1.10	0.59	4.5	1.86			120			44			25	47	

Interpretation

COMMENTS

Normal spirometry.

ANALYSIS

In flow chart 1, maximum $\dot{V}O_2$ is reduced, but the anaerobic threshold is within normal limits (Table 18-2). Proceeding next to flow chart 3, the high breathing reserve (branchpoint 3.1) and abnormal ECG that developed during exercise (branchpoint 3.3) lead us to the diagnosis of myocardial ischemia. The low O_2 pulse and the failure of $\dot{V}O_2$ and the O_2 pulse to rise appropriately for the last 2½ minutes of exercise indicate that an O_2 delivery problem developed at that time. The constant O_2 pulse indicates that the product of the arterial-mixed venous O_2 content difference and stroke volume reached their maximum value prematurely. The constant value might reflect a decreasing stroke volume while arterio-venous difference increased.

CONCLUSION

The combination of O_2 delivery abnormalities (which imply a failure of cardiac output to increase appropriately for the work rate) and ECG findings consistent with myocardial ischemia suggest that the patient had functionally important coronary artery disease. Follow-up coronary angiograms showed diffuse distal coronary artery disease.

CASE 19 *Coronary Artery Disease*

CLINICAL FINDINGS

This 57-year-old male asbestos worker was evaluated at 3-year intervals. At the time of his first evaluation he had a several-year history of diabetes mellitus treated with insulin injections, hypertension treated with hydrochlorothiazide, obesity, arthritis of the hip, and moderate exertional dyspnea. He had never smoked tobacco. Examination at that time revealed moderate obesity and minimal pleural thickening on his chest roentgenograms. The respiratory function and exercise study data of that evaluation are shown in Tables 19–1 to 19–3 and Figure 19-A. When evaluated 3 years later (Tables 19–4 to 19–6 and Figure 19-B), he had developed left-sided "gas" pains at the left sternal border, associated with exercise, which were being treated with cimetidine.

EXERCISE FINDINGS

On both occasions, the patient performed exercise on a cycle ergometer. He pedalled at 60 rpm without an added load for 2 or 3 minutes. The work rate was then increased 20 W per minute to tolerance. On the first occasion, arterial blood was sampled every second minute and intra-arterial pressure was recorded from a percutaneously placed brachial artery catheter. The patient was well motivated and cooperative and stopped exercise because of thigh pain, without chest or abdominal pain. No ECG abnormalities were noted at rest, but during high work levels, 1- to 2-mm J-point depression with upsloping ST segments was seen in a few leads.

On the second exercise test, the patient stopped exercise because of calf fatigue and an inability to maintain his cycling frequency. During the last 1 to 2 minutes of exercise he noted left parasternal non-radiating "gas" pain which subsided within 3 minutes of recovery. He denied shortness of breath. The resting ECG was entirely normal; however, at 120 W, 1.5 mm of ST segment depression was seen in leads II, III, AVF, V3 and V4; at 140 W, 2.5- to 3-mm ST segment depression was seen in the same leads plus V5 and V6. The ECG returned to normal by 3 minutes after exercise.

TABLE 19-1. *Selected Respiratory Function Data: First Study*

MEASUREMENT	PREDICTED	MEASURED
Age, yr		57
Sex		Male
Height, cm		171
Weight, kg	74	96
Hematocrit, %		46
VC, L	3.99	4.25
IC, L	2.66	3.37
TLC, L	6.03	6.00
FEV$_1$, L	3.14	3.52
FEV$_1$/VC, %	79	83
MVV, L/min	134	135
D$_{LCO}$, ml/mm Hg/min	26.4	36.4

TABLE 19-2. *Selected Exercise Data: First Study*

MEASUREMENT	PREDICTED	MEASURED
Maximum $\dot{V}O_2$, L/min	2.32	2.20
Maximum HR, beats/min	163	148
Maximum O$_2$ pulse, ml/beat	14.2	14.9
$\Delta \dot{V}O_2/\Delta WR$, ml/min/W	10.3	10.3
AT, L/min	> 1.02	1.2
Blood pressure, mm Hg (rest, max ex)		156/94,250/113
Maximum $\dot{V}E$, L/min		143
Exercise breathing reserves, L/min	> 15	−8
Pa$_{O_2}$, mm Hg (rest, max ex)		100,129
P(A−a)$_{O_2}$ mm Hg (rest, max ex)		10,3
P(a−ET)$_{CO_2}$, mm Hg (rest, max ex)		−4,−2
VD/VT (rest, max ex)		0.16,0.19
HCO$_3^-$, mEq/L (rest, 2-min recovery)		24,15

FIG. 19-A. *First Study*

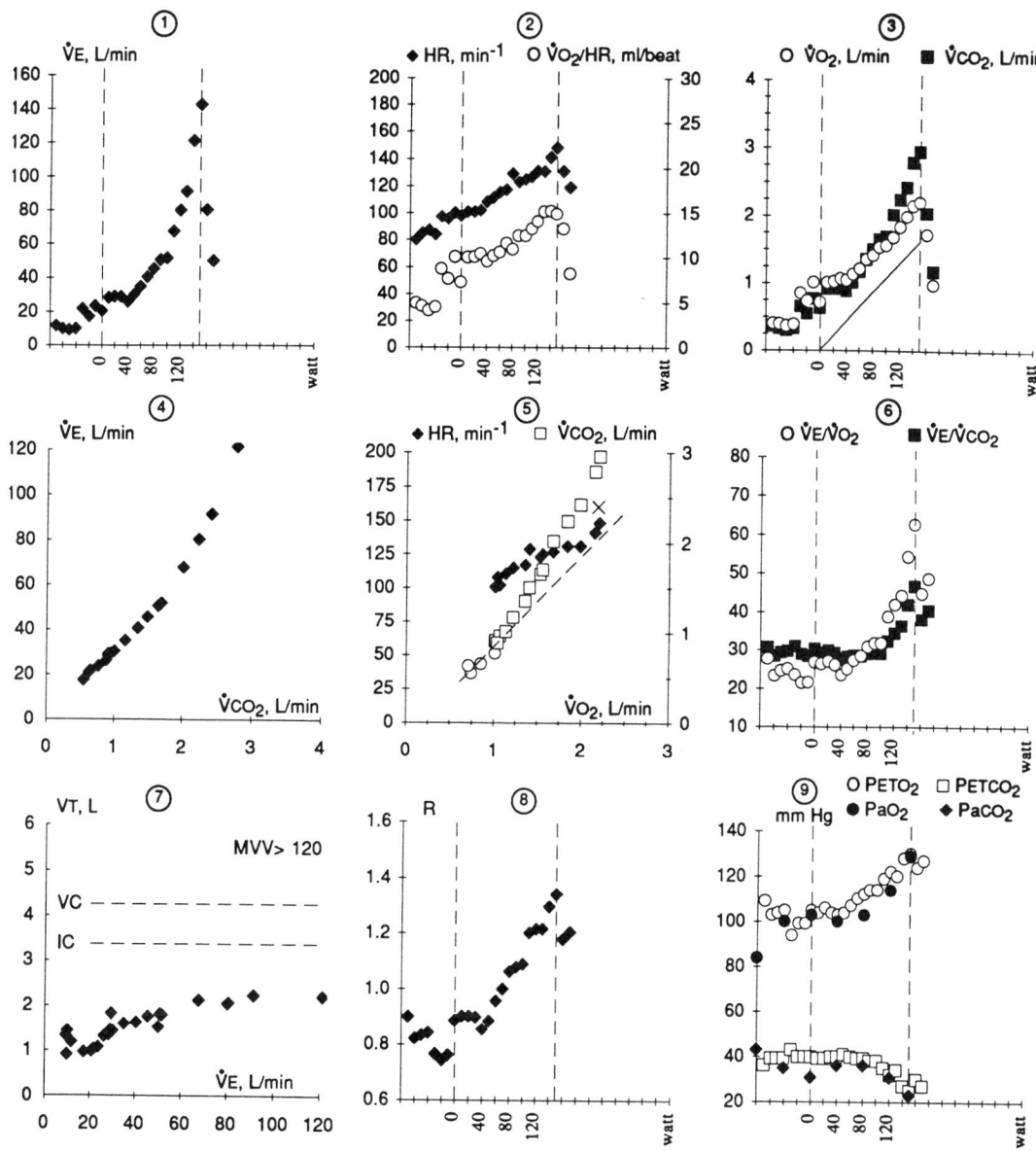

1. Vertical dashed lines in panels 1 to 3 and 6, 8, and 9 indicate the beginning and the end of increasing work period.

2. Unloaded cycling is performed for 3 minutes before the left vertical dashed line.

3. In panel 3, the diagonal line shows the increase of $\dot{V}O_2$ at a slope of 10 ml/min/W.

4. In panel 5, the diagonal dashed line has a slope of 1; the "x" in the upper right is the predicted maximum heart rate and $\dot{V}O_2$ for the subject.

TABLE 19-3. *First Study.*

Time min	Work rate watts	BP mm Hg	HR min⁻¹	f min⁻¹	V̇E L/min BTPS	V̇CO2 L/min STPD	V̇O2 L/min STPD	V̇O2/HR ml/beat	R	pH	HCO3 meq/L	PO2 ET	PO2 a	PO2 (A-a)	PCO2 ET	PCO2 a	PCO2 (a-ET)	V̇E/V̇CO2	V̇E/V̇O2	VD/VT
	Rest	156/94								7.37	24		84			43				
	Rest		80	10	11.9	0.36	0.40	5.0	0.90			109			36			31	28	
	Rest		85	11	10.0	0.32	0.39	4.6	0.82			103			39			28	23	
	Rest		87	7	9.4	0.30	0.36	4.1	0.83			104			39			29	24	
	Rest	175/100	84	7	10.1	0.32	0.38	4.5	0.84	7.40	21	105	100	10	39	35	-4	30	25	0.16
	Unloaded		97	21	21.8	0.65	0.85	8.8	0.76			94			43			31	24	
	Unloaded		96	18	17.4	0.55	0.74	7.7	0.74			99			40			29	21	
	Unloaded		100	22	23.7	0.77	1.01	10.1	0.76			99			40			28	22	
	Unloaded	206/113	98	21	20.8	0.63	0.71	7.2	0.89	7.41	19	105	103	13	40	31	-9	30	27	0.07
0.5	20		101	21	28.3	0.91	1.01	10.0	0.90			104			39			29	26	
1.0	20		101	20	29.2	0.92	1.02	10.1	0.90			106			39			30	27	
1.5	40		102	16	29.4	0.96	1.07	10.5	0.90			104			40			29	26	
2.0	40	219/106	108	20	26.3	0.89	1.04	9.6	0.86	7.39	21	103	100	9	40	36	-4	28	24	0.12
2.5	60		111	20	30.3	1.01	1.14	10.3	0.89			104			41			28	25	
3.0	60		115	22	35.2	1.17	1.22	10.6	0.96			107			40			28	27	
3.5	80		117	25	40.7	1.36	1.36	11.6	1.00			110			39			28	28	
4.0	80	238/106	129	26	45.7	1.50	1.41	10.9	1.06	7.39	21	112	103	13	39	36	-3	29	31	0.16
4.5	100		123	28	50.9	1.65	1.53	12.4	1.08			114			38			29	32	
5.0	100		125	29	51.9	1.70	1.56	12.5	1.09			114			38			29	32	
5.5	120		127	32	67.8	2.02	1.68	13.2	1.20			119			35			32	39	
6.0	120	250/113	131	39	80.3	2.24	1.84	14.0	1.22	7.41	19	122	114	9	32	31	-1	34	42	0.18
6.5	140		131	41	91.5	2.42	1.99	15.2	1.22			120			34			36	44	
7.0	140		141	55	121.3	2.79	2.15	15.2	1.30			128			27			42	54	
7.5	160	235/110	148	59	142.8	2.95	2.20	14.9	1.34	7.42	15	130	129	3	25	23	-2	47	63	0.19
	Recovery		131	39	80.8	2.04	1.73	13.2	1.18			124			30			38	45	
	Recovery		119	33	50.4	1.18	0.98	8.2	1.20			127			27			40	49	

TABLE 19-4. *Selected Respiratory Function Data: Second Study*

MEASUREMENT	PREDICTED	MEASURED
Age, yr		60
Sex		Male
Height, cm		171
Weight, kg	74	87
VC, L	3.92	4.38
IC, L	2.61	2.53
TLC, L	6.11	5.87
FEV₁, L	3.06	3.59
FEV₁/VC, %	78	81
MVV, L/min	132	158
DLCO, ml/mm Hg/min	26.4	31.8

TABLE 19-5. *Selected Exercise Data: Second Study*

MEASUREMENT	PREDICTED	MEASURED
Maximum V̇O₂, L/min	2.19	1.63
Maximum HR, beats/min	160	118
Maximum O₂ pulse, ml/beat	13.7	14.2
ΔV̇O₂/ΔWR, ml/min/W	10.3	6.8
AT, L/min	> 0.96	1.05
Blood pressure, mm Hg (rest, max ex)		140/80,210/100
Maximum V̇E, L/min		79
Exercise breathing reserve, L/min	> 15	79

Fɪɢ. 19-B. *Second Study.*

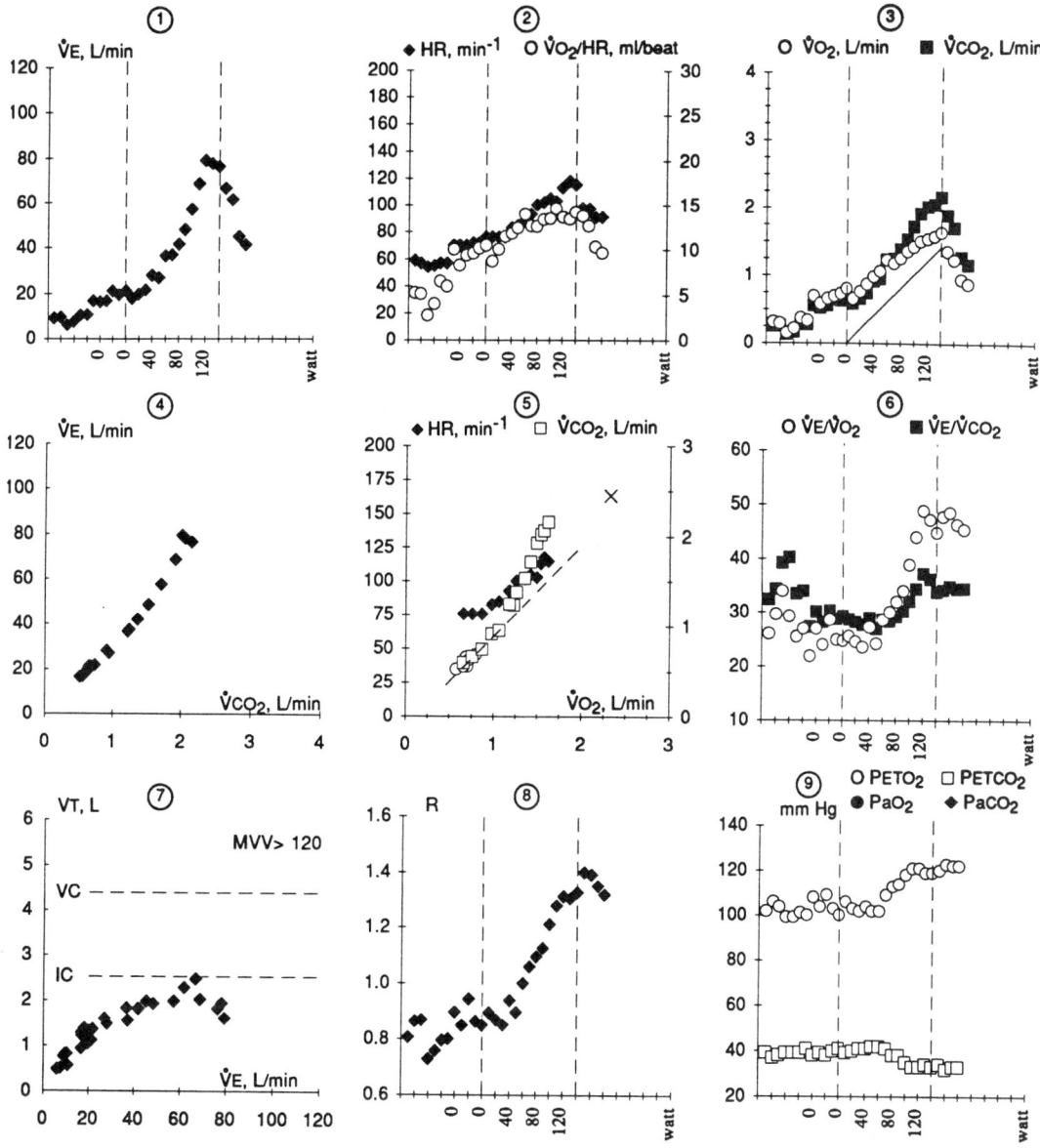

1. Vertical dashed lines in panels 1 to 3 and 6, 8, and 9 indicate the beginning and the end of increasing work period.

2. Unloaded cycling is performed for 3 minutes before the left vertical dashed line.

3. In panel 3, the diagonal line shows the increase of $\dot{V}O_2$ at a slope of 10 ml/min/W.

4. In panel 5, the diagonal dashed line has a slope of 1; the "x" in the upper right is the predicted maximum heart rate and $\dot{V}O_2$ for the subject.

TABLE 19-6. *Second Study.*

Time min	Work rate watts	BP mm Hg	HR min⁻¹	f min⁻¹	$\dot{V}_E$ L/min BTPS	$\dot{V}_{CO_2}$ L/min STPD	$\dot{V}_{O_2}$ L/min STPD	$\frac{\dot{V}_{O_2}}{HR}$ ml/beat	R	pH	HCO₃ meq/L	PO₂, mm Hg ET	a	(A-a)	PCO₂, mm Hg ET	a	(a-ET)	$\frac{\dot{V}_E}{\dot{V}_{CO_2}}$	$\frac{\dot{V}_E}{\dot{V}_{O_2}}$	$\frac{V_D}{V_T}$
	Rest	140/80																		
	Rest		59	12	9.1	0.25	0.31	5.3	0.81			102			39			32	26	
	Rest	140/90	57	12	9.6	0.25	0.29	5.1	0.86			106			37			34	30	
	Rest		54	13	6.2	0.13	0.15	2.8	0.87			104			38			39	34	
	Rest	140/90	55	15	7.7	0.16	0.22	4.0	0.73			99			39			40	29	
	Rest		57	13	10.5	0.28	0.37	6.5	0.76			99			39			34	25	
	Rest		57	19	10.8	0.27	0.34	6.0	0.79			101			39			34	27	
	Unloaded		70	18	16.8	0.56	0.70	10.0	0.80			100			41			27	22	
	Unloaded		70	13	16.7	0.52	0.58	8.3	0.90			108			38			30	27	
	Unloaded		70	14	17.0	0.56	0.66	9.4	0.85			104			39			28	24	
	Unloaded		72	19	21.3	0.65	0.69	9.6	0.94			109			38			30	29	
	Unloaded		72	19	19.8	0.63	0.73	10.1	0.86			103			40			29	25	
	Unloaded	145/90	76	16	21.2	0.68	0.80	10.5	0.85			100			41			29	25	
0.5	20		76	13	18.0	0.59	0.66	8.7	0.89			106			39			29	26	
1.0	20		76	15	19.9	0.66	0.76	10.0	0.87			103			40			28	25	
1.5	40		76	16	21.8	0.74	0.87	11.4	0.85			102			41			28	23	
2.0	40	180/90	83	19	28.2	0.92	0.98	11.8	0.94			104			41			29	27	
2.5	60		85	17	27.1	0.95	1.06	12.5	0.90			102			42			27	24	
3.0	60		88	20	36.8	1.23	1.23	14.0	1.00			102			42			29	29	
3.5	80		93	24	37.4	1.25	1.18	12.7	1.06			109			41			28	30	
4.0	80	195/85	100	23	42.1	1.38	1.26	12.6	1.10			113			38			29	32	
4.5	100		102	25	48.4	1.53	1.36	13.3	1.13			114			38			30	34	
5.0	100		105	29	57.6	1.72	1.42	13.5	1.21			118			35			32	39	
5.5	120		103	34	68.8	1.92	1.50	14.6	1.28			121			33			34	44	
6.0	120	210/100	113	49	79.3	2.02	1.54	13.6	1.31			121			33			37	49	
6.5	140		118	40	78.0	2.06	1.58	13.4	1.30			119			34			36	47	
7.0	140		115	42	76.5	2.16	1.63	14.2	1.33			119			33			34	45	
	Recovery		98	27	66.8	1.89	1.35	13.8	1.40			120			34			34	48	
	Recovery	210/90	97	27	61.9	1.71	1.23	12.7	1.39			123			32			35	48	
	Recovery		91	23	45.5	1.27	0.94	10.3	1.35			122			33			34	46	
	Recovery	180/90	91	23	41.9	1.16	0.88	9.7	1.32			122			33			34	45	

Interpretation

COMMENTS

Resting respiratory function studies including arterial blood gases and pH were normal in both tests.

ANALYSIS

In flow chart 1, in the first study all findings were normal with the exception of a negative breathing reserve, which we interpret as indicating the development of a metabolic acidosis to which the patient responded with excellent pH regulation. To maintain this normal pH, he lowered his Pa_{CO_2} from 35 to 23 mm Hg over a 3½-minute period. He had no evidence of lung or cardiovascular disease.

In the second study, 3 years later, the maximum $\dot{V}_{O_2}$ was reduced while the anaerobic threshold, although lower, remained normal (Table 19-5). In flow chart 3, the breathing reserve was normal (branchpoint 3.1). The ECG during latter exercise was clearly abnormal, leading to the diagnosis of myocardial ischemia. The low $\Delta\dot{V}_{O_2}/\Delta WR$ and flat O_2 pulse during the increasing work rate are supportive of this diagnosis.

CONCLUSION

This patient, with several risk factors for coronary artery disease, had an initially normal cardiovascular response to incremental exercise. Three years later, his O_2 flow became clearly abnormal during incremental exercise. At about the same time, he developed ECG abnormalities and chest pain, establishing the diagnosis of myocardial ischemia.

CASE 20 *Myocardial ischemia with mild interstitial and obstructive airway disease*

CLINICAL FINDINGS

This 54-year-old man was referred by a government agency for cardiopulmonary exercise testing because of his work exposure to asbestos of 15 years. He no longer smoked but had a 30 pack year history of cigarette smoking. He denied dyspnea, cough, chest pain, weight change, or ankle edema. He got little exercise and felt numbness in his legs after 20 minutes of walking. He had borderline hypertension and an elevated serum cholesterol. There were crackles at the left lung base, and a chest roentgenogram showed linear scarring in that area. Heart sounds and the resting ECGs were normal.

EXERCISE FINDINGS

The patient performed exercise on a cycle ergometer. He pedalled at 60 rpm without an added load for 3 minutes. The work rate was then increased 15 W per minute to tolerance. Heart rate and rhythm were continuously monitored; 12-lead ECGs were obtained during rest, exercise, and recovery. Blood pressure was measured with a sphygmomanometer and arterial oxygen saturation was estimated with an ear oximeter. The patient appeared to give a good effort and stopped exercise because of leg fatigue; he denied chest pain or dyspnea during or after the study. Significant ST segment depression in leads II, III, aVF, and V3 to V6 was noted beginning at the 120-W work rate with a maximum of 2.5-mm depression at end-exercise. The ST-segment abnormalities resolved after 9 minutes of recovery. No ectopy was present. Saturation as estimated by oximetry remained normal.

TABLE 20-1. *Selected Respiratory Function Data*

MEASUREMENT	PREDICTED	MEASURED
Age, yr		54
Sex		Male
Height, cm		191
Weight, kg	90	98
Hematocrit, %		47
VC, L	5.36	4.79
IC, L	3.58	3.78
FEV$_1$, L	4.25	3.05
FEV$_1$/VC, %	79	64
MVV, L/min	164	126
DL$_{CO}$, ml/mm Hg/min	29.5	27.7

TABLE 20-2. *Selected Exercise Data*

MEASUREMENT	PREDICTED	MEASURED
Maximum V̇o$_2$, L/min	2.81	2.09
Maximum HR, beats/min	166	142
Maximum O$_2$ pulse, ml/beat	16.9	14.8
ΔV̇o$_2$/ΔWR, ml/min/W	10.3	8.9
AT, L/min	> 1.21	1.4
Blood pressure, mm Hg (rest, max)		154/90, 198/78
Maximum V̇e, L/min		72
Exercise breathing reserve, L/min	> 15	54

TABLE 20-3.

Time min	Work rate watts	BP mm Hg	HR min⁻¹	f min⁻¹	V̇E L/min BTPS	V̇CO2 L/min STPD	V̇O2 L/min STPD	V̇O2/HR ml/beat	R	pH	HCO3 meq/L	PO2 mm Hg ET	a	(A-a)	PCO2 mm Hg ET	a	(a-ET)	V̇E/V̇CO2	V̇E/V̇O2	VD/VT
	Rest	154/90																		
	Rest		77	5	16.6	0.45	0.53	6.9	0.85			106			35			36	31	
	Rest		78	10	14.9	0.44	0.50	6.4	0.88			112			33			32	28	
	Rest		80	6	12.4	0.37	0.43	5.4	0.86			109			34			32	28	
	Rest	150/96	79	5	9.9	0.32	0.40	5.1	0.80			107			34			30	24	
	Rest		77	9	13.5	0.38	0.48	6.2	0.79			107			34			34	27	
	Rest		79	10	9.4	0.27	0.32	4.1	0.84			107			35			32	27	
	Unloaded		83	16	18.1	0.52	0.70	8.4	0.74			102			36			32	24	
	Unloaded		82	13	16.4	0.50	0.64	7.8	0.78			104			36			31	24	
	Unloaded		84	14	18.5	0.58	0.74	8.8	0.78			103			37			30	23	
	Unloaded		86	15	16.7	0.52	0.66	7.7	0.79			100			39			30	23	
	Unloaded		88	13	21.0	0.67	0.80	9.1	0.84			104			37			30	25	
	Unloaded	148/88	85	13	26.1	0.82	0.93	10.9	0.88			105			37			30	27	
0.5	15		87	15	22.6	0.74	0.85	9.8	0.87			103			39			29	25	
1.0	15		87	15	24.7	0.77	0.88	10.1	0.88			107			37			30	27	
1.5	30		88	12	19.9	0.65	0.75	8.5	0.87			106			37			29	25	
2.0	30	152/90	90	16	27.5	0.85	0.98	10.9	0.87			107			36			31	27	
2.5	45		92	12	22.5	0.74	0.86	9.3	0.86			100			41			29	25	
3.0	45		94	13	28.3	0.94	1.06	11.3	0.89			105			39			29	26	
3.5	60		98	16	30.9	1.02	1.17	11.9	0.87			105			39			29	25	
4.0	60	148/84	98	16	33.9	1.12	1.25	12.8	0.90			104			39			29	26	
4.5	75		99	15	35.6	1.21	1.34	13.5	0.90			103			41			28	26	
5.0	75		103	17	37.7	1.27	1.36	13.2	0.93			105			40			29	27	
5.5	90		102	18	38.3	1.31	1.39	13.6	0.94			105			41			28	26	
6.0	90	178/86	108	18	43.4	1.49	1.54	14.3	0.97			105			41			28	27	
6.5	105		112	21	49.4	1.62	1.57	14.0	1.03			110			39			29	30	
7.0	105		109	20	49.6	1.71	1.71	15.7	1.00			103			44			28	28	
7.5	120		115	22	55.1	1.83	1.69	14.7	1.08			110			40			29	31	
8.0	120	170/88	120	23	51.4	1.79	1.72	14.3	1.04			108			41			28	29	
8.5	135		128	24	60.8	2.04	1.87	14.6	1.09			111			39			29	31	
9.0	135		132	25	64.8	2.15	1.95	14.8	1.10			110			41			29	32	
9.5	150		139	27	64.4	2.17	1.98	14.2	1.10			108			43			29	31	
10.0	150	198/78	142	30	71.9	2.34	2.09	14.7	1.12			113			39			30	33	
	Recovery		137	23	68.4	2.33	2.02	14.7	1.15			113			40			29	33	
	Recovery		122	23	55.4	1.95	1.52	12.5	1.28			114			42			27	35	
	Recovery		119	22	60.1	2.02	1.29	10.8	1.57			119			40			29	45	
	Recovery		127	20	58.5	1.81	1.04	8.2	1.74			124			37			31	55	

Interpretation

COMMENTS

Resting studies showed a mild obstructive ventilatory defect.

ANALYSIS

In flow chart 1, maximum $\dot{V}O_2$ is mildly decreased, but the anaerobic threshold is normal. Proceeding next to flow chart 3, the high breathing reserve (branchpoint 3.1) and abnormal exercise ECG (branchpoint 3.3) lead to the diagnosis of myocardial ischemia, although the patient had no chest pain or distress. The $\Delta\dot{V}O_2/\Delta WR$ is within normal limits, but the plateau in the O_2 pulse for the last 4 minutes of exercise suggests the inability to further increase stroke volume and the arterio-venous O_2 difference *or* that stroke volume is decreasing as arterio-venous O_2 difference is increasing. This is coincident with the onset of abnormal ECG findings and is further supported by a slowed increase in $\dot{V}O_2$ as work rate is increased.

CONCLUSION

The patient has evidence of myocardial ischemia associated with concurrent evidence of myocar-

FIG. 20-A.

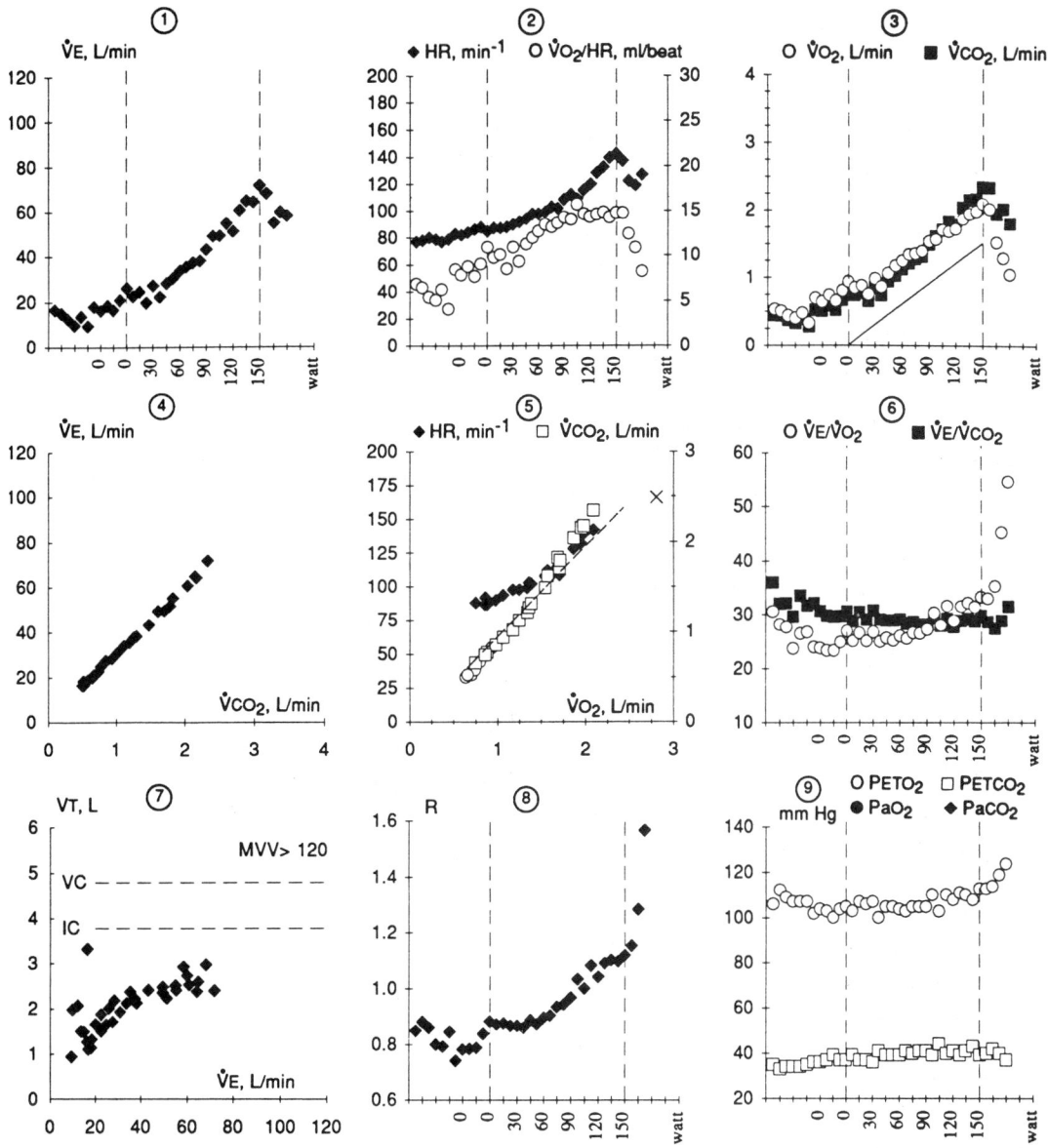

1. Vertical dashed lines in panels 1 to 3 and 6, 8, and 9 indicate the beginning and the end of increasing work period.

2. Unloaded cycling is performed for 3 minutes before the left vertical dashed line.

3. In panel 3, the diagonal line shows the increase of $\dot{V}_{O_2}$ at a slope of 10 ml/min/W.

4. In panel 5, the diagonal dashed line has a slope of 1; the "x" in the upper right is the predicted maximum heart rate and $\dot{V}_{O_2}$ for the subject.

dial dysfunction. This is most likely due to coronary artery disease with myocardial dyskinesis resulting in a falling stroke volume, further supported by ECG abnormalities. The normal ventilatory equivalents indicate satisfactory venti-lation-perfusion matching despite the mild obstructive and interstitial lung disease. The patient was referred to his private internist for further diagnostic and therapeutic evaluation of his cardiac disease.

CASE 21 *Myocardial ischemia, systemic hypertension, and mild interstitial lung disease*

CLINICAL FINDINGS

This 65-year-old man was referred for evaluation. He had retired from work in the shipyard 5 years previously. He had noted slight dyspnea on exertion beginning 6 years prior to evaluation but could still climb 2 flights of stairs without shortness of breath. He had smoked half a pack of cigarettes a day between the ages 24 and 40. He denied cough, sputum production, or wheezing. He had recently become short of breath on a fishing trip at high altitude. At age 25 he was discharged from the Army because of a "cardiac murmur," but this was not noted on later examinations. There was no history of rheumatic fever or congestive heart failure. He took no medications. Physical examination was normal except for bilateral arcus senilis. Chest roentgenograms revealed bilateral pleural plaques and possible bibasilar interstitial disease.

EXERCISE FINDINGS

The patient performed exercise on a cycle ergometer. He pedalled at 60 rpm without added load for 3 minutes. The work rate was then increased 20 W per minute. Blood was sampled every second minute, and intra-arterial blood pressure was recorded from a percutaneously placed brachial artery catheter. Resting ECG showed deep Q waves in leads 2, 3, and AVF compatible with an old inferior infarction. During exercise, occasional single ventricular premature contractions were noted. At 120 watts the ST segments were depressed 2 mm in V4 through V6 and then 4 mm before exercise was stopped at 160 W. The ST segments became isoelectric within 5 minutes of recovery. Patient experienced leg fatigue but denied any chest pain or discomfort.

TABLE 21-1. *Selected Respiratory Function Data*

MEASUREMENT	PREDICTED	MEASURED
Age, yr		65
Sex		Male
Height, cm		174
Weight, kg	77	65
Hematocrit, %		45
VC, L	3.97	3.58
IC, L	2.64	2.24
TLC, L	6.21	6.68
FEV$_1$, L	3.09	2.60
FEV$_1$/VC, %	78	73
MVV, L/min	128	117
D$_{CO}$, ml/mm Hg/min	25.6	21.7

TABLE 21-2. *Selected Exercise Data*

MEASUREMENT	PREDICTED	MEASURED
Maximum V$_{O_2}$, L/min	1.88	1.41
Maximum HR, beats/min	155	176
Maximum O$_2$ pulse, ml/beat	12.1	8.0
ΔV$_{O_2}$/ΔWR, ml/min/W	10.3	7.3
AT, L/min	> 0.84	1.05
Blood pressure, mm Hg (rest, max)		189/108,234/126
Maximum V$_E$, L/min		74
Exercise breathing reserve, L/min	> 15	43
Pa$_{O_2}$, mm Hg (rest, max ex)		93,89
P(A − a)$_{O_2}$, mm Hg (rest, max ex)		15,35
P(a − ET)$_{CO_2}$, mm Hg (rest, max ex)		3,1
V$_D$/V$_T$ (rest, heavy ex)		0.32,0.37

FIG. 21-A.

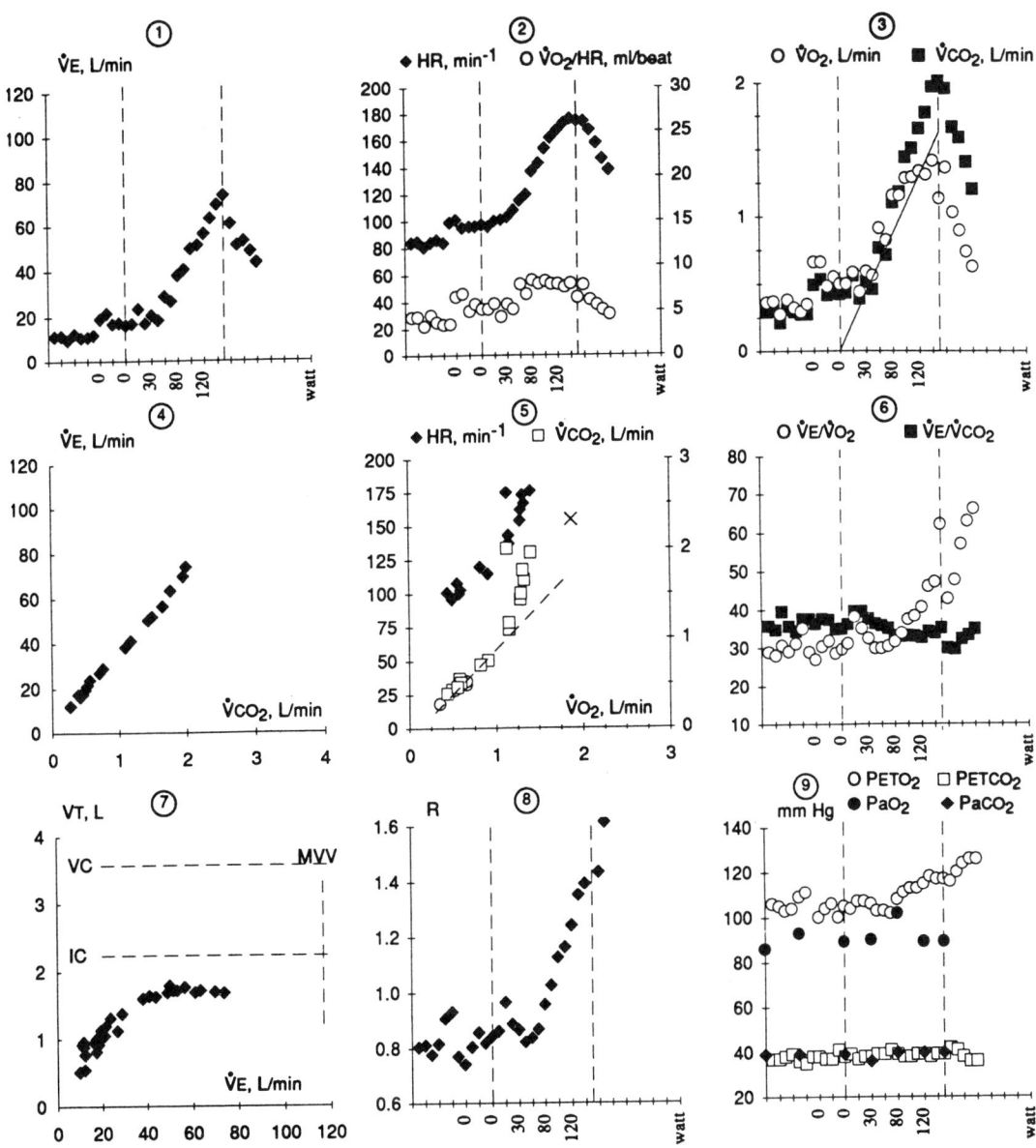

1. Vertical dashed lines in panels 1 to 3 and 6, 8, and 9 indicate the beginning and the end of increasing work period.

2. Unloaded cycling is performed for 3 minutes before the left vertical dashed line.

3. In panel 3, the diagonal line shows the increase of $\dot{V}O_2$ at a slope of 10 ml/min/W.

4. In panel 5, the diagonal dashed line has a slope of 1; the "x" in the upper right is the predicted maximum heart rate and $\dot{V}O_2$ for the subject.

Interpretation

COMMENTS

Results of the resting respiratory function studies are within normal limits (Table 21-1). The resting ECG is abnormal and suggests that the patient had an inferior wall myocardial infarction in the past.

ANALYSIS

In flow chart 1, the maximum $\dot{V}O_2$ is reduced but the anaerobic threshold is within normal limits (Table 21-2). See flow chart 3: The breathing reserve is high (branchpoint 3.1). The ECG became abnormal as the maximum work rate was approached (branchpoint 3.3). While the patient did

TABLE 21-3.

Time min	Work rate watts	BP mm Hg	HR min⁻¹	f min⁻¹	$\dot{V}E$ L/min BTPS	$\dot{V}CO_2$ L/min STPD	$\dot{V}O_2$ L/min STPD	$\dfrac{\dot{V}O_2}{HR}$ ml/beat	R	pH	HCO₃ meq/L	PO2, mm Hg ET	a	(A-a)	PCO2, mm Hg ET	a	(a-ET)	$\dfrac{\dot{V}E}{\dot{V}CO_2}$	$\dfrac{\dot{V}E}{\dot{V}O_2}$	$\dfrac{VD}{VT}$
	Rest	189/108								7.44	26		86			39				
	Rest		84	12	11.4	0.29	0.36	4.3	0.81			106			37			36	29	
	Rest		85	13	11.5	0.30	0.37	4.4	0.81			105			37			35	28	
	Rest		81	19	9.9	0.21	0.27	3.3	0.78			103			38			39	31	
	Rest		84	16	12.4	0.31	0.38	4.5	0.82			104			39			36	29	
	Rest	192/114	86	12	11.0	0.29	0.32	3.7	0.91	7.44	26	109	93	15	36	39	3	34	31	0.32
	Rest		84	12	11.2	0.27	0.29	3.5	0.93			111			35			38	35	
	Unloaded		99	22	12.0	0.27	0.35	3.5	0.77			193			38			38	29	
	Unloaded		101	17	19.2	0.49	0.66	6.5	0.74			100			38			36	27	
	Unloaded		95	18	21.5	0.53	0.66	6.9	0.80			104			37			38	30	
	Unloaded		96	18	16.8	0.41	0.48	5.0	0.85			106			37			37	32	
	Unloaded		96	19	17.3	0.45	0.55	5.7	0.82			100			41			35	29	
	Unloaded	213/120	97	17	16.2	0.42	0.50	5.2	0.84	7.43	25	105	89	16	38	39	1	35	30	0.34
0.5	20		96	17	17.0	0.43	0.50	5.2	0.86			104			39			36	31	
1.0	20		100	18	23.6	0.56	0.58	5.8	0.97			107			37			39	38	
1.5	30		101	21	17.2	0.39	0.44	4.4	0.89			107			38			40	35	
2.0	30	210/114	103	20	20.9	0.51	0.59	5.7	0.86	7.50	28	106	90	20	38	36	-2	38	33	0.33
2.5	60		108	20	18.4	0.46	0.56	5.2	0.82			103			39			36	30	
3.0	60		115	21	29.0	0.76	0.91	7.9	0.84			103			39			36	30	
3.5	80		120	24	26.9	0.71	0.82	6.8	0.87			102			41			35	30	
4.0	80	219/117	137	24	38.3	1.10	1.15	8.4	0.96	7.36	22	108	102	7	39	40	1	33	32	0.33
4.5	100		143	25	41.0	1.18	1.15	8.0	1.03			111			38			33	34	
5.0	100		154	28	50.1	1.44	1.28	8.3	1.13			113			38			33	37	
5.5	120		162	30	51.8	1.50	1.29	8.0	1.16			113			39			33	38	
6.0	120	234/126	167	32	56.6	1.65	1.33	8.0	1.24	7.35	22	115	89	27	39	40	1	33	41	0.32
6.5	140		173	37	63.5	1.77	1.31	7.6	1.35			118			38			34	46	
7.0	140		176	41	69.8	1.96	1.41	8.0	1.39			117			39			34	47	
7.5	160	234/126	175	44	73.9	2.00	1.13	6.5	1.77	7.35	22	117	89	35	39	40	1	35	62	0.37
	Recovery		174	36	61.1	1.95	1.36	7.8	1.43			116			42			30	43	
	Recovery		168	30	51.6	1.66	1.03	6.1	1.61			120			41			30	48	
	Recovery		158	31	53.3	1.58	0.89	5.6	1.78			124			38			32	57	
	Recovery	222/120	146	29	49.0	1.40	0.74	5.1	1.89			126			36			33	63	
	Recovery		138	27	44.0	1.20	0.63	4.6	1.90			126			36			35	66	

not experience chest pain, the diagnosis of myocardial ischemia is supported by the marked change in slope in $\dot{V}O_2$ in response to increasing work rate (panel 3, Fig. 21-A) and a reduced $\Delta\dot{V}O_2/\Delta WR$. The very marked increase in R starting at 80 W (Table 21-3 and panel 8, Fig. 21-A) reflects the development of a significant metabolic acidosis as the anaerobic threshold is exceeded. The steepening heart rate response with increasing oxygen uptake (panel 5, Fig. 21-A) and the failure of O_2 pulse to increase at a low work rate (panel 2, Fig. 21-A) reflect a low stroke volume and a maximal $C(a-\bar{v})_{O_2}$ being reached at a relatively low work rate.

This patient has significant systemic hypertension. We cannot therefore exclude the possibility that the myocardial ischemia and impaired cardiac function demonstrated here are due, in part, to abnormally increased myocardial work as well as coronary artery disease.

There is evidence of ventilation-perfusion mismatching (high VD/VT and positive $P(a-ET)_{CO_2}$). These abnormalities, despite normal resting respiratory function, give support to the diagnosis of interstitial lung disease, consistent with the radiologic finding.

CONCLUSION

Myocardial ischemia has limited exercise performance secondary to coronary artery disease and/or systemic hypertension. Interstitial lung disease is also present.

CASE 22 *Coronary artery disease and chronic bronchitis*

CLINICAL FINDINGS

This 65-year-old man had sustained an acute myocardial infarction 6 years ago. Since then he had required one to two nitroglycerin tablets per day and propranolol for "stable angina." He had had 30 years of asbestos exposure in the shipyards and had smoked 23 pack years of cigarettes. He could walk 2 to 3 miles before becoming dyspneic and admitted to a scantily productive morning cough. Resting ECG was normal. An exercise study was performed to evaluate the relative contributions of his pulmonary and cardiac illnesses.

EXERCISE FINDINGS

The patient performed exercise on a cycle ergometer. He pedalled at 60 rpm without added load for 3 minutes. The work rate was then increased 10 W per minute. Arterial blood was sampled every second minute, and intra-arterial blood pressure was recorded from a percutaneously placed brachial artery catheter. The incremental cycle exercise test was terminated at 70 W because of moderate substernal chest pain and the development of 3 mm of ST segment depression in leads 2, 3, and AVF, and occasional premature ventricular beats. These abnormalities resolved promptly after termination of exercise.

TABLE 22-1. *Selected Respiratory Function Data*

MEASUREMENT	PREDICTED	MEASURED
Age, yr		65
Sex		Male
Height, cm		167
Weight, kg	71	55
Hematocrit, %		41
VC, L	3.54	3.42
IC, L	2.36	1.81
TLC, L	5.57	6.16
FEV_1, L	2.75	2.33
FEV_1/VC, %	78	68
MVV, L/min	120	101
D_{LCO}, ml/mm Hg/min	22.6	26.4

TABLE 22-2. *Selected Exercise Data*

MEASUREMENT	PREDICTED	MEASURED
Maximum $\dot{V}O_2$, L/min	1.68	1.01
Maximum HR, beats/min	155	152
Maximum O_2 pulse, ml/beat	10.8	7.3
$\Delta\dot{V}O_2/\Delta WR$, ml/min/W	10.3	5.7
AT, L/min	> 0.74	0.9
Blood pressure, mm Hg (rest, max)		165/87,159/84
Maximum $\dot{V}E$, L/min		39
Exercise breathing reserve, L/min	> 15	62
PaO_2, mm Hg (rest, max ex)		94,95
$P(A-a)O_2$, mm Hg (rest, max ex)		13,18
$P(a-ET)CO_2$, mm Hg (rest, max ex)		4,2
V_D/V_T (rest, heavy ex)		0.40,0.29
HCO_3^-, mEq/L (rest, 2-min recov)		27,23

TABLE 22-3.

Time min	Work rate watts	BP mm Hg	HR min⁻¹	f min⁻¹	V̇E L/min BTPS	V̇CO2 L/min STPD	V̇O2 L/min STPD	V̇O2/HR ml/beat	R	pH	HCO3 meq/L	PO2, mm Hg			PCO2, mm Hg			V̇E/V̇CO2	V̇E/V̇O2	VD/VT
												ET	a	(A-a)	ET	a	(a-ET)			
	Rest	165/87								7.43	27		86			41				
	Rest		76	16	13.4	0.31	0.33	4.3	0.94			111			35			39	36	
	Rest		85	16	14.1	0.34	0.36	4.2	0.96			113			34			37	36	
	Rest		75	17	12.4	0.26	0.27	3.6	0.96			116			33			42	41	
	Rest	156/84	82	15	9.8	0.21	0.24	2.9	0.88	7.44	26	111	94	13	35	39	4	41	36	0.40
	Rest		84	16	9.6	0.17	0.21	2.5	0.81			110			36			48	39	
	Rest		86	15	9.2	0.17	0.20	2.3	0.85			112			34			47	40	
	Rest		84	17	12.9	0.28	0.33	3.9	0.85			111			34			41	35	
	Rest		84	17	12.8	0.28	0.31	3.7	0.90			114			33			41	37	
	Unloaded		97	19	17.5	0.40	0.52	5.4	0.77			104			39			40	31	
	Unloaded		105	22	20.3	0.52	0.73	7.0	0.71			92			39			35	25	
	Unloaded		106	24	20.4	0.55	0.71	6.7	0.77			101			38			33	26	
	Unloaded		105	23	20.6	0.55	0.65	6.2	0.85			105			37			34	29	
	Unloaded		99	24	18.8	0.50	0.61	6.2	0.82			104			39			34	27	
	Unloaded	162/84	103	23	21.1	0.58	0.68	6.6	0.85	7.44	26	107	92	14	37	39	2	33	28	0.30
0.5	10		101	27	17.4	0.44	0.50	5.0	0.88			104			39			34	30	
1.0	10		105	27	20.8	0.55	0.61	5.8	0.90			110			36			34	30	
1.5	20		109	23	24.3	0.67	0.75	6.9	0.89			106			39			33	30	
2.0	20	165/87	111	20	19.9	0.56	0.61	5.5	0.92	7.45	25	107	98	12	39	37	-2	33	30	0.26
2.5	30		117	26	28.4	0.78	0.88	7.5	0.89			105			38			34	30	
3.0	30		115	20	23.3	0.67	0.70	6.1	0.96			112			36			32	31	
3.5	40		119	23	26.0	0.75	0.82	6.9	0.91			110			37			32	29	
4.0	40	156/84	121	23	27.9	0.81	0.88	7.3	0.92	7.44	25	110	94	15	36	38	2	32	29	0.27
4.5	50		127	25	29.5	0.84	0.89	7.0	0.94			112			36			33	31	
5.0	50		135	30	25.7	0.73	0.80	5.9	0.91			101			44			32	29	
5.5	60	162/84	136	27	35.9	0.99	0.98	7.2	1.01	7.44	25	114	95	18	35	37	2	34	34	0.29
6.0	60		152	28	36.2	0.96	0.92	6.1	1.04			116			34			35	37	
6.5	70	159/84	138	30	38.9	1.03	1.01	7.3	1.02			116			34			35	36	
	Recovery		134	30	36.3	1.00	1.02	7.6	0.98			112			36			34	33	
	Recovery		121	34	38.5	1.01	0.97	8.0	1.04			114			36			35	37	
	Recovery	162/84	113	27	31.7	0.86	0.82	7.3	1.05	7.43	23	114	101	14	36	36	0	34	36	0.28
	Recovery		106	28	27.5	0.71	0.65	6.1	1.09			117			35			35	39	

Interpretation

COMMENTS

The resting respiratory function studies indicate that the patient has mild airflow obstruction (Table 22-1). The resting ECG is normal.

ANALYSIS

In flow chart 1, the maximum V̇O2 is reduced and the anaerobic threshold is normal (Table 22-2). See flow chart 3: The breathing reserve is high (branchpoint 3.1), while the exercise ECG (branchpoint 3.3) was clearly abnormal. The chest pain, low $\Delta\dot{V}O_2/\Delta WR$ and low O_2 pulse that fails to rise during exercise all add support to the primary diagnosis of myocardial ischemia. The high breathing reserve and normal indices of ventilation-perfusion matching clearly suggest that the lungs and pulmonary circulation are functioning normally. In contrast, the cardiovascular response to exercise is abnormal.

CONCLUSION

Coronary artery disease has limited exercise performance in a patient with mild airflow obstruction.

Fig. 22-A.

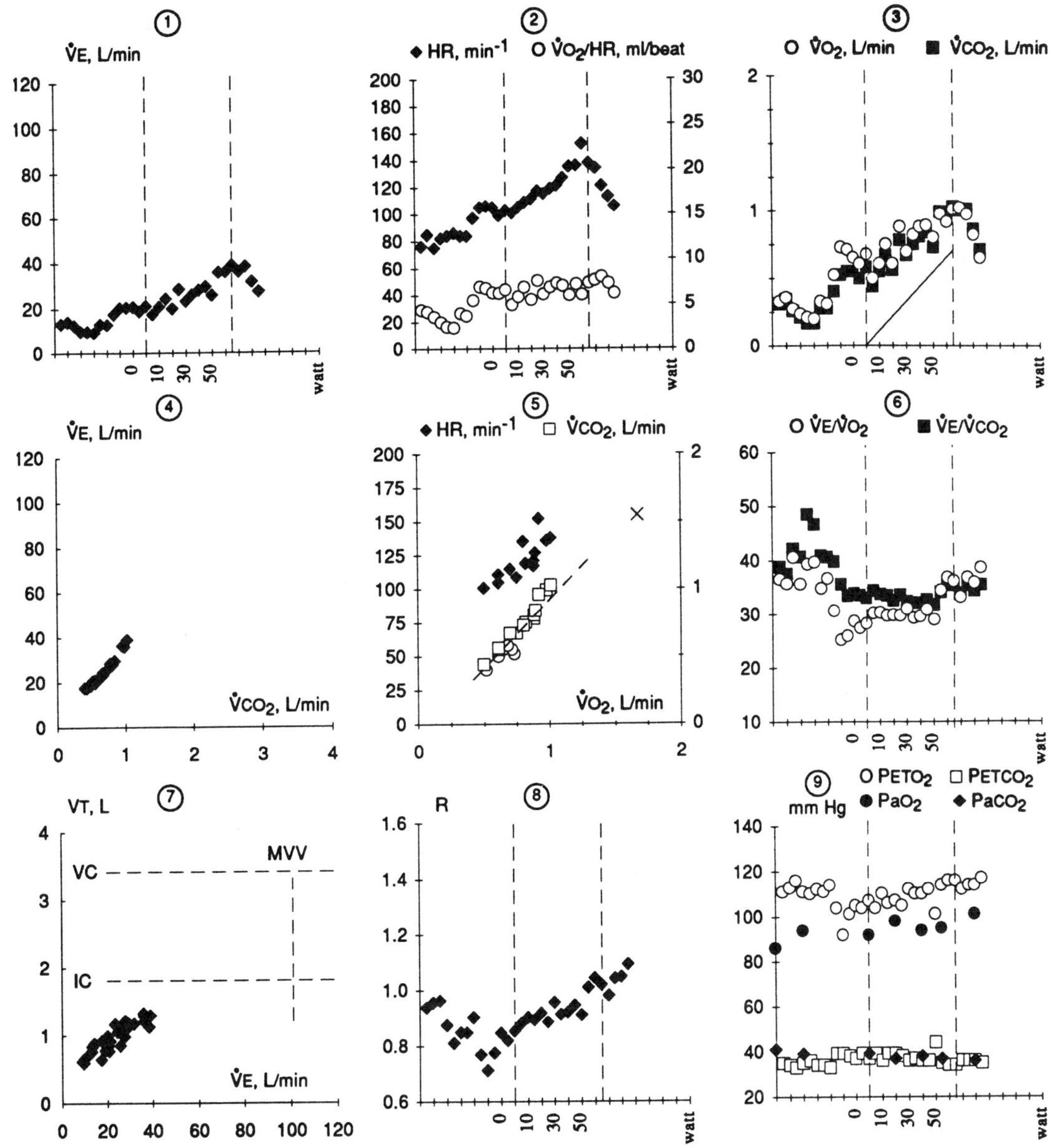

1. Vertical dashed lines in panels 1 to 3 and 6, 8, and 9 indicate the beginning and the end of increasing work period.

2. Unloaded cycling is performed for 3 minutes before the left vertical dashed line.

3. In panel 3, the diagonal line shows the increase of $\dot{V}O_2$ at a slope of 10 ml/min/W.

4. In panel 5, the diagonal dashed line has a slope of 1; the "x" in the upper right is the predicted maximum heart rate and $\dot{V}O_2$ for the subject.

CASE 23 *Cardiomyopathy*

CLINICAL FINDINGS

This 41-year-old former brickworker, woodworker, sandblaster, and security guard had been placed on disability for a back injury 9 years ago. Hypertension had been diagnosed 6 years ago. He had started complaining of dyspnea and a productive cough 3 years ago. He had been diagnosed as having "probable pulmonary asbestosis" and "asthmatic bronchitis" 2 years ago. He denied smoking but had had repeated hospitalizations for alcoholism. He was being treated with propranolol, hydrochlorothiazide, oxtriphylline, and potassium supplementation. Auscultation of the heart and lungs was entirely normal, as were posteroanterior, lateral, and oblique chest roentgenograms.

EXERCISE FINDINGS

The patient performed exercise on a cycle ergometer. He pedalled at 60 rpm without added load for 3 minutes. The work rate was then increased 20 W per minute to his symptom limited maximum. Arterial blood was sampled every second minute, and intra-arterial blood pressure was recorded from a percutaneously placed brachial artery catheter. Resting ECG was normal. He stopped exercise with complaints of shortness of breath, a feeling that he was "going to faint," and leg "tiredness." One interpolated ventricular contraction occurred during exercise, but exercise and recovery ECG were otherwise normal.

TABLE 23-1. *Selected Respiratory Function Data*

MEASUREMENT	PREDICTED	MEASURED
Age, yr		41
Sex		Male
Height, cm		170
Weight, kg	74	78
Hematocrit, %		44
VC, L	3.95	4.00
IC, L	2.63	3.30
TLC, L	5.58	5.28
FEV_1, L	3.16	3.43
FEV_1/VC, %	80	86
MVV, L/min	137	118
D_{LCO}, ml/mm Hg/min	25.8	24.7

TABLE 23-2. *Selected Exercise Data*

MEASUREMENT	PREDICTED	MEASURED
Maximum $\dot{V}O_2$, L/min	2.64	1.75
Maximum HR, beats/min	179	150
Maximum O_2 pulse, ml/beat	14.7	11.7
$\Delta\dot{V}O_2/\Delta WR$, ml/min/W	10.3	8.3
AT, L/min	> 1.11	0.85
Blood pressure, mm Hg (rest, max)		132/87,204/108
Maximum $\dot{V}E$, L/min		78
Exercise breathing reserve, L/min	> 15	40
Pa_{O_2}, mm Hg (rest, max ex)		87,117
$P(A-a)_{O_2}$, mm Hg (rest, max ex)		4,3
$P(a-ET)_{CO_2}$, mm Hg (rest, max ex)		2,−2
V_D/V_T (rest, heavy ex)		0.36,0.23
HCO_3^-, mEq/L (rest, 2-min recov)		27,18

Fig. 23-A.

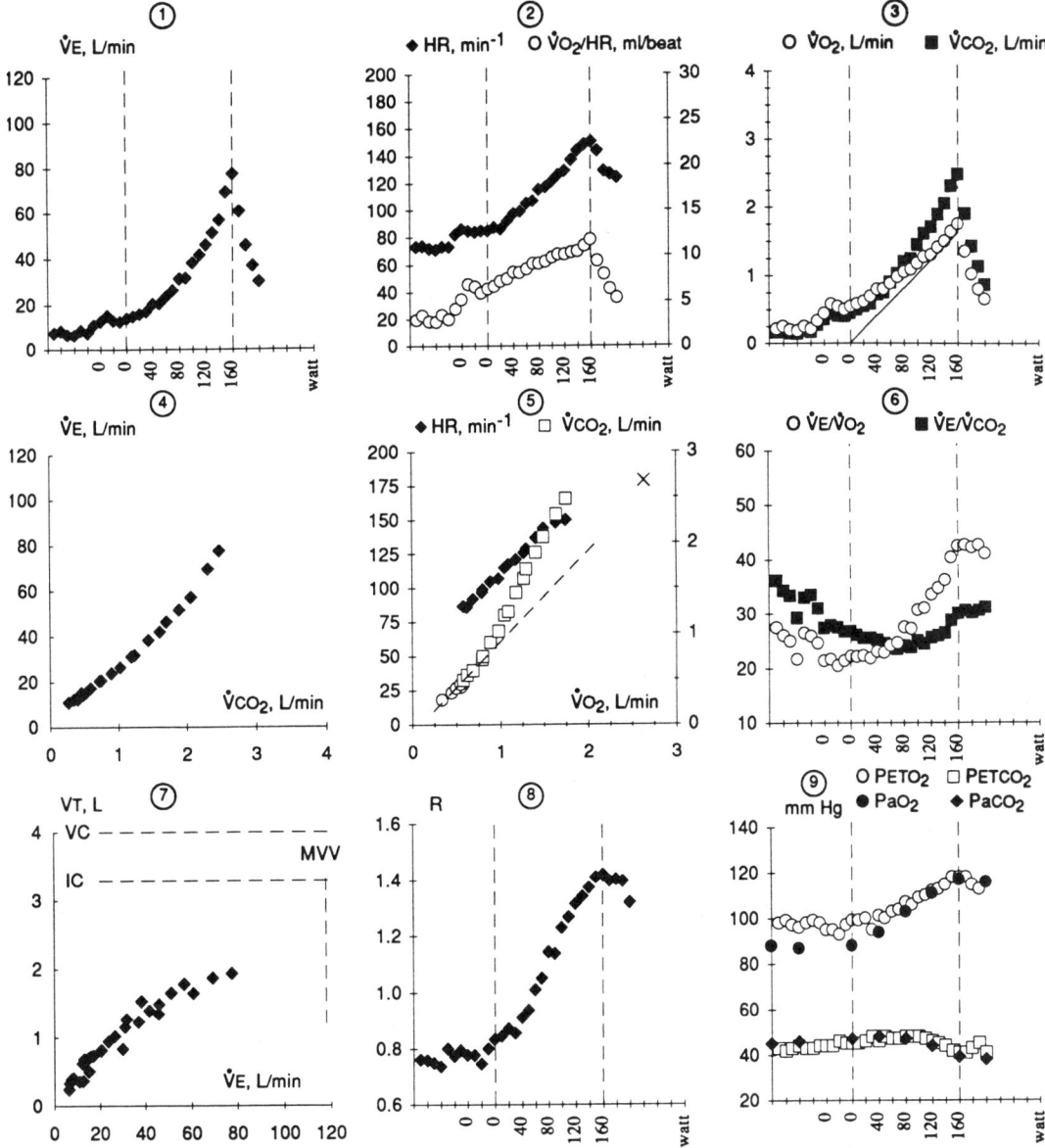

1. Vertical dashed lines in panels 1 to 3 and 6, 8, and 9 indicate the beginning and the end of increasing work period.

2. Unloaded cycling is performed for 3 minutes before the left vertical dashed line.

3. In panel 3, the diagonal line shows the increase of $\dot{V}O_2$ at a slope of 10 ml/min/W.

4. In panel 5, the diagonal dashed line has a slope of 1; the "x" in the upper right is the predicted maximum heart rate and $\dot{V}O_2$ for the subject.

TABLE 23-3.

Time min	Work rate watts	BP mm Hg	HR min^{-1}	f min^{-1}	$\dot{V}E$ L/min BTPS	$\dot{V}CO_2$ L/min STPD	$\dot{V}O_2$ L/min STPD	$\dfrac{\dot{V}O_2}{HR}$ ml/beat	R	pH	HCO$_3$ meq/L	PO2 ET	PO2 a	PO2 (A-a)	PCO2 ET	PCO2 a	PCO2 (a-ET)	$\dfrac{\dot{V}E}{\dot{V}CO_2}$	$\dfrac{\dot{V}E}{\dot{V}O_2}$	$\dfrac{VD}{VT}$
	Rest	132/87								7.39	27		88			45				
	Rest		73	19	7.4	0.16	0.21	2.9	0.76			98			43			36	28	
	Rest		74	21	8.3	0.19	0.25	3.4	0.76			99			42			34	26	
	Rest		72	20	6.7	0.15	0.20	2.8	0.75			97			43			33	25	
	Rest	126/84	71	17	6.4	0.14	0.19	2.7	0.74	7.39	27	96	87	4	44	46	2	35	26	0.36
	Rest		73	21	8.4	0.20	0.25	3.4	0.80			98			43			33	26	
	Rest		73	20	7.4	0.17	0.22	3.0	0.77			99			43			34	26	
	Unloaded		82	31	11.0	0.27	0.34	4.1	0.79			98			44			31	25	
	Unloaded		86	34	12.5	0.35	0.45	5.2	0.78			95			44			27	21	
	Unloaded		85	30	15.1	0.45	0.58	6.8	0.78			95			44			28	22	
	Unloaded		84	19	12.9	0.41	0.55	6.5	0.75			93			46			28	21	
	Unloaded		85	20	12.4	0.40	0.50	5.9	0.80			97			45			27	21	
	Unloaded	138/84	85	21	13.8	0.45	0.54	6.4	0.83	7.37	27	99	88	8	45	47	2	27	22	0.27
0.5	20		87	21	14.6	0.49	0.58	6.7	0.84			99			45			26	22	
1.0	20		86	22	15.7	0.54	0.62	7.2	0.87			100			46			26	22	
1.5	40		92	23	17.0	0.59	0.69	7.5	0.86			95			48			26	22	
2.0	40	147/90	97	25	20.3	0.72	0.79	8.1	0.91	7.38	28	101	94	4	46	48	2	25	23	0.26
2.5	60		99	25	20.5	0.75	0.80	8.1	0.94			100			48			25	23	
3.0	60		105	25	23.6	0.90	0.89	8.5	1.01			103			47			24	24	
3.5	80		107	26	26.4	1.03	0.98	9.2	1.05			104			47			23	25	
4.0	80	159/90	115	27	31.2	1.20	1.05	9.1	1.14	7.36	26	107	103	5	48	47	-1	24	28	0.22
4.5	100		117	25	31.7	1.24	1.09	9.3	1.14			106			48			24	27	
5.0	100		121	25	38.3	1.45	1.18	9.8	1.23			109			48			25	31	
5.5	120		126	30	41.9	1.61	1.27	10.1	1.27			110			47			24	31	
6.0	120	192/105	129	31	46.2	1.71	1.30	10.1	1.32	7.35	24	112	111	3	46	44	-2	25	34	0.22
6.5	140		137	31	51.5	1.89	1.41	10.3	1.34			113			45			26	35	
7.0	140		144	32	57.0	2.06	1.50	10.4	1.37			115			44			26	36	
7.5	160		148	37	69.3	2.31	1.64	11.1	1.41			118			42			29	40	
8.0	160	204/108	150	40	77.6	2.48	1.75	11.7	1.42	7.34	21	118	117	3	41	39	-2	30	42	0.25
	Recovery		144	37	61.0	1.90	1.36	9.4	1.40			118			41			30	43	
	Recovery		129	34	45.8	1.43	1.02	7.9	1.40			115			43			30	42	
	Recovery		127	30	37.0	1.13	0.81	6.4	1.40			113			45			30	43	
	Recovery	150/78	124	36	30.1	0.87	0.66	5.3	1.32	7.28	18	116	116	3	41	38	-3	31	41	0.24

Interpretation

COMMENTS

Resting pulmonary function (Table 23-1) and ECG are normal.

ANALYSIS

In flow chart 1, the maximum $\dot{V}O_2$ and anaerobic threshold are reduced (Table 23-2). See flow chart 4: The ventilatory equivalent at the anaerobic threshold (branchpoint 4.3) and the indices of ventilation-perfusion matching are normal. These findings indicate that this patient does not have primary lung or pulmonary vascular disease, but does have a nonlung disease O_2 flow problem. Because the hematocrit is normal (branchpoint 4.4), this is most likely due to cardiovascular disease. The exercise ECG is essentially normal throughout exercise. His $\Delta\dot{V}O_2/\Delta WR$ is low and he has a low but rising O_2 pulse at maximum work rate (panel 2 of Fig. 23-A). The patient's blood pressure response to exercise and heart rate reserve are normal (Table 23-2), and the patient did not have leg pain with exercise, making peripheral vascular disease unlikely. Because propranolol, itself, one of this patient's medications, ordinarily gives a high O_2 pulse during exercise, the finding of a low O_2 pulse at maximum exercise supports the diagnosis of primary heart disease. (Pulmonary vascular disease is already ruled out.)

CONCLUSION

This patient is a 41-year-old chronic alcoholic with cardiovascular limitation. Pulmonary vascular, peripheral vascular, and coronary artery disease were shown to be unlikely causes of the limitation. Two-dimensional echocardiography with exercise supported the diagnosis of cardiomyopathy.

CASE 24 *Cardiomyopathy, hypertrophic type*

CLINICAL FINDINGS

This 65-year-old female real estate broker was referred for evaluation of exertional dyspnea of 1 year's duration. She noted dyspnea without chest pain when walking half a block on the level or climbing less than one flight of stairs. She denied asthma but had smoked cigarettes until 6 years previously. She had been treated 2 decades ago for hyperthyroidism. Work-up elsewhere revealed mild airway obstruction, hypertension, and normal thyroid status. Cardiac catheterization showed 40% stenosis of one coronary artery; echocardiogram was interpreted as normal; and a wall motion study showed a left ventricular ejection fraction of 72%, decreasing slightly during exercise. Medications were clonidine, triamterene, and hydrochlorothiazide. Examination was normal except for systemic hypertension, mild obesity, and a variable systolic murmur at the third left interspace near the sternum. Resting ECG showed left ventricular hypertrophy.

EXERCISE FINDINGS

The patient performed cycle ergometer exercise on two occasions. During the first study, the murmur was loud, her O_2 pulse decreased as exercise progressed, and she was more hypertensive and became symptomatic with minimal exercise. Two weeks later she returned for the second study shortly after taking clonidine. She had less hypertension and a barely audible systolic murmur. She pedalled at 60 rpm without added load for 3 minutes. The work rate was then increased 10 W per minute to her symptom-limited maximum. Arterial blood was sampled every second minute, and intra-arterial blood pressure recorded from a percutaneously placed brachial artery catheter. The patient stopped exercise because of overall fatigue and shortness of breath. Less than 1 mm of downsloping ST segment depression developed in leads 1, AVL, and V6, while an increasing number of atrial and ventricular premature contractions developed near the end of exercise. A recording of brachial artery pressure is shown.

TABLE 24-1. *Selected Respiratory Function Data*

MEASUREMENT	PREDICTED	MEASURED
Age, yr		65
Sex		Female
Height, cm		164
Weight, kg	64	69
Hematocrit, %		40
VC, L	2.86	2.78
IC, L	1.91	2.30
TLC, L	4.93	5.45
FEV_1, L	2.26	1.88
FEV_1/VC, %	79	67
MVV, L/min	85	67
DL_{CO}, ml/mm Hg/min	21.0	19.3

TABLE 24-2. *Selected Exercise Data*

MEASUREMENT	PREDICTED	FIRST STUDY	SECOND STUDY
Maximum $\dot{V}O_2$, L/min	1.28	0.88	1.15
Maximum HR, beats/min	155	142	148
Maximum O_2 pulse, ml/beat	8.3	5.8	7.8
$\Delta\dot{V}O_2/\Delta WR$, ml/min/W	10.3		6.3
AT, L/min	> 0.63	indeterminate	1.0
Blood pressure, mm Hg (rest, max)		168/80,243/102	159/69,240/79
Maximum $\dot{V}E$, L/min		54	65
Exercise breathing reserve, L/min	> 15	13	2
Pa_{O_2}, mm Hg (rest, max ex)			84,109
$P(A-a)_{O_2}$, mm Hg (rest, max ex)			20,16
$P(a-ET)_{CO_2}$, mm Hg (rest, max ex)			5,2
VD/VT (rest, heavy ex)			0.35,0.32
HCO_3^-, mEq/L (rest, 2-min recov)			26,22

Fig. 24-A. *Second study.*

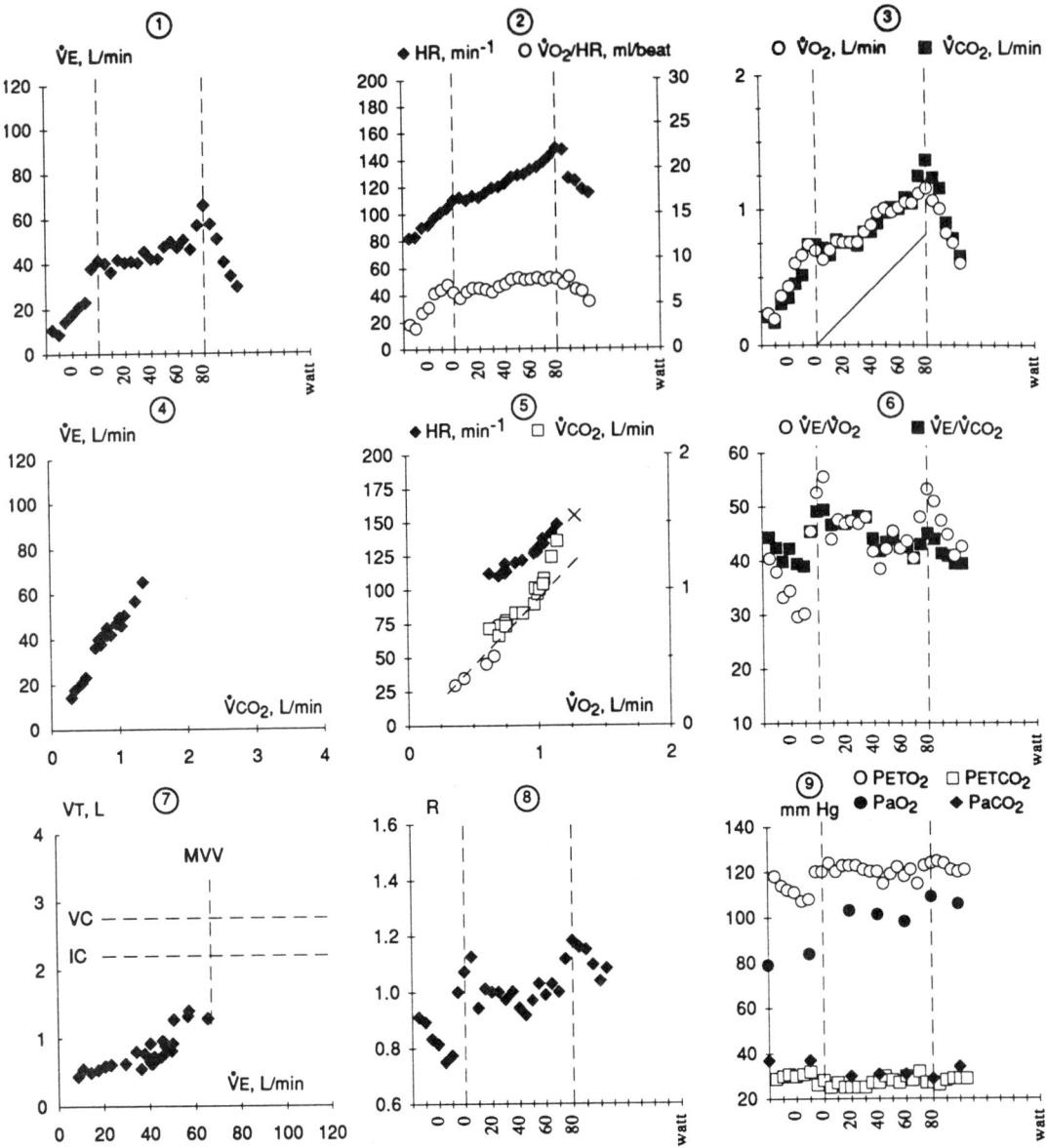

1. Vertical dashed lines in panels 1 to 3 and 6, 8, and 9 indicate the beginning and the end of increasing work period.

2. Unloaded cycling is performed for 3 minutes before the left vertical dashed line.

3. In panel 3, the diagonal line shows the increase of $\dot{V}O_2$ at a slope of 10 ml/min/W.

4. In panel 5, the diagonal dashed line has a slope of 1; the "x" in the upper right is the predicted maximum heart rate and $\dot{V}O_2$ for the subject.

TABLE 24-3. *Second study.*

Time min	Work rate watts	BP mm Hg	HR min⁻¹	f min⁻¹	$\dot{V}E$ L/min BTPS	$\dot{V}CO_2$ L/min STPD	$\dot{V}O_2$ L/min STPD	$\dfrac{\dot{V}O_2}{HR}$ ml/beat	R	pH	HCO₃ meq/L	PO2, mm Hg ET	a	(A-a)	PCO2, mm Hg ET	a	(a-ET)	$\dfrac{\dot{V}E}{\dot{V}CO_2}$	$\dfrac{\dot{V}E}{\dot{V}O_2}$	VD VT
	Rest	159/69								7.46	26		79			37				
	Rest		82	20	11.0	0.21	0.23	2.8	0.91			118			29			44	40	
	Rest		83	20	8.9	0.17	0.19	2.3	0.89			114			30			42	38	
	Unloaded		90	29	14.4	0.30	0.36	4.0	0.83			112			31			40	33	
	Unloaded		92	33	17.6	0.35	0.43	4.7	0.81			111			30			42	34	
	Unloaded		97	35	20.7	0.45	0.60	6.2	0.75			107			31			39	30	
	Unloaded	184/75	101	38	23.1	0.51	0.66	6.5	0.77	7.47	26	108	84	20	32	37	5	39	30	0.35
	Unloaded		104	49	37.8	0.74	0.74	7.1	1.00			120			26			45	45	
	Unloaded		110	58	41.2	0.74	0.69	6.3	1.07			120			28			49	53	
0.5	10		112	60	40.1	0.71	0.63	5.6	1.13			124			25			49	56	
1.0	10		110	66	36.3	0.66	0.70	6.4	0.94			120			27			47	44	
1.5	20		113	66	41.7	0.77	0.76	6.7	1.01			123			25			47	47	
2.0	20	201/90	112	63	40.4	0.75	0.75	6.7	1.00	7.52	24	123	103	17	25	30	5	47	47	0.33
2.5	30		115	65	40.9	0.75	0.75	6.5	1.00			123			25			47	47	
3.0	30		119	62	40.4	0.73	0.75	6.3	0.97			121			25			48	47	
3.5	40		120	63	45.1	0.83	0.83	6.9	1.00			120			27			48	48	
4.0	40	193/73	122	64	42.0	0.83	0.88	7.2	0.94	7.51	24	120	101	17	27	31	4	44	42	0.32
4.5	50		127	58	42.1	0.89	0.97	7.6	0.92			115			30			42	38	
5.0	50		128	60	47.1	0.97	1.00	7.8	0.97			119			28			43	42	
5.5	60		129	61	49.7	1.01	0.98	7.6	1.03			122			27			44	45	
6.0	60	220/73	132	53	47.0	1.00	1.01	7.7	0.99	7.49	23	118	98	21	30	31	1	42	42	0.31
6.5	70		134	55	50.4	1.08	1.05	7.8	1.03			121			28			42	44	
7.0	70		138	48	46.0	1.04	1.04	7.5	1.00			115			32			40	40	
7.5	80		142	43	56.8	1.24	1.11	7.8	1.12			123			27			43	48	
8.0	80	240/79	148	51	65.5	1.36	1.15	7.8	1.18	7.49	22	124	109	16	27	29	2	45	53	0.32
	Recovery		147	41	57.4	1.23	1.06	7.2	1.16			125			26			44	51	
	Recovery		126	40	50.8	1.15	1.00	7.9	1.15			124			28			41	47	
	Recovery		124	44	40.4	0.90	0.82	6.6	1.10			121			29			41	45	
	Recovery	261/92	118	43	34.3	0.78	0.75	6.4	1.04	7.42	22	120	106	11	29	34	5	39	41	0.32
	Recovery		115	47	29.5	0.65	0.60	5.2	1.08			121			29			39	43	

Interpretation

COMMENTS

The results of the resting respiratory function studies are compatible with mild airflow obstruction. A resting ECG is normal except for left ventricular hypertrophy. Her left ventricular ejection fraction at rest is 72%.

ANALYSIS

In flow chart 1, in the first study the maximum $\dot{V}O_2$ is reduced and the anaerobic threshold is indeterminate. In the second study, the maximum $\dot{V}O_2$ and anaerobic threshold are normal (Table 24-2). If we use flow chart 2 and proceed, because of the abnormal blood gases, to the right sides of branchpoint 2.1 and branchpoint 2.3 we arrive at the diagnoses of "lung or pulmonary vascular disease." Because the cardiovascular abnormalities are more striking than the evidence for ventilation-perfusion mismatching or for obstructive lung disease, we should refer to flow chart 5. Addressing the question of branchpoint 5.1, VD/VT, and $P(a-ET)_{CO_2}$ are mildly abnormal, but $P(A-a)_{O_2}$ is normal (Tables 24-2 and 24-3). Taking the abnormal branch of branchpoint 5.1, we address the question of the breathing reserve (branchpoint 5.3). In this patient it is slightly reduced, in part because of her lung disease and, to a greater degree, to the hyperventilation that she develops during exercise. Because of the normal heart rate reserve and the absence of respiratory acidosis at maximal exercise, we must examine the other side of branchpoint 5.1.

In this study the prominent disorders are a low $\Delta\dot{V}O_2/\Delta WR$ and a low O_2 pulse that fails to increase with increasing work rate (Table 24-2 and panel 2 of Fig. 24-A). Therefore, it seems more likely that this patient has a cardiovascular defect. Taking the left sides of branchpoint 5.1, 5.2, and 5.4, we should conclude that this patient has heart

FIG. 24-B. *Four tracings of ECG (upper) and brachial artery blood pressure (lower) during and immediately after cycle ergometer exercise: (1) unloaded pedalling; (2) 30 W; (3) 80 W; and (4) early recovery. Each tracing is 4 seconds in duration. Note premature contractions at unloaded pedalling and early recovery and their effect on the contour of the following pulse.*

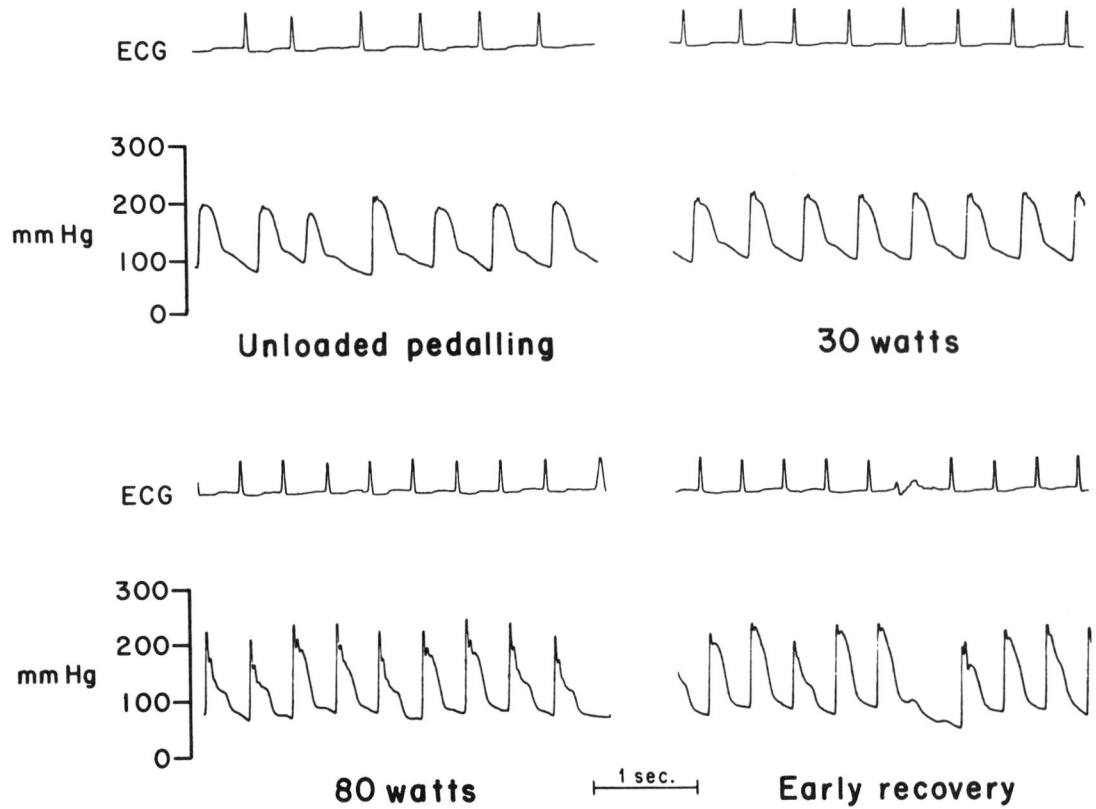

disease limiting her exercise performance. To support this diagnosis are the observations that the $\dot{V}O_2$ does not rise normally in response to increasing work rate (panel 3, Fig. 24-A), the O_2 pulse is flat (panel 2, Fig. 24-A), and her heart rate becomes steeper with increasing $\dot{V}O_2$ (panel 5, Fig. 24-A). During her more symptomatic test (not shown here), not only was her limitation greater, but her O_2 pulse actually decreased with increasing work rate.

The directly recorded arterial pressures are unusual and provide a clue to her cardiac diagnosis. The upstrokes in arterial pressure during systole are steep and abruptly stop increasing. Thus, the pressure wave takes on a spike and dome pattern. This pattern becomes more prominent with increasing work rate and remains so during early recovery (Fig. 24-B), characteristic of idiopathic hypertrophic cardiomyopathy. Premature ventricular contractions in recovery were followed by heart beats with a reduced, rather than increased, systolic and pulse pressure, a finding also characteristic of this disorder.

CONCLUSION

Idiopathic hypertrophic cardiomyopathy has limited exercise performance.

CASE 25 *Congestive heart failure: Before and after therapy*

CLINICAL FINDINGS

This 64-year-old retired man had recurrent episodic shortness of breath for 11 years, initially diagnosed as "asthma," and hypertension. He had recently been hospitalized repeatedly for congestive heart failure without evidence of prior myocardial infarction or valvular heart disease. He had been a cigarette smoker and was being treated with digoxin, furosemide, hydralazine, KCl, prednisone, ranitidine, occasional albuterol, and diazepam. Examination revealed a heavy-set man without peripheral edema, an increased posterior-anterior chest diameter, and decreased breath sounds without rales or rhonchi. Chest roentgenograms showed cardiomegaly and Kerley B lines; resting ECG showed left atrial enlargement and probable left ventricular hypertrophy. Exercise studies were performed after stabilization and every several weeks during 3 months of a drug study. The patient had progressive improvement; the first and final exercise tests of this period are presented.

EXERCISE FINDINGS

On both occasions, the patient performed exercise on a cycle ergometer. He pedalled at 60 rpm without an added load for 3 minutes. The work rate was then increased in a ramp fashion 10 W per minute to tolerance. Blood pressure was measured with a sphygmomanometer. On both occasions, the patient was well motivated and cooperative and stopped exercise because of generalized fatigue. The patient had no chest pain, arrhythmia, or abnormal ST-T wave changes.

TABLE 25-1. *Selected Respiratory Function Data*

MEASUREMENT	PREDICTED	MEASURED
Age, yr		64
Sex		Male
Height, cm		170
Weight, kg	73	82
VC, L	3.65	2.70 (2.80*)
IC, L	2.43	1.92
TLC, L	5.95	4.33
FEV_1, L	2.92	2.01 (2.30*)
FEV_1/VC, %	80	74
MVV, L/min, indirect	117	80 (92*)
DL_{CO}, ml/mm Hg/min	23.4	22
Hematocrit		44

* After 4 breaths of aerosolized albuterol.

TABLE 25-2. *Selected Exercise Data*

MEASUREMENT	PREDICTED	FIRST STUDY	FINAL STUDY
Maximum $\dot{V}O_2$, L/min	2.03	0.91	1.34
Maximum HR, beats/min	156	131	160
Maximum O_2 pulse, ml/beat	13.0	7.0	9.0
$\Delta\dot{V}O_2/\Delta WR$, ml/min/W	10.3	8.0	9.2
AT, L/min	> 0.89	0.6	1.0
Blood pressure, mm Hg (rest, max ex)		112/95,139/88	139/88,204/104
Maximum $\dot{V}E$, L/min		44	55
Exercise breathing reserve, L/min	> 15	36	25

FIG. 25-A. *First study.*

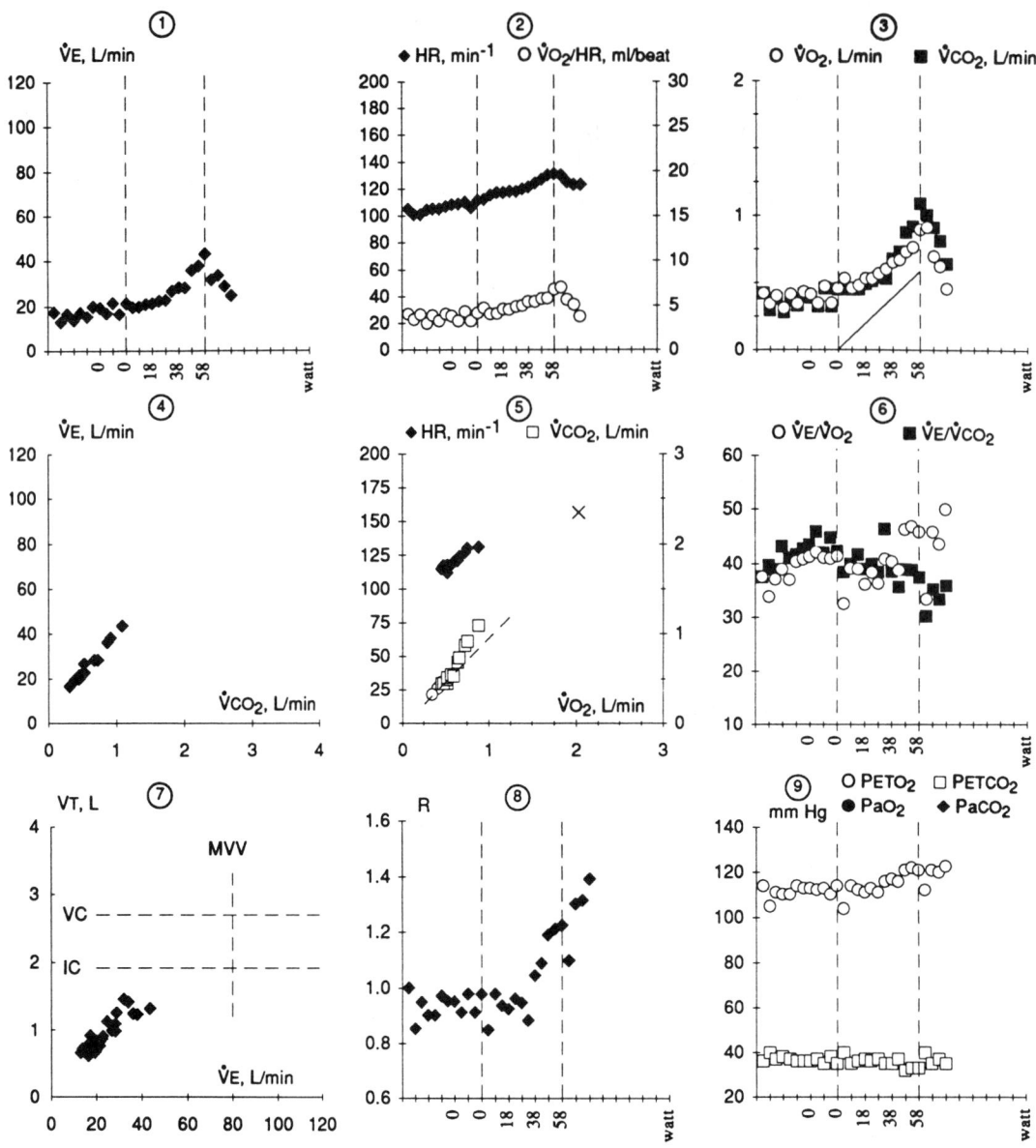

1. Vertical dashed lines in panels 1 to 3 and 6, 8, and 9 indicate the beginning and the end of increasing work period.
2. Unloaded cycling is performed for 3 minutes before the left vertical dashed line.
3. In panel 3, the diagonal line shows the increase of $\dot{V}O_2$ at a slope of 10 ml/min/W.
4. In panel 5, the diagonal dashed line has a slope of 1; the "x" in the upper right is the predicted maximum heart rate and $\dot{V}O_2$ for the subject.

Fɪɢ. 25-B. *First study.*

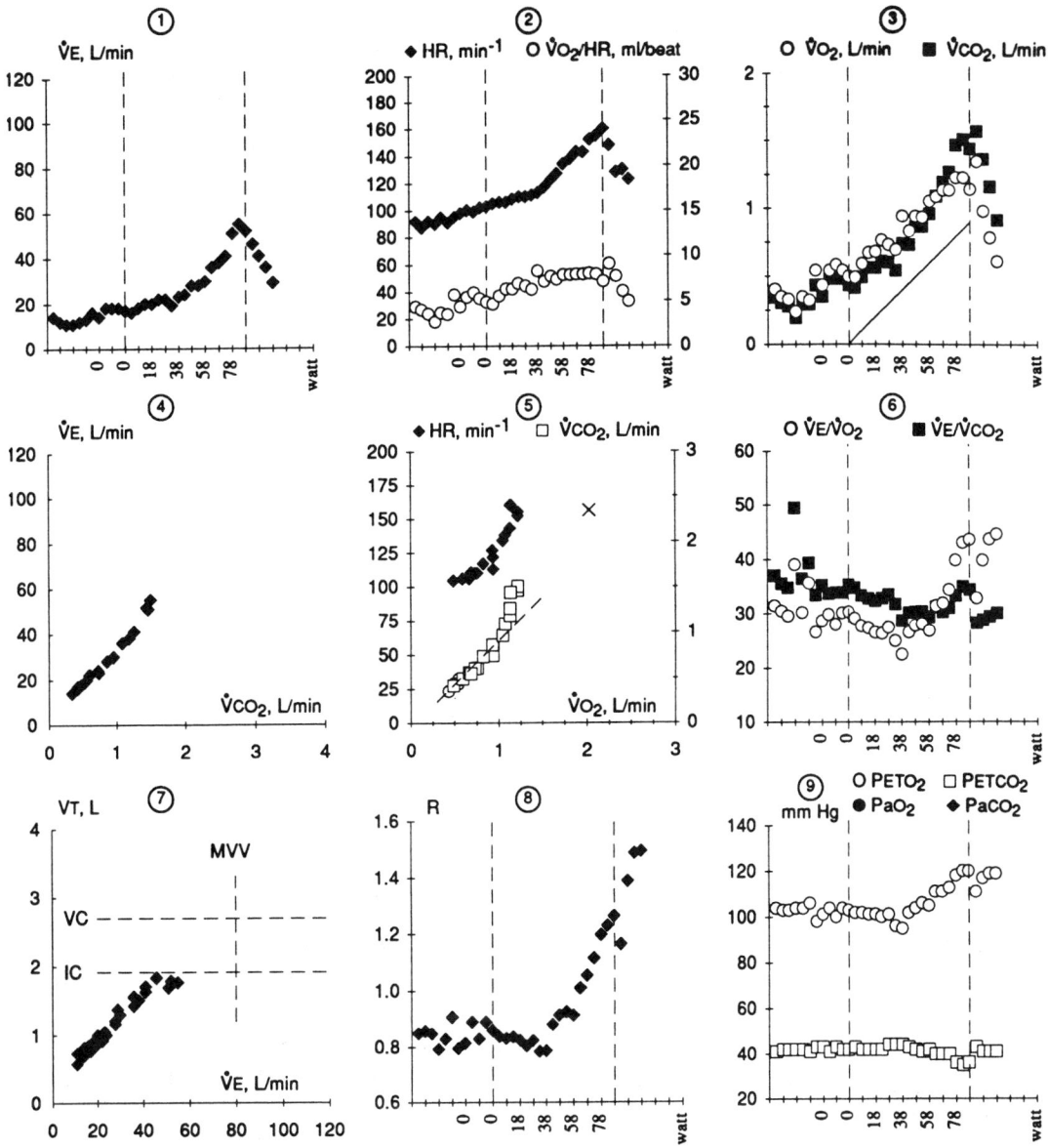

1. Vertical dashed lines in panels 1 to 3 and 6, 8, and 9 indicate the beginning and the end of increasing work period.

2. Unloaded cycling is performed for 3 minutes before the left vertical dashed line.

3. In panel 3, the diagonal line shows the increase of $\dot{V}O_2$ at a slope of 10 ml/min/W.

4. In panel 5, the diagonal dashed line has a slope of 1; the "x" in the upper right is the predicted maximum heart rate and $\dot{V}O_2$ for the subject.

Table 25-3. *First study.*

Time min	Work rate watts	BP mm Hg	HR min⁻¹	f min⁻¹	V̇E L/min BTPS	V̇CO2 L/min STPD	V̇O2 L/min STPD	V̇O2/HR ml/beat	R	pH	HCO3 meq/L	PO2, mm Hg ET	a	(A-a)	PCO2, mm Hg ET	a	(a-ET)	V̇E/V̇CO2	V̇E/V̇O2	VD/VT
	Rest	112/95	105	19	17.4	0.42	0.42	4.0	1.00			114			36			38	38	
	Rest		101	20	13.2	0.29	0.34	3.4	0.85			105			40			40	34	
	Rest		101	21	16.6	0.38	0.40	4.0	0.95			111			37			39	37	
	Rest		104	19	13.7	0.28	0.31	3.0	0.90			110			38			43	39	
	Rest		105	24	17.2	0.37	0.41	3.9	0.90			110			37			41	37	
	Rest		105	22	15.6	0.33	0.34	3.2	0.97			114			36			42	40	
	Unloaded		107	28	19.9	0.41	0.43	4.0	0.95			113			36			43	41	
	Unloaded		108	29	19.4	0.39	0.41	3.8	0.95			113			36			43	41	
	Unloaded		109	26	16.9	0.32	0.35	3.2	0.91			112			37			46	42	
	Unloaded		110	26	21.5	0.46	0.47	4.3	0.98			113			35			42	41	
	Unloaded		106	27	16.6	0.32	0.35	3.3	0.91			110			38			45	41	
	Unloaded		111	28	21.4	0.45	0.46	4.1	0.98			114			35			42	41	
0.5	3		112	29	19.7	0.45	0.53	4.7	0.85			104			40			38	33	
1.0	8		115	24	20.0	0.45	0.46	4.0	0.98			114			35			40	39	
1.5	13		117	28	21.1	0.45	0.48	4.1	0.94			112			36			42	39	
2.0	18		117	25	21.2	0.49	0.53	4.5	0.92			111			37			39	36	
2.5	23		118	26	22.5	0.51	0.53	4.5	0.96			113			36			40	38	
3.0	28		118	25	22.8	0.54	0.57	4.8	0.95			111			37			38	36	
3.5	33		120	27	26.8	0.53	0.60	5.0	0.88			116			35			46	41	
4.0	38		121	26	28.4	0.68	0.65	5.4	1.05			117			35			39	40	
4.5	43		124	29	28.4	0.73	0.67	5.4	1.09			116			37			36	39	
5.0	48		127	29	36.2	0.87	0.73	5.7	1.19			121			32			39	46	
5.5	53		130	31	38.2	0.92	0.76	5.8	1.21			122			33			39	47	
6.0	58	139/88	131	33	43.5	1.09	0.89	6.8	1.22			121			33			37	46	
	Recovery		130	22	32.1	1.00	0.91	7.0	1.10			112			40			30	33	
	Recovery		125	24	34.0	0.91	0.70	5.6	1.30			121			35			35	46	
	Recovery		123	23	29.0	0.81	0.62	5.0	1.31			120			37			33	44	
	Recovery		123	22	24.8	0.64	0.46	3.7	1.39			123			35			36	50	

Interpretation

COMMENTS

Initial resting respiratory function studies showed respiratory restriction and mild airway obstruction with some response to inhaled albuterol, typical of congestive heart disease. The resting respiratory function tests were not repeated 3 months later.

ANALYSIS

In flow chart 1, in the first study the patient has a reduced maximum V̇O2 and anaerobic threshold (Table 25-2 and Fig. 25-A). In flow chart 4, the breathing reserve is high (branchpoint 4.1), and the VE/V̇CO2 is high (branchpoint 4.3), suggesting an abnormal pulmonary circulation. Because the vital capacity is low, however, we are directed to consider lung disease with impaired peripheral oxygenation. The patient has physiologic features of this problem including low O2 pulse and low ΔV̇O2/ΔWR. In view of this patient's clinical back-ground, his bronchospasm and reduced lung volumes could be secondary to congestive heart failure. The low and slowly increasing O2 pulse during exercise and the increase when exercise stopped are consistent with left ventricular dysfunction.

Three months after treatment (Table 25-4 and Fig. 25-B), the maximum work rate, maximum V̇O2, maximum O2 pulse, anaerobic threshold, and ΔV̇O2/ΔWR findings are considerably improved.

CONCLUSION

This study is presented to show the findings of severe left ventricular dysfunction, as may be seen with cardiomyopathy of any cause, and the response over a 3-month period to effective medical management. This analysis demonstrates the value of exercise testing in demonstrating the pathophysiology and the effectiveness of specific therapy.

TABLE 25-4. *Final study.*

Time min	Work rate watts	BP mm Hg	HR min⁻¹	f min⁻¹	V̇E L/min BTPS	V̇CO2 L/min STPD	V̇O2 L/min STPD	V̇O2/HR ml/beat	R	pH	HCO3 meq/L	PO2, mm Hg ET	a	(A-a)	PCO2, mm Hg ET	a	(a-ET)	V̇E/V̇CO2	V̇E/V̇O2	VD/VT
	Rest	139/88	92	17	14.0	0.34	0.40	4.3	0.85			104			41			37	31	
	Rest		87	16	12.0	0.30	0.35	4.0	0.86			103			42			35	30	
	Rest		92	15	11.0	0.28	0.33	3.6	0.85			103			42			35	29	
	Rest		90	19	11.0	0.19	0.24	2.7	0.79			104			42			49	39	
	Rest		95	17	12.0	0.29	0.35	3.7	0.83			104			42			36	30	
	Rest		91	19	13.0	0.29	0.32	3.5	0.91			106			41			39	36	
	Unloaded		95	19	16.0	0.43	0.54	5.7	0.80			98			43			33	27	
	Unloaded		98	20	14.0	0.35	0.43	4.4	0.81			101			43			35	29	
	Unloaded		100	22	18.0	0.48	0.54	5.4	0.89			104			41			34	30	
	Unloaded		99	21	18.0	0.48	0.58	5.9	0.83			100			43			34	28	
	Unloaded		102	21	18.0	0.48	0.54	5.3	0.89			104			42			34	30	
	Unloaded		103	22	17.0	0.43	0.50	4.9	0.86			103			42			35	30	
0.5	3		105	21	16.0	0.41	0.49	4.7	0.84			102			43			35	29	
1.0	8		106	20	18.0	0.49	0.59	5.6	0.83			102			42			33	28	
1.5	13		106	20	20.0	0.56	0.67	6.3	0.84			101			42			33	27	
2.0	18		108	23	20.0	0.56	0.68	6.3	0.82			101			42			32	27	
2.5	23		110	24	22.0	0.61	0.76	6.9	0.80			100			42			33	26	
3.0	28		110	23	22.0	0.60	0.73	6.6	0.82			101			44			33	27	
3.5	33		111	22	19.0	0.54	0.69	6.2	0.78			96			44			32	25	
4.0	38		113	22	23.0	0.74	0.94	8.3	0.79			95			44			29	22	
4.5	43		117	24	24.0	0.73	0.83	7.1	0.88			102			43			30	26	
5.0	48		122	24	28.0	0.86	0.94	7.7	0.91			104			42			30	28	
5.5	53		127	23	28.0	0.86	0.93	7.3	0.92			106			41			30	28	
6.0	58		134	23	30.0	0.96	1.05	7.8	0.91			105			42			29	27	
6.5	63		138	25	36.0	1.09	1.08	7.8	1.01			111			40			31	31	
7.0	68		143	25	38.0	1.19	1.13	7.9	1.05			111			40			30	32	
7.5	73		143	25	41.0	1.26	1.13	7.9	1.12			113			40			31	34	
8.0	78		152	30	51.0	1.46	1.22	8.0	1.20			118			36			33	40	
8.5	83		155	31	55.0	1.50	1.22	7.9	1.23			120			35			35	43	
9.0	88	204/104	160	29	52.0	1.44	1.14	7.1	1.26			120			36			34	43	
	Recovery		148	25	46.0	1.56	1.34	9.1	1.16			111			43			28	33	
	Recovery		128	24	41.0	1.36	0.98	7.7	1.39			117			41			29	40	
	Recovery		130	23	36.0	1.16	0.78	6.0	1.49			119			41			29	44	
	Recovery		123	21	29.0	0.91	0.61	5.0	1.49			119			41			30	45	

CASE 26 *Cardiomyopathy with oscillatory function*

CLINICAL FINDINGS

This 35-year-old former truck driver with idiopathic cardiomyopathy underwent exercise testing as part of his evaluation for a study using new pharmaceutical agents. He had developed loss of energy and shortness of breath over the past 3 years and had been hospitalized twice for "pneumonia." He used alcohol occasionally but denied use of tobacco or other oral or intravenous drugs. He had no history of angina, hypertension, rheumatic fever, or edema. An endocardial biopsy 2 years previously was nondiagnostic. The patient was taking 40 mg furosemide, 0.25 mg digoxin, and 60 mg isosorbide daily. Resting heart rate was 104 and blood pressure 122/86. On physical examination there was cardiomegaly, an audible S-3, and fine basilar rales, but no peripheral edema. Chest roentgenograms were normal except for left ventricular enlargement. Resting ECG revealed sinus rhythm, left ventricular hypertrophy, and diffuse ST-T wave depression, more marked in the anterolateral leads.

EXERCISE FINDINGS

The patient performed exercise on a cycle ergometer. After 2 minutes of rest, he pedalled at 60 rpm without added load for 3 minutes. The work rate was then increased in ramp pattern 15 W per minute to his symptom-limited maximum. Arm blood pressure was measured with a sphygmomanometer. Exercise was stopped because of lightheadedness. No further ECG abnormalities were noted.

TABLE 26-1. *Selected Respiratory Function Data*

MEASUREMENT	PREDICTED	MEASURED
Age, yr		35
Sex		Male
Height, cm		178
Weight, kg	80	82
Hematocrit, %		45
VC, L	5.23	4.72
IC, L	3.47	3.10
FEV_1, L	4.29	3.78
FEV_1/VC, %	82	80
MVV, L/min	172	148

TABLE 26-2. *Selected Exercise Data*

MEASUREMENT	PREDICTED	MEASURED
Maximum $\dot{V}O_2$, L/min	3.02	1.71
Maximum HR, beats/min	185	157
Maximum O_2 pulse, ml/beat	16.3	10.9
$\Delta \dot{V}O_2/\Delta WR$, ml/min/W	10.3	10.8
AT, L/min	> 1.27	1.0
Maximum $\dot{V}E$, L/min		81
Exercise breathing reserve, L/min	> 15	67

Fig. 26-A.

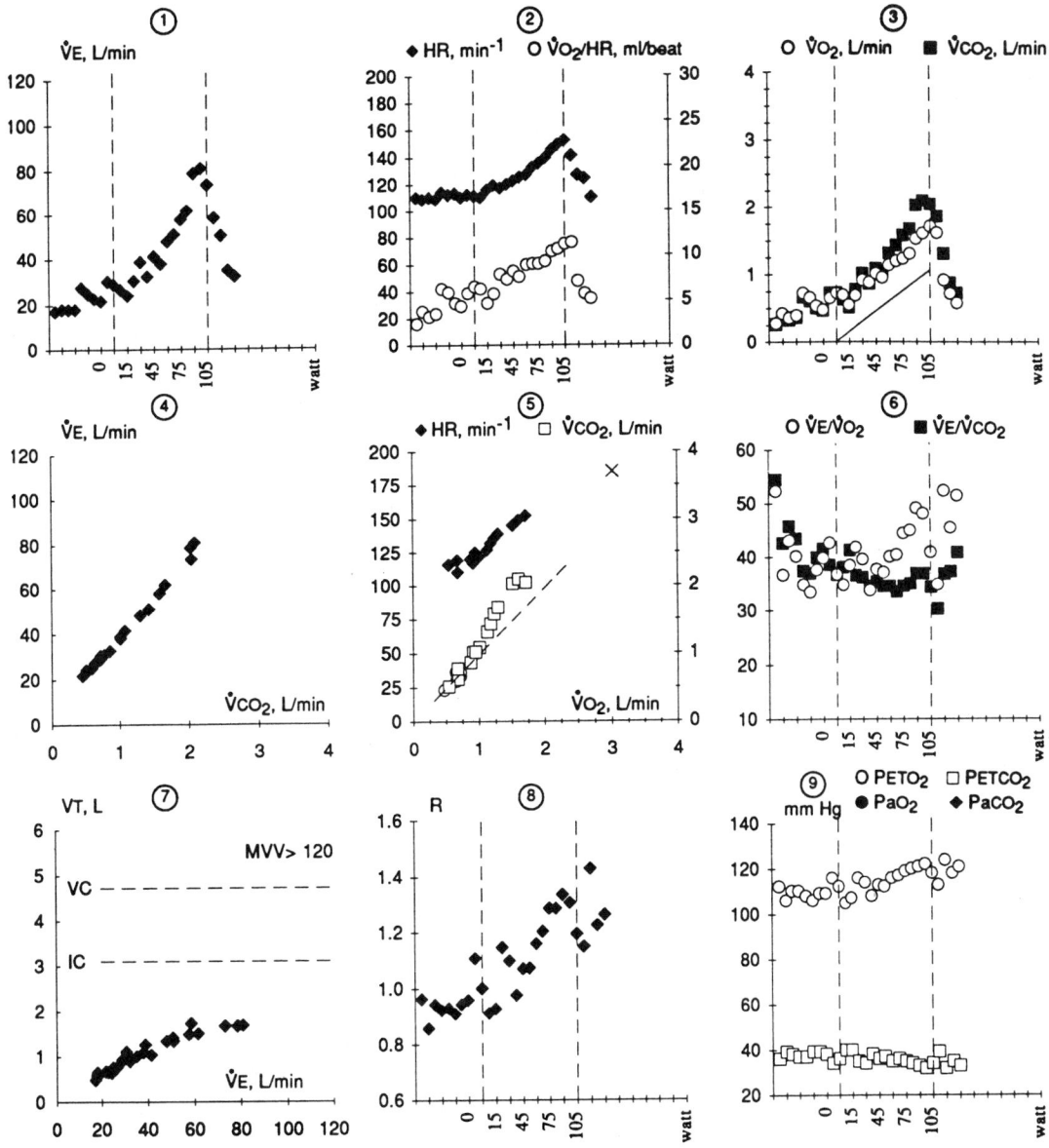

1. Vertical dashed lines in panels 1 to 3 and 6, 8, and 9 indicate the beginning and the end of increasing work period.

2. Unloaded cycling is performed for 3 minutes before the left vertical dashed line.

3. In panel 3, the diagonal line shows the increase of $\dot{V}O_2$ at a slope of 10 ml/min/W.

4. In panel 5, the diagonal dashed line has a slope of 1; the "x" in the upper right is the predicted maximum heart rate and $\dot{V}O_2$ for the subject.

TABLE 26-3.

Time min	Work rate watts	BP mm Hg	HR min⁻¹	f min⁻¹	$\dot{V}E$ L/min BTPS	$\dot{V}CO_2$ L/min STPD	$\dot{V}O_2$ L/min STPD	$\dfrac{\dot{V}O_2}{HR}$ ml/beat	R	pH	HCO₃ meq/L	PO2, mm Hg ET	a	(A-a)	PCO2, mm Hg ET	a	(a-ET)	$\dfrac{\dot{V}E}{\dot{V}CO_2}$	$\dfrac{\dot{V}E}{\dot{V}O_2}$	$\dfrac{VD}{VT}$
	Rest	119/81																		
	Rest		110	36	17.2	0.26	0.27	2.5	0.96			112			36			54	52	
	Rest		109	30	17.9	0.36	0.42	3.9	0.86			106			39			43	37	
	Rest		110	33	17.9	0.33	0.35	3.2	0.94			110			38			46	43	
	Rest		109	28	18.0	0.36	0.39	3.6	0.92			110			37			43	40	
	Unloaded		114	33	27.8	0.67	0.72	6.3	0.93			108			37			37	35	
	Unloaded		112	33	24.9	0.60	0.66	5.9	0.91			106			39			37	33	
	Unloaded		113	34	22.8	0.50	0.53	4.7	0.94			109			39			40	38	
	Unloaded		110	32	21.8	0.46	0.48	4.4	0.96			109			38			41	40	
	Unloaded		112	31	30.3	0.72	0.65	5.8	1.11			116			34			38	43	
	Unloaded		111	31	29.0	0.72	0.72	6.5	1.00			112			36			37	37	
0.5	7.5	122/87	110	35	26.9	0.63	0.69	6.3	0.91			105			40			38	35	
1.0	15		116	38	24.3	0.51	0.55	4.7	0.93			107			40			41	38	
1.5	22.5		119	28	30.8	0.78	0.68	5.7	1.15			116			35			36	42	
2.0	30		117	31	39.0	1.01	0.92	7.9	1.10			114			34			36	40	
2.5	37.5	140/92	120	34	32.5	0.86	0.88	7.3	0.98			108			38			34	34	
3.0	45		122	40	41.4	1.08	1.01	8.3	1.07			113			36			35	38	
3.5	52.5		125	35	38.1	1.02	0.95	7.6	1.07			112			37			34	37	
4.0	60		127	36	48.2	1.31	1.13	8.9	1.16			116			35			34	40	
4.5	67	154/85	132	38	51.1	1.43	1.19	9.0	1.20			117			36			33	40	
5.0	75		135	39	57.8	1.58	1.23	9.1	1.28			119			35			34	44	
5.5	82		139	41	61.8	1.67	1.30	9.4	1.28			120			34			35	45	
6.0	90		145	47	78.7	2.03	1.52	10.5	1.34			121			33			37	49	
6.5	97	156/87	149	48	80.9	2.09	1.60	10.7	1.31			122			32			37	48	
7.0	105		152	44	73.4	2.04	1.71	11.3	1.19			118			34			34	41	
	Recovery	144/83	141	34	58.7	1.85	1.61	11.4	1.15			113			39			30	35	
	Recovery		127	36	50.7	1.30	0.91	7.2	1.43			124			32			37	52	
	Recovery		124	35	35.2	0.87	0.71	5.7	1.23			118			35			37	45	
	Recovery		110	36	32.3	0.72	0.57	5.2	1.26			121			33			41	51	
		137/85																		

Interpretation

COMMENTS

This patient has an idiopathic cardiomyopathy, New York Heart Association Class II. Respiratory function is normal. An oscillatory pattern of change in $\dot{V}O_2$, $\dot{V}CO_2$, and $\dot{V}E$ is seen during exercise testing in some patients with cardiomyopathy and is well illustrated in this patient in Figure 26-B, which uses an 8-second rolling average of the breath-by-breath values.

ANALYSIS

In flow chart 1, the maximum $\dot{V}O_2$ and anaerobic threshold are reduced (Table 26-2). The breathing reserve is normal (branchpoint 4.1), whereas the ventilatory equivalents are high at the anaerobic threshold (branchpoint 4.3). The rightward direction takes us to the diagnostic box "abnormal pulmonary circulation." We do not have confirmatory blood gas or oximetry measures for this diagnosis, but we do have a low O_2 pulse, strong evidence for a circulatory problem. Undoubtedly, the cardiomyopathy has led to abnormalities in the pulmonary circulation.

If we take the leftward direction from branchpoint 4.3, through branchpoint 4.4, (normal hematocrit) and branchpoint 4.6, we find confirmatory evidence for heart disease (abnormal ECG) and none for peripheral vascular disease. Finally, we should consider in this analysis the most striking finding, i.e., the oscillatory pattern of the $\dot{V}O_2$, $\dot{V}CO_2$, depicted in Figure 26-B, and the accompanying oscillatory pattern of $\dot{V}E$ and R, which are not displayed here. The oscillations have a frequency of about 40 seconds from peak to peak and are greatest for mild to moderate exercise. This phenomenon is typical for some patients

Fig. 26-B. *Tracings of* $\dot{V}_{O_2}$ *(left) and* $\dot{V}_{CO_2}$ *(right) using an 8-second rolling average of breath-by-breath data during 2 minutes of rest, 3 minutes of unloaded pedalling, 7 minutes of ramp (incremental) exercise, and 2 minutes of recovery. The vertical dashed lines indicate the onset and end of exercise. Although oscillations can be seen throughout this 14-minute period, they are most marked during mild and moderate exercise. It is thought that the increased catecholamine response that occurs with heavy exercise obliterates the changing vasomotor tone from the central nervous system (Traube-Hering's waves in blood pressure).[1] When data are plotted with less temporal resolution, i.e., every half minute, the oscillations become indistinct.*

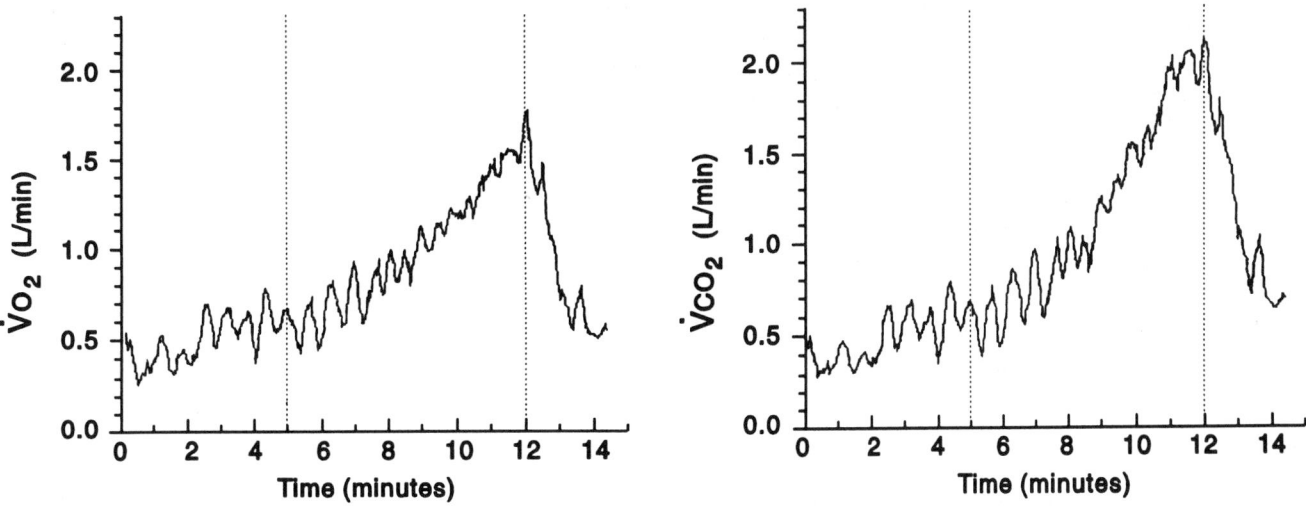

with congestive heart failure and appears to be from cyclic changes in cardiac output rather than secondary to cyclic changes in ventilation.[1]

CONCLUSION

This patient is presented to illustrate the oscillatory pattern in O_2 uptake and other accompanying parameters that frequently occur in patients with congestive heart failure, especially during mild to moderate exercise.

Reference

1. Ben-Dov, I., Sietsema, K.E., Casaburi, R., and Wasserman, K.: Evidence that circulatory oscillations accompany ventilatory oscillations during exercise in patients with heart failure. Am. Rev. Respir. Dis., 145:776–781, 1992.

CASE 27 *Mitral insufficiency*

CLINICAL FINDINGS

This 43-year-old female electronics assembler had rheumatic fever at age 10. In the last 6 months she developed increasing dyspnea and orthopnea, with intermittent atrial fibrillation and pleural effusion, requiring repeated hospitalizations. There was no evidence of mitral stenosis or coronary artery disease on catheterization, angiography, or echocardiography. At the time of exercise study she had a sinus rhythm, findings of mitral regurgitation with left atrial and left ventricular enlargement, but no pleural effusion or dependent edema. Her medications were digoxin, furosemide, and potassium chloride.

EXERCISE FINDINGS

The patient performed exercise on a cycle ergometer. She pedalled at 60 rpm without added load for 3 minutes. The work rate was then increased 5 W per minute to her symptom-limited maximum. She stopped cycling because of general fatigue. There were no ST segment changes or arrhythmia.

TABLE 27-1. *Selected Respiratory Function Data*

MEASUREMENT	PREDICTED	MEASURED
Age, yr		43
Sex		Female
Height, cm		160
Weight, kg	61	56
Hematocrit, %		40
VC, L	2.88	2.03
IC, L	1.92	1.49
TLC, L	4.33	3.32
FEV$_1$, L	2.36	1.81
FEV$_1$/VC, %	82	89
MVV, L/min	90	90
D$_{LCO}$, ml/mm Hg/min	21.7	23.5

TABLE 27-2. *Selected Exercise Data*

MEASUREMENT	PREDICTED	MEASURED
Maximum V̇o$_2$, L/min	1.57	0.79
Maximum HR, beats/min	177	186
Maximum O$_2$ pulse, ml/beat	8.9	4.2
ΔV̇o$_2$/ΔWR, ml/min/W	10.3	5.6
AT, L/min	> 0.74	0.65
Maximum V̇E, L/min		31
Exercise breathing reserve, L/min	> 15	59

Fig. 27-A.

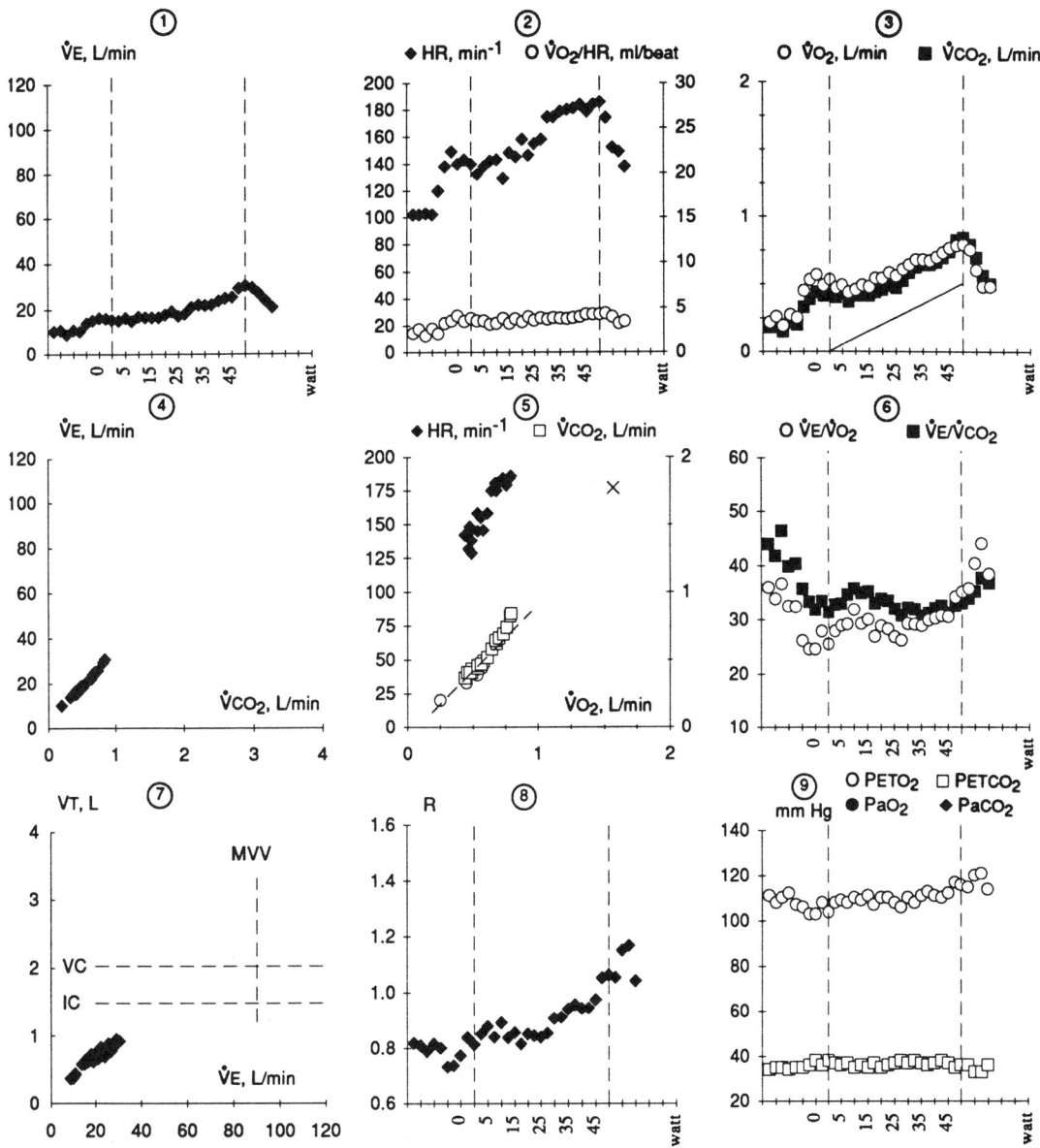

1. Vertical dashed lines in panels 1 to 3 and 6, 8, and 9 indicate the beginning and the end of increasing work period.

2. Unloaded cycling is performed for 3 minutes before the left vertical dashed line.

3. In panel 3, the diagonal line shows the increase of $\dot{V}O_2$ at a slope of 10 ml/min/W.

4. In panel 5, the diagonal dashed line has a slope of 1; the "x" in the upper right is the predicted maximum heart rate and $\dot{V}O_2$ for the subject.

TABLE 27-3.

Time min	Work rate watts	BP mm Hg	HR min⁻¹	f min⁻¹	$\dot{V}E$ L/min BTPS	$\dot{V}CO_2$ L/min STPD	$\dot{V}O_2$ L/min STPD	$\frac{\dot{V}O_2}{HR}$ ml/beat	R	pH	HCO₃ meq/L	PO2, mm Hg ET	a	(A-a)	PCO2, mm Hg ET	a	(a-ET)	$\frac{\dot{V}E}{\dot{V}CO_2}$	$\frac{\dot{V}E}{\dot{V}O_2}$	$\frac{VD}{VT}$
	Rest		102	27	10.2	0.18	0.22	2.2	0.82			111			34			44	36	
	Rest		102	26	11.0	0.21	0.26	2.5	0.81			108			35			42	34	
	Rest		103	24	9.0	0.15	0.19	1.8	0.79			110			35			46	37	
	Rest		102	25	10.9	0.22	0.27	2.6	0.81			112			34			40	33	
	Unloaded		120	25	10.2	0.20	0.25	2.1	0.80			107			35			40	32	
	Unloaded		138	24	13.8	0.33	0.45	3.3	0.73			106			35			36	26	
	Unloaded		149	25	15.1	0.39	0.53	3.6	0.74			103			36			33	24	
	Unloaded		140	26	16.2	0.44	0.57	4.1	0.77			103			38			32	25	
	Unloaded		143	26	15.9	0.41	0.49	3.4	0.84			108			36			33	28	
	Unloaded		140	24	15.5	0.43	0.53	3.8	0.81			104			38			31	25	
0.5	5		132	25	15.2	0.40	0.47	3.6	0.85			108			37			33	28	
1.0	5		138	26	16.4	0.43	0.49	3.6	0.88			109			36			33	29	
1.5	10		142	26	15.0	0.37	0.44	3.1	0.84			108			37			35	29	
2.0	10		143	27	16.9	0.41	0.46	3.2	0.89			110			35			36	32	
2.5	15		129	27	16.6	0.41	0.49	3.8	0.84			109			36			35	29	
3.0	15		148	26	16.6	0.41	0.48	3.2	0.85			111			35			35	30	
3.5	20		145	26	16.7	0.44	0.54	3.7	0.81			107			37			33	27	
4.0	20		158	27	17.8	0.46	0.54	3.4	0.85			110			35			34	29	
4.5	25		146	31	19.0	0.49	0.58	4.0	0.84			110			36			33	28	
5.0	25		155	25	17.1	0.47	0.56	3.6	0.84			108			37			32	27	
5.5	30		158	25	18.1	0.52	0.61	3.9	0.85			106			38			31	26	
6.0	30		175	28	21.0	0.58	0.64	3.7	0.91			110			37			32	29	
6.5	35		175	29	22.2	0.62	0.68	3.9	0.91			108			38			32	29	
7.0	35		179	27	21.9	0.64	0.68	3.8	0.94			111			37			31	29	
7.5	40		180	27	22.3	0.64	0.67	3.7	0.96			113			36			31	30	
8.0	40		181	30	23.7	0.66	0.70	3.9	0.94			111			37			32	30	
8.5	45		184	30	24.9	0.69	0.73	4.0	0.95			110			38			32	31	
9.0	45		179	29	25.6	0.74	0.76	4.2	0.97			112			37			31	30	
9.5	50		184	31	29.2	0.82	0.78	4.2	1.05			117			35			32	34	
10.0	50		186	33	30.5	0.84	0.79	4.2	1.06			116			36			33	35	
	Recovery		174	33	29.6	0.79	0.75	4.3	1.05			115			36			34	36	
	Recovery		152	35	27.2	0.69	0.60	3.9	1.15			120			33			35	40	
	Recovery		149	35	24.1	0.56	0.48	3.2	1.17			121			33			38	44	
	Recovery		138	32	21.1	0.50	0.48	3.5	1.04			114			36			37	38	

Interpretation

COMMENTS

Respiratory function at rest is compatible with a restrictive defect but the diffusing capacity (D_{LCO}) is normal (Table 27-1).

ANALYSIS

In flow chart 1, the maximum $\dot{V}O_2$ and anaerobic threshold are low (Table 27-2). See flow chart 4. The breathing reserve is high (branchpoint 4.1). The ventilatory equivalent for CO_2 is slightly elevated at the anaerobic threshold. By referring to the insert in Figure 27-13 and the P_{ETCO_2} values in Table 27-3, the slightly elevated $\dot{V}E/\dot{V}CO_2$ appears to be due to a mild degree of hyperventilation of the pulmonary blood flow, rather than an increase in VD/VT (branchpoint 4.3). This indicates that the abnormality is an O_2 flow problem of nonpulmonary origin. The hematocrit is normal (branchpoint 4.4). The striking finding is the low and flat O_2 pulse throughout exercise (panel 2, Fig. 27-A) (branchpoint 4.6) leading to the diagnosis of heart disease. The steep heart rate-$\dot{V}O_2$ relationship (panel 5, Fig. 27-A), low heart rate reserve and low $\Delta\dot{V}O_2/\Delta WR$ confirm the diagnosis of heart disease. The low and unchanging O_2 pulse suggests that the patient's effective stroke volume is low and the arterial-mixed venous O_2 difference is maximized at a low work rate.

CONCLUSION

Valvular heart disease, as suggested by the patient's history, has caused marked exercise intolerance because of an inadequate cardiac output response to exercise.

Case 28 *Mitral stenosis: Pre- and post-β-adrenergic blockade*

Clinical Findings

This 57-year-old former receptionist had had rheumatic fever at age 16. She had had orthopnea during pregnancy at age 24. She was otherwise well except for gradually increasing dyspnea of 6 years' duration and exertional dull substernal aching radiating to the jaw and left arm of 3 months' duration. Examination revealed a grade II pre-systolic murmur and an opening snap. The mitral valve area was mildly decreased and the left atrium was moderately dilated. Coronary arteriography was normal. The second exercise study was performed 17 months after the first while the patient was receiving propranolol 3 times daily. At that time she complained of increasing dyspnea, even at rest, associated with lightheadedness, sweating, numbness of the fingers, and perioral tingling.

Exercise Findings

On both occasions the patient exercised on a cycle ergometer to her symptom-limited maximum. She pedalled at 60 rpm without added load for 3 minutes. During the first test the work rate was increased 10 W per minute, and during the second test (17 months later), it was increased 5 W per minute. Arterial blood was sampled every second minute, and intra-arterial blood pressure was recorded from a percutaneously placed brachial artery catheter. Resting ECGs showed left atrial enlargement and sinus rhythm; there were no abnormal ST segment changes, nor arrhythmia during exercise. She stopped exercise in both studies complaining of leg fatigue, not dyspnea or chest pain.

TABLE 28-1. *Selected Respiratory Function Data*

MEASUREMENT	PREDICTED	BEFORE BLOCKADE	AFTER BLOCKADE
Age, yr		57	59
Sex		Female	
Height, cm		166	
Weight, kg	65	67	
Hematocrit, %		40	
VC, L	3.10	3.16	2.73
IC, L	2.07	2.26	2.19
TLC, L	5.15	5.01	4.62
FEV$_1$, L	2.48	2.58	2.26
FEV$_1$/VC, %	80	82	83
MVV, L/min	93	96	81
D$_{LCO}$, ml/mm Hg/min	21.9	20.3	18.7

TABLE 28-2. *Selected Exercise Data*

MEASUREMENT	PREDICTED	BEFORE BLOCKADE	AFTER BLOCKADE
Maximum V̇o$_2$, L/min	1.42	0.74	0.91
Maximum HR, beats/min	162	120	108
Maximum O$_2$ pulse, ml/beat	8.7	6.2	8.4
ΔV̇o$_2$/ΔWR, ml/min/W	10.3		7.4
AT, L/min	> 0.70	indeterminate	indeterminate
Blood pressure, mm Hg (rest, max)		128/62,164/83	153/72,168/78
Maximum V̇E, L/min		43	47
Exercise breathing reserve, L/min	> 15	53	34
Pa$_{O_2}$, mm Hg (rest, max ex)		97,125	87,122
P(A−a)$_{O_2}$, mm Hg (rest, max ex)		10,2	11,5
P(a−ET)$_{CO_2}$, mm Hg (rest, max ex)		0,−1	3,−1
V$_D$/V$_T$ (rest, heavy ex)		0.26,0.25	0.28,0.19
HCO$_3^-$, mEq/L (rest, 2-min recov)		24,18	24,18

Fɪɢ. 28-A. *Pre-β-adrenergic blockade.*

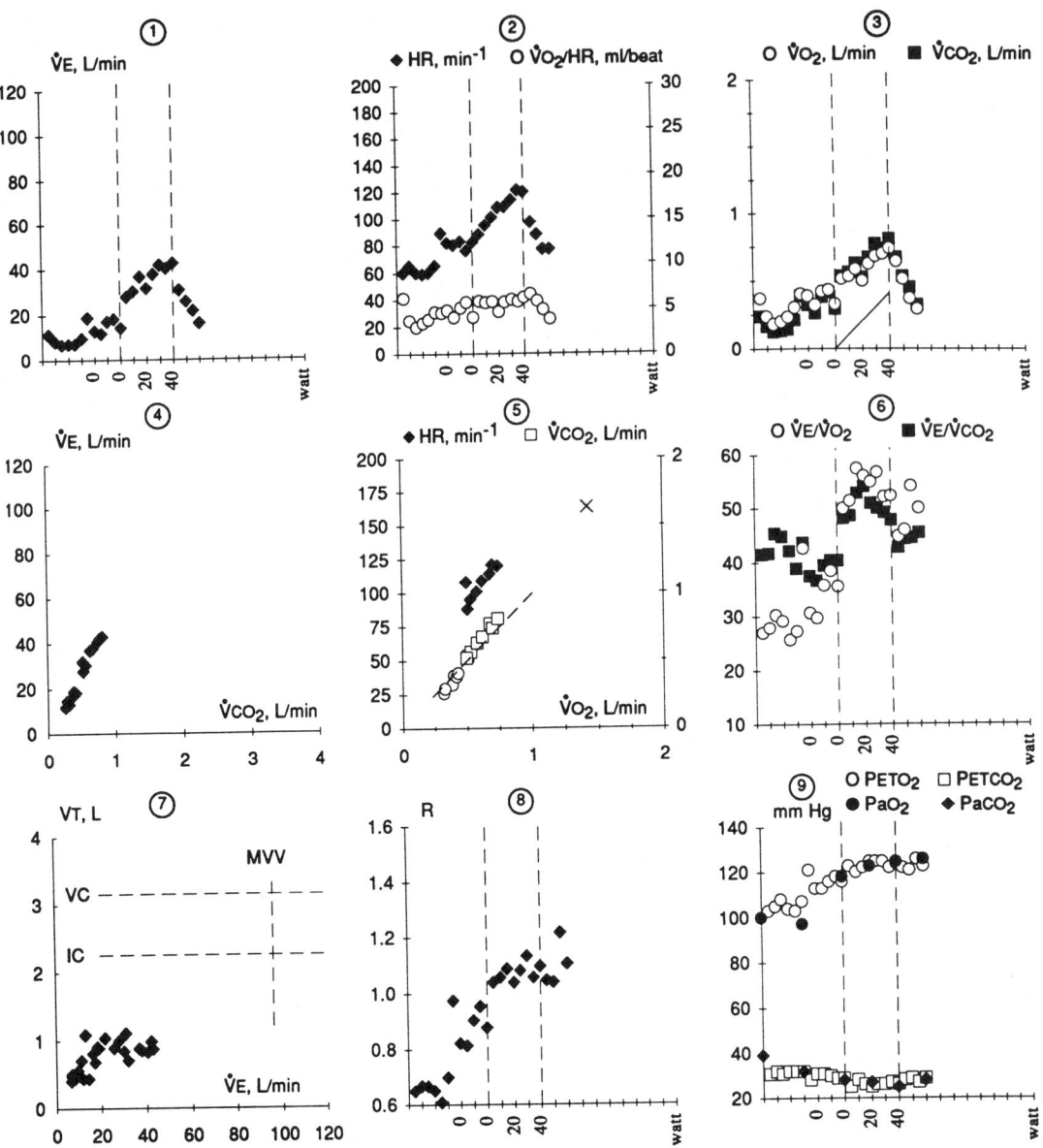

1. Vertical dashed lines in panels 1 to 3 and 6, 8, and 9 indicate the beginning and the end of increasing work period.

2. Unloaded cycling is performed for 3 minutes before the left vertical dashed line.

3. In panel 3, the diagonal line shows the increase of $\dot{V}O_2$ at a slope of 10 ml/min/W.

4. In panel 5, the diagonal dashed line has a slope of 1; the "x" in the upper right is the predicted maximum heart rate and $\dot{V}O_2$ for the subject.

FIG. 28-B. *Post-β-adrenergic blockade.*

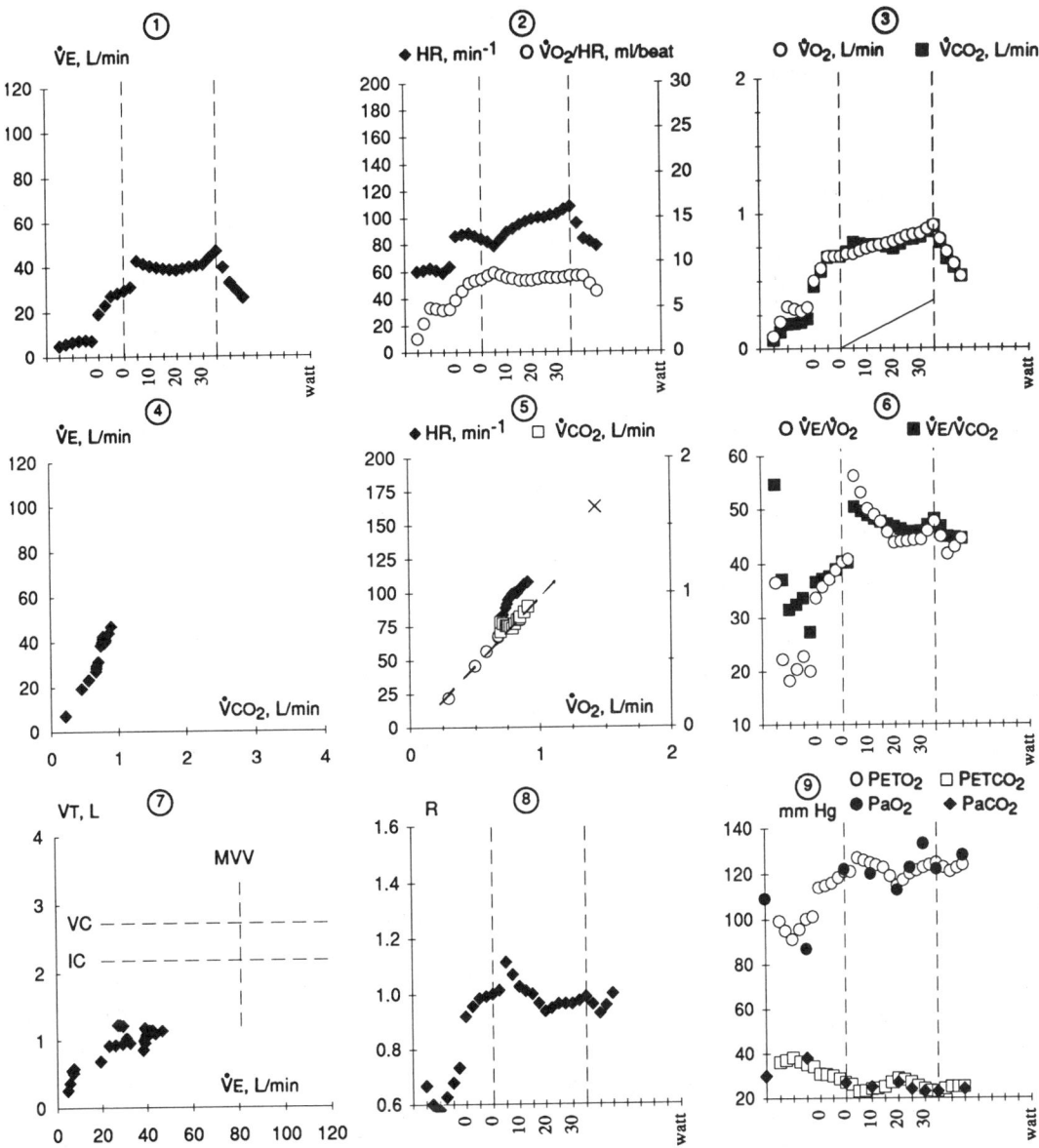

1. Vertical dashed lines in panels 1 to 3 and 6, 8, and 9 indicate the beginning and the end of increasing work period.

2. Unloaded cycling is performed for 3 minutes before the left vertical dashed line.

3. In panel 3, the diagonal line shows the increase of $\dot{V}_{O_2}$ at a slope of 10 ml/min/W.

4. In panel 5, the diagonal dashed line has a slope of 1; the "x" in the upper right is the predicted maximum heart rate and $\dot{V}_{O_2}$ for the subject.

TABLE 28-3. *Pre-β-adrenergic blockade.*

Time min	Work rate watts	BP mm Hg	HR min⁻¹	f min⁻¹	$\dot{V}_E$ L/min BTPS	$\dot{V}_{CO_2}$ L/min STPD	$\dot{V}_{O_2}$ L/min STPD	$\dfrac{\dot{V}_{O_2}}{HR}$ ml/beat	R	pH	HCO₃ meq/L	PO₂ ET	PO₂ a	PO₂ (A-a)	PCO₂ ET	PCO₂ a	PCO₂ (a-ET)	$\dfrac{\dot{V}_E}{\dot{V}_{CO_2}}$	$\dfrac{\dot{V}_E}{\dot{V}_{O_2}}$	$\dfrac{V_D}{V_T}$
	Rest	128/62								7.40	24		100			39				
	Rest		60	16	11.3	0.24	0.37	6.2	0.65			103			31			41	27	
	Rest		65	18	8.2	0.16	0.24	3.7	0.67			105			32			42	28	
	Rest		60	17	6.9	0.12	0.18	3.0	0.67			108			31			45	30	
	Rest		59	15	7.1	0.13	0.20	3.4	0.65			104			32			45	29	
	Rest		60	14	7.1	0.14	0.23	3.8	0.61			103			32			42	26	
	Rest	140/77	65	17	9.6	0.21	0.30	4.6	0.70	7.43	21	107	97	10	32	32	0	39	27	0.26
	Unloaded		89	21	18.8	0.39	0.40	4.5	0.98			121			28			44	43	
	Unloaded		82	12	13.0	0.32	0.39	4.8	0.82			113			31			37	31	
	Unloaded		80	27	11.8	0.26	0.32	4.0	0.81			113			31			37	30	
	Unloaded		83	25	17.1	0.38	0.42	5.1	0.90			116			30			39	36	
	Unloaded		76	20	18.2	0.41	0.43	5.7	0.95			118			29			40	38	
	Unloaded	146/80	82	33	14.5	0.29	0.33	4.0	0.88	7.47	20	116	118	1	29	28	-1	40	35	0.19
0.5	10		88	28	27.9	0.53	0.51	5.8	1.04			123			25			48	50	
1.0	10		95	36	30.3	0.56	0.53	5.6	1.06			120			28			49	51	
1.5	20		101	42	36.9	0.63	0.58	5.7	1.09			122			26			53	57	
2.0	20	152/80	108	45	31.9	0.52	0.50	4.6	1.04	7.50	21	125	123	1	25	27	2	54	56	0.36
2.5	30		109	44	37.8	0.67	0.62	5.7	1.08			125			26			51	55	
3.0	30		114	43	42.2	0.77	0.68	6.0	1.13			125			26			50	57	
3.5	40		121	49	40.6	0.74	0.70	5.8	1.06			122			27			49	52	
4.0	40	164/83	120	49	42.9	0.81	0.74	6.2	1.09	7.49	19	124	125	2	26	25	-1	48	52	0.25
	Recovery		97	28	31.0	0.67	0.64	6.6	1.05			122			28			43	45	
	Recovery		88	29	25.9	0.53	0.51	5.8	1.04			121			29			44	46	
	Recovery		77	21	21.8	0.45	0.37	4.8	1.22			126			27			44	54	
	Recovery	149/71	77	20	16.2	0.32	0.29	3.8	1.10	7.42	18	123	126	-2	29	28	-1	45	50	0.29

Interpretation

COMMENTS

Resting pulmonary function is normal on both occasions of study (Table 28-1). The ECG is normal except for evidence of left atrial enlargement. This case is presented because it illustrates the abnormalities of mitral stenosis and changes in O_2 pulse with propranolol. Moreover, it is presented because the development of respiratory alkalosis during exercise is unusual.

ANALYSIS

During exercise, the maximum $\dot{V}_{O_2}$ is decreased and the anaerobic threshold is indeterminate (Table 28-2). See flow chart 5. The indices of distribution of ventilation relative to perfusion are normal at maximum exercise, making lung disease and pulmonary vascular disease unlikely diagnoses (branchpoint 5.1). The heart rate reserve was high, but because the patient was taking a β-adrenergic blocking drug this is an unreliable index for separating heart diseases from other disorders (branchpoint 5.2). If considered to have a normal heart rate reserve and normal hematocrit (branchpoint 5.4), then heart disease is the likely primary disorder. Consistent with heart disease as the primary diagnosis is the low O_2 pulse that fails to rise as the work rate increases.

Commonly, an anticipatory respiratory alkalosis occurs at rest, but disappears with the start of

TABLE 28-4. *Post-β-adrenergic blockade.*

Time min	Work rate watts	BP mm Hg	HR min⁻¹	f min⁻¹	$\dot{V}_E$ L/min BTPS	$\dot{V}_{CO_2}$ L/min STPD	$\dot{V}_{O_2}$ L/min STPD	$\dfrac{\dot{V}_{O_2}}{HR}$ ml/beat	R	pH	HCO₃ meq/L	PO2, mm Hg ET	a	(A-a)	PCO2, mm Hg ET	a	(a-ET)	$\dfrac{\dot{V}_E}{\dot{V}_{CO_2}}$	$\dfrac{\dot{V}_E}{\dot{V}_{O_2}}$	$\dfrac{V_D}{V_T}$
	Rest	153/72								7.48	22	109			30					
	Rest																			
	Rest		60	19	4.9	0.06	0.09	1.5	0.67			99			36			55	37	
	Rest		61	16	5.8	0.12	0.20	3.3	0.60			95			37			37	22	
	Rest		62	12	6.7	0.18	0.31	5.0	0.58			91			38			32	18	
	Rest		61	13	7.1	0.19	0.30	4.8	0.63			96			37			32	20	
	Rest	159/72	59	13	7.5	0.19	0.28	4.7	0.68	7.41	24	100	87	11	35	38	3	34	23	0.28
	Unloaded		63	14	7.2	0.22	0.30	4.8	0.73			101			34			27	20	
	Unloaded		86	28	19.2	0.46	0.50	5.8	0.92			114			31			37	34	
	Unloaded		87	25	23.2	0.57	0.59	6.8	0.96			115			31			37	36	
	Unloaded		88	22	27.1	0.67	0.68	7.7	0.99			116			30			38	37	
	Unloaded		86	23	28.3	0.68	0.68	7.9	0.99			119			29			39	39	
	Unloaded	162/78	84	24	29.4	0.68	0.68	8.1	1.00	7.50	21	121	122	1	27	27	0	40	40	0.19
0.5	5		82	30	31.1	0.71	0.70	8.5	1.01			121			26			40	41	
1.0	5		79	37	42.5	0.78	0.70	8.9	1.11			127			23			50	56	
1.5	10		84	36	41.3	0.77	0.72	8.6	1.07			126			24			50	53	
2.0	10	168/78	89	35	40.1	0.76	0.74	8.3	1.03	7.52	20	125	120	6	24	25	1	49	50	0.27
2.5	15		92	34	39.6	0.76	0.75	8.2	1.01			124			25			48	49	
3.0	15		95	33	39.1	0.76	0.76	8.0	1.00			123			25			48	48	
3.5	20		97	39	38.8	0.75	0.78	8.0	0.97			119			27			47	46	
4.0	20	171/81	99	45	38.4	0.74	0.79	8.0	0.94	7.49	20	115	113	9	29	27	-2	47	44	0.28
4.5	25		100	41	39.1	0.77	0.81	8.1	0.95			118			28			46	44	
5.0	25	168/78	100	37	39.8	0.80	0.83	8.3	0.96	7.51	19	120	123	2	27	24	-3	46	44	0.20
5.5	30		102	38	40.4	0.81	0.84	8.2	0.96			122			26			46	44	
6.0	30	168/78	103	38	40.9	0.82	0.85	8.3	0.96	7.51	18	123	133	-7	24	23	-1	46	44	0.17
6.5	35		106	40	43.9	0.86	0.88	8.3	0.98			124			24			47	46	
7.0	35	168/78	108	41	46.8	0.90	0.91	8.4	0.99	7.50	18	125	122	5	23	23	0	48	48	0.20
	Recovery		96	38	39.7	0.78	0.81	8.4	0.96			123			24			47	45	
	Recovery		84	34	32.5	0.66	0.71	8.5	0.93			121			25			45	42	
	Recovery		82	31	29.3	0.60	0.62	7.6	0.96			123			25			45	43	
	Recovery	156/72	79	28	26.0	0.53	0.53	6.7	1.00	7.49	18	124	128	-2	25	24	-1	45	45	0.18

exercise. The respiratory alkalosis in response to exercise as observed in this patient on both study occasions is unusual and probably abnormal.

In the post-propranolol study (Fig. 28-B), after an initial elevation, $\dot{V}_E$ remains relatively unchanged (panel 1, Fig. 28-B) while R remains high (panel 8, Fig. 28-B) and Pa_{CO_2} falls further as work rate is increased (panel 9, Fig. 28-B and Table 28-4). The further hyperventilation of the arterial blood (decrease in Pa_{CO_2}) without an increase in $\dot{V}_E$ probably results from an inordinately small pulmonary blood flow increase in response to increasing work rate. This also accounts for the shallow $\dot{V}_{O_2}$ response as work rate is increased (panel 3, Fig. 28-B) and the low flat O₂-pulse response (panel 2, Fig. 28-B).

CONCLUSION

This patient has mitral stenosis with and without β-adrenergic blockade. This is a rare occurrence of exercise-induced respiratory alkalosis.

CASE 29 *Congenital heart disease*

CLINICAL FINDINGS

This 18-year-old young woman was referred to evaluate exercise dyspnea. She had a known history of dextrocardia and had had a pulmonic valve replacement as a child. Pulmonary hypertension and pulmonic valve insufficiency were recently diagnosed. She had had dyspnea from climbing less than one flight of stairs. She had smoked cigarettes for 1 year. Examination revealed normal breath sounds and a grade II diastolic murmur over the upper sternum.

EXERCISE FINDINGS

Exercise studies with the patient breathing room air and 100% O_2 were performed twice in the same morning on a cycle ergometer with an intermediate rest period. On both occasions, arterial blood was sampled every second minute and intra-arterial pressure was recorded from a percutaneously placed brachial artery catheter. The patient pedalled at 60 rpm without an added load for 3 minutes. The work rate was then increased in a ramp of 7 W per minute to tolerance. The patient was cooperative, appeared to give good efforts, and stopped exercise on both occasions because of dyspnea. Resting and repeated ECGs during exercise (taken with reversed limb and right chest leads) did not reveal arrhythmias or evidence of ischemia. Arterial saturation by ear oximetry fell from 97% at rest to 87% at maximal exercise, but direct arterial blood gas measurements did not support this change.

TABLE 29-1. *Selected Respiratory Function Data*

MEASUREMENT	PREDICTED	MEASURED
Age, yr		18
Sex		Female
Height, cm		160
Weight, kg	61	49
Hematocrit, %		39
VC, L	3.38	2.20
IC, L	2.25	1.61
TLC, L	4.81	3.62
FEV_1, L	2.97	1.91
FEV_1/VC, %	88	87
MVV, L/min		
direct	118	58
indirect	119	76
DL_{CO}, ml/mm Hg/min	25.1	12.6

TABLE 29-2. *Selected Exercise Data*

MEASUREMENT	PREDICTED	ROOM AIR	OXYGEN
Maximum $\dot{V}O_2$, L/min	1.93	0.76	
Maximum HR, beats/min	202	111	113
Maximum O_2 pulse, ml/beat	9.6	6.8	
$\Delta\dot{V}O_2/\Delta WR$, ml/min/W	10.3	6.3	
AT, L/min	> 0.87	< 0.65	
Work rate, max, W		< 35	35
Blood pressure, mm Hg (rest, max ex)		96/60,126/66	102/60,114/66
Maximum $\dot{V}E$, L/min		47	38
Exercise breathing reserve, L/min			
using direct MVV	> 15	11	20
using indirect MVV	> 15	19	38
O_2 saturation, oximeter (rest, max ex)		97,87	
Pa_{O_2}, mm Hg (rest, max ex)		75,81	479,532
$P(A - a)_{O_2}$ mm Hg (rest, max ex)		40,42	203,150
$P(a - ET)_{CO_2}$, mm Hg (rest, max ex)		5,6	3,4
V_D/V_T (rest, max ex)		0.31,0.37	0.35,0.35
HCO_3^-, mEq/L (rest, recovery)		20,19	21,20

Fig. 29-A. *Air breathing.*

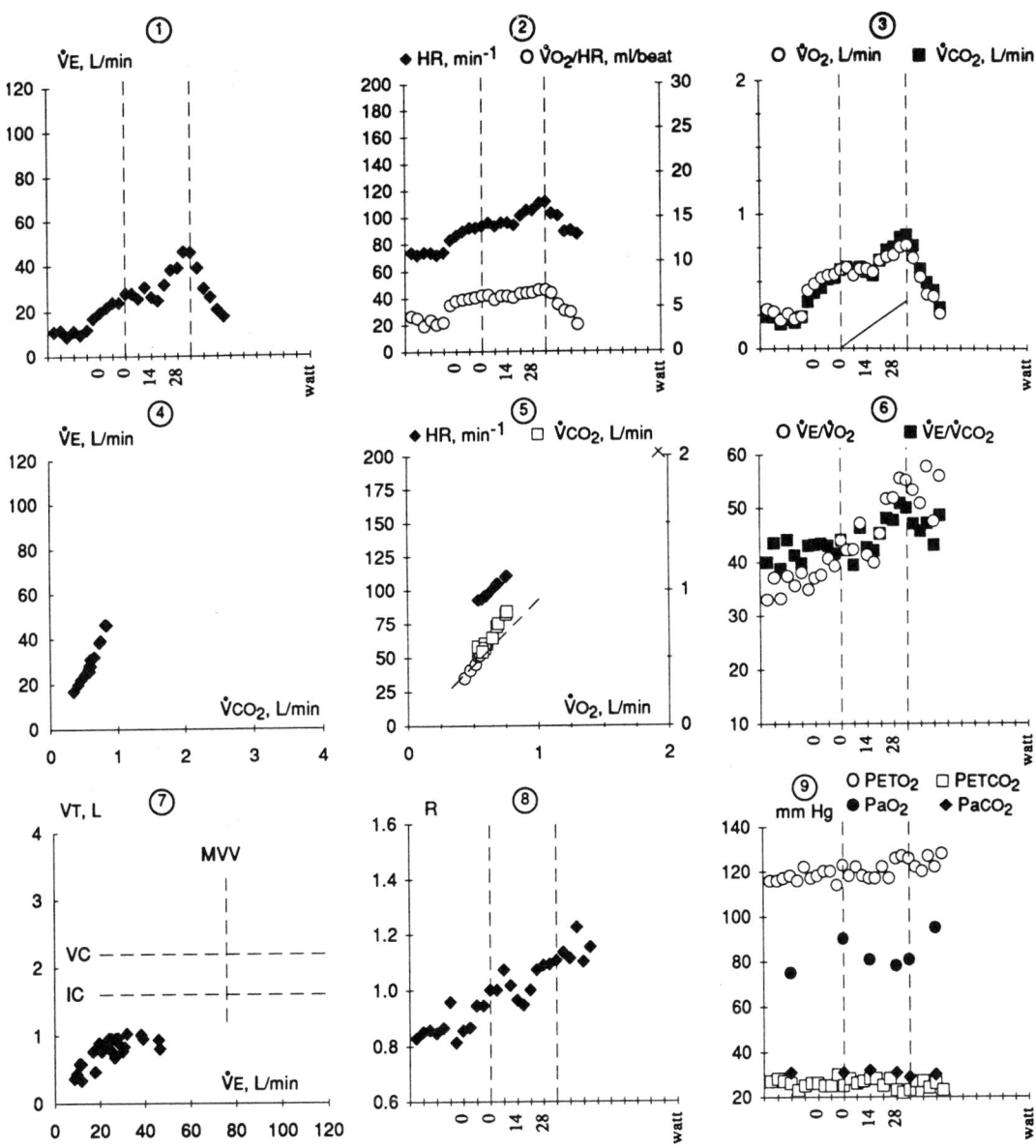

1. Vertical dashed lines in panels 1 to 3 and 6, 8, and 9 indicate the beginning and the end of increasing work period.

2. Unloaded cycling is performed for 3 minutes before the left vertical dashed line.

3. In panel 3, the diagonal line shows the increase of $\dot{V}O_2$ at a slope of 10 ml/min/W.

4. In panel 5, the diagonal dashed line has a slope of 1; the ''x'' in the upper right is the predicted maximum heart rate and $\dot{V}O_2$ for the subject.

FIG. 29-B. *Oxygen breathing.*

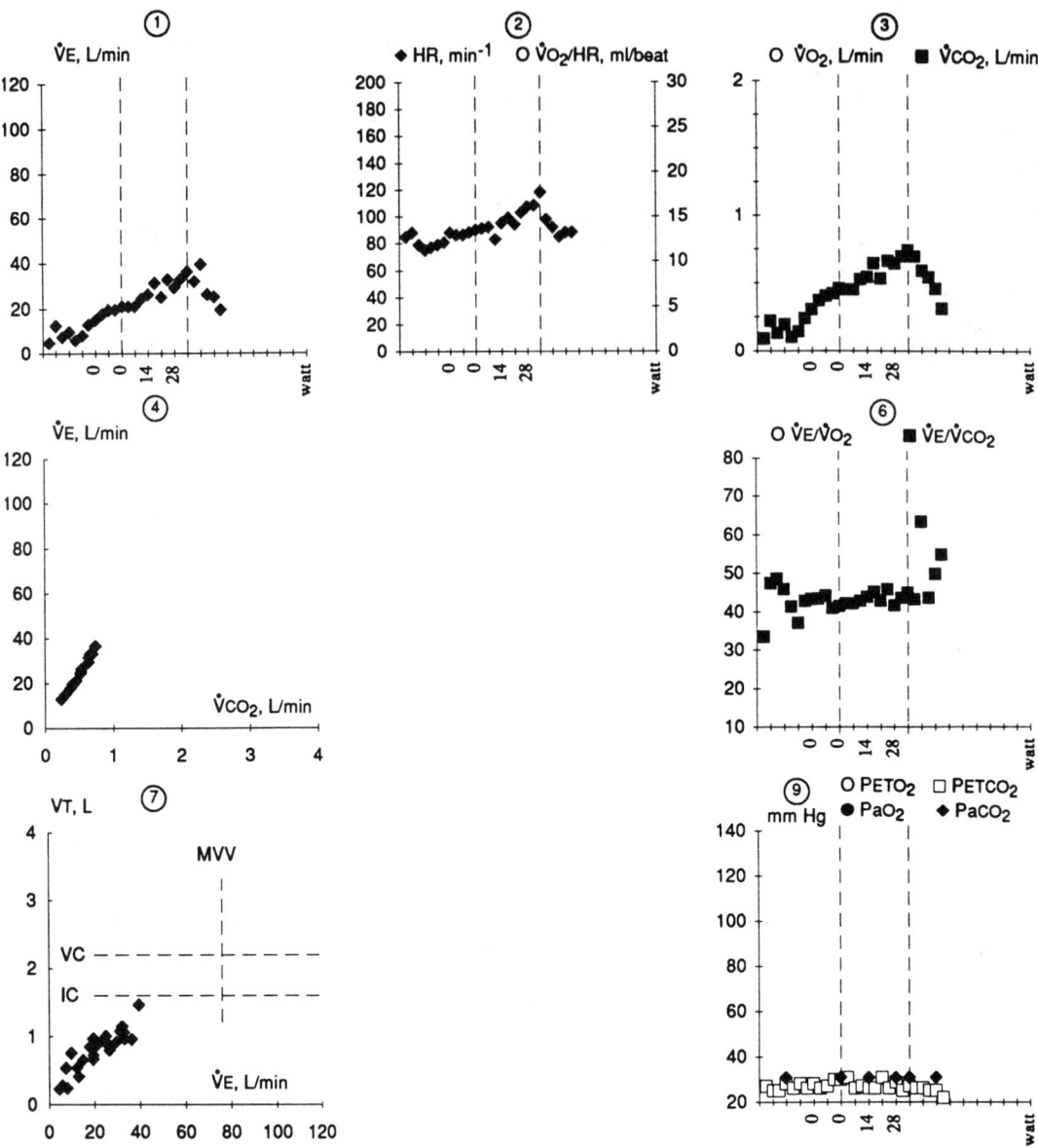

1. Vertical dashed lines in panels 1 to 3 and 6 and 9 indicate the beginning and the end of increasing work period.
2. Unloaded cycling is performed for 3 minutes before the left vertical dashed line.

TABLE 29-3. *Air breathing.*

Time min	Work rate watts	BP mm Hg	HR min⁻¹	f min⁻¹	V̇E L/min BTPS	V̇CO2 L/min STPD	V̇O2 L/min STPD	V̇O2/HR ml/beat	R	pH	HCO3 meq/L	PO2, mm Hg ET	a	(A-a)	PCO2, mm Hg ET	a	(a-ET)	V̇E/V̇CO2	V̇E/V̇O2	VD/VT
	Rest		74	19	11.2	0.24	0.29	3.9	0.83			116			27			40	33	
	Rest		72	20	11.7	0.23	0.27	3.8	0.85			116			28			43	37	
	Rest		74	24	9.0	0.18	0.21	2.8	0.86			117			27			39	33	
	Rest	96/60	74	20	11.4	0.22	0.26	3.5	0.85	7.43	20	118	75	40	26	31	5	44	37	0.31
	Rest		72	22	9.7	0.19	0.22	3.1	0.86			116			23			41	36	
	Rest		74	35	12.1	0.23	0.24	3.2	0.96			122			25			40	38	
	Unloaded		83	22	16.9	0.35	0.43	5.2	0.81			117			26			43	35	
	Unloaded		86	22	19.6	0.41	0.48	5.6	0.85			118			26			43	37	
	Unloaded		89	27	21.8	0.45	0.52	5.8	0.87			120			25			43	38	
	Unloaded		92	25	24.0	0.51	0.54	5.9	0.94			120			25			43	41	
	Unloaded		92	29	24.0	0.52	0.55	6.0	0.95			114			30			41	39	
	Unloaded	102/66	93	29	28.0	0.58	0.58	6.2	1.00	7.46	22	123	90	29	25	31	6	44	44	0.34
0.5	4		96	31	27.9	0.60	0.60	6.3	1.00			118			28			42	42	
1.0	7		93	34	25.7	0.58	0.54	5.8	1.07			122			26			39	42	
1.5	11		96	37	30.9	0.60	0.59	6.1	1.02			118			27			46	47	
2.0	14	114/66	96	28	26.7	0.57	0.59	6.1	0.97	7.43	21	117	81	36	28	32	4	43	41	0.34
2.5	18		94	26	24.9	0.54	0.57	6.1	0.95			117			28			42	40	
3.0	21		101	31	32.0	0.65	0.65	6.4	1.00			122			25			45	45	
3.5	25		105	38	38.3	0.73	0.68	6.5	1.07			117			28			48	52	
4.0	28	126/66	105	41	39.2	0.75	0.69	6.6	1.09	7.43	20	126	78	43	23	31	8	48	52	0.38
4.5	32		110	57	46.5	0.82	0.75	6.8	1.09			127			22			51	56	
5.0	35		111	49	46.1	0.84	0.76	6.8	1.11	7.45	20	126	81	42	23	29	6	50	55	0.37
	Recovery		103	41	39.2	0.76	0.67	6.5	1.13			122			27			47	53	
	Recovery		101	39	30.2	0.59	0.53	5.2	1.11			120			27			46	51	
	Recovery		89	39	26.4	0.49	0.40	4.5	1.23			127			24			47	58	
	Recovery	108/60	90	27	20.8	0.43	0.39	4.3	1.10	7.41	19	122	95	27	26	30	4	43	47	0.29
	Recovery		87	38	17.8	0.30	0.26	3.0	1.15			128			23			49	56	

Interpretation

COMMENTS

This is a patient with known congenital heart disease, previously surgically repaired, with recent deterioration, and mild restrictive lung disease. The arterial oxyhemoglobin saturation did not fall during the brief exercise period when directly measured, but ear oximetry saturation declined 10% during the same time.

ANALYSIS

In flow chart 1, in the room air study the maximum V̇O2 was reduced while the anaerobic threshold was also low (Table 29-2). This directs us to flow chart 4, which leads us through branchpoints 4.1 and 4.2 to lung disease with impaired peripheral oxygenation. Although this is correct, it is incomplete. More appropriate is flow chart 5. The VD/VT, $P(A-a)_{O_2}$, and $P(a-ET)_{CO_2}$ are abnormal (branchpoint 5.1), whereas the breathing reserve is normal (branchpoint 5.3). Evidence of a reduced cardiac output response and of a reduced $\Delta V̇O_2/\Delta WR$ is indicative of a circulatory limitation. Despite the patient's symptoms of dyspnea on air and O_2 breathing, no good evidence indicates ventilatory limitation. The breathing reserve is borderline normal on air and O_2 breathing. O_2 breathing provided no benefit to the patient with respect to work capacity or the

TABLE 29-4. *Oxygen breathing.*

Time min	Work rate watts	BP mm Hg	HR min⁻¹	f min⁻¹	$\dot{V}E$ L/min BTPS	$\dot{V}CO_2$ L/min STPD	$\dot{V}O_2$ L/min STPD	$\frac{\dot{V}O_2}{HR}$ ml/beat	R	pH	HCO₃ meq/L	PO2, mm Hg ET	a	(A-a)	PCO2, mm Hg ET	a	(a-ET)	$\frac{\dot{V}E}{\dot{V}CO_2}$	$\frac{\dot{V}E}{\dot{V}O_2}$	VD VT
	Rest		85	20	4.7	0.09									27			33		
	Rest		88	23	12.4	0.22									25			47		
	Rest		79	14	7.5	0.13									25			49		
	Rest	102/60	75	13	9.8	0.19				7.45	21		479	203	28	31	3	46		0.35
	Rest		77	22	6.0	0.10									26			41		
	Rest		79	33	8.0	0.14									28			37		
	Unloaded		81	31	12.9	0.24									26			43		
	Unloaded		88	23	14.9	0.30									28			43		
	Unloaded		86	21	17.8	0.37									26			43		
	Unloaded		86	20	19.4	0.40									27			44		
	Unloaded		88	27	19.5	0.42									30			41		
	Unloaded	114/66	90	23	21.0	0.46				7.42	20		533	149	30	31	1	41		0.30
0.5	4		91	24	21.0	0.45									31			42		
1.0	7		92	24	21.0	0.45									26			42		
1.5	11		83	26	24.4	0.52									27			43		
2.0	14	120/72	95	33	26.4	0.54				7.44	21		536	146	26	31	5	44		0.32
2.5	18		99	29	31.3	0.64									26			45		
3.0	21		94	28	25.1	0.53									31			43		
3.5	25		103	31	32.8	0.66									26			46		
4.0	28	114/72	107	32	29.4	0.64				7.42	20		534	148	29	31	2	42		0.30
4.5	32		108	34	33.0	0.69									25			44		
5.0	35	114/66	118	38	36.4	0.74				7.43	20		532	150	27	31	4	45		0.35
	Recovery		98	28	32.1	0.69									26			43		
	Recovery		92	27	39.6	0.59									26			63		
	Recovery		85	30	26.1	0.54									25			44		
	Recovery	90/48	88	25	25.0	0.46				7.42	20		543	139	25	31	6	50		0.40
	Recovery		88	29	19.4	0.31									22			55		

ventilatory response. This suggests that the sensation of dyspnea may be due to her known pulmonary hypertension (perhaps via J-receptor stimulation), which is worsened by exercise. Neither the breathing frequency nor the VT/IC is abnormally high on either test. The high heart rate reserve suggests chronotropic insufficiency. The high Pa_{O_2} during O_2 breathing excludes a significant right to left shunt.

CONCLUSION

This patient demonstrates a severe cardiovascular limitation to exercise, secondary to congenital heart disease, subjectively experienced as dyspnea. For some reason, the patient regulates her Pa_{CO_2} at a low level (has a low set-point), thereby requiring a high ventilation to eliminate the metabolic CO_2 of exercise (see the high $\dot{V}E/\dot{V}CO_2$ at the anaerobic threshold in panel 6 of Fig. 29-A). This high ventilatory requirement is likely the main factor stimulating dyspnea and limiting exercise tolerance.

As is not uncommonly seen in patients with cardiovascular limitation to exercise, the ear oximeter values were falsely decreased at maximal exercise, probably because of inadequate cardiac output and reduced perfusion of the ear lobe.[1]

Reference

1. Hansen, J.E., and Casaburi, R.: Validity of ear oximetry in clinical exercise testing. Chest, 91:333–337, 1987.

CASE 30 *Peripheral vascular disease*

CLINICAL FINDINGS

This 65-year-old cigarette-smoking man was evaluated as part of a research study looking for coronary artery calcification. He had been overweight and a known diabetic for approximately 6 years. He had continued to lead an active life, but had been limited in his speed of walking for approximately 5 years, with pain in his thighs and calves, especially on the right side. He had had some cough and sputum production for a decade. He denied chest pain, shortness of breath, wheezing, edema, or skin problems. Pulses could not be palpated in the legs except for a faint right femoral artery pulse. The patient had no edema; skin warmth and color were good. The coronary arteries were free of calcification.

EXERCISE FINDINGS

The patient performed exercise on a cycle ergometer. He pedalled at 60 rpm without an added load for 3 minutes. The work rate was then increased 15 W per minute to tolerance. Heart rate and rhythm were continuously monitored; 12-lead ECGs were obtained during rest, exercise, and recovery. Blood pressure was measured with a sphygmomanometer every minute. The patient appeared to give an excellent effort and stopped exercise because of bilateral thigh and calf pain. He denied chest pain or discomfort during or after the study. The ECGs showed occasional premature ventricular contractions both at rest and during exercise, but were otherwise normal. No abnormal ST segments or T waves were noted before, during, or after exercise.

TABLE 30-1. *Selected Respiratory Function Data*

MEASUREMENT	PREDICTED	MEASURED
Age, yr		65
Sex		Male
Height, cm		170
Weight, kg	74	88
Hematocrit, %		42
VC, L	3.43	3.65
IC, L	2.44	3.20
FEV$_1$, L	2.74	2.48
FEV$_1$/VC, %	79	68
MVV, L/min	110	92

TABLE 30-2. *Selected Exercise Data*

MEASUREMENT	PREDICTED	MEASURED
Maximum $\dot{V}O_2$, L/min	2.04	1.06
Maximum HR, beats/min	155	135
Maximum O_2 pulse, ml/beat	13.2	7.9
$\Delta\dot{V}O_2/\Delta WR$, ml/min/W	10.3	6.9
AT, L/min	> 0.95	0.8
Blood pressure, mm Hg (rest, max)		164/88,278/110
Maximum $\dot{V}E$, L/min		33
Exercise breathing reserve, L/min	> 15	59

TABLE 30-3.

Time min	Work rate watts	BP mm Hg	HR min^{-1}	f min^{-1}	$\dot{V}E$ L/min BTPS	$\dot{V}CO_2$ L/min STPD	$\dot{V}O_2$ L/min STPD	$\dfrac{\dot{V}O_2}{HR}$ ml/beat	R	pH	HCO$_3$ meq/L	PO2, mm Hg ET	a	(A-a)	PCO2, mm Hg ET	a	(a-ET)	$\dfrac{\dot{V}E}{\dot{V}CO_2}$	$\dfrac{\dot{V}E}{\dot{V}O_2}$	VD VT
	Rest	164/88																		
	Rest		95	22	12.8	0.36	0.36	3.8	1.00			111			38			30	30	
	Rest	188/80	93	21	11.1	0.32	0.36	3.9	0.89			106			41			29	26	
	Rest		95	19	11.2	0.32	0.35	3.7	0.91			110			38			30	27	
	Rest	218/80	94	20	10.6	0.30	0.33	3.5	0.91			108			39			30	27	
	Rest		97	22	8.0	0.20	0.23	2.4	0.87			105			40			31	27	
	Rest	198/82	98	20	10.3	0.29	0.35	3.6	0.83			105			40			30	25	
	Unloaded		110	20	14.1	0.46	0.52	4.7	0.88			104			41			27	24	
	Unloaded	214/100	110	20	13.5	0.44	0.54	4.9	0.81			100			42			27	22	
	Unloaded		113	20	13.4	0.39	0.49	4.3	0.80			108			37			30	24	
	Unloaded	238/96	112	20	17.3	0.62	0.72	6.4	0.86			100			43			25	22	
	Unloaded		113	19	17.8	0.63	0.72	6.4	0.88			101			44			26	22	
	Unloaded	254/90	111	22	17.1	0.59	0.68	6.1	0.87			101			44			26	22	
0.5	7.5		115	20	19.2	0.69	0.75	6.5	0.92			102			44			25	23	
1.0	15	255/100	117	20	19.2	0.70	0.76	6.5	0.92			103			43			25	23	
1.5	22.5		119	22	20.6	0.74	0.79	6.6	0.94			103			43			25	24	
2.0	30	245/114	121	19	23.7	0.88	0.94	7.8	0.94			103			43			25	23	
2.5	37.5		122	21	23.7	0.88	0.91	7.5	0.97			103			44			25	24	
3.0	45	252/110	125	21	24.7	0.91	0.94	7.5	0.97			103			44			25	24	
3.5	52.5		127	19	24.8	0.92	0.92	7.2	1.00			105			44			25	25	
4.0	60	256/114	130	21	29.7	1.08	1.04	8.0	1.04			107			43			26	27	
4.5	67.5		131	21	32.7	1.15	1.07	8.2	1.07			109			42			27	29	
5.0	75	278/110	135	24	32.6	1.13	1.06	7.9	1.07			111			42			27	29	
	Recovery		126	21	28.4	1.02	0.95	7.5	1.07			108			44			26	28	
	Recovery	268/90	124	20	26.5	0.95	0.86	6.9	1.10			109			44			26	29	
	Recovery		119	26	22.6	0.71	0.63	5.3	1.13			115			40			29	32	
	Recovery	241/86	113	23	21.2	0.72	0.64	5.7	1.13			111			42			27	30	

Interpretation

COMMENTS

The patient has mild, asymptomatic airways obstruction, diabetes mellitus, obesity, and clinical evidence of peripheral vascular disease without heart disease.

ANALYSIS

In flow chart 1, maximum $\dot{V}O_2$ and the anaerobic threshold are reduced (Table 30-2). Proceeding next to flow chart 4, the high breathing reserve (branchpoint 4.1) and normal VE/$\dot{V}CO_2$ at the anaerobic threshold (branchpoint 4.3) lead us to "O$_2$ flow problem of non-pulmonary origin." The normal hematocrit (branchpoint 4.4) indicates a cardiovascular disorder with a low unchanging O$_2$ pulse (branchpoint 4.6). The findings of exercise-induced systemic hypertension, leg pain, low $\Delta\dot{V}O_2/\Delta WR$, and high heart rate reserve all support the diagnosis of peripheral vascular disease. The absence of ECG changes of myocardial ischemia suggests that the coronary vessels are relatively uninvolved.

CONCLUSION

The exercise-induced hypertension is especially typical of peripheral vascular disease. Although many such patients are limited by associated coronary artery disease, this does not seem to be true for this man.

Fɪɢ. 30-A.

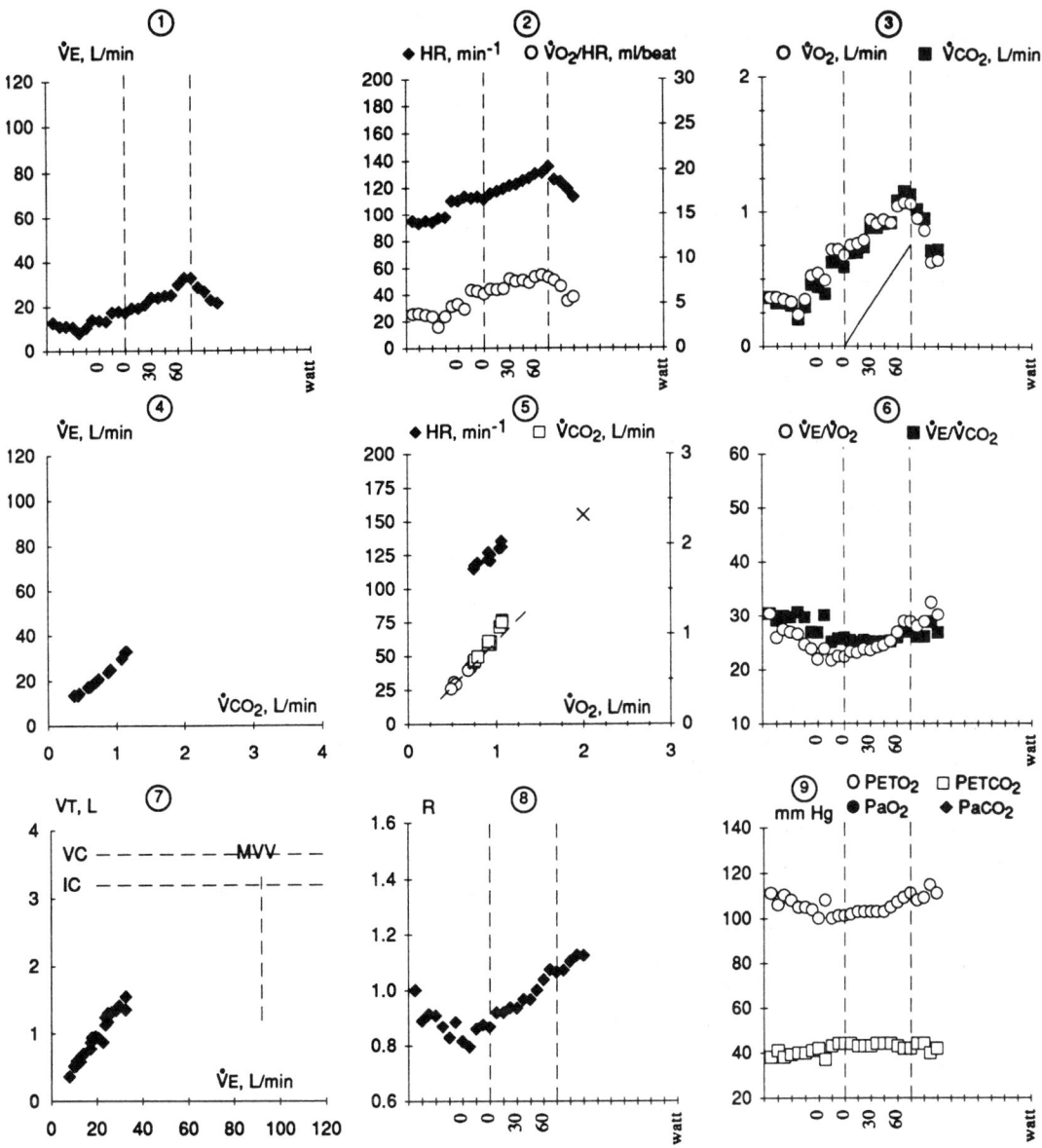

1. Vertical dashed lines in panels 1 to 3 and 6, 8, and 9 indicate the beginning and the end of increasing work period.
2. Unloaded cycling is performed for 3 minutes before the left vertical dashed line.
3. In panel 3, the diagonal line shows the increase of $\dot{V}O_2$ at a slope of 10 ml/min/W.
4. In panel 5, the diagonal dashed line has a slope of 1; the "x" in the upper right is the predicted maximum heart rate and $\dot{V}O_2$ for the subject.

CASE 31 *Peripheral vascular disease, accompanied by pulmonary vascular and obstructive airway diseases*

CLINICAL FINDINGS

This 69-year-old retired shipyard worker had been a heavy cigarette smoker until 5 years before. For more than a decade he had noted excessive shortness of breath on climbing one flight of stairs. For the last several years his activity had been limited by cramps in the calves after walking approximately 100 yards; they were relieved by rest. He took no medication. Examination revealed a left cataract and reduced arterial pulsations in the legs, but no rales, wheezing, or edema. Chest x-ray studies showed pleural thickening on the right, an elevated left leaf of the diaphragm, and normal heart size.

EXERCISE FINDINGS

The patient performed exercise on a cycle ergometer. He pedalled at 60 rpm without added load for 3 minutes. The work rate was then increased 10 W per minute to his symptom-limited maximum. Blood was sampled every second minute, and intra-arterial blood pressure was recorded from a percutaneously placed brachial artery catheter. The patient stopped exercise because of pain in both calves. He developed frequent premature ventricular contractions and hypertension during exercise that resolved during recovery. Resting, exercise, and recovery ECG tracings were otherwise normal.

TABLE 31-1. *Selected Respiratory Function Data*

MEASUREMENT	PREDICTED	MEASURED
Age, yr		69
Sex		Male
Height, cm		165
Weight, kg	70	76
Hematocrit, %		40
VC, L	3.68	3.25
IC, L	2.45	2.69
TLC, L	6.11	6.05
FEV_1, L	2.87	1.92
FEV_1/VC, %	78	59
MVV, L/min	113	87
D_{LCO}, ml/mm Hg/min	21.8	17.5

TABLE 31-2. *Selected Exercise Data*

MEASUREMENT	PREDICTED	MEASURED
Maximum $\dot{V}O_2$, L/min	1.78	0.83
Maximum HR, beats/min	151	155
Maximum O_2 pulse, ml/beat	11.8	7.2
$\Delta\dot{V}O_2/\Delta WR$, ml/min/W	10.3	5.2
AT, L/min	> 0.80	not reached
Blood pressure, mm Hg (rest, max)		198/84,264/120
Maximum $\dot{V}E$, L/min		30
Exercise breathing reserve, L/min	> 15	57
Pa_{O_2}, mm Hg (rest, max ex)		87,80
$P(A-a)_{O_2}$, mm Hg (rest, max ex)		11,28
$P(a-ET)_{CO_2}$, mm Hg (rest, max ex)		5,1
V_D/V_T (rest, heavy ex)		0.47,0.38
HCO_3^-, mEq/L (rest, 2-min recov)		24,23

Fig. 31-A.

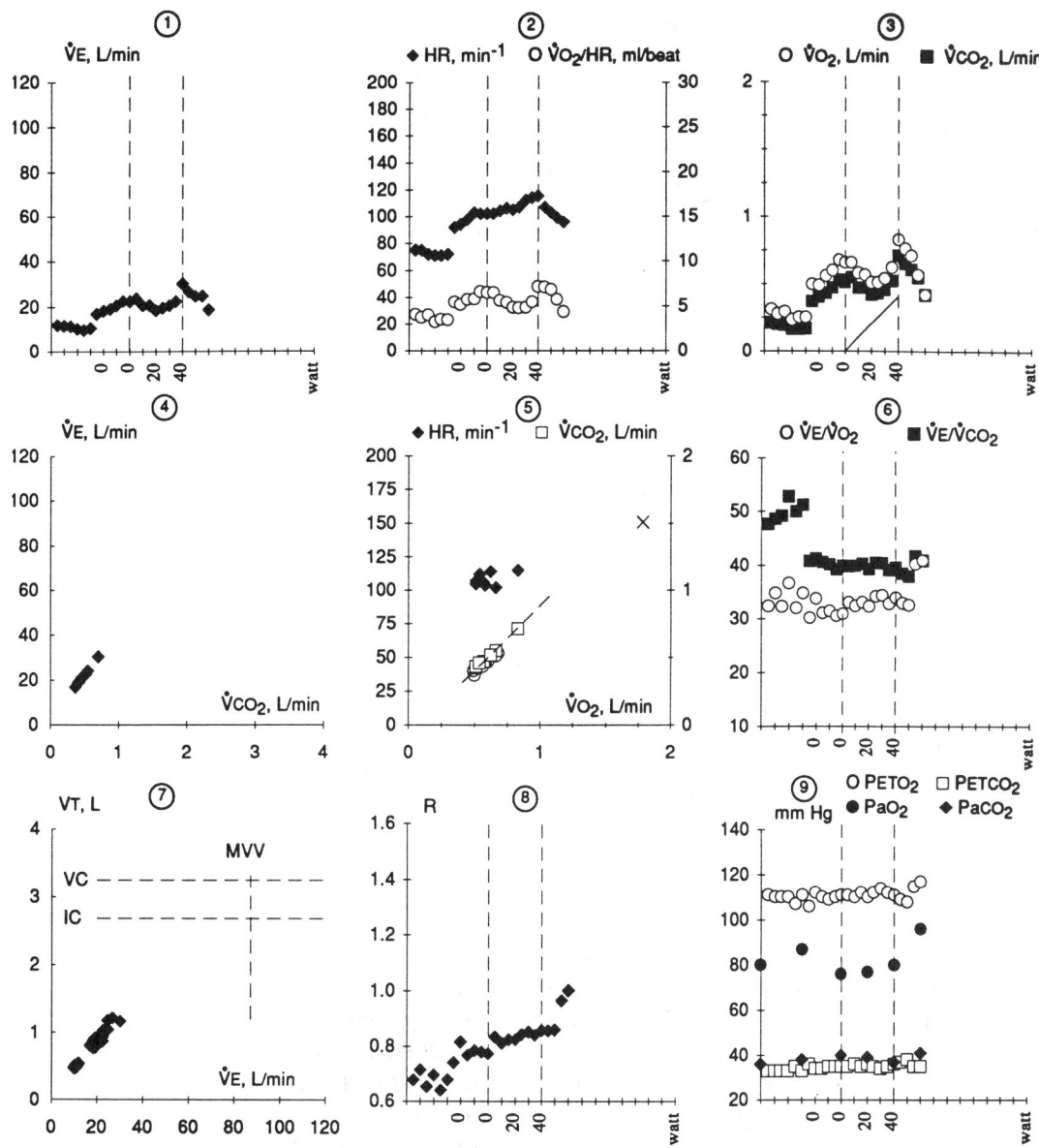

1. Vertical dashed lines in panels 1 to 3 and 6, 8, and 9 indicate the beginning and the end of increasing work period.
2. Unloaded cycling is performed for 3 minutes before the left vertical dashed line.
3. In panel 3, the diagonal line shows the increase of $\dot{V}O_2$ at a slope of 10 ml/min/W.
4. In panel 5, the diagonal dashed line has a slope of 1; the "x" in the upper right is the predicted maximum heart rate and $\dot{V}O_2$ for the subject.

Interpretation

COMMENTS

Resting respiratory function studies show the patient to have moderate airflow obstruction (Table 31-1). The resting electrocardiogram is normal.

ANALYSIS

In flow chart 1, the maximum $\dot{V}O_2$ is reduced while the anaerobic threshold is borderline normal. (Table 31-2), If we were to consider the anaerobic threshold normal, we would proceed through branchpoints 1.1, 1.2, and 1.3 to flow chart 3. The

TABLE 31-3.

Time min	Work rate watts	BP mm Hg	HR min^{-1}	f min^{-1}	$\dot{V}_E$ L/min BTPS	$\dot{V}CO_2$ L/min STPD	$\dot{V}O_2$ L/min STPD	$\dfrac{\dot{V}O_2}{HR}$ ml/beat	R	pH	HCO$_3$ meq/L	PO2, mm Hg ET	a	(A-a)	PCO2, mm Hg ET	a	(a-ET)	$\dfrac{\dot{V}_E}{\dot{V}CO_2}$	$\dfrac{\dot{V}_E}{\dot{V}O_2}$	$\dfrac{V_D}{V_T}$
	Rest	210/84								7.43	23		80			36				
	Rest		75	22	11.9	0.21	0.31	4.1	0.68			111			33			48	32	
	Rest		75	22	11.6	0.20	0.28	3.7	0.71			110			33			49	35	
	Rest		72	23	11.3	0.19	0.29	4.0	0.66			110			33			49	32	
	Rest		71	22	10.3	0.16	0.23	3.2	0.70			110			33			53	37	
	Rest		71	20	9.7	0.16	0.25	3.5	0.64			107			35			50	32	
	Rest	198/84	72	20	10.4	0.17	0.25	3.5	0.68	7.41	24	111	87	11	33	38	5	51	35	0.47
	Unloaded		92	21	16.9	0.37	0.50	5.4	0.74			106			36			41	30	
	Unloaded		94	21	18.3	0.40	0.49	5.2	0.82			112			34			41	34	
	Unloaded		98	21	19.2	0.43	0.56	5.7	0.77			110			34			41	31	
	Unloaded		103	22	20.7	0.47	0.60	5.8	0.78			109			35			40	31	
	Unloaded		102	22	22.6	0.53	0.68	6.7	0.78			110			35			39	30	
	Unloaded	246/93	102	24	22.4	0.51	0.66	6.5	0.77	7.40	24	111	76	25	35	40	5	40	31	0.42
0.5	10		102	23	23.8	0.55	0.66	6.5	0.83			111			35			40	33	
1.0	10		104	23	20.7	0.47	0.58	5.6	0.81			110			36			40	32	
1.5	20		106	24	20.9	0.47	0.57	5.4	0.82			112			35			40	33	
2.0	20	252/114	105	24	18.5	0.42	0.51	4.9	0.82	7.40	24	110	77	27	36	39	3	39	32	0.39
2.5	30		107	25	19.5	0.43	0.51	4.8	0.84			112			35			40	34	
3.0	30		112	25	20.7	0.46	0.54	4.8	0.85			114			34			40	34	
3.5	40		114	26	22.5	0.52	0.62	5.4	0.84			112			35			39	33	
4.0	40	264/120	115	26	30.3	0.71	0.83	7.2	0.86	7.40	23	111	80	28	36	37	1	40	34	0.38
	Recovery		107	22	26.8	0.65	0.76	7.1	0.86			109			37			38	33	
	Recovery		103	21	24.8	0.61	0.71	6.9	0.86			108			38			38	32	
	Recovery		99	24	24.9	0.55	0.57	5.8	0.96			115			35			42	40	
	Recovery	210/96	96	21	18.9	0.42	0.42	4.4	1.00	7.37	23	117	96	13	35	41	6	41	41	0.44

breathing reserve (branchpoint 3.1) is normal, but frequent premature ventricular contractions occur during exercise (branchpoint 3.3). There may well be some myocardial ischemia, but this is an unsatisfactory final end-point, considering the other abnormalities noted. Therefore, we consider the anaerobic threshold to be indeterminate and use flow chart 5. While the maximum work rate performed is quite low, the maximum exercise V_D/V_T is high, and $P(a-\text{ET})_{CO_2}$ and $P(A-a)_{O_2}$ are at the borderline of abnormality (branchpoint 5.1). The breathing reserve is high (branchpoint 5.3). This suggests that the disease process is either that of pulmonary vascular or circulatory origin. Pa_{O_2} becomes slightly abnormal with exercise (Table 31-3 and panel 9, Fig. 31-A). Other measurements listed under pulmonary vascular diseases are consistent with this diagnosis; however, the high heart rate reserve is inconsistent with pulmonary vascular disease being the symptom limiting diagnosis. Returning to consider branchpoints 5.1, 5.2, and 5.5, we reach branchpoint 5.8. The patient has

systemic hypertension, reduced arterial pulses in the legs and lower extremity pain with exercise suggesting that peripheral vascular disease is the diagnosis limiting exercise performance. Supporting this is the very low value of $\Delta \dot{V}O_2/\Delta WR$ (branchpoint 5.8). ($\dot{V}O_2$ could increase only slightly above that required for unloaded cycling).

CONCLUSION

Both peripheral and pulmonary vascular disease are present, with the former being the primary limiting disorder. The exercise-induced arrhythmia also suggests the presence of myocardial ischemia, perhaps from the high cardiac afterload induced by systemic hypertension. The poor perfusion of the exercising muscles probably prevented the cellular metabolic acidosis from being reflected in the arterial blood. Note that while this patient has moderate airflow obstruction, it does not appear to be important in this patient's exercise limitation.

CASE 32 *Circulatory disease: Heart and peripheral vascular, with anemia and carboxyhemoglobinemia*

CLINICAL FINDINGS

This 54-year-old male bartender was referred for preoperative study to evaluate his exercise capacity. He occasionally had calf pain at rest and always after walking one block. He had smoked at least 60 pack years but denied cardiac or respiratory symptoms. The right iliac and superficial femoral arteries were demonstrated to be obstructed on angiography. He was moderately anemic (hematocrit = 34) with occult blood in the stool.

EXERCISE FINDINGS

The patient performed exercise on a cycle ergometer. He pedalled at 60 rpm without added load for 3 minutes. The work rate was then increased 15 W per minute to his symptom-limited maximum. Blood was sampled every second minute, and intra-arterial blood pressure was recorded from a percutaneously placed brachial artery catheter. Resting and exercise ECGs were normal. He stopped exercise because of severe leg pain, which was more prominent on the left. Carboxyhemoglobin was 5.6% in his resting arterial blood.

TABLE 32-1. *Selected Respiratory Function Data*

MEASUREMENT	PREDICTED	MEASURED
Age, yr		59
Sex		Male
Height, cm		168
Weight, kg	72	60
Hematocrit, %		34
VC, L	3.94	3.84
IC, L	2.63	3.64
TLC, L	5.86	7.16
FEV_1, L	3.12	3.07
FEV_1/VC, %	79	80
MVV, L/min	136	110
D_{LCO}, ml/mm Hg/min	23.0	22.9

TABLE 32-2. *Selected Exercise Data*

MEASUREMENT	PREDICTED	MEASURED
Maximum $\dot{V}_{O_2}$, L/min	1.90	0.82
Maximum HR, beats/min	161	141
Maximum O_2 pulse, ml/beat	11.8	5.8
$\Delta\dot{V}_{O_2}/\Delta WR$, ml/min/W	10.3	6.2
AT, L/min	> 0.84	0.7
Blood pressure, mm Hg (rest, max)		168/72,255/114
Maximum $\dot{V}_E$, L/min		60
Exercise breathing reserve, L/min	> 15	50
Pa_{O_2}, mm Hg (rest, max ex)		94,117
$P(A-a)_{O_2}$, mm Hg (rest, max ex)		20,11
$P(a-ET)_{CO_2}$, mm Hg (rest, max ex)		3,2
V_D/V_T (rest, heavy ex)		0.45,0.38
HCO_3^-, mEq/L (rest, 2-min recov)		20,16

TABLE 32-3.

Time min	Work rate watts	BP mm Hg	HR min⁻¹	f min⁻¹	$\dot{V}E$ L/min BTPS	$\dot{V}CO_2$ L/min STPD	$\dot{V}O_2$ L/min STPD	$\dfrac{\dot{V}O_2}{HR}$ ml/beat	R	pH	HCO3 meq/L	PO2, mm Hg			PCO2, mm Hg			$\dfrac{\dot{V}E}{\dot{V}CO_2}$	$\dfrac{\dot{V}E}{\dot{V}O_2}$	$\dfrac{VD}{VT}$
												ET	a	(A-a)	ET	a	(a-ET)			
	Rest	168/72								7.43	20		90			31				
	Rest		93	18	12.0	0.20	0.24	2.6	0.83			116			27			52	44	
	Rest		94	15	14.0	0.25	0.29	3.1	0.86			117			28			51	44	
	Rest		92	16	14.3	0.19	0.23	2.5	0.83			116			28			68	56	
	Rest	168/72	95	14	11.7	0.19	0.23	2.4	0.83	7.42	20	116	94	20	28	31	3	55	46	0.45
	Rest		93	16	12.6	0.22	0.29	3.1	0.76			113			29			51	39	
	Rest		92	16	11.1	0.19	0.23	2.5	0.83			115			29			51	42	
	Unloaded		100	19	15.7	0.27	0.32	3.2	0.84			117			28			52	44	
	Unloaded		108	20	17.9	0.31	0.35	3.2	0.89			119			27			52	46	
	Unloaded		109	20	19.1	0.34	0.39	3.6	0.87			118			27			51	45	
	Unloaded		110	20	20.5	0.38	0.43	3.9	0.88			117			28			49	44	
	Unloaded		110	22	22.5	0.45	0.50	4.5	0.90			118			28			46	41	
	Unloaded	231/93	111	21	22.3	0.46	0.52	4.7	0.88	7.43	20	117	97	20	28	30	2	45	39	0.33
0.5	15		114	22	25.2	0.54	0.59	5.2	0.92			118			28			43	40	
1.0	15		116	24	27.1	0.57	0.61	5.3	0.93			120			27			44	41	
1.5	30		118	24	26.8	0.56	0.59	5.0	0.95			119			28			44	42	
2.0	30	245/102	121	24	32.3	0.68	0.69	5.7	0.99	7.43	19	121	106	15	27	29	2	45	44	0.31
2.5	45		127	28	37.4	0.74	0.69	5.4	1.07			124			25			47	51	
3.0	45		128	31	40.1	0.78	0.72	5.6	1.08			124			26			48	52	
3.5	60		134	36	48.6	0.86	0.72	5.4	1.19			129			23			53	63	
4.0	60	255/114	141	38	59.7	1.02	0.82	5.8	1.24	7.44	17	128	117	11	24	26	2	55	69	0.38
	Recovery		123	30	43.9	0.83	0.72	5.9	1.15			137			25			50	57	
	Recovery		113	25	38.6	0.74	0.61	5.4	1.21			127			25			49	60	
	Recovery		110	28	35.9	0.66	0.52	4.7	1.27			128			25			51	64	
	Recovery	258/102	107	26	31.7	0.59	0.46	4.3	1.28	7.39	16	127	117	11	26	27	1	50	64	0.34

Interpretation

COMMENTS

The resting respiratory function is normal, including the diffusing capacity (Table 32-1).

ANALYSIS

In flow chart 1, maximum $\dot{V}O_2$ and anaerobic threshold are reduced during exercise testing (Table 32-2). See flow chart 4 for further analysis. The breathing reserve is high (branchpoint 4.1). This patient has a combination of abnormalities that fit the major diagnoses leading from both branches of branchpoint 4.3. Mildly elevated values of VD/VT and $P(a-ET)_{CO_2}$, and normal $P(A-a)_{O_2}$ and Pa_{O_2} at maximal exercise suggest mild ventilation-perfusion mismatching such as might be seen in the case of minimal disease involving pulmonary circulation (right branch of branchpoint 4.3). The low $\Delta\dot{V}O_2/\Delta WR$, and low and flat O_2-pulse are marked, implicating an O_2 flow problem of nonpulmonary origin (left branch of branchpoint 4.3), however. While these major abnormalities point to a dominant cardiovascular disturbance, the patient's anemia and carboxyhemoglobinemia (branchpoint 4.4) may contribute to the abnormality in peripheral oxygenation. The steep heart rate versus $\dot{V}O_2$ relationship and low O_2 pulse noted with increasing work rate is consistent with either a cardiac abnormality, anemia, or a combination of both disorders.

CONCLUSION

Although the patient has ischemic peripheral vascular disease as documented by angiography and reflected by his leg pain in response to exercise, the flat O_2 pulse pattern as work rate is increased and the steep heart rate response to exercise suggest that heart disease, the patient's anemia, and carboxyhemoglobinemia are also major factors contributing to exercise limitation.

FIG. 32-A.

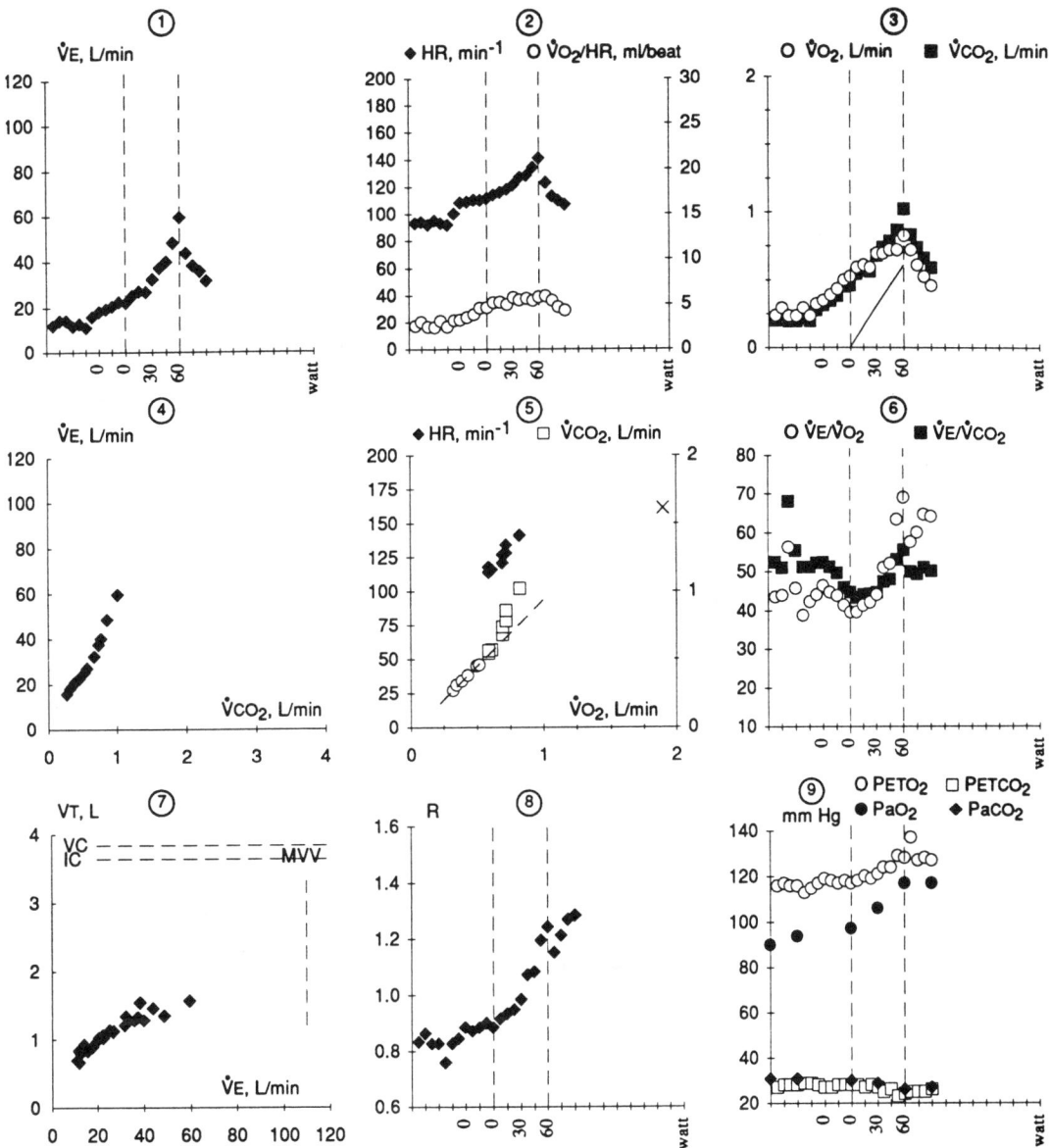

1. Vertical dashed lines in panels 1 to 3 and 6, 8, and 9 indicate the beginning and the end of increasing work period.

2. Unloaded cycling is performed for 3 minutes before the left vertical dashed line.

3. In panel 3, the diagonal line shows the increase of $\dot{V}O_2$ at a slope of 10 ml/min/W.

4. In panel 5, the diagonal dashed line has a slope of 1; the "x" in the upper right is the predicted maximum heart rate and $\dot{V}O_2$ for the subject.

CASE 33 *Hypertensive cardiovascular disease and carboxyhemoglobinemia*

CLINICAL FINDINGS

This 46-year-old current shipyard worker was referred for evaluation of shortness of breath. He complained of chronic cough and sputum production of 8 to 10 years' duration. He dated the shortness of breath to a hospitalization for a leg fracture 6 years before. He had previously abused alcohol, but his history of cigarette smoking was contradictory. Physical examination revealed a smooth liver edge 5 cm below the right costal margin without other evidence of liver disease. There were no physical signs of cardiovascular or pulmonary disease. Chest roentgenogram showed small bilateral pleural plaques. ECG showed a left anterior hemiblock.

EXERCISE FINDINGS

The patient performed exercise on a cycle ergometer. He pedalled at 60 rpm without added load for 3 minutes. The work rate was then increased 20 W per minute to his symptom-limited maximum. Arterial blood was sampled every second minute, and intra-arterial blood pressure was recorded from a percutaneously placed brachial artery catheter. He stopped exercise complaining of shortness of breath and exhaustion. Carboxyhemoglobin level was 7.5% at the start of exercise, suggesting that the patient had recently smoked. There was no chest pain or abnormal ECG changes.

TABLE 33-1. *Selected Respiratory Function Data*

MEASUREMENT	PREDICTED	MEASURED
Age, yr		46
Sex		Male
Height, cm		161
Weight, kg	67	70
Hematocrit, %		43
VC, L	3.32	3.23
IC, L	2.22	2.24
TLC, L	4.77	4.77
FEV_1, L	2.65	2.62
FEV_1/VC, %	80	81
MVV, L/min	122	104
DL_{CO}, ml/mm Hg/min	22.3	22.1

TABLE 33-2. *Selected Exercise Data*

MEASUREMENT	PREDICTED	MEASURED
Maximum $\dot{V}O_2$, L/min	2.26	1.17
Maximum HR, beats/min	174	149
Maximum O_2 pulse, ml/beat	13.0	8.1
$\Delta\dot{V}O_2/\Delta WR$, ml/min/W	10.3	7.6
AT, L/min	> 0.97	0.9
Blood pressure, mm Hg (rest, max)		168/108,228/126
Maximum $\dot{V}E$, L/min		45
Exercise breathing reserve, L/min	> 15	59
PaO_2, mm Hg (rest, max ex)		93,101
$P(A-a)O_2$, mm Hg (rest, max ex)		12,21
$P(a-ET)CO_2$, mm Hg (rest, max ex)		0,−2
VD/VT (rest, heavy ex)		0.25,0.19
HCO_3^-, mEq/L (rest, 2-min recov)		23,18

Fig. 33-A.

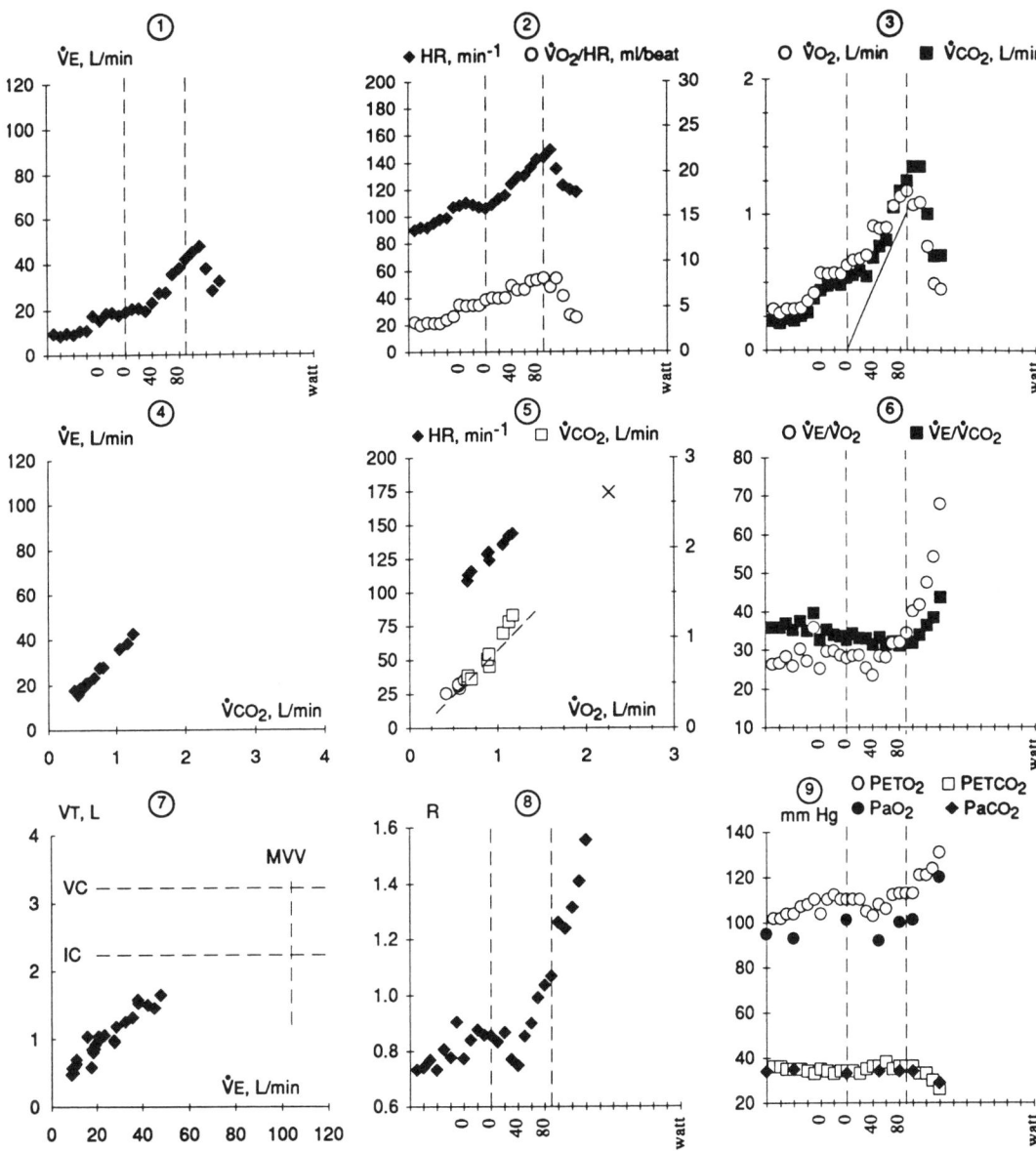

1. Vertical dashed lines in panels 1 to 3 and 6, 8, and 9 indicate the beginning and the end of increasing work period.

2. Unloaded cycling is performed for 3 minutes before the left vertical dashed line.

3. In panel 3, the diagonal line shows the increase of $\dot{V}_{O_2}$ at a slope of 10 ml/min/W.

4. In panel 5, the diagonal dashed line has a slope of 1; the "x" in the upper right is the predicted maximum heart rate and $\dot{V}_{O_2}$ for the subject.

TABLE 33-3.

Time min	Work rate watts	BP mm Hg	HR min^{-1}	f min^{-1}	$\dot{V}E$ L/min BTPS	$\dot{V}CO_2$ L/min STPD	$\dot{V}O_2$ L/min STPD	$\dfrac{\dot{V}O_2}{HR}$ ml/beat	R	pH	HCO$_3$ meq/L	PO2, mm Hg			PCO2, mm Hg			$\dfrac{\dot{V}E}{\dot{V}CO_2}$	$\dfrac{\dot{V}E}{\dot{V}O_2}$	$\dfrac{VD}{VT}$
												ET	a	(A-a)	ET	a	(a-ET)			
	Rest	168/108								7.44	23	95			34					
	Rest		90	19	9.5	0.22	0.30	3.3	0.73			102			36			36	26	
	Rest		92	18	8.7	0.20	0.27	2.9	0.74			102			36			36	27	
	Rest		92	17	9.9	0.23	0.30	3.3	0.77			104			35			37	28	
	Rest	168/108	95	16	9.1	0.22	0.30	3.2	0.73	7.41	22	104	93	12	35	35	0	35	26	0.25
	Rest		98	17	10.8	0.25	0.31	3.2	0.81			107			35			37	30	
	Rest		99	16	11.1	0.28	0.36	3.6	0.78			108			34			35	27	
	Unloaded		107	30	17.6	0.38	0.42	3.9	0.90			110			33			40	36	
	Unloaded		108	15	15.6	0.44	0.57	5.3	0.77			104			35			33	25	
	Unloaded		110	23	18.5	0.47	0.56	5.1	0.84			110			34			35	30	
	Unloaded		109	22	18.8	0.50	0.57	5.2	0.88			112			33			34	30	
	Unloaded		107	21	17.8	0.48	0.56	5.2	0.86			110			34			33	29	
	Unloaded	186/111	106	21	19.1	0.53	0.62	5.8	0.85	7.45	23	110	101	12	34	33	-1	33	28	0.18
0.5	20		109	21	20.5	0.55	0.66	6.1	0.83			110			34			34	28	
1.0	20		113	20	20.8	0.58	0.67	5.9	0.87			110			33			33	29	
1.5	40		116	21	19.5	0.54	0.70	6.0	0.77			105			35			33	25	
2.0	40		124	22	23.2	0.68	0.91	7.3	0.75			103			36			31	23	
2.5	60	204/120	129	28	27.5	0.76	0.89	6.9	0.85	7.43	22	108	92	19	36	34	-2	33	28	0.21
3.0	60		130	29	27.8	0.81	0.90	6.9	0.90			106			38			31	28	
3.5	80		136	27	35.8	1.05	1.06	7.8	0.99			112			35			32	32	
4.0	80	225/123	142	25	38.3	1.17	1.13	8.0	1.04	7.41	21	113	100	17	36	34	-2	31	32	0.17
4.5	100		144	28	42.4	1.25	1.17	8.1	1.07			113			36			32	34	
	Recovery	228/126	149	31	45.3	1.35	1.07	7.2	1.26	7.40	21	113	101	21	36	34	-2	32	40	0.19
	Recovery		135	29	47.9	1.35	1.09	8.1	1.24			121			33			34	42	
	Recovery		123	24	38.1	1.00	0.76	6.2	1.32			121			33			36	47	
	Recovery		120	24	28.5	0.69	0.49	4.1	1.41			124			30			38	54	
	Recovery	183/111	118	26	32.7	0.70	0.45	3.8	1.56	7.41	18	131	120	9	26	29	3	44	68	0.30

Interpretation

COMMENTS

Respiratory function at rest is normal (Table 33-1). Resting ECG is consistent with a left anterior hemiblock.

ANALYSIS

In flow chart 1, the maximum $\dot{V}O_2$ and anaerobic threshold are reduced during exercise (Table 33-2). See flow chart 4: The breathing reserve is high (Table 33-2) (branchpoint 4.1). The ventilatory equivalent for CO_2 at the anaerobic threshold is normal (see Fig. 33-A), and the indices of distribution of ventilation relative to perfusion are normal (branchpoint 4.3), supporting the diagnosis of an O_2 flow problem of nonpulmonary origin. The

hematocrit is normal (branchpoint 4.4). The O_2 pulse is low at the reduced maximum work rate. $\Delta\dot{V}O_2/\Delta WR$ is significantly decreased. The patient did not experience chest pain and his ECG remained normal throughout the exercise test. He has resting and exercise hypertension.

CONCLUSION

The patient evidently has exercise intolerance secondary to cardiovascular disease. This is possibly secondary to combined peripheral vascular dysfunction with systemic hypertension and failure of the heart to respond adequately to the increased after load; however, the reduced O_2 capacity of the blood and shift to the left of the oxyhemoglobin dissociation curve, caused by the elevated carboxyhemoglobin concentration, may also contribute to the patient's circulatory dysfunction.

CASE 34 *Patent ductus arteriosus*

CLINICAL FINDINGS

This 25-year-old man recently developed exertional dyspnea. He was found to have a patent ductus arteriosus. Cardiac angiography demonstrated normal coronary arteries, a left ventricular ejection fraction of 56%, a large flow from the aorta through the patent ductus to the pulmonary artery, and normal pulmonary artery pressures at rest. The surgeon desired a pre-operative cycle ergometer study with a pulmonary artery catheter in place to assess pulmonary artery pressures during exercise. The patient was sent to the exercise laboratory with a right radial artery catheter and pulmonary artery catheter placed via the right subclavian vein. Resting 12-lead ECGs showed left atrial enlargement and left ventricular hypertrophy.

EXERCISE FINDINGS

The patient performed exercise on a cycle ergometer. He pedalled at 60 rpm without an added load for 3 minutes. The work rate was then increased 15 W per minute to tolerance. Intra-arterial pressures were recorded continuously except when blood was simultaneously sampled every 2 minutes from the systemic and pulmonary arterial catheters. The patient stopped exercise because of calf and thigh fatigue. The patient had no chest pain and no further ECG abnormalities.

TABLE 34-1. *Selected Respiratory Function Data*

MEASUREMENT	PREDICTED	MEASURED
Age, yr		25
Sex		Male
Height, cm		170
Weight, kg	74	56
Hemoglobin, g/100 ml		14.6
VC, L	4.39	4.27
IC, L	2.93	2.42
TLC, L	5.81	6.62
FEV_1, L	3.57	3.62
FEV_1/VC, %	81	85
MVV, L/min	156	158
DL_{CO}, ml/mm Hg/min	29.6	35.6

TABLE 34-2. *Selected Exercise Data*

MEASUREMENT	PREDICTED	MEASURED
Maximum $\dot{V}O_2$, L/min	2.68	1.68
Maximum HR, beats/min	195	166
Maximum O_2 pulse, ml/beat	13.7	10.1
$\Delta\dot{V}O_2/\Delta WR$, ml/min/W	10.3	8.2
AT, L/min	> 1.09	< 1.0
Systemic blood pressure, mm Hg (rest, max)		154/70,228/105
Pulmonary artery pressure, mm Hg (rest, max)		20/10,30/15
Maximum $\dot{V}E$, L/min		54
Exercise breathing reserve, L/min	> 15	104
Pa_{O_2}, mm Hg (rest, max ex)		103,95
$P(A-a)_{O_2}$ mm Hg (rest, max ex)		6,17
$P(a-ET)_{CO_2}$, mm Hg (rest, max ex)		0,−3
V_D/V_T (rest, max ex)		0.39,0.20
HCO_3^-, mEq/L (rest, 2-min recov)		25,18

TABLE 34-3.

Time min	Work rate watts	BP mm Hg	HR min⁻¹	f min⁻¹	V̇E L/min BTPS	V̇CO2 L/min STPD	V̇O2 L/min STPD	V̇O2/HR ml/beat	R	pH	HCO3 meq/L	PO2 ET	PO2 a	PO2 (A-a)	PCO2 ET	PCO2 a	PCO2 (a-ET)	V̇E/V̇CO2	V̇E/V̇O2	VD/VT
	Rest	154/69								7.32	23	108			46					
	Rest		80	20	10.5	0.26	0.36	4.5	0.72			91			44			34	24	
	Rest		85	19	9.8	0.24	0.35	4.1	0.69			93			43			34	23	
	Rest		84	18	7.1	0.17	0.22	2.6	0.77			97			43			33	25	
	Rest	180/87	80	25	10.0	0.18	0.19	2.4	0.95	7.42	25	110	103	6	39	39	0	44	41	0.39
	Rest		87	18	12.3	0.36	0.45	5.2	0.80			95			44			30	24	
	Rest		90	37	23.9	0.37	0.46	5.1	0.80			100			43			56	45	
	Unloaded		100	25	13.5	0.37	0.45	4.5	0.82			101			42			31	25	
	Unloaded		100	32	15.5	0.40	0.49	4.9	0.82			98			42			32	26	
	Unloaded		101	33	13.3	0.36	0.57	5.6	0.63			88			46			29	18	
	Unloaded		99	29	19.2	0.56	0.77	7.8	0.73			92			44			30	22	
	Unloaded		101	29	20.2	0.62	0.79	7.8	0.78			93			46			29	22	
	Unloaded		101	33	27.1	0.81	0.88	8.7	0.92			104			41			30	28	
0.5	15		99	32	19.5	0.56	0.67	6.8	0.84			97			45			30	25	
1.0	15		104	29	25.4	0.82	0.89	8.6	0.92			103			43			28	26	
1.5	30		109	33	24.7	0.81	0.90	8.3	0.90			101			44			27	24	
2.0	30	222/102	106	33	22.7	0.71	0.76	7.2	0.93	7.39	26	98	99	6	47	43	-4	28	26	0.25
2.5	45		109	30	25.4	0.58	0.94	8.6	0.62			99			47			39	24	
3.0	45		115	29	28.0	1.01	1.02	8.9	0.99			102			47			25	25	
3.5	60		121	29	30.0	1.12	1.07	8.8	1.05			104			47			25	26	
4.0	60	231/96	121	30	27.9	1.04	1.01	8.3	1.03	7.35	25	103	93	12	48	46	-2	24	25	0.21
4.5	75		126	38	27.4	1.07	1.04	8.3	1.03			101			50			23	23	
5.0	75		132	32	34.1	1.29	1.19	9.0	1.08			106			47			24	26	
5.5	90		141	35	38.9	1.47	1.27	9.0	1.16			109			46			24	28	
6.0	90		151	36	42.8	1.60	1.36	9.0	1.18			108			46			25	29	
6.5	105		162	37	49.8	1.83	1.48	9.1	1.24			111			45			25	32	
7.0	105	246/108	165	40	49.6	1.82	1.51	9.2	1.21	7.34	22	111	105	9	45	42	-3	25	31	0.18
7.5	120		166	40	49.0	1.75	1.47	8.9	1.19			111			44			26	31	
8.0	120	228/105	166	39	53.5	1.97	1.68	10.1	1.17	7.30	21	108	95	17	46	43	-3	25	30	0.20
	Recovery		157	37	51.1	1.73	1.28	8.2	1.35			114			43			28	37	
	Recovery		150	34	40.8	1.30	0.85	5.7	1.53			120			41			29	45	
	Recovery		146	37	47.0	1.32	0.80	5.5	1.65			121			39			33	55	
	Recovery	171/90	144	32	32.2	0.95	0.75	5.2	1.27	7.29	18	117	111	7	40	38	-2	31	39	0.25

Interpretation

COMMENTS

Resting respiratory function studies were normal with a high normal $D_{L_{CO}}$, suggestive of an increase in pulmonary capillary blood volume. For the level of $\dot{V}O_2$, the left ventricular output at rest and exercise, as calculated from the Fick equation, was considerably elevated. The exercise systemic blood pressure was high, but the pulmonary artery pressure was normal. The breathing reserve was high and gas exchange measures were normal.

ANALYSIS

In flow chart 1, maximum $\dot{V}O_2$ and the anaerobic threshold are decreased. If one goes next to flow chart 4, the high breathing reserve (branchpoint 4.1), normal $\dot{V}E/\dot{V}CO_2$ (branchpoint 4.3), normal hematocrit (branchpoint 4.4), and low, unchanging O_2 pulse (branchpoint 4.6) lead us to the diagnosis of heart disease. The ECG does not show evidence of myocardial ischemia, but the low $\Delta\dot{V}O_2/\Delta WR$ and steep HR versus $\dot{V}O_2$ response confirm the presence of cardiovascular dysfunction.

CONCLUSION

The patient's large left to right shunt through the patent ductus arteriosus requires an increased left ventricular output to support the peripheral O_2 flow requirements. That this output is not adequate at the time of this study is evident from the

FIG. 34-A.

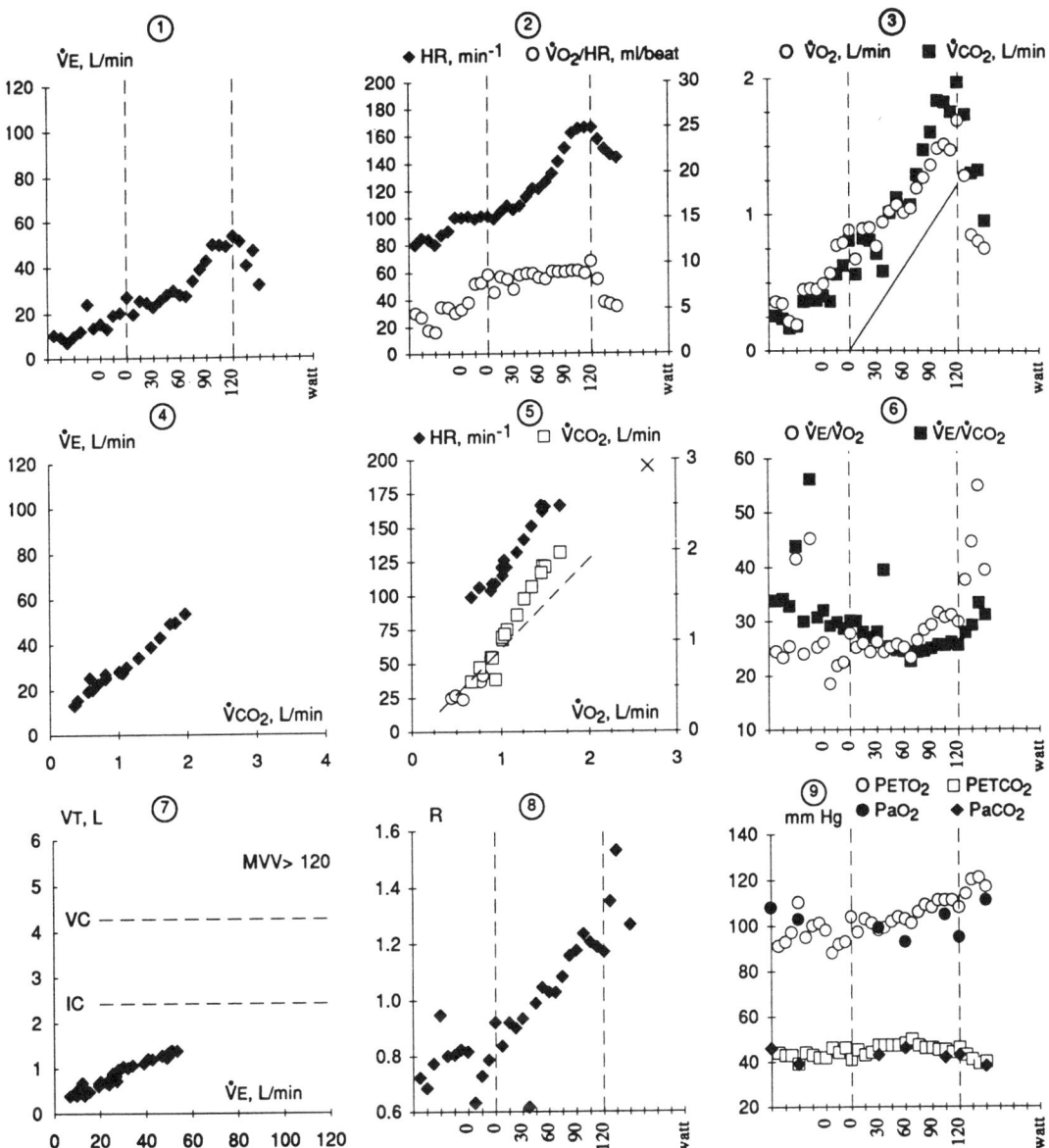

1. Vertical dashed lines in panels 1 to 3 and 6, 8, and 9 indicate the beginning and the end of increasing work period.
2. Unloaded cycling is performed for 3 minutes before the left vertical dashed line.
3. In panel 3, the diagonal line shows the increase of $\dot{V}O_2$ at a slope of 10 ml/min/W.
4. In panel 5, the diagonal dashed line has a slope of 1; the "x" in the upper right is the predicted maximum heart rate and $\dot{V}O_2$ for the subject.

low anaerobic threshold and $\dot{V}O_2$max. In addition, the noninvasively measured low and relatively unchanging O_2 pulse throughout incremental exercise indicates that the patient reached maximum stroke volume and maximum arterial-mixed venous O_2 extraction early in the exercise study.

Presumably, by removing the pulmonary steal of systemic blood flow by closing the ductus, these abnormalities would be corrected. Following surgical correction of the patent ductus arteriosus, the patient's dyspnea and exercise tolerance improved considerably.

CASE 35 *Vasoregulatory asthenia*

CLINICAL FINDINGS

This 31-year-old woman was referred for exercise testing because of the insidious and progressive fatigability of 10 months' duration. She had formerly been active as a homemaker, had worked frequent 12-hour shifts as an ICU nurse, and had done 2 to 3 hours of vigorous exercise daily. At this time, she recognized dyspnea on walking two blocks and often experienced rapid, forceful palpitations with exertion or emotion. Her sleep requirements had increased markedly and she had gained 17 pounds in weight. She frequently woke from sleep diaphoretic and with palpitations, but did not snore. She had had hypertension only during her two pregnancies. She did not smoke or use drugs. Work-up elsewhere revealed a normal physical examination, chest roentgenograms, ECG, spirometry, echocardiograms, ejection fraction, resting blood gases, and thyroid function. Exercise studies elsewhere, including cardiac catheterization, showed tachycardia, normal ear oximetry, normal right- and left-sided arterial pressures, and an increasing mixed venous P_{O_2} during exercise. Examination here revealed a healthy-looking, animated woman with resting tachycardia and normal peripheral pulses. The oxyhemoglobin dissociation curve was normal, as assessed by measuring the P_{50}.

EXERCISE FINDINGS

The patient performed exercise on a cycle ergometer. She pedalled at 60 rpm without an added load for 3 minutes. The work rate was then increased 15 W per minute to tolerance. Heart rate and rhythm were continuously monitored; 12-lead ECGs were obtained during rest, exercise, and recovery. Blood pressure was measured with a sphygmomanometer and oxygen saturation with an ear oximeter. The patient appeared to give an excellent effort and stopped exercise because of generalized and thigh fatigue. She denied chest pain during or after the study. No arrhythmias or ischemic changes were noted on ECGs.

TABLE 35-1. *Selected Respiratory Function Data*

MEASUREMENT	PREDICTED	MEASURED
Age, yr		31
Sex		Female
Height, cm		167
Weight, kg	66	63
Hematocrit, %		40
VC, L	3.75	4.81
IC, L	2.50	3.34
TLC, L	5.51	6.64
FEV$_1$, L	3.08	4.27
FEV$_1$/VC, %	82	89
MVV, L/min	116	146
D$_{L_{CO}}$, ml/mm Hg/min	27.1	28.8

TABLE 35-2. *Selected Exercise Data*

MEASUREMENT	PREDICTED	MEASURED
Maximum V̇$_{O_2}$, L/min	1.88	1.73
Maximum HR, beats/min	189	195
Maximum O$_2$ pulse, ml/beat	10.1	8.9
ΔV̇$_{O_2}$/ΔWR, ml/min/W	10.3	10.3
AT, L/min	> 0.86	0.8
Blood pressure, mm Hg (rest, max)		115/90,155/90
Maximum V̇$_E$, L/min		67
Exercise breathing reserve, L/min	> 15	79
O$_2$ saturation, oximeter (rest, max)		99,100

FIG. 35-A.

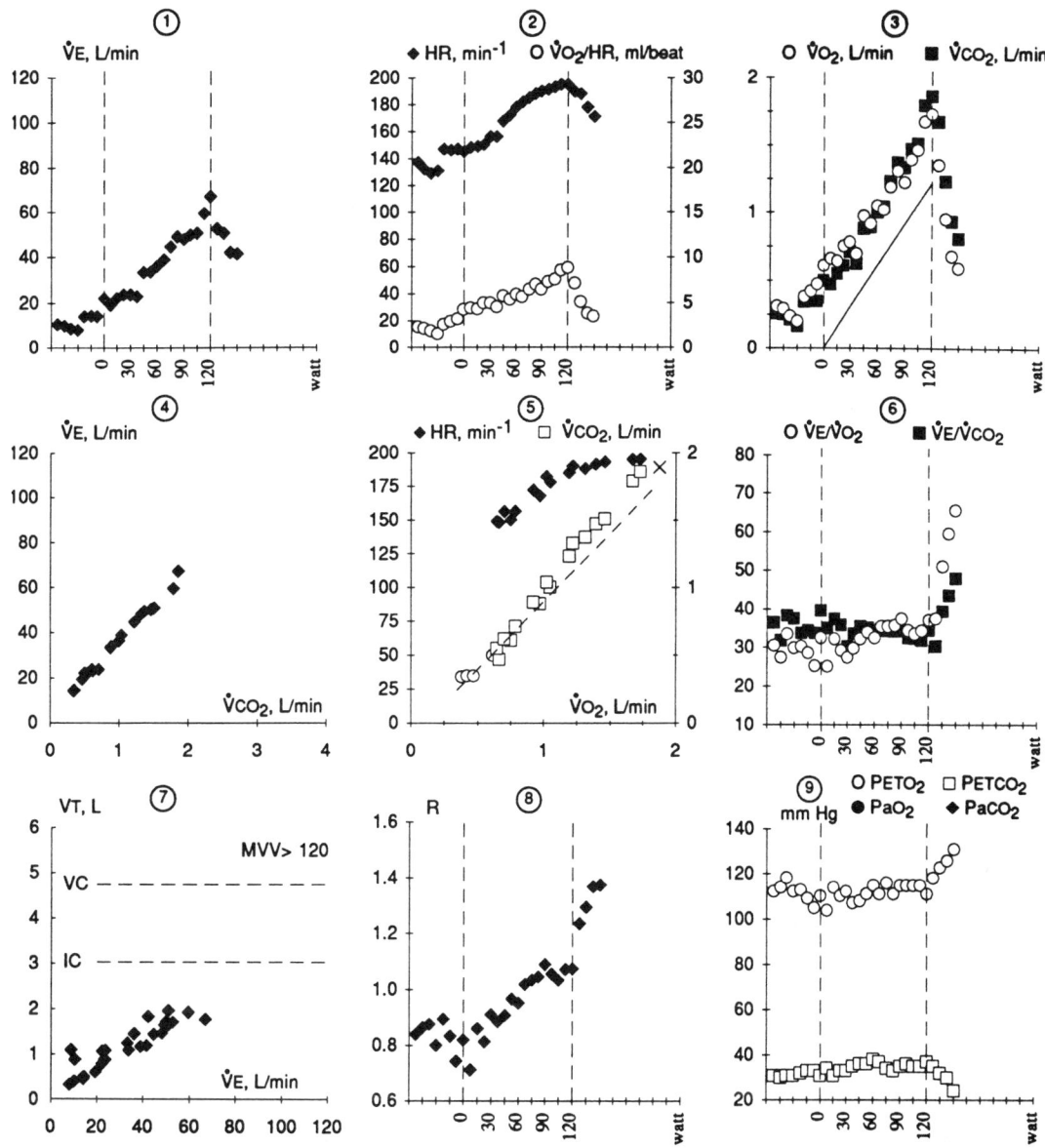

1. Vertical dashed lines in panels 1 to 3 and 6, 8, and 9 indicate the beginning and the end of increasing work period.

2. Unloaded cycling is performed for 3 minutes before the left vertical dashed line.

3. In panel 3, the diagonal line shows the increase of $\dot{V}O_2$ at a slope of 10 ml/min/W.

4. In panel 5, the diagonal dashed line has a slope of 1; the "x" in the upper right is the predicted maximum heart rate and $\dot{V}O_2$ for the subject.

TABLE 35-3.

Time min	Work rate watts	BP mm Hg	HR min⁻¹	f min⁻¹	$\dot{V}_E$ L/min BTPS	$\dot{V}_{CO_2}$ L/min STPD	$\dot{V}_{O_2}$ L/min STPD	$\frac{\dot{V}_{O_2}}{HR}$ ml/beat	R	pH	HCO₃ meq/L	PO₂, mm Hg ET	a	(A-a)	PCO₂, mm Hg ET	a	(a-ET)	$\frac{\dot{V}_E}{\dot{V}_{CO_2}}$	$\frac{\dot{V}_E}{\dot{V}_{O_2}}$	$\frac{V_D}{V_T}$
	Rest		137	12	10.5	0.26	0.31	2.3	0.84			112			31			36	31	
	Rest		132	25	10.1	0.25	0.29	2.2	0.86			114			30			32	28	
	Rest		129	8	8.7	0.21	0.24	1.9	0.88			118			31			38	33	
	Rest	115/90	131	25	8.1	0.16	0.20	1.5	0.80			112			31			37	30	
	Unloaded		147	31	14.1	0.34	0.38	2.6	0.89			113			32			34	30	
	Unloaded		146	29	14.5	0.35	0.42	2.9	0.83			109			33			34	29	
	Unloaded		147	28	14.2	0.35	0.47	3.2	0.74			105			33			34	25	
	Unloaded	140/95	145	28	22.1	0.50	0.61	4.2	0.82			110			31			39	32	
0.5	15		148	32	19.2	0.47	0.66	4.5	0.71			104			34			35	25	
1.0	15		149	21	22.3	0.55	0.64	4.3	0.86			114			31			37	32	
1.5	30		150	22	23.7	0.61	0.75	5.0	0.81			110			33			36	29	
2.0	30		156	27	23.7	0.71	0.78	5.0	0.91			112			33			30	27	
2.5	45		156	26	23.0	0.62	0.70	4.5	0.89			107			35			34	30	
3.0	45		168	27	33.4	0.88	0.97	5.8	0.91			108			36			35	32	
3.5	60		172	31	33.8	0.89	0.92	5.3	0.97			111			36			35	34	
4.0	60	155/90	178	25	36.3	1.00	1.05	5.9	0.95			115			38			34	33	
4.5	75		182	33	38.9	1.04	1.02	5.6	1.02			111			37			35	35	
5.0	75		185	31	44.7	1.23	1.19	6.4	1.03			116			34			34	35	
5.5	90		188	30	49.2	1.37	1.31	7.0	1.05			111			33			34	36	
6.0	90		190	33	48.2	1.33	1.22	6.4	1.09			115			35			34	37	
6.5	105		191	29	50.1	1.47	1.39	7.3	1.06			115			36			32	34	
7.0	105		193	26	51.0	1.51	1.46	7.6	1.03			115			35			32	33	
7.5	120		195	31	59.7	1.79	1.67	8.6	1.07			115			35			32	34	
8.0	120		195	38	67.1	1.86	1.73	8.9	1.08			111			37			34	37	
	Recovery		190	31	53.0	1.67	1.35	7.1	1.24			118			35			30	37	
	Recovery		188	31	50.9	1.23	0.95	5.1	1.29			123			32			39	51	
	Recovery		178	23	42.3	0.93	0.68	3.8	1.37			126			30			43	59	
	Recovery	125/60	171	35	41.6	0.81	0.59	3.5	1.37			131			24			48	65	

Interpretation

COMMENTS

Resting respiratory function studies were better than average. The predicted exercise values in Table 35-2 are for a sedentary person rather than a physically active person such as this patient.

ANALYSIS

In flow chart 1, the maximum $\dot{V}_{O_2}$ is normal for a sedentary person (which this patient is not), but the anaerobic threshold is low (Table 35-2). We are directed through branchpoints 1.1, 1.2, and 1.3 to flow chart 4. The breathing reserve was high (branchpoint 4.1). Although the $\dot{V}_E/\dot{V}_{CO_2}$ at the anaerobic threshold is high, the $P_{ET_{CO_2}}$ is reduced; therefore, we cannot determine whether the V_D/V_T is elevated. We then go to the box labelled "O_2 flow problem of non-pulmonary origin." We are moderately confident that the patient does not have appreciable widening of the $P(A - a)_{O_2}$ because of the normal ear oximetry. The hematocrit is normal (branchpoint 4.4). The O_2 pulse is not low and nonchanging (branchpoint 4.6), leading us to the box labelled "peripheral vascular disease." This does not fit this patient well, considering her resting tachycardia, negative heart rate reserve, absence of hypertension, and good peripheral pulses. Exploring further, she does not fit well the diagnosis of "anemia" or "heart disease," but she does have a steep HR versus $\dot{V}_{O_2}$ and a low heart rate reserve. Knowing from prior studies that she did not have a low mixed venous P_{O_2} during heavy exercise, we can presume that the exercising muscles have difficulty extracting oxygen from their capillaries. These findings fit the diagnosis of vasoregulatory asthenia,[1-3] which appears to be characterized by an inability to vasodilate the exercising muscle vascular beds and to vasoconstrict non-exercising organs. This may represent a specific defect in the autonomic nervous system.

CONCLUSION

The patient's findings were consistent with vasoregulatory asthenia, but follow-up evaluation was recommended. The patient was placed on a physical training program with some objective and subjective improvement in exercise tolerance, but there was no improvement with β-blockade. As the pathophysiologic mechanisms underlying vasoregulatory asthenia are unclear, a subsequent exercise test was performed in which serial venous blood samples were drawn. Blood lactate levels were markedly increased during exercise (reaching a peak of 8.2 mEq/L), ruling out McArdle's syndrome[4] as the cause of her exercise intolerance. Other muscle disorders (e.g., electron transport chain defects) cannot be excluded, however.[5,6] Further, blood epinephrine and norepinephrine values rose appropriately with exercise, which seems inconsistent with generalized autonomic dysfunction.

References

1. Holmgren, A., Jonsson, B., Levander, M., Linderholm, H., Sjöstrand, T., and Ström, G.: Low physical work capacity in suspected heart cases due to inadequate adjustment of peripheral blood flow (vasoregulatory asthenia). Acta Med. Scand., 158:413–436, 1957.
2. Holmgren, A., Jonsson, B., Levander, M., Linderholm, H., Mossfeld, F., Sjöstrand, T., and Ström, G.: Physical training of patients with vasoregulatory asthenia. Acta Med. Scand., 158:437–446, 1957.
3. Gillum, R.F., Teicholz, L.E., Herman, M.V., and Gorlin, R.: The idiopathic hyperkinetic heart syndrome: clinical course and long-term prognosis. Am. Heart J., 102: 728–734, 1981.
4. McArdle, B.: Myopathy due to a defect in muscle glycogen breakdown. Clin. Sci., 10:13–18, 1951.
5. Carroll, J.E., Hagberg, J.H., Brooke, M.H., and Shumate, J.B.: Bicycle ergometry and gas exchange measurements in neuromuscular diseases. Arch. Neurol., 36:457–461, 1979.
6. DiMauro, S., Bonilla, E., Zevina, M., Nakagawa, M., and DeVivo, D.C.: Mitochondrial myopathies. Ann. Neurol., 17:521–538, 1985.

CASE 36 *Chronic bronchitis, mild, without exercise limitation*

CLINICAL FINDINGS

This 55-year-old shipyard worker complained of dyspnea after walking up one flight of stairs or a few blocks on a level surface. He had had morning cough several months of each year and had noted occasional retrosternal pain unrelated to exertion or emotional upset. He had 35 pack years of smoking until stopping 12 years ago. He exercised regularly. The physical examination was normal except for mild obesity. Chest x-ray studies showed bilateral pleural thickening in the mid lung zones and old granulomatous disease in the right upper lobe. Resting ECG was normal.

EXERCISE FINDINGS

The patient performed exercise on a cycle ergometer. He first pedalled at 60 rpm, without added load, for 3 minutes. The work rate was then increased 20 W per minute to his symptom-limited maximum. Arterial blood was sampled every second minute and intra-arterial blood pressure was recorded from a percutaneously placed brachial artery catheter. The patient stopped exercise because of "exhaustion." ECG remained normal throughout exercise.

TABLE 36-1. *Selected Respiratory Function Data*

MEASUREMENT	PREDICTED	MEASURED
Age, yr		54
Sex		Male
Height, cm		174
Weight, kg	77	88
Hematocrit, %		45
VC, L	4.28	3.59
IC, L	2.86	3.12
TLC, L	6.38	6.15
FEV$_1$, L	3.39	2.40
FEV$_1$/VC, %	79	67
MVV, L/min	142	112
D$_{LCO}$, ml/mm Hg/min	28.8	29.8

TABLE 36-2. *Selected Exercise Data*

MEASUREMENT	PREDICTED	MEASURED
Maximum V̇$_{O_2}$, L/min	2.42	2.66
Maximum HR, beats/min	166	169
Maximum O$_2$ pulse, ml/beat	14.6	15.7
ΔV̇$_{O_2}$/ΔWR, ml/min/W	10.3	9.9
AT, L/min	> 1.04	1.3
Blood pressure, mm Hg (rest, max)		141/93,225/117
Maximum V̇$_E$, L/min		86
Exercise breathing reserve, L/min	> 15	26
Pa$_{O_2}$, mm Hg (rest, max ex)		81,92
P(A−a)$_{O_2}$, mm Hg (rest, max ex)		18,21
P(a−ET)$_{CO_2}$, mm Hg (rest, max ex)		5,−3
V$_D$/V$_T$ (rest, heavy ex)		0.41,0.23
HCO$_3^-$, mEq/L (rest, 2-min recov)		26,16

Fig. 36-A.

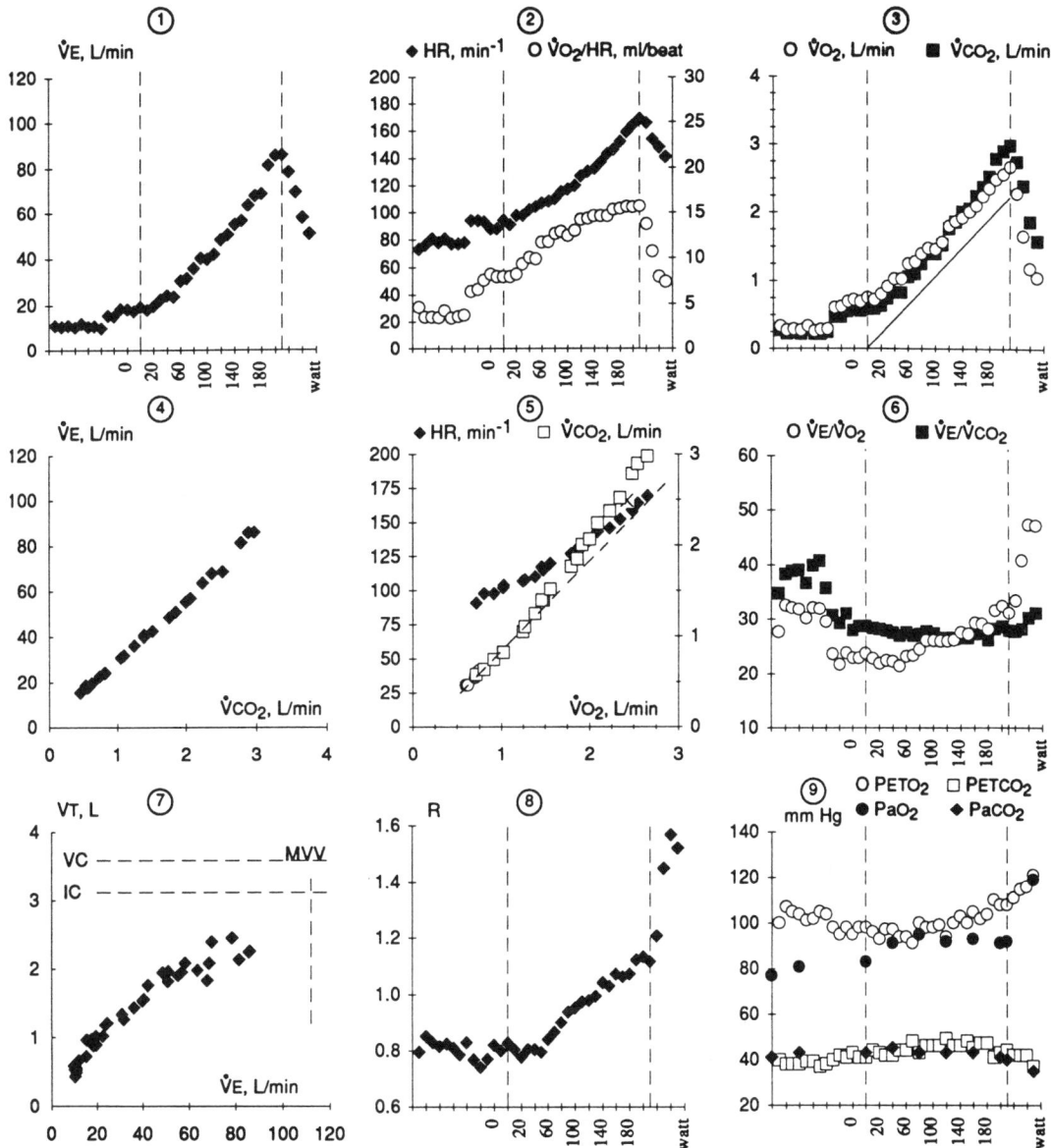

1. Vertical **dashed** lines in panels 1 to 3 and 6, 8, and 9 indicate the beginning and the end of increasing work period.

2. Unloaded cycling is performed for 3 minutes before the left vertical dashed line.

3. In panel 3, the diagonal line shows the increase of $\dot{V}_{O_2}$ at a slope of 10 ml/min/W.

4. In panel 5, the diagonal dashed line has a slope of 1; the "x" in the upper right is the predicted maximum heart rate and $\dot{V}_{O_2}$ for the subject.

TABLE 36-3.

Time min	Work rate watts	BP mm Hg	HR min⁻¹	f min⁻¹	$\dot{V}E$ L/min BTPS	$\dot{V}CO_2$ L/min STPD	$\dot{V}O_2$ L/min STPD	$\dfrac{\dot{V}O_2}{HR}$ ml/beat	R	pH	HCO₃ meq/L	PO2, mm Hg ET	a	(A-a)	PCO2, mm Hg ET	a	(a-ET)	$\dfrac{\dot{V}E}{\dot{V}CO_2}$	$\dfrac{\dot{V}E}{\dot{V}O_2}$	VD VT
	Rest	141/93								7.42	26		77			41				
	Rest		73	20	11.1	0.27	0.34	4.7	0.79			100			40			35	28	
	Rest		76	20	10.5	0.23	0.27	3.6	0.85			107			38			38	33	
	Rest		81	21	11.1	0.24	0.29	3.6	0.83			105			38			39	32	
	Rest	141/90	78	19	10.2	0.22	0.27	3.5	0.81	7.40	26	104	81	18	38	43	5	39	32	0.41
	Rest		81	18	11.8	0.28	0.34	4.2	0.82			101			39			37	30	
	Rest		77	24	10.4	0.21	0.26	3.4	0.81			102			39			40	32	
	Rest		77	22	10.8	0.22	0.28	3.6	0.79			105			37			41	32	
	Rest		78	17	10.0	0.24	0.29	3.7	0.83			104			38			36	30	
	Unloaded		94	16	15.5	0.46	0.60	6.4	0.77			98			40			31	24	
	Unloaded		94	21	15.2	0.46	0.62	6.6	0.74			95			42			29	22	
	Unloaded		93	21	18.5	0.54	0.70	7.5	0.77			98			41			31	24	
	Unloaded		88	20	18.2	0.59	0.72	8.2	0.82			95			43			28	23	
	Unloaded		88	18	17.6	0.56	0.70	8.0	0.80			98			41			29	23	
	Unloaded	162/99	94	19	19.4	0.62	0.75	8.0	0.83	7.39	26	98	83	17	41	43	2	29	24	0.28
0.5	20		91	19	18.0	0.58	0.72	7.9	0.81			96			44			28	23	
1.0	20		98	22	19.6	0.63	0.81	8.3	0.78			93			43			28	22	
1.5	40		98	22	22.5	0.74	0.92	9.4	0.80			97			42			28	22	
2.0	40	174/96	102	20	24.3	0.82	1.02	10.0	0.80	7.37	26	97	91	5	42	45	3	28	22	0.28
2.5	60		104	20	23.8	0.82	1.03	9.9	0.80			94			44			27	21	
3.0	60		107	23	30.9	1.05	1.25	11.7	0.84			94			44			28	23	
3.5	80		108	25	31.8	1.10	1.27	11.8	0.87			91			48			27	23	
4.0	80	174/93	110	25	36.1	1.25	1.39	12.6	0.90	7.37	24	100	95	8	43	43	0	27	24	0.25
4.5	100		115	26	40.6	1.39	1.48	12.9	0.94			98			46			28	26	
5.0	100		117	26	40.1	1.39	1.46	12.5	0.95			98			46			27	26	
5.5	120		120	24	42.4	1.52	1.56	13.0	0.97			99			46			27	26	
6.0	120	204/99	127	25	48.7	1.76	1.80	14.2	0.98	7.36	24	94	92	14	49	43	-6	26	26	0.23
6.5	140		130	28	51.0	1.85	1.86	14.3	0.99			100			46			26	26	
7.0	140		132	29	55.4	2.00	1.92	14.5	1.04			103			46			26	28	
7.5	160		137	29	56.9	2.06	2.00	14.6	1.03			100			48			26	27	
8.0	160	210/105	143	32	63.7	2.24	2.09	14.6	1.07	7.35	23	105	93	16	45	43	-2	27	29	0.25
8.5	180		146	37	67.9	2.37	2.23	15.3	1.06			102			47			27	29	
9.0	180		152	33	68.8	2.52	2.35	15.5	1.07			104			47			26	28	
9.5	200		159	38	81.4	2.78	2.48	15.6	1.12			110			41			28	32	
10.0	200	228/114	164	38	85.7	2.89	2.55	15.5	1.13	7.33	21	108	91	22	43	41	-2	29	32	0.25
10.5	220	225/117	169	38	86.0	2.97	2.66	15.7	1.12	7.31	20	108	92	21	44	40	-4	28	31	0.22
	Recovery		166	32	78.5	2.74	2.27	13.7	1.21			111			42			28	33	
	Recovery		154	29	69.7	2.39	1.65	10.7	1.45			115			42			28	41	
	Recovery		148	28	58.3	1.85	1.18	8.0	1.57			116			42			30	47	
	Recovery	183/96	141	26	51.2	1.58	1.04	7.4	1.52	7.27	16	121	119	5	37	35	-2	31	47	0.20

Interpretation

COMMENTS

Resting respiratory function is compatible with mild airflow obstruction (Table 36-1). The resting ECG is normal.

ANALYSIS

In flow chart 1, the maximum oxygen uptake and anaerobic threshold are normal (Table 36-2). See flow chart 2: Arterial blood gases and ECG at maximum $\dot{V}O_2$ are normal (branchpoint 2.1). The patient is about 14% overweight (branchpoint 2.2). This is not a serious obesity problem but does contribute toward the additional metabolic cost of work. The patient also has mild airflow obstruction, however, causing a characteristic obstructive pattern at high exercise levels.

CONCLUSION

This shows normal exercise performance in a mildly obese man with airflow obstruction.

Case 37 *Chronic bronchitis, moderate*

Clinical Findings

This 69-year-old former shipyard worker had first noted dyspnea on exertion 16 years ago, later accompanied by cough, sputum production, and frequent wheezing. He had been receiving bronchodilators and antibiotics intermittently for 16 years. Physical examination revealed obesity, bilaterally decreased breath sounds, and fine expiratory wheezes. There was no evidence of cardiovascular disease. Chest x-ray study revealed moderate pleural thickening bilaterally and scattered parenchymal calcifications compatible with inactive granulomatous disease. The heart was not enlarged. ECG was compatible with left atrial enlargement and left ventricular hypertrophy. He admitted to a 15 pack year history of cigarette smoking.

Exercise Findings

The patient performed exercise on a cycle ergometer. He first pedalled at 60 rpm, without added load, for 3 minutes. The work rate was then increased 10 W per minute to his symptom-limited maximum. Arterial blood was sampled every second minute, and intra-arterial blood pressure was recorded from a percutaneously placed brachial artery catheter. The patient stopped exercising complaining of shortness of breath and chest tightness. There were no ST segment changes or arrhythmia.

TABLE 37-1. *Selected Respiratory Function Data*

MEASUREMENT	PREDICTED	MEASURED
Age, yr		69
Sex		Male
Height, cm		166
Weight, kg	70	98
Hematocrit, %		45
VC, L	3.31	2.91 (2.15*)
IC, L	2.21	2.35 (1.89*)
TLC, L	5.38	7.32
FEV$_1$, L	2.55	1.47 (1.30*)
FEV$_1$/VC, %	77	51 (60*)
MVV, L/min	112	56 (44*)
D$_{LCO}$, ml/mm Hg/min	22.6	26.0

* On day of exercise study

TABLE 37-2. *Selected Exercise Data*

MEASUREMENT	PREDICTED	MEASURED
Maximum V̇$_{O_2}$, L/min	1.93	1.50
Maximum HR, beats/min	151	125
Maximum O$_2$ pulse, ml/beat	12.8	12.0
ΔV̇$_{O_2}$/ΔWR, ml/min/W	10.3	10.4
AT, L/min	> 0.87	1.35
Blood pressure, mm Hg (rest, max)		142/72,234/99
Maximum V̇$_E$, L/min		55
Exercise breathing reserve, L/min	> 15	1
Pa$_{O_2}$, mm Hg (rest, max ex)		73,92
P(A−a)$_{O_2}$, mm Hg (rest, max ex)		32,17
P(a−ET)$_{CO_2}$, mm Hg (rest, max ex)		6,1
V$_D$/V$_T$ (rest, heavy ex)		0.40,0.35
HCO$_3^-$, mEq/L (rest, 2-min recov)		26,22

TABLE 37-3.

Time min	Work rate watts	BP mm Hg	HR min⁻¹	f min⁻¹	$\dot{V}E$ L/min BTPS	$\dot{V}CO_2$ L/min STPD	$\dot{V}O_2$ L/min STPD	$\dfrac{\dot{V}O_2}{HR}$ ml/beat	R	pH	HCO₃ meq/L	PO2, mm Hg ET	a	(A-a)	PCO2, mm Hg ET	a	(a-ET)	$\dfrac{\dot{V}E}{\dot{V}CO_2}$	$\dfrac{\dot{V}E}{\dot{V}O_2}$	$\dfrac{VD}{VT}$
	Rest	142/72								7.40	26	75			43					
	Rest		78	24	12.4	0.27	0.35	4.5	0.77			103			36			38	30	
	Rest		76	18	10.7	0.27	0.36	4.7	0.75			100			39			34	25	
	Rest		79	24	11.4	0.23	0.30	3.8	0.77			100			38			41	31	
	Rest	156/81	77	21	12.8	0.27	0.31	4.0	0.87	7.42	25	110	73	32	34	40	6	41	36	0.41
	Rest		79	21	13.3	0.30	0.35	4.4	0.86			109			34			38	33	
	Rest		80	22	12.9	0.24	0.28	3.5	0.86			110			34			46	39	
	Unloaded		90	36	18.0	0.29	0.38	4.2	0.76			107			34			52	39	
	Unloaded		98	50	28.0	0.53	0.66	6.7	0.80			108			34			45	36	
	Unloaded		98	56	29.5	0.57	0.65	6.6	0.88			101			40			43	38	
	Unloaded		101	43	31.8	0.79	0.89	8.8	0.89			99			42			36	32	
	Unloaded		104	49	29.1	0.69	0.77	7.4	0.90			107			38			36	32	
	Unloaded	198/93	105	47	34.6	0.76	0.85	8.1	0.89	7.40	26	106	82	22	39	42	3	40	36	0.43
0.5	10		102	55	41.2	0.90	0.96	9.4	0.94			110			36			41	38	
1.0	10		103	53	37.6	0.85	0.93	9.0	0.91			107			38			39	36	
1.5	20		105	58	46.3	0.98	0.99	9.4	0.99			114			34			42	42	
2.0	20	204/87	107	47	34.5	0.82	0.91	8.5	0.90	7.37	26	106	84	17	40	45	5	37	34	0.43
2.5	30		108	40	36.6	0.94	1.05	9.7	0.90			104			40			35	32	
3.0	30		109	50	39.8	0.95	0.95	9.6	0.90			105			39			37	34	
3.5	40		109	45	40.1	1.02	1.16	10.6	0.88			106			38			36	31	
4.0	40	207/87	110	46	42.2	1.11	1.28	11.6	0.87	7.38	24	106	80	23	38	42	4	34	30	0.37
4.5	50		113	47	42.1	1.09	1.23	10.9	0.89			105			39			35	31	
5.0	50		114	44	38.7	1.02	1.16	10.2	0.88			103			41			34	30	
5.5	60		117	45	47.1	1.26	1.39	11.9	0.91			107			39			34	31	
6.0	60	219/90	120	54	48.3	1.24	1.34	11.2	0.93	7.38	23	107	87	22	39	39	0	35	33	0.34
6.5	70		124	49	53.0	1.38	1.45	11.7	0.95			108			39			35	34	
7.0	70	234/99	125	50	55.0	1.43	1.50	12.0	0.95	7.37	22	110	92	17	38	39	1	35	34	0.35
	Recovery		128	59	51.3	1.50	1.51	11.8	0.99			109			38			31	31	
	Recovery		117	41	47.1	1.30	1.30	11.1	1.00			112			37			34	34	
	Recovery		117	52	48.5	1.20	1.22	10.4	0.98			112			36			37	36	
	Recovery		110	51	45.1	0.98	0.94	8.5	1.04			113			36			42	43	
	Recovery	204/84	107	42	31.0	0.61	0.56	5.2	1.09	7.37	22	115	95	19	36	39	3	45	49	0.45

Interpretation

COMMENTS

Respiratory function studies indicate that this patient has a moderate obstructive defect (Table 37-1). The ECG is interpreted to demonstrate left ventricular hypertrophy and left atrial enlargement.

ANALYSIS

In flow chart 1, maximum $\dot{V}O_2$ is low and anaerobic threshold is normal. See flow chart 3: The breathing reserve is low (branchpoint 3.1) indicating that this patient has lung disease. Confirming this diagnosis is the finding that the indices of ventilation-perfusion matching (VD/VT, $P(A-a)_{O_2}$ and $P(a-ET)_{CO_2}$) are abnormal and the heart rate reserve is high.

The actual maximum work rate performed by the patient is quite low, despite a mildly reduced maximum $\dot{V}O_2$, because he has an exceptionally high oxygen cost for unloaded cycling ($\dot{V}O_2 = .85$ L/min). This is most likely due to his obesity (added metabolic cost of moving his lower extremities). The fall in $P(A-a)_{O_2}$ and rise in Pa_{O_2}, when changing activity from rest to exercise, suggest that the resting hypoxemia in this patient is attributable to obesity-related basilar micro-atelectasis at rest that disappears with the increased ventilation accompanying exercise.

The elevated dead space fraction of the tidal volume (VD/VT) and high metabolic cost of exercise

FIG. 37-A.

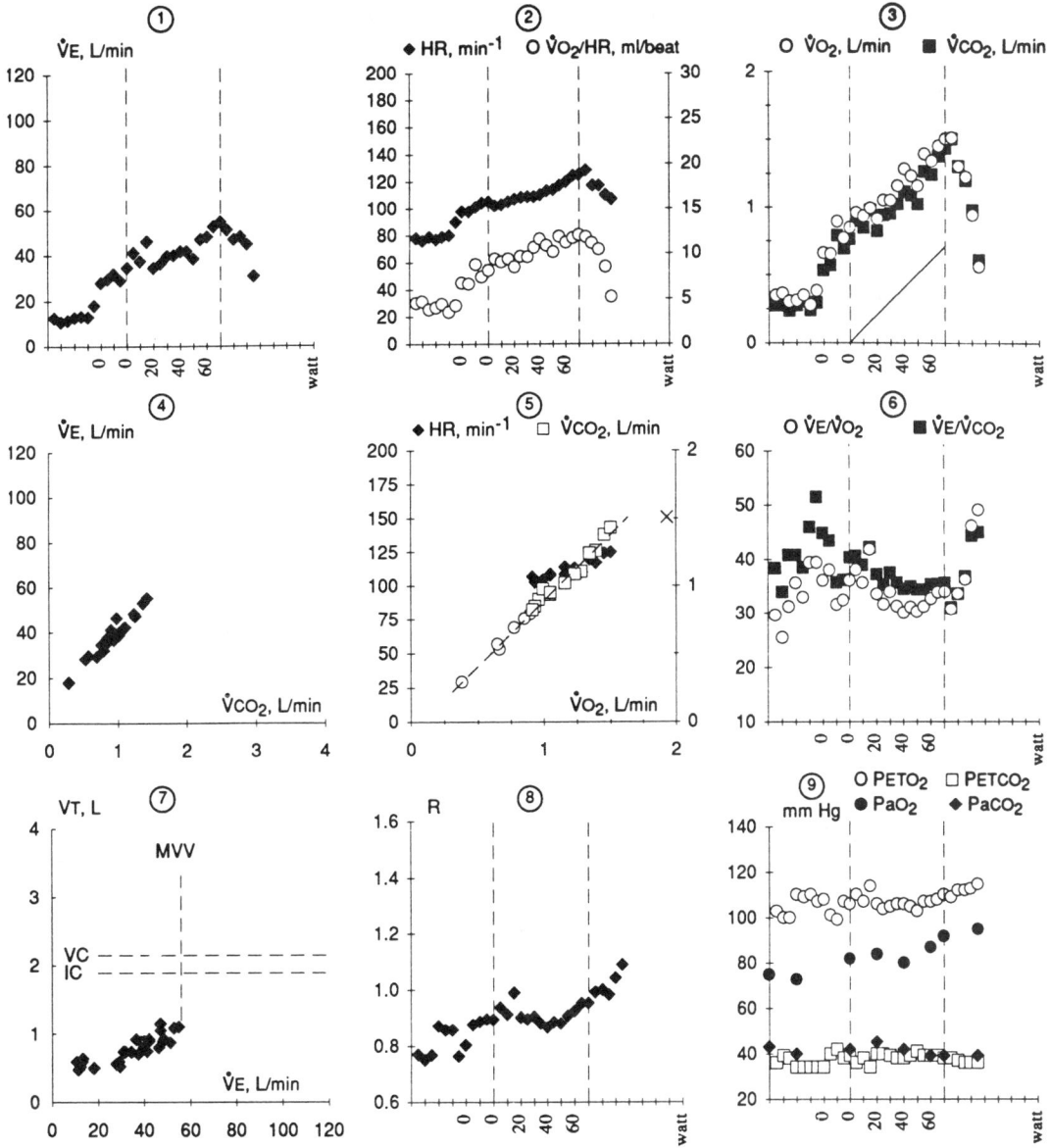

1. Vertical dashed lines in panels 1 to 3 and 6, 8, and 9 indicate the beginning and the end of increasing work period.

2. Unloaded cycling is performed for 3 minutes before the left vertical dashed line.

3. In panel 3, the diagonal line shows the increase of $\dot{V}_{O_2}$ at a slope of 10 ml/min/W.

4. In panel 5, the diagonal dashed line has a slope of 1; the "x" in the upper right is the predicted maximum heart rate and $\dot{V}_{O_2}$ for the subject.

caused by obesity, combined with mechanical limitation to breathe caused by moderate obstructive lung disease are all likely contributors to the patient's exertional dyspnea. Evidence against primary heart disease causing this patient's symptom is the absence of myocardial ischemia on the 12-lead ECG, the high heart rate reserve at maximum exercise, the normal anaerobic threshold, and the normal $\Delta\dot{V}_{O_2}/\Delta WR$.

CONCLUSION

Exertional dyspnea is secondary to moderate obstructive lung disease and obesity.

CASE 38 *Chronic bronchitis and obesity*

CLINICAL FINDINGS

This 50-year-old shipyard worker was referred for evaluation. He had a 65 pack year history of smoking and had complained of shortness of breath and frequent chest colds with cough and sputum production for the last 7 years. He had been told that he had borderline hypertension but took no medications for this or his pulmonary symptoms. Examination was normal except for obesity, blood pressure of 140/100, and expiratory wheezes on forced expiration. Chest roentgenograms showed focal pleural plaques.

EXERCISE FINDINGS

The patient performed exercise on a cycle ergometer. He pedalled at 60 rpm without added load for 3 minutes. The work rate was then increased 20 W per minute to his symptom-limited maximum. Arterial blood was sampled every second minute, and intra-arterial blood pressure was recorded from a percutaneously placed brachial artery catheter. Resting carboxyhemoglobin level was 9.4%. He stopped exercise complaining of shortness of breath. After exercise, while sitting quietly on the cycle, he became lightheaded and hypotensive. He was put in the supine position and his legs elevated; this provided immediate relief of his lightheadedness and return of his systemic blood pressure to pre-exercise levels. Resting, exercise, and recovery ECGs showed no abnormalities.

TABLE 38-1. *Selected Respiratory Function Data*

MEASUREMENT	PREDICTED	BEFORE BRONCHODILATOR	AFTER BRONCHODILATOR
Age, yr		50	
Sex		Male	
Height, cm		174	
Weight, kg	77	113	
Hematocrit, %		45	
VC, L	4.40	3.95	4.36
IC, L	2.94	3.30	3.75
TLC, L	6.44	6.08	
FEV$_1$, L	3.49	2.53	2.96
FEV$_1$/VC, %	79	64	
MVV, L/min	147	96	101
DL$_{CO}$, ml/mm Hg/min	28.6	30.6	

TABLE 38-2. *Selected Exercise Data*

MEASUREMENT	PREDICTED	MEASURED
Maximum V̇$_{O_2}$, L/min	2.68	1.84
Maximum HR, beats/min	170	131
Maximum O$_2$ pulse, ml/beat	15.8	14.3
ΔV̇$_{O_2}$/ΔWR, ml/min/W	10.3	10.2
AT, L/min	> 1.15	1.0
Blood pressure, mm Hg (rest, max)		131/88,206/106
Maximum V̇$_E$, L/min		93
Exercise breathing reserve, L/min	> 15	3
Pa$_{O_2}$, mm Hg (rest, max ex)		73,97
P(A − a)$_{O_2}$, mm Hg (rest, max ex)		34,23
P(a − ET)$_{CO_2}$, mm Hg (rest, max ex)		7,2
V$_D$/V$_T$ (rest, heavy ex)		0.41,0.31

FIG. 38-A.

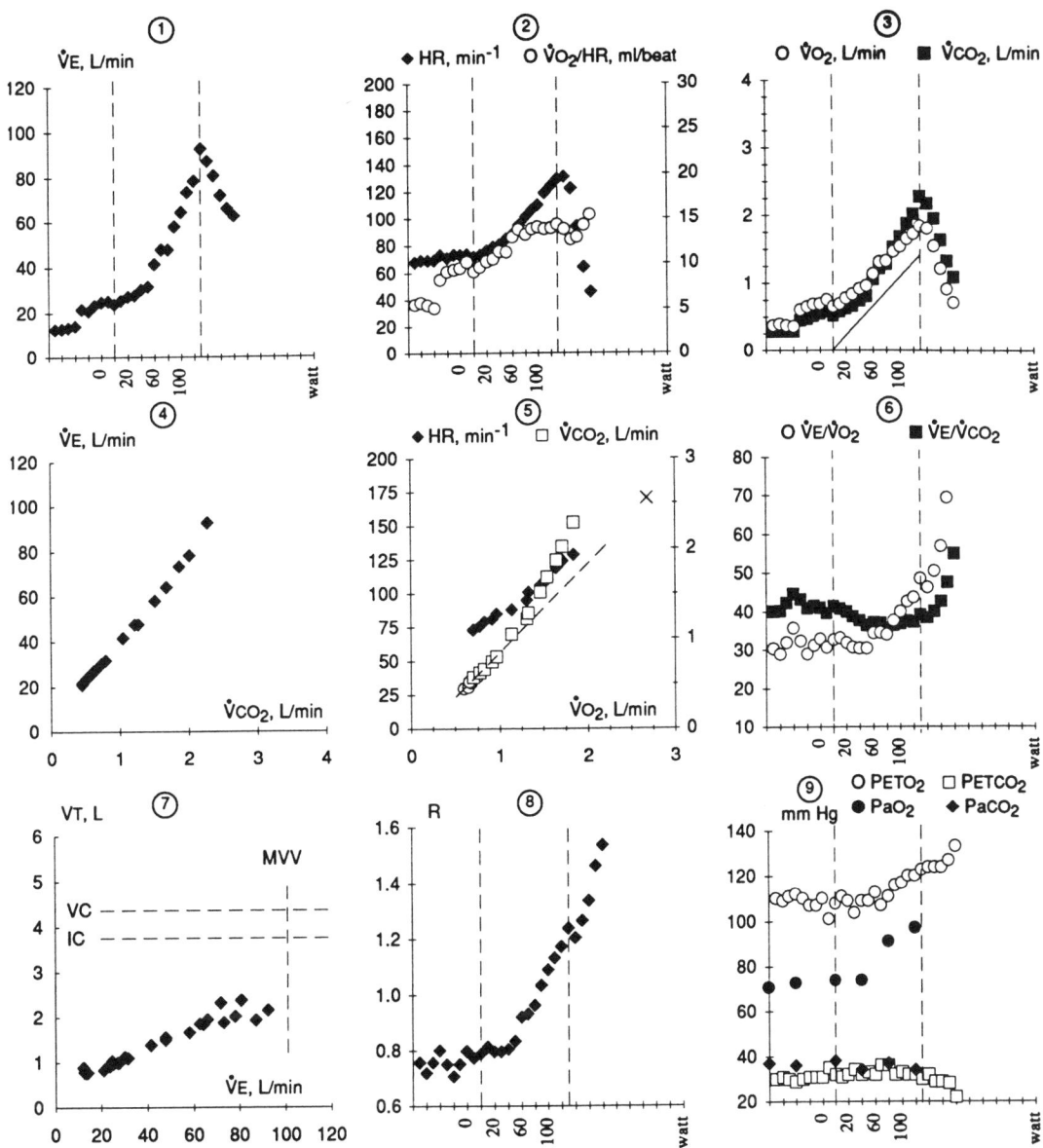

1. Vertical dashed lines in panels 1 to 3 and 6, 8, and 9 indicate the beginning and the end of increasing work period.

2. Unloaded cycling is performed for 3 minutes before the left vertical dashed line.

3. In panel 3, the diagonal line shows the increase of $\dot{V}O_2$ at a slope of 10 ml/min/W.

4. In panel 5, the diagonal dashed line has a slope of 1; the "x" in the upper right is the predicted maximum heart rate and $\dot{V}O_2$ for the subject.

Interpretation

COMMENTS

Resting respiratory function studies reveal mild airflow obstruction that improves following treatment with an aerosolized bronchodilator (Table 38-1). The patient is 36 kg overweight. His resting carboxyhemoglobin is 9.4% (normal < 2.0%). The patient's resting ECG is normal. This case is also presented because of the orthostasis that the patient developed when stopping exercise; this phenomenon is occasionally observed when heavy, upright exercise is abruptly terminated. To avoid this, we usually ask the patient who exercised

TABLE 38-3.

Time min	Work rate watts	BP mm Hg	HR min⁻¹	f min⁻¹	V̇E L/min BTPS	V̇CO2 L/min STPD	V̇O2 L/min STPD	V̇O2/HR ml/beat	R	pH	HCO3 meq/L	PO2, mm Hg ET	a	(A-a)	PCO2, mm Hg ET	a	(a-ET)	V̇E/V̇CO2	V̇E/V̇O2	VD/VT
	Rest	131/88								7.41	23		71			37				
	Rest		68	14	12.4	0.28	0.37	5.4	0.76			110			30			40	30	
	Rest		69	16	12.6	0.28	0.39	5.7	0.72			109			31			40	29	
	Rest		69	17	13.3	0.28	0.37	5.4	0.76			111			30			42	32	
	Rest	138/88	69	18	14.0	0.28	0.35	5.1	0.80	7.38	21	112	73	34	29	36	7	45	36	0.41
	Unloaded		73	25	21.5	0.45	0.60	8.2	0.75			110			30			43	32	
	Unloaded		71	25	20.9	0.46	0.65	9.2	0.71			107			31			41	29	
	Unloaded		73	25	23.3	0.51	0.68	9.3	0.75			107			31			42	31	
	Unloaded		73	24	24.6	0.55	0.69	9.5	0.80			110			31			41	33	
	Unloaded		74	26	25.2	0.58	0.75	10.1	0.77			101			35			40	31	
	Unloaded	150/88	72	26	23.7	0.52	0.66	9.2	0.79	7.39	23	108	74	30	32	38	6	41	33	0.41
0.5	20		73	26	25.4	0.57	0.70	9.6	0.81			111			31			41	33	
1.0	20		76	27	27.0	0.62	0.78	10.3	0.79			109			32			40	32	
1.5	40		79	28	27.8	0.66	0.83	10.5	0.80			104			34			39	31	
2.0	40	156/88	81	27	30.2	0.74	0.92	11.4	0.80	7.42	22	109	74	35	32	34	2	38	30	0.30
2.5	60		85	29	31.6	0.80	0.96	11.3	0.83			109			33			36	30	
3.0	60		88	30	41.5	1.05	1.14	13.0	0.92			113			32			37	34	
3.5	80		95	32	47.8	1.22	1.31	13.8	0.93			107			36			37	34	
4.0	80	169/94	101	31	47.8	1.28	1.33	13.2	0.96	7.36	21	111	91	21	36	37	1	35	34	0.32
4.5	100		106	35	58.1	1.52	1.47	13.9	1.03			116			32			36	38	
5.0	100		110	35	64.4	1.68	1.54	14.0	1.09			117			33			37	40	
5.5	120		119	39	73.3	1.87	1.65	13.9	1.13			120			32			37	42	
6.0	120	200/100	124	39	78.3	2.02	1.72	13.9	1.17	7.35	18	120	97	23	32	34	2	37	44	0.30
6.5	140		129	43	92.6	2.28	1.84	14.3	1.24			123			30			39	48	
	Recovery		131	45	87.3	2.18	1.81	13.8	1.20			124			32			38	46	
	Recovery	131/72	122	34	80.9	1.96	1.55	12.7	1.26			124			29			40	50	
	Recovery	113/63	94	31	71.9	1.63	1.22	13.0	1.34			124			29			42	57	
	Recovery	88/44	64	34	66.1	1.33	0.91	14.2	1.46			127			28			48	69	
	Recovery	75/31	46	34	62.7	1.09	0.71	15.4	1.54			133			22			55	84	

hard to continue very light exercise (unloading cycle or slow walking) after completing the maximum work rate.

ANALYSIS

In flow chart 1, the maximum V̇O2 and anaerobic threshold are reduced (Table 38-2), which directs us through branchpoints 1.1, 1.2, and 1.3 to flow chart 4. The breathing reserve is low (branchpoint 4.1) and the VD/VT is high (branchpoint 4.2). The diagnosis of "lung disease with impaired peripheral oxygenation" is not fully satisfactory, although the patient does have a positive $P(a - ET)_{CO_2}$ as evidence for ventilation-perfusion mismatching and mild obstructive lung disease. The resting oxyhemoglobin saturation is reduced because of carboxyhemoglobinemia and a low Pa_{O_2}, but the improvement in resting hypoxemia with exercise is typical of obesity. The heart rate

reserve is also high, consistent with ventilatory limitation to exercise.

The development of a metabolic acidosis at a low V̇O2 (i.e., a low AT) also contributed to the exercise limitation, because it stimulated ventilation at all work rates above the AT, evidenced by the steep rise in V̇E/V̇O2 in panel 6 of Fig. 38-A. This response is in contrast to that seen in cases 37, 40, and 42, where the V̇E/V̇O2 does not rise as steeply towards the end of exercise and where a circulatory-induced metabolic acidosis did not contribute to a low breathing reserve and ventilatory limitation.

CONCLUSION

Mild airflow obstruction, obesity, and cigarette smoking all contribute to ventilatory limitation to exercise.

CASE 39 *Emphysema with mild airway obstruction*

CLINICAL FINDINGS

This 50-year-old male long-term smoker was referred for cardiopulmonary exercise testing for evaluation of his exertional dyspnea. He became symptomatic after walking one block. He had mild obstructive lung disease of long duration consistent with emphysema. His only current medication was a frequently used inhaled β agonist. The study was done to determine whether his exercise limitation was due to his lung disease.

EXERCISE FINDINGS

The patient performed exercise on a cycle ergometer. He pedalled at 60 rpm without an added load for 3 minutes. The work rate was then increased 15 W per minute to tolerance. Heart rate and rhythm were continuously monitored; 12-lead ECGs were obtained during rest, exercise, and recovery. Blood pressure was measured with a sphygmomanometer and oxygen saturation with an ear oximeter. The patient appeared to give an excellent effort and stopped exercise because of shortness of breath. He denied chest pain during or after the study. Resting, exercise, and recovery ECGs were not remarkable except for occasional multifocal premature ventricular contractions during exercise and recovery.

TABLE 39-1. *Selected Respiratory Function Data*

MEASUREMENT	PREDICTED	MEASURED
Age, yr		50
Sex		Male
Height, cm		168
Weight, kg	72	66
Hematocrit, %		46
VC, L	4.06	4.10
IC, L	2.71	3.30
TLC, L	5.92	7.07
FEV_1, L	3.22	2.57
FEV_1/VC, %	79	63
MVV, L/min	141	91
D_{LCO}, ml/mm Hg/min	25.4	14.7

TABLE 39-2. *Selected Exercise Data*

MEASUREMENT	PREDICTED	MEASURED
Maximum $\dot{V}_{O_2}$, L/min	2.22	1.39
Maximum HR, beats/min	170	126
Maximum O_2 pulse, ml/beat	13.1	11.0
$\Delta \dot{V}_{O_2}/\Delta WR$, ml/min/W	10.3	7.3
AT, L/min	> 0.95	0.9
Blood pressure, mm Hg (rest, max)		120/80,160/100
Maximum $\dot{V}_E$, L/min		89
Exercise breathing reserve, L/min	> 15	2
O_2 saturation (oximeter) (rest, max)		93,88

TABLE 39-3.

Time min	Work rate watts	BP mm Hg	HR min^-1	f min^-1	$\dot{V}_E$ L/min BTPS	$\dot{V}CO_2$ L/min STPD	$\dot{V}O_2$ L/min STPD	$\dfrac{\dot{V}O_2}{HR}$ ml/beat	R	pH	HCO₃ meq/L	PO2, mm Hg ET	a	(A-a)	PCO2, mm Hg ET	a	(a-ET)	$\dfrac{\dot{V}_E}{\dot{V}CO_2}$	$\dfrac{\dot{V}_E}{\dot{V}O_2}$	$\dfrac{V_D}{V_T}$
	Rest	120/80																		
	Rest		72	22	16.9	0.26	0.32	4.4	0.81			123			22			58	47	
	Rest		73	23	19.0	0.28	0.36	4.9	0.78			122			22			61	47	
	Rest		66	21	17.9	0.27	0.34	5.2	0.79			121			23			60	47	
	Rest	120/80	70	19	15.0	0.23	0.29	4.1	0.79			121			23			58	46	
	Rest		70	19	15.6	0.24	0.31	4.4	0.77			122			22			58	45	
	Rest		77	18	17.8	0.27	0.33	4.3	0.82			123			22			60	49	
	Unloaded		84	19	23.9	0.43	0.53	6.3	0.81			119			24			52	42	
	Unloaded		87	21	29.1	0.49	0.58	6.7	0.84			122			23			56	47	
	Unloaded		83	23	30.6	0.51	0.59	7.1	0.86			123			23			56	49	
	Unloaded		84	22	28.8	0.51	0.61	7.3	0.84			121			24			53	44	
	Unloaded		88	23	31.1	0.55	0.64	7.3	0.86			123			23			53	46	
	Unloaded	140/90	88	22	31.9	0.57	0.67	7.6	0.85			122			23			53	45	
0.5	8		86	23	33.0	0.60	0.68	7.9	0.88			123			24			52	46	
1.0	15		88	22	33.2	0.60	0.67	7.6	0.90			123			24			52	47	
1.5	23		88	23	42.5	0.73	0.74	8.4	0.99			126			22			56	55	
2.0	30	140/90	91	25	40.9	0.68	0.69	7.6	0.99			125			22			57	56	
2.5	38		95	26	45.0	0.78	0.83	8.7	0.94			122			24			55	52	
3.0	45		93	25	44.9	0.80	0.86	9.2	0.93			123			24			53	50	
3.5	53		101	26	50.3	0.92	0.93	9.2	0.99			124			24			52	52	
4.0	60	150/92	105	28	55.3	1.01	0.99	9.4	1.02			124			24			52	53	
4.5	68		108	31	63.5	1.13	1.07	9.9	1.06			126			23			54	57	
5.0	75		111	31	66.8	1.21	1.12	10.1	1.08			126			24			53	57	
5.5	83		115	34	72.7	1.30	1.17	10.2	1.11			127			23			54	60	
6.0	90	160/100	117	37	75.2	1.35	1.22	10.4	1.11			127			24			53	59	
6.5	98		120	39	83.5	1.47	1.29	10.8	1.14			127			24			55	62	
7.0	105		124	41	87.9	1.54	1.34	10.8	1.15			128			24			55	63	
7.5	113		126	41	89.3	1.60	1.39	11.0	1.15			128			23			54	62	
	Recovery		109	37	80.1	1.42	1.20	11.0	1.18			129			23			54	64	
	Recovery	140/90	105	36	73.4	1.22	1.08	10.3	1.13			129			23			58	65	
	Recovery		99	30	57.9	1.01	0.85	8.6	1.19			128			24			55	65	
	Recovery	140/80	92	28	51.5	0.87	0.71	7.7	1.23			130			23			56	69	

Interpretation

COMMENTS

Resting respiratory function studies showed mild obstruction, an insignificant bronchodilator response to inhaled β agonist, and a moderately reduced D$_{LCO}$.

ANALYSIS

In flow chart 1, maximum $\dot{V}O_2$ and the anaerobic threshold are low (Table 39-2). Going next to flow chart 4, the breathing reserve (branchpoint 4.1) is clearly low, confirming the diagnosis that airway obstruction is limiting exercise tolerance. Although blood gases are not available, the high ventilatory equivalents indicate increased dead space ventilation or hyperventilation. Blood gas measurements would have been helpful in the differentiation, because the low P$_{ETCO_2}$ is compatible with either. Because the R is normal at rest and at low work rates, the unusually low P$_{ETCO_2}$ is chronic and therefore is not accounted for by acute hyperventilation. It indicates that the patient requires an inordinately high ventilatory response to exercise. The high heart rate reserve is also consistent with ventilation limiting exercise. The low $\Delta\dot{V}O_2/\Delta WR$ and multifocal beats might be due to pulmonary vascular disease secondary to the patient's obstructive lung disease or the result of reduced venous return during exercise resulting from high intrapleural pressure consequent to air trapping and hyperinflation.

CONCLUSION

This patient has mild to moderate obstructive lung disease with high ventilatory requirements probably secondary to ventilation-perfusion mismatching causing ventilatory limitation to exercise.

FIG. 39-A.

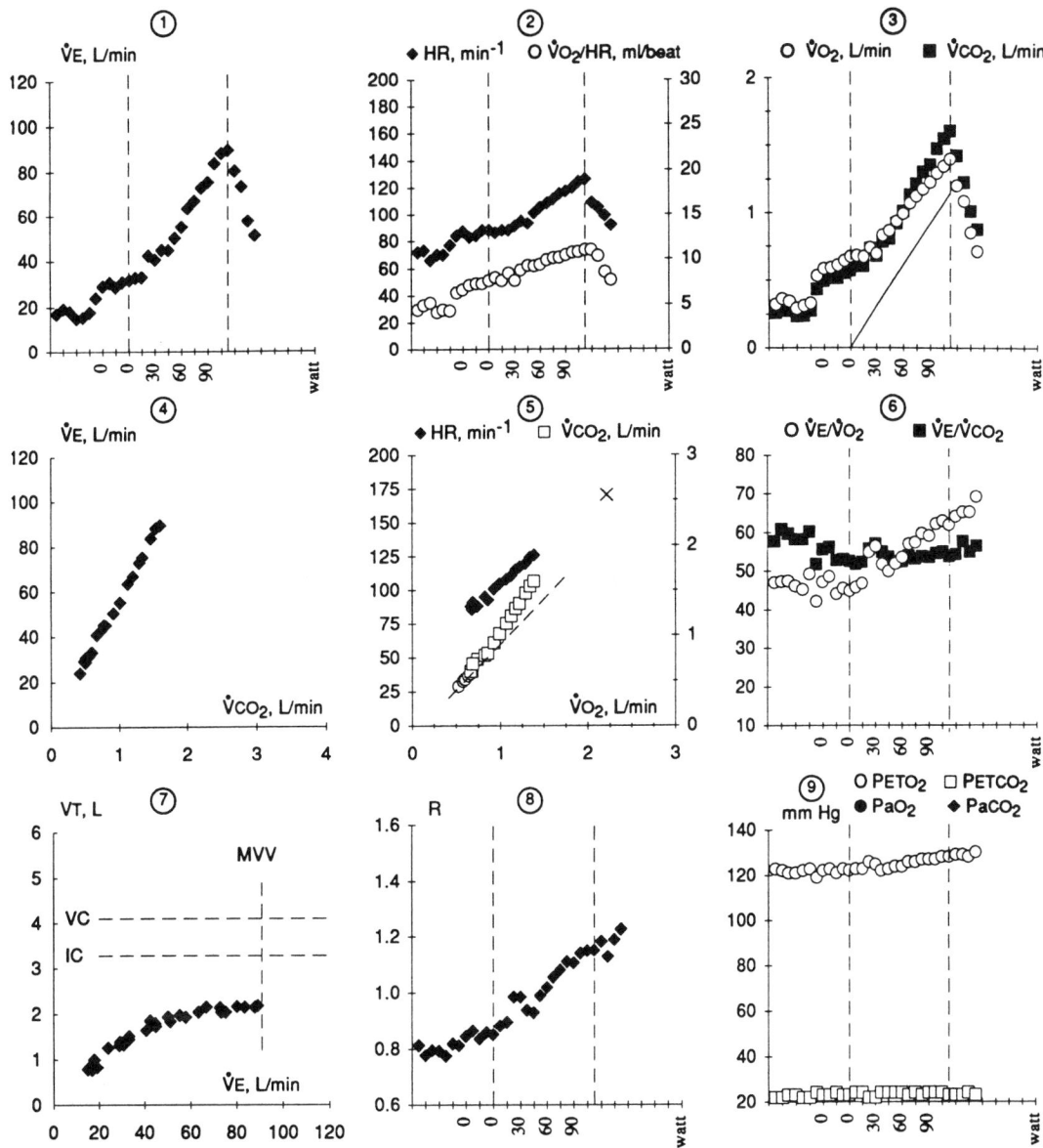

1. Vertical dashed lines in panels 1 to 3 and 6, 8, and 9 indicate the beginning and the end of increasing work period.

2. Unloaded cycling is performed for 3 minutes before the left vertical dashed line.

3. In panel 3, the diagonal line shows the increase of $\dot{V}O_2$ at a slope of 10 ml/min/W.

4. In panel 5, the diagonal dashed line has a slope of 1; the "x" in the upper right is the predicted maximum heart rate and $\dot{V}O_2$ for the subject.

CASE 40 *Emphysema, severe*

CLINICAL FINDINGS

This 65-year-old man had a long history of asbestos exposure and heavy cigarette smoking. He was being treated with aminophylline, inhaled bronchodilators, and home oxygen therapy. He was also receiving chlorothiazide for treatment of hypertension. He had stopped smoking 12 years previously. Resting ECG suggested left atrial enlargement. The question was raised with respect to the role of the patient's circulatory disease in his ventilatory impairment.

EXERCISE FINDINGS

The patient performed exercise on a cycle ergometer. He first pedalled at 60 rpm, without added load, for 3 minutes. The work rate was then increased 10 W per minute to his symptom-limited maximum. Blood was sampled every second minute and intra-arterial blood pressure was recorded from a brachial artery catheter. There were no abnormal ST segment changes at rest or during exercise. He stopped exercise complaining of shortness of breath.

TABLE 40-1. *Selected Respiratory Function Data*

MEASUREMENT	PREDICTED	MEASURED
Age, yr		65
Sex		Male
Height, cm		170
Weight, kg	74	99
Hematocrit, %		53
VC, L	3.72	2.17
IC, L	2.48	1.31
TLC, L	5.85	8.22
FEV_1, L	2.89	0.56
FEV_1/VC, %	78	26
MVV, L/min	123	31
D_{LCO}, ml/mm Hg/min	25.1	13.2

TABLE 40-2. *Selected Exercise Data*

MEASUREMENT	Predicted	MEASURED
Maximum $\dot{V}_{O_2}$, L/min	2.11	0.90
Maximum HR, beats/min	155	129
Maximum O_2 pulse, ml/beat	13.6	7.0
$\Delta\dot{V}_{O_2}/\Delta WR$, ml/min/W	10.3	8.9
AT, L/min	> 0.93	not reached
Blood pressure, mm Hg (rest, max)		175/94,256/138
Maximum $\dot{V}_E$, L/min		28
Exercise breathing reserve, L/min	> 15	3
Pa_{O_2}, mm Hg (rest, max ex)		56,46
$P(A-a)_{O_2}$, mm Hg (rest, max ex)		39,48
$P(a-ET)_{CO_2}$, mm Hg (rest, max ex)		4,6
V_D/V_T (rest, heavy ex)		0.40,0.41
HCO_3^-, mEq/L (rest, 2-min recov)		28,27

TABLE 40-3.

Time min	Work rate watts	BP mm Hg	HR min⁻¹	f min⁻¹	$\dot{V}_E$ L/min BTPS	$\dot{V}_{CO_2}$ L/min STPD	$\dot{V}_{O_2}$ L/min STPD	$\frac{\dot{V}_{O_2}}{HR}$ ml/beat	R	pH	HCO3 meq/L	PO2 ET	PO2 a	PO2 (A-a)	PCO2 ET	PCO2 a	PCO2 (a-ET)	$\frac{\dot{V}_E}{\dot{V}_{CO_2}}$	$\frac{\dot{V}_E}{\dot{V}_{O_2}}$	$\frac{V_D}{V_T}$
	Rest	175/94																		
	Rest		107	18	13.2	0.32	0.40	3.7	0.80			91			44			36	29	
	Rest	175/94	102	15	11.1	0.28	0.36	3.5	0.78	7.41	28	87	56	39	46	45		35	27	0.40
	Unloaded	194/100	111	23	17.0	0.42	0.52	4.7	0.81	7.41	28	97	54	43	41	45	4	36	29	0.41
	Unloaded		110	23	17.5	0.42	0.52	4.7	0.81			92			44			37	30	
0.5	10		109	25	18.6	0.47	0.59	5.4	0.80			95			43			35	28	
1.0	10		112	24	19.4	0.51	0.62	5.5	0.82			97			41			34	28	
1.5	20		115	27	20.5	0.53	0.65	5.7	0.82			95			43			34	28	
2.0	20	225/113	119	27	21.3	0.57	0.69	5.8	0.83	7.40	29	97	49	45	42	48	6	33	28	0.41
2.5	30		123	30	23.4	0.62	0.74	6.0	0.84			96			43			34	28	
3.0	30		125	29	24.0	0.66	0.78	6.2	0.85			95			44			33	28	
3.5	40		129	32	25.4	0.68	0.80	6.2	0.85			97			43			33	28	
4.0	40	250/131	129	31	25.8	0.72	0.83	6.4	0.87	7.37	27	92	47	49	47	48	1	32	28	0.40
4.5	50	256/138	129	33	26.2	0.73	0.85	6.6	0.86	7.37	28	92	46	48	44	50	6	32	28	0.41
	Recovery		122	34	28.0	0.79	0.90	7.4	0.88			95			45			32	28	
	Recovery		120	32	26.3	0.70	0.79	6.6	0.89			100			42			34	30	
	Recovery		114	32	23.5	0.62	0.70	6.1	0.89			98			43			34	30	
	Recovery	194/94	112	29	21.3	0.55	0.61	5.4	0.90	7.38	27	101	49	51	42	46	4	34	31	0.40
	Recovery		107	27	20.8	0.54	0.59	5.5	0.92			95			47			34	31	

FIG. 40-A.

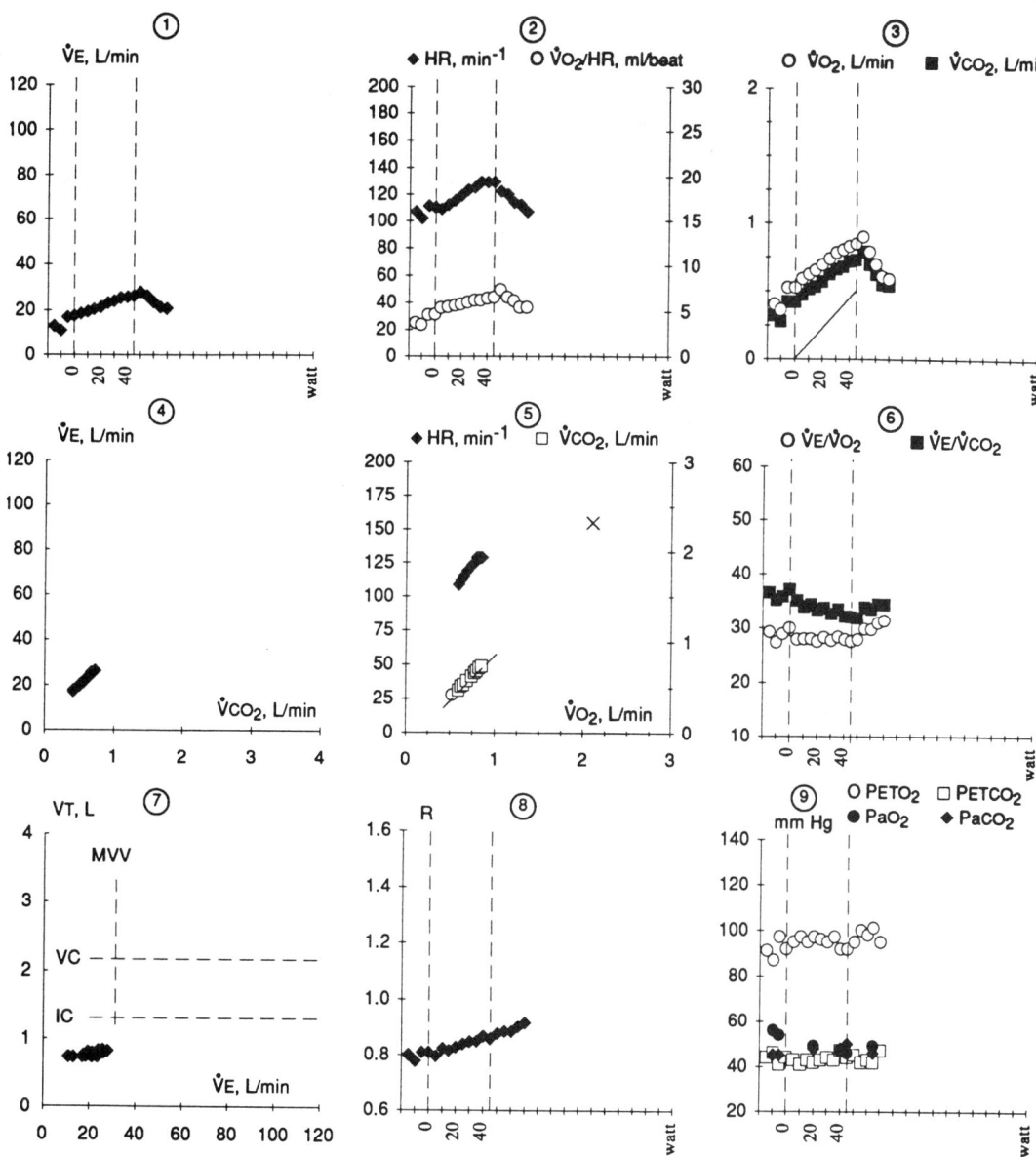

1. Vertical dashed lines in panels 1 to 3 and 6, 8, and 9 indicate the beginning and the end of increasing work period.

2. Unloaded cycling is performed for 3 minutes before the left vertical dashed line.

3. In panel 3, the diagonal line shows the increase of $\dot{V}O_2$ at a slope of 10 ml/min/W.

4. In panel 5, the diagonal dashed line has a slope of 1; the "x" in the upper right is the predicted maximum heart rate and $\dot{V}O_2$ for the subject.

Interpretation

COMMENTS

This patient clearly has evidence of very severe obstructive lung disease (Table 40-1). His resting ECG suggests left atrial enlargement.

ANALYSIS

In flow chart 1, the maximum $\dot{V}O_2$ is reduced while the anaerobic threshold is not reached, but is above lower limits of normal (Table 40-2), which directs us through branchpoints 1.1, 1.2, and 1.3 to flow chart 3. The breathing reserve is low (branchpoint 3.1), and strong evidence for ventilation-perfusion mismatching (increased V_D/V_T, $P(A-a)_{O_2}$, $P(a-ET)_{O_2}$) is found. The heart rate reserve is also high, consistent with ventilatory limitation to exercise. The maximal ventilatory frequency is low (branchpoint 3.2), typical of obstructive lung disease demonstrated during the patient's resting respiratory function tests. The mild respiratory acidosis during exercise and the high $\dot{V}E$ during recovery also confirm a diagnosis of ventilatory limitation.

CONCLUSION

The patient, while having ECG evidence of left atrial enlargement and significant systemic hypertension during exercise, clearly is limited by his obstructive lung disease and not by cardiac dysfunction. The presence of a high heart rate reserve and the absence of a ventilatory reserve, along with the development of a mild respiratory acidosis at this patient's maximum $\dot{V}O_2$, support the conclusion that he has ventilatory limitation. Circulatory limitation was not severe enough to cause a metabolic acidosis over the low range of work rates the patient was able to tolerate. Thus, lactic acidosis did not contribute to ventilatory drive.

CASE 41 *Emphysema with pulmonary vascular disease*

CLINICAL FINDINGS

This 61-year-old man with bullous emphysema and right middle lobe scarring on roentgenograms was referred for evaluation regarding the need for oxygen supplementation. The patient had a 35 pack year history of cigarette smoking. He had not sought medical care until 4 months previously when he was hospitalized for pneumonia, severe dyspnea, and hemoptysis. Bronchoscopy, transbronchial biopsy, cytology, and mycobacterial studies were negative. Resting ECG showed poor R-wave progression.

EXERCISE FINDINGS

The patient performed exercise on a cycle ergometer. He pedalled at 60 rpm without an added load for 3 minutes. The work rate was then increased 10 W per minute to tolerance. Arterial blood was sampled every second minute and intra-arterial pressure was recorded from a percutaneously placed brachial artery catheter. The patient stopped exercise because of leg fatigue. The patient had no chest pain or further ECG abnormalities.

TABLE 41-1. *Selected Respiratory Function Data*

MEASUREMENT	PREDICTED	MEASURED
Age, yr		61
Sex		Male
Height, cm		173
Weight, kg	76	63
Hematocrit, %		45
VC, L	4.00	4.37
IC, L	2.67	2.62
TLC, L	6.15	9.11
FEV_1, L	3.13	2.11
FEV_1/VC, %	78	48
MVV, L/min	131	87
D_{LCO}, ml/mm Hg/min	26.0	8.4

TABLE 41-2. *Selected Exercise Data*

MEASUREMENT	PREDICTED	MEASURED
Maximum $\dot{V}O_2$, L/min	1.95	1.25
Maximum HR, beats/min	159	149
Maximum O_2 pulse, ml/beat	12.3	8.4
$\Delta \dot{V}O_2/\Delta WR$, ml/min/W	10.3	8.5
AT, L/min	> 0.86	0.7
Blood pressure, mm Hg (rest, max)		129/75, 190/96
Maximum $\dot{V}E$, L/min		85
Exercise breathing reserve, L/min	> 15	2
Pa_{O_2}, mm Hg (rest, max ex)		83, 72
$P(A-a)_{O_2}$ mm Hg (rest, max ex)		32, 52
$P(a-ET)_{CO_2}$, mm Hg (rest, max ex)		4, 8
V_D/V_T (rest, max ex)		0.28, 0.41
HCO_3^-, mEq/L (rest, 2-min recov)		22, 13

TABLE 41-3.

Time min	Work rate watts	BP mm Hg	HR min⁻¹	f min⁻¹	V̇E L/min BTPS	V̇CO2 L/min STPD	V̇O2 L/min STPD	V̇O2/HR ml/beat	R	pH	HCO3 meq/L	PO2, mm Hg ET	a	(A-a)	PCO2, mm Hg ET	a	(a-ET)	V̇E/V̇CO2	V̇E/V̇O2	VD/VT
	Rest	129/75								7.44	22	86			33					
	Rest		77	15	13.9	0.30	0.28	3.6	1.07			122			30			42	45	
	Rest		75	13	10.8	0.23	0.23	3.1	1.00			121			31			42	42	
	Rest		76	14	9.9	0.21	0.21	2.8	1.00			118			32			41	41	
	Rest	129/75	75	15	10.8	0.27	0.26	3.5	1.04	7.41	22	118	83	32	32	36	4	35	37	0.28
	Rest		74	12	10.4	0.22	0.20	2.7	1.10			123			29			43	47	
	Rest		75	11	10.4	0.25	0.24	3.2	1.04			120			31			38	39	
	Unloaded		83	20	17.8	0.40	0.38	4.6	1.05			117			32			40	42	
	Unloaded	138/41	86	19	18.6	0.43	0.41	4.8	1.05	7.41	22	121	91	25	30	35	5	40	41	0.34
	Unloaded		89	16	19.6	0.48	0.46	5.2	1.04			120			30			38	40	
	Unloaded		94	17	21.2	0.52	0.51	5.4	1.02			120			31			38	39	
	Unloaded		94	18	24.4	0.59	0.57	6.1	1.04			121			30			39	40	
	Unloaded	168/90	95	18	25.0	0.62	0.59	6.2	1.05	7.40	21	121	78	38	30	35	5	38	40	0.33
0.5	10		97	17	25.3	0.64	0.59	6.1	1.08			120			31			37	40	
1.0	10	168/90	98	20	29.0	0.71	0.65	6.6	1.09	7.41	22	122	77	40	29	35	6	38	42	0.34
1.5	20		101	22	28.5	0.70	0.64	6.3	1.09			119			32			38	42	
2.0	20	174/90	102	21	32.5	0.78	0.70	6.9	1.11	7.40	21	123	74	45	29	34	5	39	44	0.34
2.5	30		104	24	28.9	0.73	0.67	6.4	1.09			120			32			37	40	
3.0	30	174/40	110	21	40.1	0.96	0.83	7.5	1.16	7.40	21	124	71	48	28	35	7	40	46	0.37
3.5	40		115	20	38.7	0.97	0.84	7.3	1.15			122			30			38	44	
4.0	40	180/90	119	23	44.4	1.08	0.92	7.7	1.17	7.39	20	123	71	49	29	34	5	39	46	0.34
4.5	50		123	22	47.7	1.16	0.95	7.7	1.22			125			28			40	48	
5.0	50	182/88	126	25	51.7	1.22	0.97	7.7	1.26	7.38	19	125	70	52	28	33	5	41	51	0.34
5.5	60		130	25	56.9	1.35	1.05	8.1	1.29			126			28			41	52	
6.0	60	189/93	132	26	58.7	1.40	1.08	8.2	1.30	7.36	18	125	72	51	29	33	4	40	52	0.34
6.5	70		138	26	62.3	1.47	1.12	8.1	1.31			127			28			41	54	
7.0	70	190/90	140	31	68.1	1.54	1.14	8.1	1.35	7.32	17	128	72	51	27	34	7	43	57	0.39
7.5	80		144	32	71.4	1.62	1.19	8.3	1.36			127			28			42	58	
8.0	80	190/96	149	38	80.2	1.73	1.24	8.3	1.40	7.32	17	129	72	52	26	34	8	44	62	0.41
8.5	90		148	39	85.2	1.80	1.25	8.4	1.44			129			26			45	66	
	Recovery		141	27	66.6	1.49	1.07	7.6	1.39			129			26			43	60	
	Recovery		140	26	63.3	1.38	0.90	6.4	1.53			130			26			44	68	
	Recovery		133	22	54.5	1.19	0.74	5.6	1.61			131			26			44	71	
	Recovery	174/87	126	22	51.3	1.07	0.65	5.2	1.65	7.26	13	132	115	14	25	30	5	46	76	0.36
	Recovery		120	24	45.5	0.88	0.54	4.5	1.63			133			24			49	80	

Interpretation

COMMENTS

Resting studies showed a moderate obstructive ventilatory defect, increased total lung capacity, and low DLCO. The ECG showed poor R-wave progression.

ANALYSIS

In flow chart 1, maximum V̇O2 and anaerobic threshold are decreased. Proceeding next to flow chart 4, the low breathing reserve (branchpoint 4.1) and high VD/VT (branchpoint 4.2) lead to the diagnosis of lung disease with impaired peripheral oxygenation. The high VT/IC and low arterial saturation are confirmatory, whereas the low breathing frequency is typical for obstructive lung disease, which was evident prior to exercise testing. Although the patient stated that he stopped exercise because of leg fatigue, his low breathing reserve indicated that he also had ventilatory limitation. The abnormal gas exchange (high ventilatory equivalents, high VD/VT, low Pa_{O_2}, high $P(A-a)_{O_2}$, and positive $P(a-ET)_{CO_2}$) are consistent with obliterative pulmonary vascular disease secondary to obstructive lung disease. The severity of the metabolic acidodis (decrease in HCO_3^- from 22 to 13 mEq/L) is consistent with the low anaerobic threshold and suggests poor O_2 flow to the exercising muscle, most likely because the patient's pulmonary vascular disease limited his ability to increase cardiac output.

FIG. 41-A.

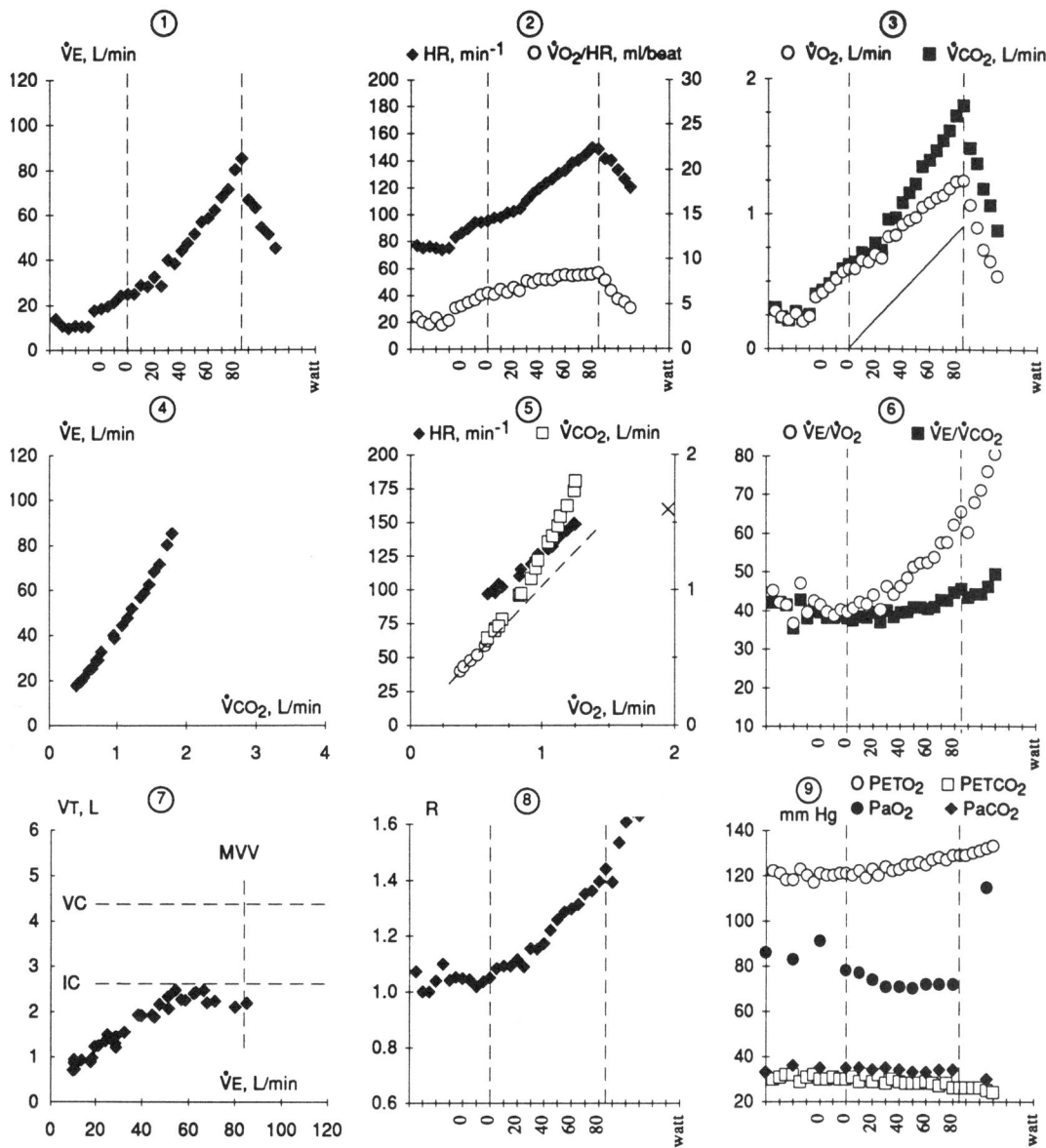

1. Vertical dashed lines in panels 1 to 3 and 6, 8, and 9 indicate the beginning and the end of increasing work period.

2. Unloaded cycling is performed for 3 minutes before the left vertical dashed line.

3. In panel 3, the diagonal line shows the increase of $\dot{V}O_2$ at a slope of 10 ml/min/W.

4. In panel 5, the diagonal dashed line has a slope of 1; the "x" in the upper right is the predicted maximum heart rate and $\dot{V}O_2$ for the subject.

CONCLUSION

This patient has physiologic evidence of pulmonary vascular disease, secondary to obvious obstructive lung disease. The mild degree of hypoxemia does not qualify for O_2 supplementation under current federal funding guidelines, but dyspnea may well be less with O_2 supplementation. This is an example of lung disease causing secondary cardiovascular disease, which in turn results in a high ventilatory requirement as compensation for the exercise-induced lactic acidosis. This makes the patient more exercise limited than predicted from his moderate defect in spirometry.

CASE 42 *Emphysema and bronchitis, severe: Air and oxygen breathing*

CLINICAL FINDINGS

This 62-year-old retired accountant had a long history of heavy cigarette smoking but had stopped 4 years previously. He had a chronic cough and shortness of breath. He had gradually increased his activity by physical training and rode his bicycle many miles daily. There was no history of congestive failure. He took oral aminophylline but no other medications. He participated in a study evaluating the effects of oxygen supplementation.

EXERCISE FINDINGS

The patient performed exercise on a cycle ergometer. He pedalled at 60 rpm without added load for 3 minutes while breathing humidified compressed air. The work rate was then increased 10 W per minute to his symptom-limited maximum. Blood was sampled every second minute, and intra-arterial blood pressure was recorded from a percutaneously placed brachial artery catheter. He stopped exercise complaining of shortness of breath. Following 30 minutes of rest, he was given humidified 100% O_2 to breathe while the exercise study was repeated. He again stopped exercise complaining of shortness of breath. The 12-lead ECG showed no ST segment changes or arrhythmia.

TABLE 42-1. *Selected Respiratory Function Data*

MEASUREMENT	PREDICTED	MEASURED
Age, yr		62
Sex		Male
Height, cm		173
Weight, kg	76	78
Hematocrit, %		51
VC, L	4.30	1.67
IC, L	2.87	1.22
TLC, L	6.87	8.30
FEV_1, L	3.40	0.54
FEV_1/VC, %	79	32
MVV, L/min	131	32
DL_{CO}, ml/mm Hg/min	30.9	18.5

TABLE 42-2. *Selected Exercise Data*

MEASUREMENT	PREDICTED	ROOM AIR	100% O_2
Maximum WR, W		80	120
Maximum $\dot{V}O_2$, L/min	2.11	0.96	
Maximum HR, beats/min	158	140	165
Maximum O_2 pulse, ml/beat	13.4	6.9	
$\Delta\dot{V}O_2/\Delta WR$, ml/min/W	10.3	8.3	
AT, L/min	> 0.93	not reached	
Blood pressure, mm Hg (rest, max)		169/106,250/125	144/94,234/119
Maximum $\dot{V}E$, L/min		32	40
Exercise breathing reserve, L/min	> 15	0	−8
Pa_{O_2}, mm Hg (rest, max ex)		78,53	587,583
$P(A-a)_{O_2}$, mm Hg (rest, max ex)		21,51	77,66
$P(a-ET)_{CO_2}$, mm Hg (rest, max ex)		6,5	8,3
VD/VT (rest, heavy ex)		0.42,0.38	0.48,0.37
HCO_3^-, mEq/L (rest, 2-min recov)		25,24	27,22

FIG. 42-A. *Air breathing.*

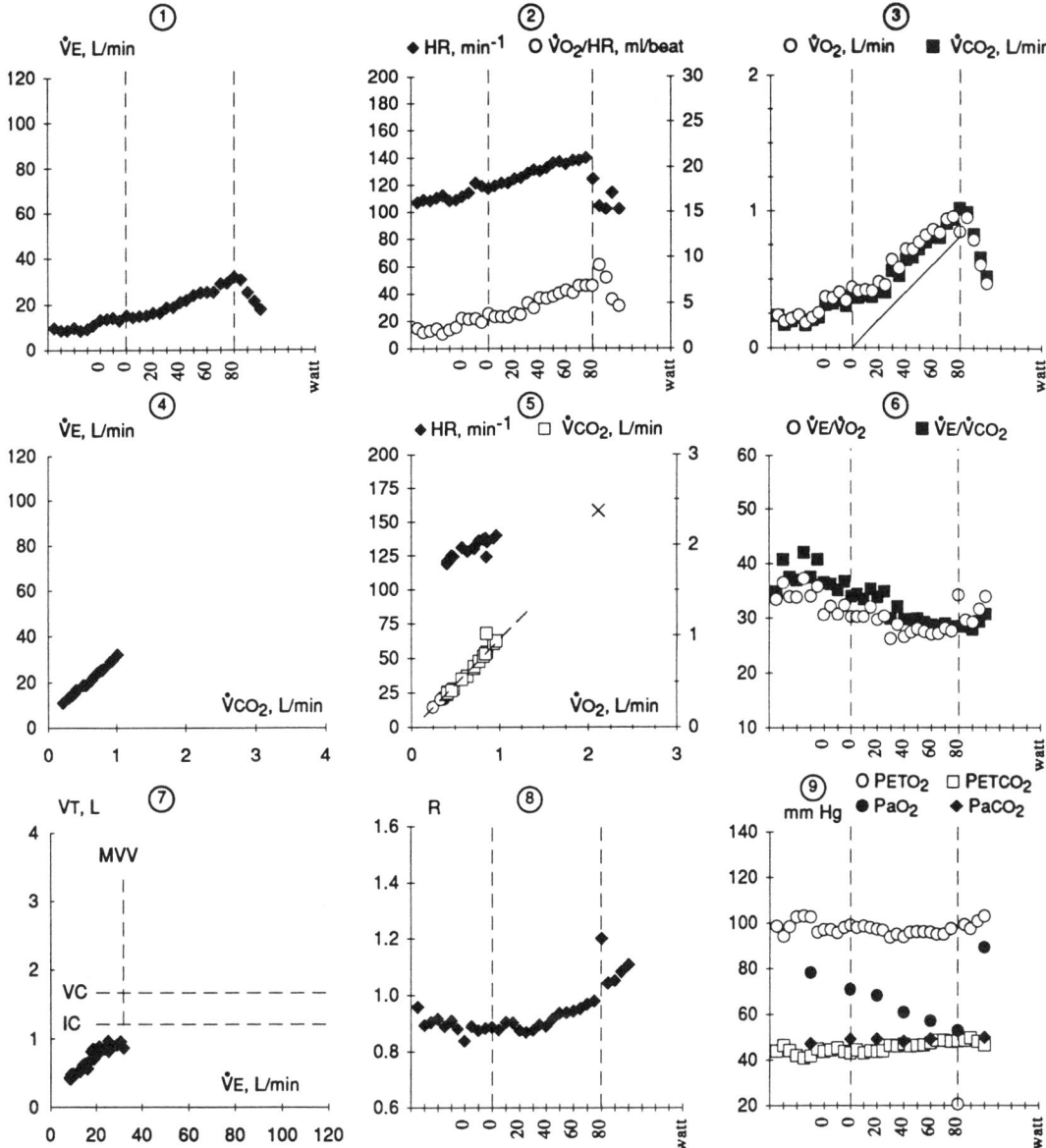

1. Vertical dashed lines in panels 1 to 3 and 6, 8, and 9 indicate the beginning and the end of increasing work period.

2. Unloaded cycling is performed for 3 minutes before the left vertical dashed line.

3. In panel 3, the diagonal line shows the increase of $\dot{V}_{O_2}$ at a slope of 10 ml/min/W.

4. In panel 5, the diagonal dashed line has a slope of 1; the "x" in the upper right is the predicted maximum heart rate and $\dot{V}_{O_2}$ for the subject.

FIG. 42-B. *Oxygen breathing.*

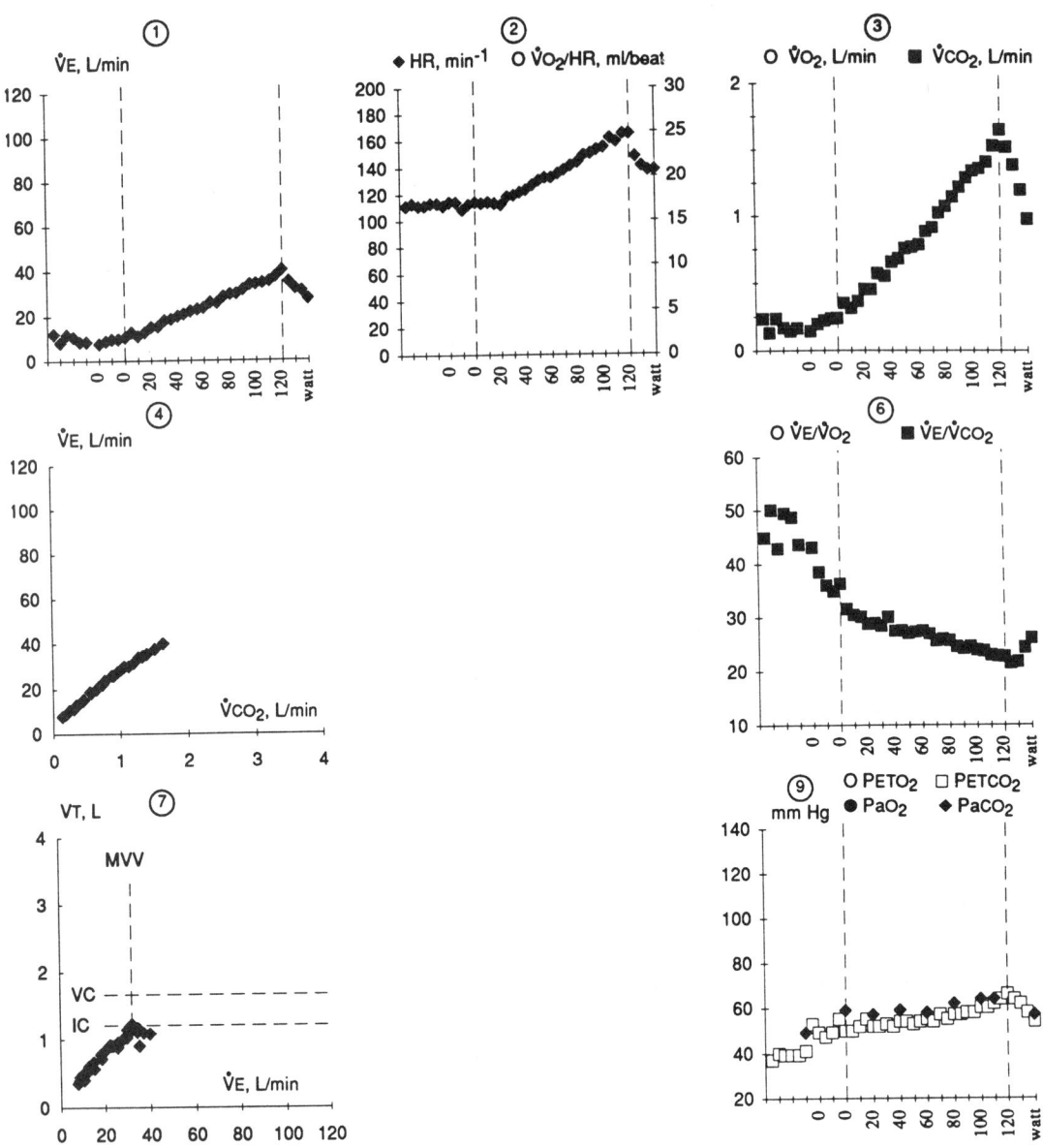

1. Vertical dashed lines in panels 1 to 3 and 6 and 9 indicate the beginning and the end of increasing work period.
2. Unloaded cycling is performed for 3 minutes before the left vertical dashed line.

TABLE 42-3. *Air breathing.*

Time min	Work rate watts	BP mm Hg	HR min⁻¹	f min⁻¹	V̇E L/min BTPS	V̇CO2 L/min STPD	V̇O2 L/min STPD	V̇O2/HR ml/beat	R	pH	HCO3 meq/L	PO2, mm Hg ET	a	(A-a)	PCO2, mm Hg ET	a	(a-ET)	V̇E/V̇CO2	V̇E/V̇O2	VD/VT
	Rest		107	20	9.7	0.23	0.24	2.2	0.96			99			44			35	33	
	Rest		109	21	8.7	0.17	0.19	1.7	0.89			94			46			41	36	
	Rest		108	20	8.8	0.19	0.21	1.9	0.90			98			44			37	34	
	Rest		110	20	9.8	0.22	0.24	2.2	0.92			102			42			37	34	
	Rest		112	20	8.4	0.16	0.18	1.6	0.89			103			41			42	37	
	Rest	169/106	108	19	9.1	0.20	0.22	2.0	0.91	7.35	25	102	78	21	42	47	6	37	34	0.42
	Unloaded		109	23	10.9	0.22	0.25	2.3	0.88			96			45			41	36	
	Unloaded		111	25	13.4	0.31	0.37	3.3	0.84			97			44			36	30	
	Unloaded		114	24	13.6	0.32	0.36	3.2	0.89			97			44			36	32	
	Unloaded		121	23	14.2	0.35	0.40	3.3	0.88			96			45			35	31	
	Unloaded		119	25	13.1	0.30	0.34	2.9	0.88			98			44			37	32	
	Unloaded	181/100	117	24	15.3	0.39	0.44	3.8	0.89	7.35	27	99	71	25	43	49	6	34	30	0.42
0.5	10		119	24	14.4	0.36	0.41	3.4	0.88			98			44			34	30	
1.0	10		121	25	14.8	0.38	0.42	3.5	0.90			99			43			33	30	
1.5	20		121	24	15.1	0.37	0.41	3.4	0.90			98			44			35	32	
2.0	20	187/106	124	25	16.3	0.42	0.48	3.9	0.88	7.35	27	97	68	27	44	49	6	34	30	0.42
2.5	30		125	29	16.4	0.40	0.46	3.7	0.87			97			44			35	30	
3.0	30		128	22	18.6	0.56	0.64	5.0	0.88			94			46			30	26	
3.5	40		131	27	18.9	0.52	0.58	4.4	0.90			95			46			32	29	
4.0	40	213/113	130	24	21.1	0.64	0.72	5.5	0.89	7.35	26	94	61	36	47	48	1	30	26	0.36
4.5	50		132	27	21.9	0.66	0.72	5.5	0.92			96			46			30	27	
5.0	50		136	28	23.9	0.72	0.77	5.7	0.94			96			46			30	28	
5.5	60		137	30	25.0	0.77	0.82	6.0	0.94			96			47			29	27	
6.0	60	225/119	135	28	25.6	0.81	0.86	6.4	0.94	7.35	27	96	57	42	48	49	1	29	27	0.35
6.5	70		138	31	25.4	0.80	0.84	6.1	0.95			95			49			28	27	
7.0	70		138	32	29.0	0.91	0.94	6.8	0.97			95			48			29	28	
7.5	80		140	32	29.2	0.94	0.96	6.9	0.98			98			48			28	28	
8.0	80	250/125	124	37	32.1	1.02	0.85	6.9	1.20	7.32	27	21	53	51	48	53	5	28	34	0.38
	Recovery		104	32	30.7	0.99	0.95	9.1	1.04			99			48			28	29	
	Recovery		102	26	25.2	0.83	0.79	7.7	1.05			98			50			28	29	
	Recovery		114	24	21.3	0.66	0.61	5.4	1.08			101			48			29	32	
	Recovery		102	22	17.8	0.52	0.47	4.6	1.11	7.30	24	103	89	15	47	50	3	31	34	0.39

Interpretation

COMMENTS

Resting respiratory function studies indicate that this patient has severe obstructive lung disease (Table 42-1); he also had significant systemic hypertension at rest.

ANALYSIS

In flow chart 1, maximum $\dot{V}O_2$ is moderately severely reduced and the anaerobic threshold is not reached (Table 42-2). We could satisfactorily use flow chart 3, but we use flow chart 5 because it is more detailed. The indices of ventilation-perfusion mismatching (V_D/V_T, $P(a-ET)_{CO_2}$ and $P(A-a)_{O_2}$) are abnormal (branchpoint 5.1). The breathing reserve is zero (branchpoint 5.3) indicating that the patient's exercise limitation is a result of lung disease. The breathing frequency (f) is less than 50 at the maximum work rate (branchpoint 5.7) consistent with the diagnosis of lung disease of the obstructive type. Other abnormal findings are an obstructive expiratory flow pattern (not shown), arterial oxygen tension, and $P(A-a)_{O_2}$ normal at rest but abnormal with exercise, a high heart rate reserve, and a respiratory acidosis at the maximum $\dot{V}O_2$.

As a result of breathing 100% O_2, the patient was able to increase his maximal work rate by 40 W and the maximum heart rate by 25 beats per minute (i.e., from 140 during air breathing to 165 during 100% oxygen breathing). These results demonstrate that the increased heart rate reserve, during the air breathing test, results from his ventilatory limitation. Moreover, the maximum exercise ventilation increases during oxygen breathing

TABLE 42-4. *Oxygen breathing.*

Time min	Work rate watts	BP mm Hg	HR min⁻¹	f min⁻¹	V̇E L/min BTPS	V̇CO2 L/min STPD	V̇O2 L/min STPD	V̇O2/HR ml/beat	R	pH	HCO3 meq/L	PO2 ET	PO2 a	PO2 (A-a)	PCO2 ET	PCO2 a	PCO2 (a-ET)	V̇E/V̇CO2	V̇E/V̇O2	VD/VT
	Rest		111	23	12.3	0.23									37			45		
	Rest		113	21	8.3	0.13									40			50		
	Rest		111	23	11.8	0.23									39			43		
	Rest		111	26	10.6	0.17									39			49		
	Rest		113	22	8.7	0.14									39			49		
	Rest	144/94	113	19	8.6	0.16				7.35	27	587	77		41	49	8	44		0.48
	Unloaded		111	11											53					
	Unloaded		114	22	7.9	0.14									49			43		
	Unloaded		114	20	9.0	0.19									47			38		
	Unloaded		108	20	9.6	0.22									49			36		
	Unloaded		112	22	9.9	0.23									55			35		
	Unloaded	181/106	114	21	10.5	0.24				7.29	28	587	67		50	59	9	36		0.50
0.5	10		113	21	12.8	0.35									50			31		
1.0	10		114	21	11.2	0.31									52			30		
1.5	20		113	21	12.6	0.36									55			30		
2.0	20	194/106	112	22	14.8	0.45				7.30	28	584	72		52	57	5	29		0.41
2.5	30		118	27	15.3	0.45									52			29		
3.0	30		119	23	18.1	0.57									53			28		
3.5	40		121	26	18.7	0.55									52			30		
4.0	40	200/106	123	24	19.9	0.65				7.29	28	580	74		54	59	5	27		0.42
4.5	50		127	24	20.8	0.68									54			28		
5.0	50		130	24	22.2	0.75									53			27		
5.5	60		132	25	22.8	0.76									54			27		
6.0	60	206/100	132	26	23.6	0.78				7.29	27	595	60		55	58	3	27		0.41
6.5	70		135	27	25.9	0.88									54			27		
7.0	70		138	29	25.8	0.91									57			26		
7.5	80		141	28	28.7	1.02									55			26		
8.0	80	213/106	144	29	29.8	1.07				7.27	28	601	50		57	62	5	26		0.42
8.5	90		149	26	30.0	1.14									57			24		
9.0	90		150	28	31.5	1.21									58			24		
9.5	100		153	30	33.8	1.28									58			24		
10.0	100	231/106	155	29	34.2	1.33				7.24	27	606	43		60	64	4	24		0.40
10.5	110		162	31	34.5	1.35									60			24		
11.0	110	234/119	159	39	35.4	1.40				7.23	26	583	66		62	64	2	23		0.37
11.5	120		165	34	37.3	1.52									64			23		
12.0	120		165	37	40.1	1.64									66			23		
	Recovery		148	30	35.0	1.51									64			21		
	Recovery		141	26	32.1	1.38									62			22		
	Recovery		138	26	31.1	1.19									58			24		
	Recovery	214/100	138	28	27.6	0.97				7.21	22	587	69		54	57	3	26		0.38

at the maximum work rate from 32 L/min, the value of his resting MVV, to 40 L/min.

The increased work rate achieved during O_2 breathing is primarily the result of depression in the ventilatory response to exercise. Consequently, the patient develops a more significant respiratory and metabolic acidoses as compared to the air breathing test (increase in Pa_{CO_2} of 6 mm Hg above rest during air breathing, as compared to 15 mm Hg for oxygen breathing). Pa_{O_2} remains above 580 mm Hg when he breathes oxygen, indicating that no significant right to left shunt devel-

ops during exercise. Bicarbonate does not decrease in either study until 2 minutes after the exercise is terminated, because of the rising Pa_{CO_2} during exercise.

CONCLUSION

Exercise performance is limited by severe obstructive lung disease. Oxygen breathing results in an increased work capacity, despite a normal resting Pa_{O_2}.

CASE 43 *Lung cancer and chronic bronchitis: Preoperative evaluation*

CLINICAL FINDINGS

This 62-year-old man with a long history of chronic obstructive pulmonary disease was referred for exercise testing to assess operative risk because of the finding of a malignant pulmonary nodule. The patient had quit smoking approximately 3 months before and was being treated aggressively with bronchodilator therapy including oral corticosteroids. He had no known history of cardiovascular disease and stated he could walk 2 miles.

EXERCISE FINDINGS

The patient performed exercise on a cycle ergometer. He pedalled at 60 rpm without an added load for 3 minutes. The work rate was then increased 10 W per minute to tolerance. Heart rate and rhythm were continuously monitored and ECGs were repeatedly obtained. Blood pressure was measured with a sphygmomanometer and arterial saturation estimated with an ear oximeter. The patient gave an excellent effort and stopped exercise because of shortness of breath and leg fatigue. Resting and exercise ECGs and oximetry were normal.

TABLE 43-1. *Selected Respiratory Function Data*

MEASUREMENT	PREDICTED	MEASURED
Age, yr		62
Sex		Male
Height, cm		170
Weight, kg	74	68
Hematocrit		49
VC, L	3.35	2.76
IC, L	2.23	2.07
TLC, L	5.20	5.46
FEV_1, L	2.62	1.28
FEV_1/VC, %	78	46
MVV, L/min	113	62
$D_{L_{CO}}$, ml/mm Hg/min	22.9	20.2

TABLE 43-2. *Selected Exercise Data*

MEASUREMENT	PREDICTED	MEASURED
Maximum $\dot{V}_{O_2}$, L/min	1.98	1.22
Maximum HR, beats/min	158	175
Maximum O_2 pulse, ml/beat	12.5	7.1
$\Delta \dot{V}_{O_2}/\Delta$WR, ml/min/W	10.3	6.7
AT, L/min	> 0.87	0.6
Blood pressure, mm Hg (rest, max)		130/80,220/110
Maximum $\dot{V}_E$, L/min		48
Exercise breathing reserve, L/min	> 15	14
O_2 saturation, oximeter (rest, max)		96,96

TABLE 43-3.

Time min	Work rate watts	BP mm Hg	HR min⁻¹	f min⁻¹	V̇E L/min BTPS	V̇CO2 L/min STPD	V̇O2 L/min STPD	V̇O2/HR ml/beat	R	pH	HCO3 meq/L	PO2 ET	PO2 a	PO2 (A-a)	PCO2 ET	PCO2 a	PCO2 (a-ET)	V̇E/V̇CO2	V̇E/V̇O2	VD/VT
	Rest	130/80																		
	Rest		108	15	9.7	0.26	0.28	2.6	0.93			108			37			32	30	
	Rest		110	16	10.3	0.27	0.30	2.7	0.90			109			36			33	30	
	Rest		110	13	10.1	0.27	0.29	2.6	0.93			109			36			33	31	
	Rest	130/80	106	11	9.2	0.23	0.25	2.4	0.92			108			37			36	33	
	Rest		108	9	9.7	0.26	0.29	2.7	0.90			108			37			34	31	
	Rest		110	15	9.6	0.24	0.26	2.4	0.92			110			36			35	32	
	Unloaded		118	13	14.8	0.41	0.43	3.6	0.95			109			37			33	32	
	Unloaded		112	12	16.1	0.47	0.50	4.5	0.94			107			38			32	30	
	Unloaded		118	10	15.3	0.51	0.56	4.7	0.91			103			41			28	26	
	Unloaded		126	12	19.0	0.59	0.61	4.8	0.97			104			40			30	29	
	Unloaded		128	13	18.3	0.59	0.57	4.5	1.04			109			40			29	30	
	Unloaded	140/80	120	13	20.6	0.65	0.64	5.3	1.02			106			41			30	30	
0.5	10		120	15	20.9	0.65	0.64	5.3	1.02			108			39			30	31	
1.0	10		124	13	20.3	0.66	0.65	5.2	1.02			107			41			29	30	
1.5	20		124	15	22.5	0.72	0.70	5.6	1.03			108			39			29	30	
2.0	20	150/90	126	16	24.1	0.76	0.73	5.8	1.04			108			39			30	31	
2.5	30		124	15	23.5	0.77	0.74	6.0	1.04			105			42			29	30	
3.0	30		130	15	26.2	0.86	0.80	6.2	1.08			108			41			29	31	
3.5	40		132	16	27.4	0.93	0.87	6.6	1.07			107			41			28	30	
4.0	40	150/90	140	16	28.8	1.00	0.91	6.5	1.10			108			42			27	30	
4.5	50		139	18	32.1	1.06	0.93	6.7	1.14			108			42			29	33	
5.0	50		148	17	30.4	1.05	0.93	6.3	1.13			108			42			28	31	
5.5	60		150	19	34.0	1.14	1.01	6.7	1.13			110			41			28	32	
6.0	60	200/100	152	21	36.5	1.21	1.08	7.1	1.12			110			41			29	32	
6.5	70		160	23	39.3	1.29	1.16	7.3	1.11			110			40			29	32	
7.0	70		160	20	37.5	1.31	1.18	7.4	1.11			107			43			27	30	
7.5	80		170	24	41.6	1.39	1.19	7.0	1.17			109			42			28	33	
8.0	80	200/100	170	25	42.2	1.43	1.20	7.1	1.19			110			43			28	33	
8.5	90		175	28	46.5	1.52	1.22	7.0	1.25			112			42			29	36	
9.0	90		175	31	48.2	1.60	1.19	6.8	1.34			109			42			28	38	
	Recovery		170	22	42.6	1.55	1.16	6.8	1.34			112			44			26	35	
	Recovery		170	22	42.5	1.40	0.97	5.7	1.44			117			41			29	42	
	Recovery		160	22	31.3	0.97	0.71	4.4	1.37			116			40			30	41	
	Recovery	220/110	154	19	32.6	0.98	0.74	4.8	1.32			118			37			32	42	

Interpretation

COMMENTS

Resting studies showed a moderately severe obstructive ventilatory defect. The anaerobic threshold is low. During unloaded pedalling, the R rose over 1.0 and persisted thereafter, evidence of excess CO_2 production because of lactic acid buffering at that low $\dot{V}O_2$.

ANALYSIS

The most distinctive abnormalities are the exercise tachycardia, low and early plateau of the $\dot{V}O_2$ and the O_2 pulse, and the low $\Delta\dot{V}O_2/\Delta WR$. Maximum $\dot{V}O_2$ and the anaerobic threshold are decreased (Table 43-2) leading us to flow chart 4, which is confusing in this case. The breathing reserve is borderline low (branchpoint 4.1), the $\dot{V}E/\dot{V}CO_2$ at the anaerobic threshold is slightly increased (branchpoint 4.2), and oximetry is within normal limits. The high ratio of tidal volume to inspiratory capacity and the borderline breathing reserve are compatible with obstructive lung disease. We know from panels 2, 3, 5, and 8 of the exercise test that the patient has a significant circulatory problem, but it is difficult to say whether it is exclusively pulmonary vascular disease secondary to the obstructive lung disease or whether the patient has additional peripheral vascular disease or a primary cardiac disorder.

FIG. 43-A.

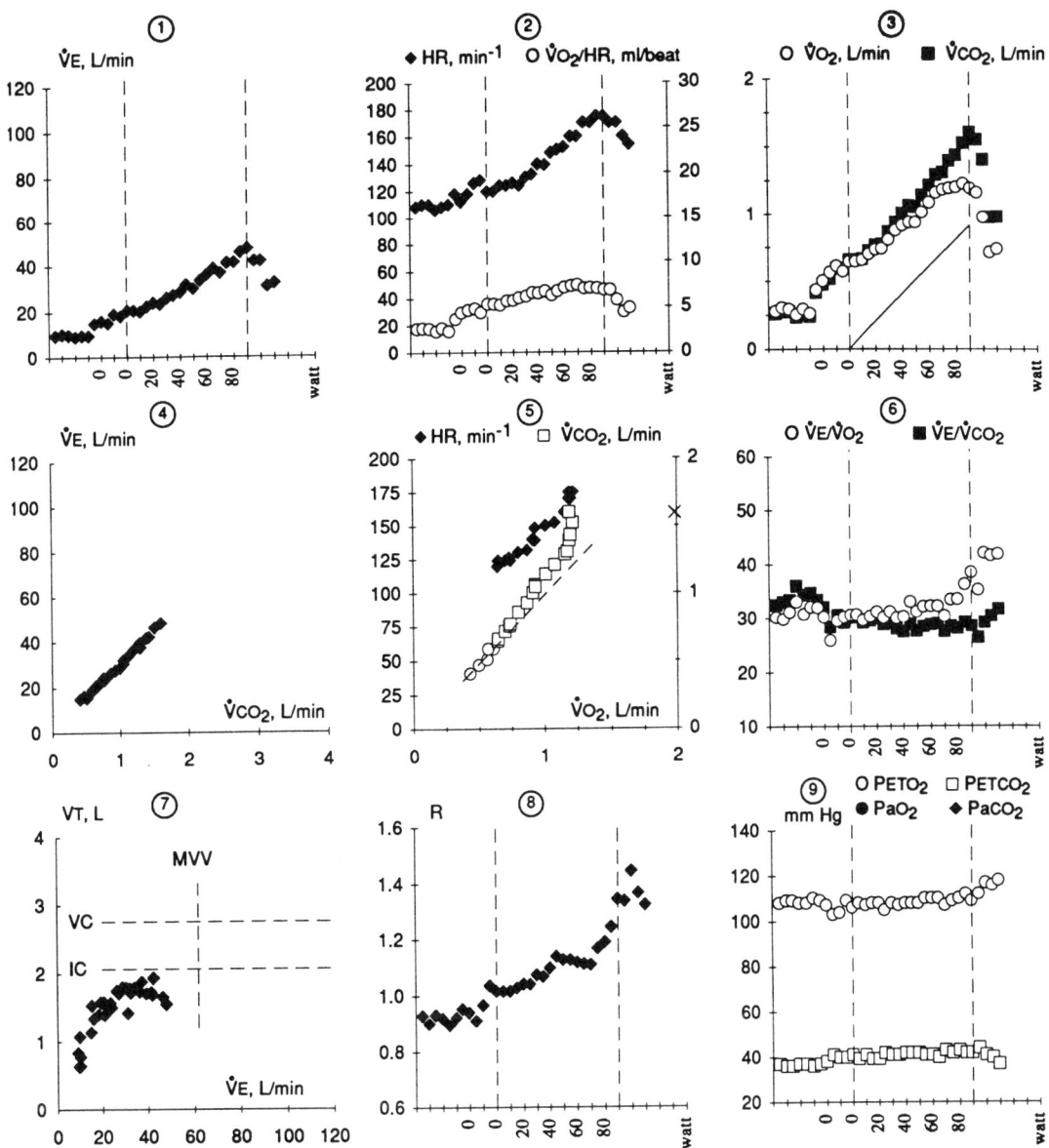

1. Vertical dashed lines in panels 1 to 3 and 6, 8, and 9 indicate the beginning and the end of increasing work period.

2. Unloaded cycling is performed for 3 minutes before the left vertical dashed line.

3. In panel 3, the diagonal line shows the increase of $\dot{V}O_2$ at a slope of 10 ml/min/W.

4. In panel 5, the diagonal dashed line has a slope of 1; the "x" in the upper right is the predicted maximum heart rate and $\dot{V}O_2$ for the subject.

CONCLUSION

The patient's $\dot{V}O_2$max of 18 ml/min/kg is associated with an intermediate risk for morbidity and mortality for lung resection. Values below 15 ml/min/kg indicate a higher risk. Unfortunately, the patient was found to have an enlarged axillary lymph node with metastatic malignant cells a few days later and was no longer a potential operative candidate.

CASE 44 *Bullous Emphysema: Pre- and post-bullectomy*

CLINICAL FINDINGS

This 50-year-old computer technician had retired approximately 10 years prior to initial evaluation because of progressive dyspnea. He denied cough, sputum production, wheezing, or chest pain. There was no family history of lung disease. Chest x-ray studies showed large bullous lesions in the right mid and upper lung fields. Flow rates did not improve following four breaths of nebulized isoproterenol. Perfusion scan demonstrated no perfusion in the right mid and upper hemithorax or at the left apex. α-1-Antitrypsin levels were normal. One month after the first exercise test, the patient's right upper lobe and portions of the right middle lobe were resected. The resected lung showed bullous and centriacinar emphysema with patchy atelectasis; a small squamous cell scar carcinoma was found in the upper lobe. He continued to smoke heavily.

EXERCISE FINDINGS

Preoperatively, the patient performed exercise on a cycle ergometer breathing room air, and following a 90-minute rest, breathing 100% oxygen. Three months postoperatively, only an air breathing study was performed. On each occasion, he pedalled at 60 rpm, on an unloaded cycle, for 2, 3, or 4 minutes. The work rate was then increased 20 W every minute. Arterial blood was sampled every second minute, and intra-arterial blood pressure was recorded from a percutaneous brachial artery catheter. Resting ECGs were normal. Preoperatively, the patient stopped exercise because of dyspnea without an exercise-induced abnormality in the ECG. He stopped during the postoperative test because of dyspnea and pressure-like right-sided chest pain. There were multifocal, back-to-back, and salvos of premature ventricular contractions at the end of exercise and for 2 minutes of recovery without abnormal ST segment changes.

TABLE 44-1. *Selected Respiratory Function Data*

MEASUREMENT	PREDICTED	PREOPERATIVE	POSTOPERATIVE
Age, yr		50	
Sex		Male	
Height, cm		170	
Weight, kg	74	71	
Hematocrit, %		46	
VC, L	3.89	3.01	3.57
IC, L	2.59	2.03	2.46
TLC, L	5.69	7.05	5.56
FEV_1, L	3.09	1.93	2.44
FEV_1/VC, %	79	64	68
MVV, L/min	131	90	110
D_{LCO}, ml/mm Hg/min	26.5	10.0	13.0

TABLE 44-2. *Selected Exercise Data*

MEASUREMENT	PREDICTED	PREOPERATIVE	POSTOPERATIVE
Maximum $\dot{V}_{O_2}$, L/min	2.32	0.99	1.06
Maximum HR, beats/min	170	144	144
Maximum O_2 pulse, ml/beat	13.7	7.5	7.9
$\Delta\dot{V}_{O_2}/\Delta WR$, ml/min/W	10.3	5.1	5.8
AT, L/min	> 1.00	0.6	0.75
Blood pressure, mm Hg (rest, max)		144/90,187/100	144/88,238/94
Maximum $\dot{V}_E$, L/min		84	80
Exercise breathing reserve, L/min	> 15	6	30
Pa_{O_2}, mm Hg (rest, max ex)		67,54	74,74
$P(A-a)_{O_2}$, mm Hg (rest, max ex)		47,72	34,52
$P(a-ET)_{CO_2}$, mm Hg (rest, max ex)		4,8	4,3
V_D/V_T (rest, heavy ex)		0.39,0.47	0.41,0.40
HCO_3^-, mEq/L (rest, 2-min recov)		21,14	21,14

TABLE 44-3. *Pre-bullectomy study.*

Time min	Work rate watts	BP mm Hg	HR min⁻¹	f min⁻¹	$\dot{V}_E$ L/min BTPS	$\dot{V}_{CO_2}$ L/min STPD	$\dot{V}_{O_2}$ L/min STPD	$\dfrac{\dot{V}_{O_2}}{HR}$ ml/beat	R	pH	HCO₃ meq/L	PO2, mm Hg ET	a	(A-a)	PCO2, mm Hg ET	a	(a-ET)	$\dfrac{\dot{V}_E}{\dot{V}_{CO_2}}$	$\dfrac{\dot{V}_E}{\dot{V}_{O_2}}$	$\dfrac{V_D}{V_T}$
	Rest									7.41	21		63			34				
	Rest		69	21	9.7	0.12	0.14	2.0	0.86			120			25			66	57	
	Rest		69	17	10.3	0.16	0.20	2.9	0.80			117			26			55	44	
	Rest		70	15	8.5	0.14	0.18	2.6	0.78			115			27			52	40	
	Rest		70	19	10.7	0.18	0.22	3.1	0.82			117			27			50	41	
	Rest		70	14	10.0	0.18	0.21	3.0	0.86			119			26			49	42	
	Rest	144/90	69	15	10.1	0.17	0.21	3.0	0.81	7.41	19	119	67	47	26	30	4	52	42	0.39
	Unloaded		76	31	29.2	0.45	0.49	6.4	0.92			124			23			59	54	
	Unloaded		80	32	30.5	0.48	0.52	6.5	0.92			125			23			58	53	
	Unloaded		80	32	31.4	0.50	0.52	6.5	0.96			125			23			57	55	
	Unloaded		84	29	28.3	0.47	0.50	6.0	0.94			124			24			55	52	
	Unloaded		88	33	29.8	0.46	0.48	5.5	0.96			124			24			59	56	
	Unloaded	156/94	87	28	28.9	0.48	0.51	5.9	0.94	7.41	18	125	62	58	24	29	5	55	52	0.42
0.5	20		91	32	32.6	0.53	0.57	6.3	0.93			125			24			56	52	
1.0	20		93	30	32.8	0.55	0.57	6.1	0.96			125			24			55	53	
1.5	40		93	32	35.0	0.57	0.59	6.3	0.97			124			24			57	55	
2.0	40	162/94	96	32	37.4	0.62	0.62	6.5	1.00	7.40	17	125	59	63	24	28	4	56	56	0.42
2.5	60		100	35	42.9	0.70	0.68	6.8	1.03			156			24			57	59	
3.0	60		104	40	50.8	0.80	0.76	7.3	1.05			156			24			59	62	
3.5	80		111	43	57.5	0.91	0.82	7.4	1.11			159			22			59	66	
4.0	80	181/96	116	45	62.7	1.00	0.87	7.5	1.15	7.40	18	159	51	72	22	30	8	59	68	0.48
4.5	100		120	58	77.3	1.13	0.95	7.9	1.19			131			20			64	76	
5.0	100		132	60	84.2	1.20	0.97	7.3	1.24			132			20			66	82	
5.5	120	187/100	144	57	78.6	1.19	0.99	6.9	1.20	7.39	17	133	54	72	20	28	8	62	75	0.47
	Recovery		138	55	76.5	1.23	1.01	7.3	1.22			132			21			58	71	
	Recovery		132	47	70.3	1.12	0.92	7.0	1.22			132			20			59	72	
	Recovery		120	44	66.2	1.08	0.83	6.9	1.30			133			20			58	75	
	Recovery	196/99	109	40	56.5	0.92	0.64	5.9	1.44	7.31	14	133	66	62	21	29	8	58	83	0.46

TABLE 44-4. *Post-bullectomy study.*

Time min	Work rate watts	BP mm Hg	HR min⁻¹	f min⁻¹	$\dot{V}_E$ L/min BTPS	$\dot{V}_{CO_2}$ L/min STPD	$\dot{V}_{O_2}$ L/min STPD	$\dfrac{\dot{V}_{O_2}}{HR}$ ml/beat	R	pH	HCO₃ meq/L	PO2, mm Hg ET	a	(A-a)	PCO2, mm Hg ET	a	(a-ET)	$\dfrac{\dot{V}_E}{\dot{V}_{CO_2}}$	$\dfrac{\dot{V}_E}{\dot{V}_{O_2}}$	$\dfrac{V_D}{V_T}$
	Rest	150/94								7.44	21		76			32				
	Rest		74	15	10.6	0.19	0.25	3.4	0.76			112			30			49	37	
	Rest	144/88	77	16	12.1	0.23	0.30	3.9	0.77	7.42	22	112	74	34	30	34		47	36	0.41
	Unloaded		94	21	23.3	0.46	0.57	6.1	0.81			111			30			47	38	
	Unloaded		93	19	22.0	0.45	0.54	5.8	0.83			113			30			45	38	
	Unloaded		91	19	21.9	0.46	0.56	6.2	0.82			115			29			44	36	
	Unloaded	163/88	92	19	22.2	0.47	0.49	5.3	0.96	7.42	21		68	48	31	33	2	44	42	0.37
0.5	20		103	22	24.2	0.49	0.58	5.6	0.84			116			29			46	39	
1.0	20		95	20	24.3	0.51	0.61	6.4	0.84			114			30			44	37	
1.5	40		99	21	28.3	0.60	0.69	7.0	0.87			114			30			44	38	
2.0	40	175/94	100	26	33.7	0.69	0.75	7.5	0.92	7.42	21	117	64	51	29	33	4	46	42	0.40
2.5	60		107	28	40.1	0.83	0.81	7.6	1.02			120			28			45	47	
3.0	60		112	32	47.2	0.98	0.88	7.9	1.11			121			28			45	51	
3.5	80		119	36	54.9	1.10	0.94	7.9	1.17			120			30			47	55	
4.0	80	225/94	130	42	62.4	1.25	1.03	7.9	1.21	7.39	20	123	66	55	28	34	6	47	57	0.43
4.5	100		134	44	69.9	1.40	1.06	7.9	1.32			125			28			47	62	
5.0	100	238/94	138	48	75.7	1.48	1.06	7.7	1.40	7.35	17	126	74	52	28	31	3	48	68	0.40
5.5	120		144	57	79.5	1.52	1.06	7.4	1.43			128			26			49	70	
	Recovery		144	45	74.5	1.49	1.00	6.9	1.49			129			26			47	71	
	Recovery		132	39	69.8	1.41	1.00	7.6	1.41			128			27			47	66	
	Recovery		114	36	63.5	1.26	0.85	7.5	1.48			130			26			48	71	
	Recovery	231/100	102	31	53.2	1.01	0.65	6.4	1.55	7.31	14	131	88	41	25	29	4	50	78	0.39

Fig. 44-A. *Pre-bullectomy study.*

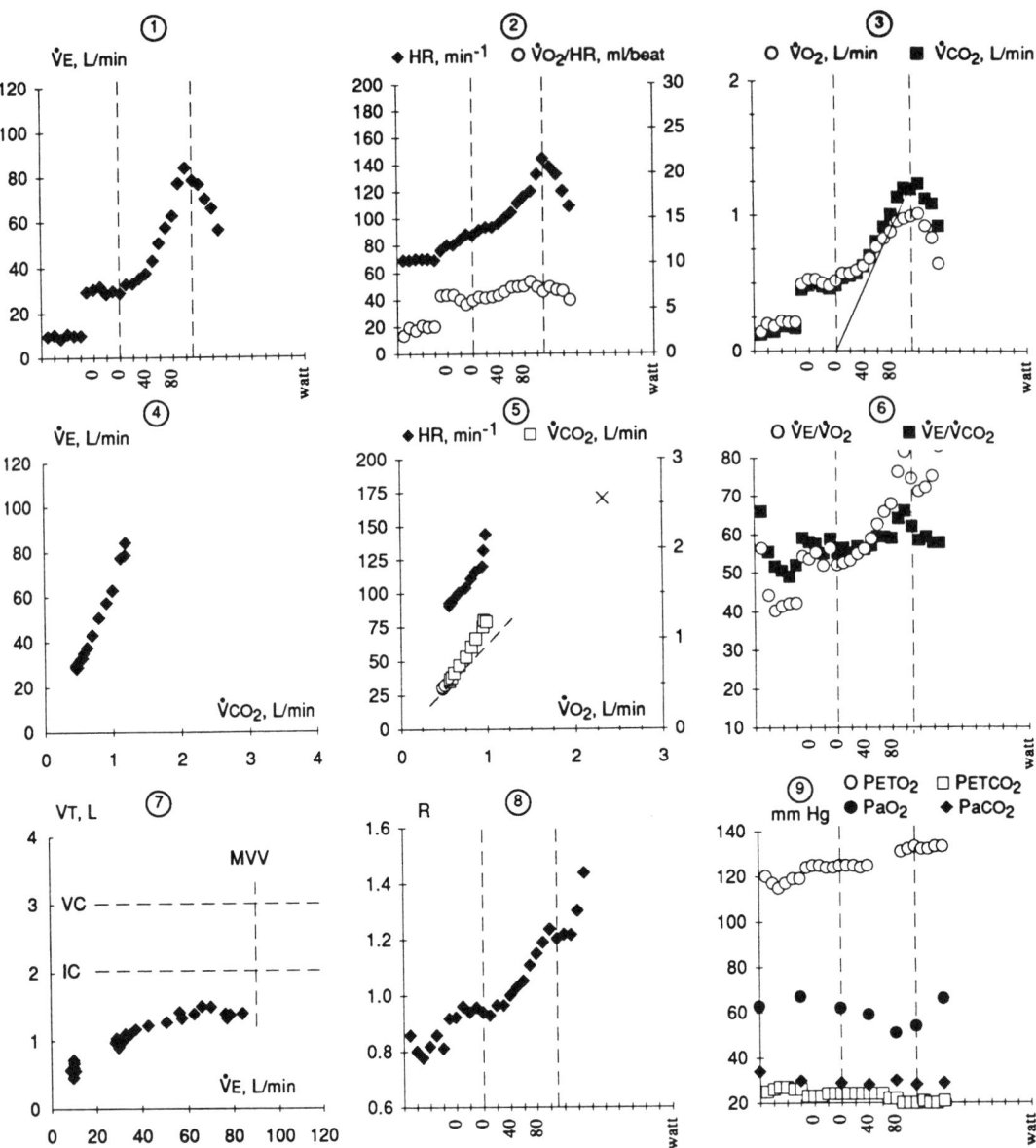

1. Vertical dashed lines in panels 1 to 3 and 6, 8, and 9 indicate the beginning and the end of increasing work period.
2. Unloaded cycling is performed for 3 minutes before the left vertical dashed line.
3. In panel 3, the diagonal line shows the increase of $\dot{V}O_2$ at a slope of 10 ml/min/W.
4. In panel 5, the diagonal dashed line has a slope of 1; the "x" in the upper right is the predicted maximum heart rate and $\dot{V}O_2$ for the subject.

FIG. 44-B. *Post-bullectomy study.*

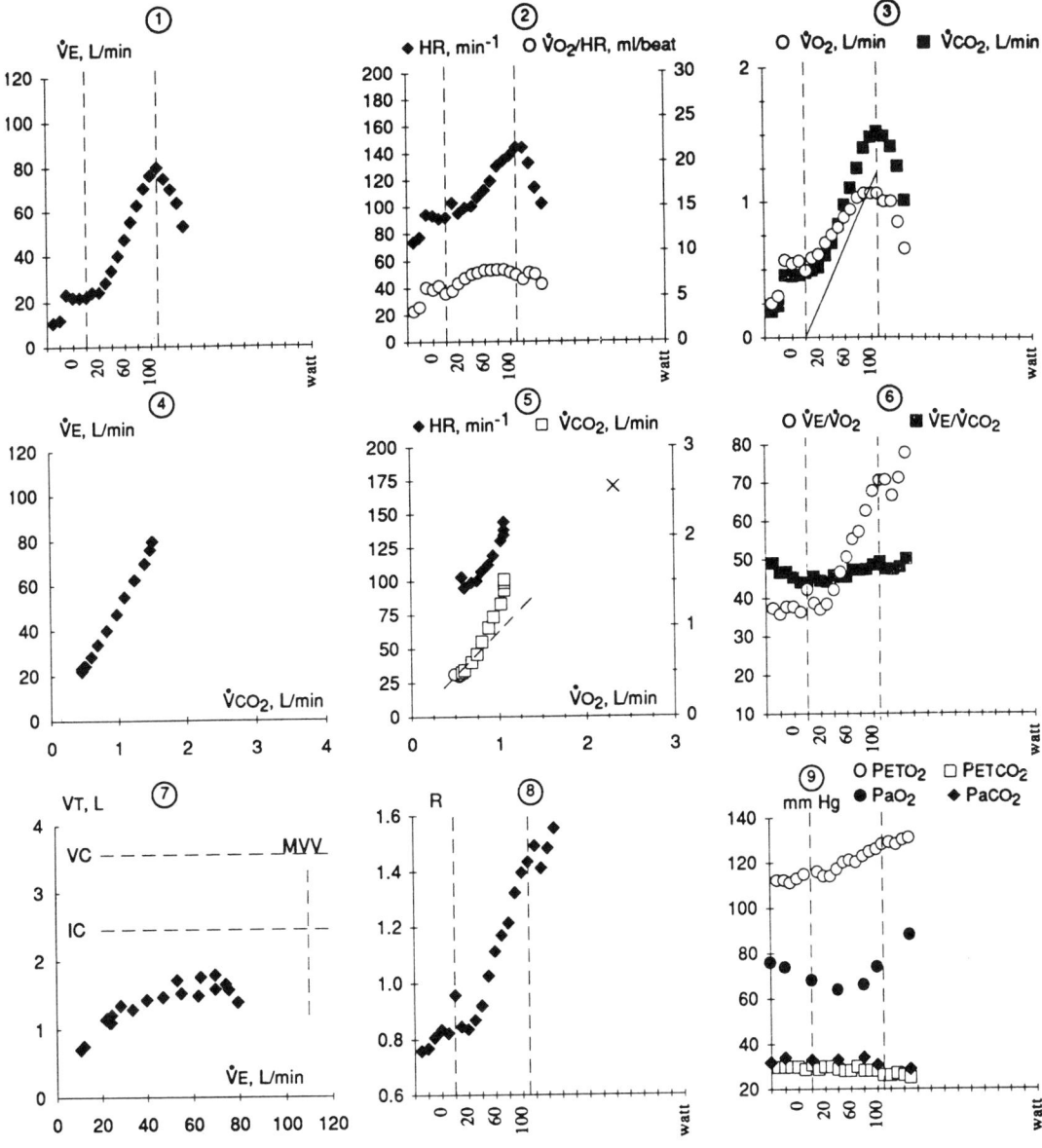

1. Vertical dashed lines in panels 1 to 3 and 6, 8, and 9 indicate the beginning and the end of increasing work period.

2. Unloaded cycling is performed for 2 minutes before the left vertical dashed line.

3. In panel 3, the diagonal line shows the increase of $\dot{V}O_2$ at a slope of 10 ml/min/W.

4. In panel 5, the diagonal dashed line has a slope of 1; the "x" in the upper right is the predicted maximum heart rate and $\dot{V}O_2$ for the subject.

Interpretation

COMMENTS

Resting respiratory function studies show moderate obstructive lung disease with marked reduction in diffusing capacity (D_{LCO}). Following a bullectomy, the vital capacity increased, and the residual volume decreased with improvement in expiratory flow (Table 44-1). Although the diffusing capacity is slightly improved, it is still disproportionately reduced compared to the flow rate impairment. For example, postoperatively the MVV is 84% of predicted, whereas the diffusing capacity measurement is 50% of predicted. Exercise tolerance, surprisingly, is only slightly improved postoperatively.

ANALYSIS

In flow chart 1, the maximum $\dot{V}O_2$ and anaerobic threshold are significantly reduced pre- and postoperatively (Table 44-2). See flow chart 4: Preoperatively the exercise breathing reserve is low, but postoperatively the breathing reserve is normal (branchpoint 4.1). Taking the low breathing reserve branch directed by the preoperative study, V_D/V_T is high, consistent with lung disease with an O_2 flow problem (branchpoint 4.2). The confirmatory abnormalities noted in that diagnostic box are found in Table 44-3.

Taking the normal breathing reserve branch at branchpoint 4.1, consistent with the post-bullectomy study, the ventilatory equivalent for CO_2 is high and the indices of ventilation-perfusion mismatching are abnormal, supporting the diagnosis of an abnormal pulmonary circulation (branchpoint 4.3). The abnormality of the pulmonary circulation is also suggested by the low resting D_{LCO}. There is no abrupt reduction in Pa_{O_2}, postoperatively, as might be expected with a right to left shunt. This was confirmed by a repeat exercise test with the patient breathing 100% oxygen (not shown). Referring to the diagnostic box under abnormal pulmonary circulation, confirmatory observations are: (1) a steep heart rate response to the increase in $\dot{V}O_2$, becoming steeper as the maximum $\dot{V}O_2$ is approached (panel 5); (2) a low O_2 pulse with a flat contour as work rate is increased (panel 2); and (3) a decreasing $\Delta\dot{V}O_2/\Delta WR$ as work rate is increased (panel 3) for both the pre- (Fig. 44-A) and postoperative (Fig. 44-B) studies. All these findings are consistent with an oxygen flow problem of the type seen with functionally important pulmonary vascular disease. The latter is most likely related to this patient's lung disease. Although postoperatively, respiratory mechanics are improved, exercise performance did not improve significantly, and pulmonary vascular disease appears to be the predominant limiting factor. The ectopy noted during exercise, after bullectomy, might be secondary to the development of critically important pulmonary hypertension.

CONCLUSION

The patient has bullous emphysema. Pulmonary vascular occlusive disease has limited exercise performance, after bullectomy.

CASE 45 *Obstructive airway disease: Before and after rehabilitation*

CLINICAL FINDINGS

This 69-year-old man with known chronic obstructive lung disease was evaluated before and after a pulmonary rehabilitation program of 2 months' duration, which featured (among other components) a program of vigorous cycle ergometer exercise. The patient exercised for 45 minutes per day, 3 days per week on a stationery bicycle at exercise intensities approaching his maximum tolerance. Resting respiratory and exercise testing data for both occasions are shown. The patient had recently stopped smoking, though he had a 51 pack year history of cigarette smoking. His medications included theophylline and inhaled β agonist and anticholinergic agents.

EXERCISE FINDINGS

The patient performed exercise on a cycle ergometer before and after a 2-month training period. He pedalled at 60 rpm without an added load for 3 minutes. The work rate was then increased 5 W per minute to tolerance. Heart rate and rhythm were continuously monitored; 12-lead ECGs were obtained during rest, exercise, and recovery. Every 2 minutes, blood pressure was measured by a sphygmomanometer, and a sample of blood was drawn from a venous catheter placed in the back of the hand. Blood samples were assayed for blood lactate concentration. The patient was well motivated and cooperative and stopped exercise on both occasions because of dyspnea. No ECG abnormalities at rest or during exercise were noted.

TABLE 45-1. *Selected Respiratory Function Data*

MEASUREMENT	PREDICTED	MEASURED	
Age, yr		69	
Sex		Male	
Height, cm		170	
Weight, kg	60	74	
Hematocrit, %		40	
		BEFORE	AFTER*
VC, L	3.60	1.99	2.19
IC, L	2.40	1.50	1.65
FEV_1, L	2.78	0.99	1.11
FEV_1/VC, %	77	50	51
MVV, indirect, L/min	111	40	44
$D_{L_{CO}}$, ml/mm Hg/min	22.4	10.6	12.7

* After training.

TABLE 45-2. *Selected Exercise Data*

MEASUREMENT	PREDICTED	BEFORE	AFTER
Maximum $\dot{V}_{O_2}$, L/min	1.67	0.90	1.00
Maximum HR, beats/min	151	136	140
Work rate, max, W		30	50
Maximum O_2 pulse, ml/beat	11.1	6.6	7.6
$\Delta \dot{V}_{O_2}/\Delta WR$, ml/min/W	10.3		8.2
AT, L/min	> 0.75	0.75	indeterminate*
Maximum $\dot{V}_E$, L/min		40	42
Exercise breathing reserve, L/min, using indirect MVV	> 15	0	2
Peak lactate, mEq/L		3.0	2.3

* Apparently, because of the small increase in lactate after training, a breakpoint in the V-slope plot (panel 5) is not observed.

FIG. 45-A. *Before training.*

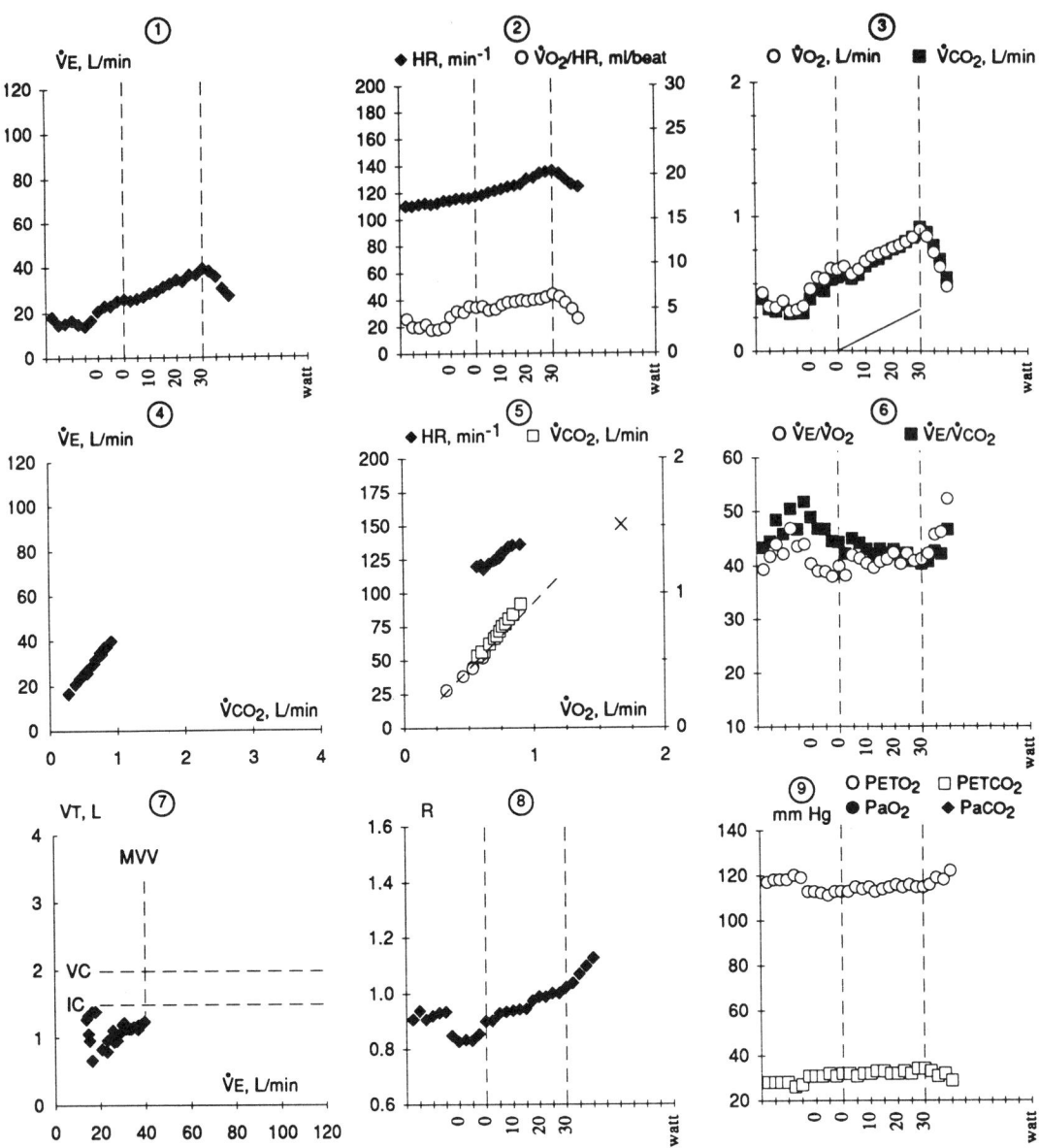

1. Vertical dashed lines in panels 1 to 3 and 6, 8, and 9 indicate the beginning and the end of increasing work period.

2. Unloaded cycling is performed for 3 minutes before the left vertical dashed line.

3. In panel 3, the diagonal line shows the increase of $\dot{V}O_2$ at a slope of 10 ml/min/W.

4. In panel 5, the diagonal dashed line has a slope of 1; the "x" in the upper right is the predicted maximum heart rate and $\dot{V}O_2$ for the subject.

Fig. 45-B. *After training.*

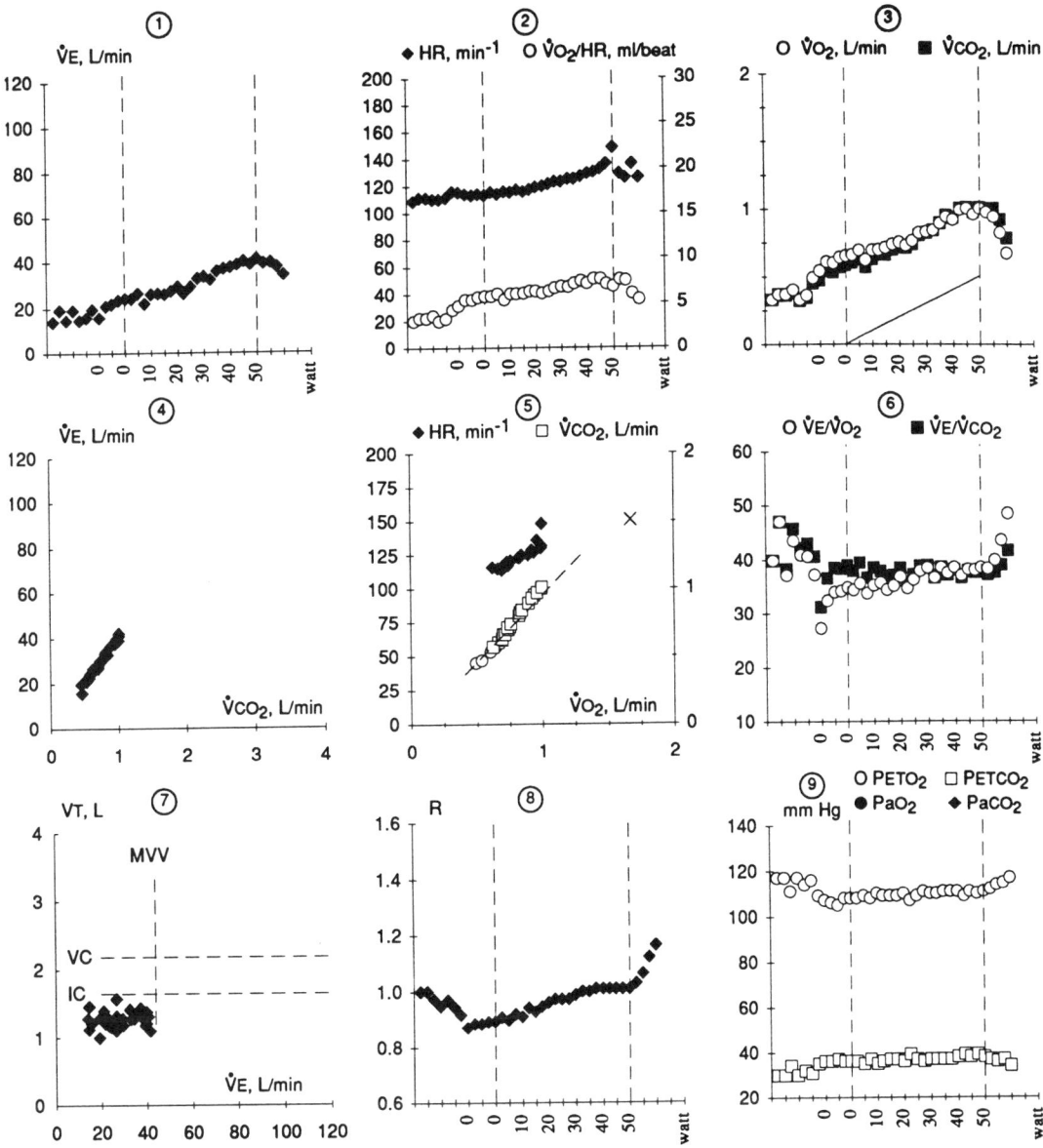

1. Vertical dashed lines in panels 1 to 3 and 6, 8, and 9 indicate the beginning and the end of increasing work period.

2. Unloaded cycling is performed for 3 minutes before the left vertical dashed line.

3. In panel 3, the diagonal line shows the increase of $\dot{V}O_2$ at a slope of 10 ml/min/W.

4. In panel 5, the diagonal dashed line has a slope of 1; the "x" in the upper right is the predicted maximum heart rate and $\dot{V}O_2$ for the subject.

TABLE 45-3. *Before training.*

Time min	Work rate watts	BP mm Hg	HR min⁻¹	f min⁻¹	$\dot{V}E$ L/min BTPS	$\dot{V}CO_2$ L/min STPD	$\dot{V}O_2$ L/min STPD	$\frac{\dot{V}O_2}{HR}$ ml/beat	R	pH	HCO₃ meq/L	PO2, mm Hg ET	a	(A-a)	PCO2, mm Hg ET	a	(a-ET)	$\frac{\dot{V}E}{\dot{V}CO_2}$	$\frac{\dot{V}E}{\dot{V}O_2}$	$\frac{VD}{VT}$
	Rest		110	13	18.0	0.39	0.43	3.9	0.91			117			28			43	39	
	Rest		110	11	14.7	0.31	0.33	3.0	0.94			118			28			44	42	
	Rest		111	16	15.4	0.29	0.32	2.9	0.91			118			28			48	44	
	Rest		112	12	16.6	0.34	0.37	3.3	0.92			118			28			46	42	
	Rest		111	14	14.8	0.27	0.29	2.6	0.93			120			26			50	47	
	Rest		112	11	14.0	0.28	0.30	2.7	0.93			119			27			47	44	
	Unloaded		114	25	16.6	0.28	0.33	2.9	0.85			113			31			52	44	
	Unloaded		114	25	20.7	0.38	0.46	4.0	0.83			113			31			49	40	
	Unloaded		115	24	23.1	0.45	0.54	4.7	0.83			112			31			47	39	
	Unloaded		116	29	23.0	0.44	0.53	4.6	0.83			111			32			47	39	
	Unloaded		116	25	25.2	0.52	0.61	5.3	0.85			113			31			44	38	
	Unloaded		117	25	26.0	0.54	0.60	5.1	0.90			113			32			44	40	
0.5	5		118	23	25.6	0.56	0.62	5.3	0.90			113			32			42	38	
1.0	5		120	28	26.2	0.53	0.57	4.8	0.93			115			31			45	42	
1.5	10		121	27	27.0	0.56	0.60	5.0	0.93			114			32			44	41	
2.0	10		122	27	28.9	0.62	0.66	5.4	0.94			115			32			43	40	
2.5	15		124	25	29.8	0.66	0.70	5.6	0.94			113			33			42	40	
3.0	15		125	28	31.6	0.68	0.72	5.8	0.94			114			33			43	41	
3.5	20		126	29	32.8	0.72	0.74	5.9	0.97			115			32			42	41	
4.0	20		130	30	34.7	0.75	0.76	5.8	0.99			116			32			43	42	
4.5	25		131	30	33.9	0.77	0.78	6.0	0.99			115			33			41	40	
5.0	25		134	33	36.9	0.81	0.81	6.0	1.00			116			32			42	42	
5.5	30		135	31	36.9	0.84	0.84	6.2	1.00			115			34			41	41	
6.0	30		136	32	39.7	0.92	0.90	6.6	1.02			115			34			40	41	
	Recovery		134	32	38.5	0.88	0.85	6.3	1.04			116			33			41	42	
	Recovery		130	31	35.9	0.78	0.73	5.6	1.07			119			31			43	46	
	Recovery		126	25	30.7	0.68	0.62	4.9	1.10			118			32			42	46	
	Recovery		124	29	27.6	0.54	0.48	3.9	1.13			122			29			47	52	

Interpretation

COMMENTS

This case shows the effects of a training program on resting respiratory function, work capacity, and maximum $\dot{V}O_2$. Resting studies show moderate obstructive lung disease, with severe loss of effective pulmonary capillary bed.

ANALYSIS

In flow chart 1, on the initial study the maximum $\dot{V}O_2$ was low, whereas the anaerobic threshold was at the lower limits of normal (Table 45-2). Regardless of which flow chart is used, we would arrive at the diagnosis of obstructive lung disease for both studies. Using flow chart 3 for the first study, we would go through branchpoints 3.1 and 3.2 to that diagnosis. Using flow chart 4, the low breathing reserve (branchpoint 4.1) and presumed high VD/VT because of the high VE/$\dot{V}CO_2$ (branchpoint 4.2) lead us to the diagnosis of "lung disease with impaired peripheral oxygenation." If we had used flow chart 5.1, we would have arrived at the diagnosis of obstructive lung disease through branchpoints 5.1, 5.3, and 5.7.

CONCLUSION

Comparing the studies performed before and after pulmonary rehabilitation, it is apparent that this patient's exercise tolerance has improved appreciably. This can be explained only in part by the small improvement in airways obstruction. Insight into the cause of the improvement can be gained by comparing the physiologic responses at identical work rates in the two studies.

TABLE 45-4. *After training.*

Time min	Work rate watts	BP mm Hg	HR min⁻¹	f min⁻¹	V̇E L/min BTPS	V̇CO₂ L/min STPD	V̇O₂ L/min STPD	V̇O₂/HR ml/beat	R	pH	HCO₃ meq/L	PO2, mm Hg ET	a	(A-a)	PCO2, mm Hg ET	a	(a-ET)	V̇E/V̇CO2	V̇E/V̇O2	VD/VT
	Rest		109	11	14.1	0.33	0.33	3.0	1.00			117			30			40	40	
	Rest		111	19	19.0	0.37	0.37	3.3	1.00			117			30			47	47	
	Rest		111	10	14.6	0.36	0.37	3.3	0.97			111			34			38	37	
	Rest		110	19	19.0	0.38	0.40	3.6	0.95			117			30			46	43	
	Rest		110	13	14.6	0.32	0.33	3.0	0.97			114			32			42	41	
	Rest		111	13	15.7	0.34	0.36	3.2	0.94			116			31			43	41	
	Unloaded		116	15	19.5	0.45	0.49	4.2	0.92			109			35			41	37	
	Unloaded		115	13	15.8	0.47	0.54	4.7	0.87			107			36			31	27	
	Unloaded		114	15	21.0	0.54	0.61	5.4	0.89			106			36			37	32	
	Unloaded		113	18	21.9	0.53	0.60	5.3	0.88			105			37			38	34	
	Unloaded		114	20	23.5	0.57	0.64	5.6	0.89			108			36			38	34	
	Unloaded		113	21	24.4	0.58	0.65	5.8	0.89			108			36			39	35	
0.5	5		115	20	24.4	0.60	0.66	5.7	0.91			108			36			38	34	
1.0	5		114	24	26.5	0.62	0.69	6.1	0.90			109			35			39	35	
1.5	10		116	17	22.3	0.57	0.62	5.3	0.92			108			37			37	34	
2.0	10		115	23	26.2	0.63	0.69	6.0	0.91			110			35			38	35	
2.5	15		117	20	26.6	0.66	0.70	6.0	0.94			109			36			38	36	
3.0	15		116	21	26.1	0.66	0.71	6.1	0.93			109			37			37	34	
3.5	20		117	22	27.8	0.70	0.74	6.3	0.95			109			37			37	35	
4.0	20		119	25	29.7	0.72	0.75	6.3	0.96			110			36			38	37	
4.5	25		120	17	26.7	0.71	0.73	6.1	0.97			107			39			36	35	
5.0	25		121	23	29.5	0.74	0.76	6.3	0.97			109			37			37	36	
5.5	30		123	26	33.2	0.80	0.82	6.7	0.98			111			36			39	38	
6.0	30		123	26	34.0	0.82	0.83	6.7	0.99			110			37			39	38	
6.5	35		125	23	32.6	0.84	0.84	6.7	1.00			110			37			36	36	
7.0	35		125	26	36.4	0.89	0.89	7.1	1.00			111			37			38	38	
7.5	40		127	26	37.4	0.95	0.94	7.4	1.01			111			37			37	37	
8.0	40		129	29	37.8	0.93	0.92	7.1	1.01			111			38			38	38	
8.5	45		130	29	39.0	1.00	0.99	7.6	1.01			109			39			37	37	
9.0	45		132	31	40.8	1.01	1.00	7.6	1.01			111			38			38	38	
9.5	50		136	33	39.3	0.97	0.96	7.1	1.01			110			39			38	38	
10.0	50		148	38	41.7	1.01	1.00	6.8	1.01			111			38			38	38	
	Recovery		129	33	39.9	1.00	0.97	7.5	1.03			112			37			37	38	
	Recovery		126	29	40.0	1.00	0.94	7.5	1.06			114			36			38	40	
	Recovery		136	29	38.2	0.92	0.82	6.0	1.12			115			37			39	44	
	Recovery		126	27	34.7	0.78	0.67	5.3	1.16			117			34			42	48	

TABLE 45-5. *Selected comparisons.*

	RESPONSES TO 30 WATTS	
	BEFORE REHABILITATION	AFTER REHABILITATION
V̇E, L/min	40	34
V̇O₂, L/min	0.9	0.83
V̇CO₂, L/min	0.92	0.82
Heart rate, beats/min	136	123
Lactate, mEq/L	3.0	1.7

The reduction in lactate at a given work rate is characteristic of a physiologic training effect. This is also reflected in a lower V̇CO₂ (less CO_2 release from HCO_3^- buffering). The reduction in V̇E is likely a consequence of the reduced acid stimulus to breathing. The improvement in exercise tolerance is based, at least in part, on the reduced ventilatory requirement.

CASE 46 *Early asbestosis and chronic bronchitis*

CLINICAL FINDINGS

This 48-year-old shipyard worker denied having breathing difficulties and could climb 3 to 4 flights of stairs before noting shortness of breath. He had been treated for pneumonia 14 years before and for a pleural effusion 12 years ago. Two years previously, a benign "calcified mass" attached to a left lower rib had been removed. He had smoked a pack of cigarettes daily for 25 years and had a morning cough with small amounts of yellow sputum. No deformity, rhonchi, rales, or clubbing were noted on physical examination. Chest roentgenograms, including computerized tomographic views, showed bilateral pleural plaques and marked coarse parenchymal scarring at both bases.

EXERCISE FINDINGS

The patient performed exercise on a cycle ergometer. He pedalled at 60 rpm without added load for 3 minutes. The work rate was then increased 20 W per minute to his symptom-limited maximum. Arterial blood was sampled every second minute, and intra-arterial blood pressure was recorded from a percutaneously placed brachial artery catheter. The patient stopped exercise because of chest discomfort. Resting and exercise ECG were normal. Carboxyhemoglobin was 8.3%.

TABLE 46-1. *Selected Respiratory Function Data*

MEASUREMENT	PREDICTED	MEASURED
Age, yr		48
Sex		Male
Height, cm		180
Weight, kg	82	97
Hematocrit, %		49
VC, L	4.87	4.84 (5.04*)
IC, L	3.25	3.12
TLC, L	7.06	7.12
FEV_1, L	3.88	3.23 (3.59*)
FEV_1/VC, %	80	67
MVV, L/min	158	183 (172*)
D_{LCO}, ml/mm Hg/min	31.8	20.0

* After 4 breaths of aerosolized isoproterenol

TABLE 46-2. *Selected Exercise Data*

MEASUREMENT	PREDICTED	MEASURED
Maximum $\dot{V}O_2$, L/min	2.77	2.37
Maximum HR, beats/min	172	149
Maximum O_2 pulse, ml/beat	16.1	15.9
$\Delta\dot{V}O_2$/ΔWR, ml/min/W	10.3	10.3
AT, L/min	> 1.19	1.3
Blood pressure, mm Hg (rest, max)		120/81,213/84
Maximum $\dot{V}E$, L/min		98
Exercise breathing reserve, L/min	> 15	85
Pa_{O_2}, mm Hg (rest, max ex)		96,72
$P(A-a)_{O_2}$, mm Hg (rest, max ex)		17,47
$P(a-ET)_{CO_2}$, mm Hg (rest, max ex)		3,1
V_D/V_T (rest, heavy ex)		0.41,0.29
HCO_3^-, mEq/L (rest, 2-min recov)		25,18

Fig. 46-A.

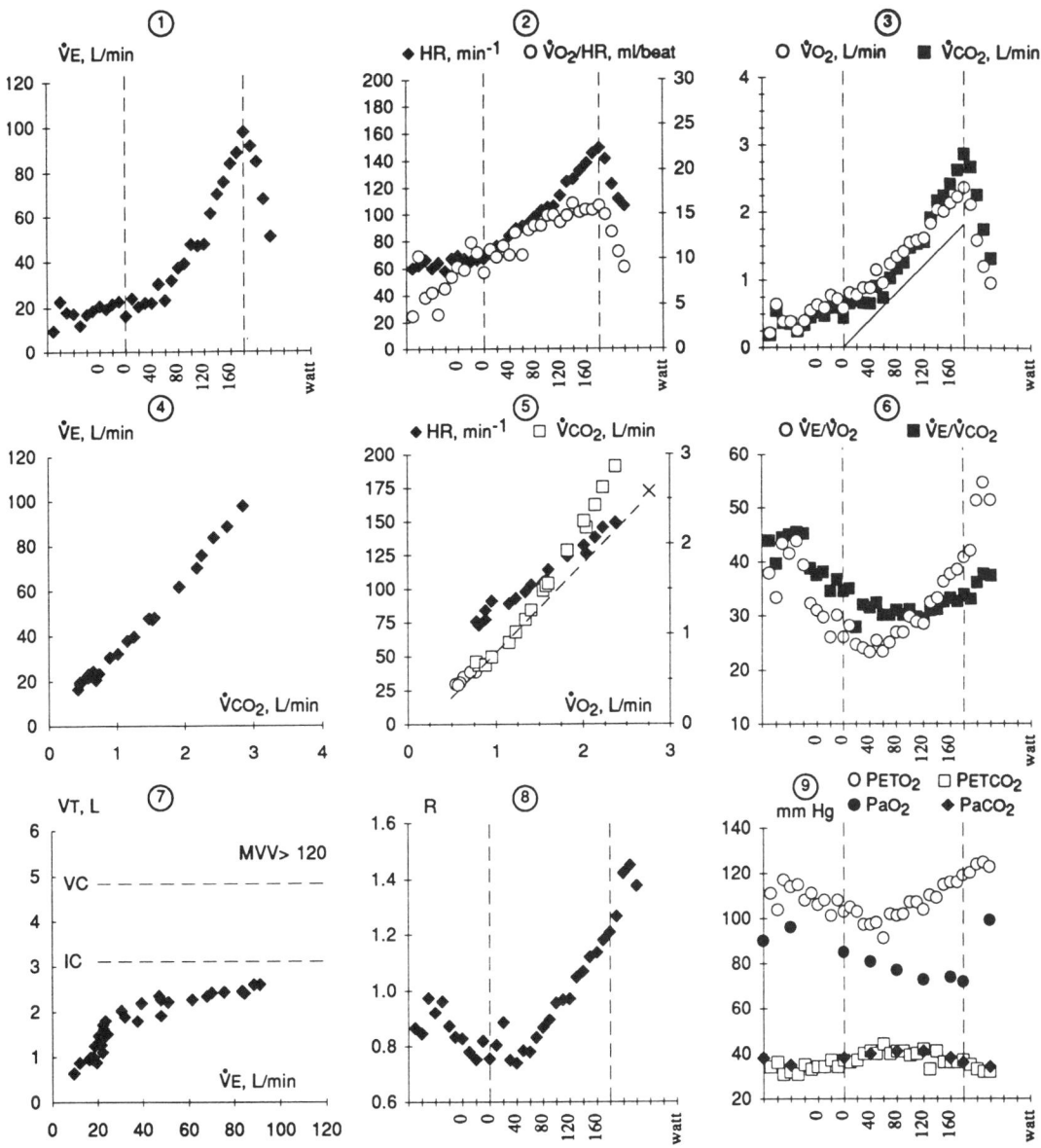

1. Vertical dashed lines in panels 1 to 3 and 6, 8, and 9 indicate the beginning and the end of increasing work period.

2. Unloaded cycling is performed for 3 minutes before the left vertical dashed line.

3. In panel 3, the diagonal line shows the increase of $\dot{V}O_2$ at a slope of 10 ml/min/W.

4. In panel 5, the diagonal dashed line has a slope of 1; the "x" in the upper right is the predicted maximum heart rate and $\dot{V}O_2$ for the subject.

Interpretation

COMMENTS

The results of the resting respiratory function studies indicate that this patient has mild, reversible airflow obstruction and a moderate reduction in diffusing capacity (Table 46-1). His resting and exercise ECGs are normal. The man is a cigarette smoker with a high carboxyhemoglobin level in his blood.

ANALYSIS

In flow chart 1, the maximum $\dot{V}O_2$ and anaerobic threshold are at the lower limits of normal (Table 46-2). (See flow chart 2.) Even though these values are within the normal range and the ECG at the

TABLE 46-3.

Time min	Work rate watts	BP mm Hg	HR min⁻¹	f min⁻¹	$\dot{V}E$ L/min BTPS	$\dot{V}CO_2$ L/min STPD	$\dot{V}O_2$ L/min STPD	$\dfrac{\dot{V}O_2}{HR}$ ml/beat	R	pH	HCO₃ meq/L	PO2, mm Hg ET	a	(A-a)	PCO2, mm Hg ET	a	(a-ET)	$\dfrac{\dot{V}E}{\dot{V}CO_2}$	$\dfrac{\dot{V}E}{\dot{V}O_2}$	$\dfrac{VD}{VT}$
	Rest	120/81								7.43	25		90			38				
	Rest		60	15	9.6	0.19	0.22	3.7	0.86			111			34			44	38	
	Rest		62	14	22.6	0.54	0.64	10.3	0.84			104			36			40	33	
	Rest		66	18	18.0	0.37	0.38	5.8	0.97			117			31			45	43	
	Rest	120/78	60	18	17.3	0.35	0.38	6.3	0.92	7.45	24	114	96	17	32	35	3	45	42	0.41
	Rest		64	14	12.1	0.24	0.25	3.9	0.96			115			31			46	44	
	Rest		58	17	16.8	0.34	0.39	6.7	0.87			108			35			45	39	
	Unloaded		67	15	18.7	0.45	0.54	8.1	0.83			111			33			39	32	
	Unloaded		69	14	20.7	0.52	0.63	9.1	0.83			106			34			38	31	
	Unloaded		67	22	19.4	0.46	0.59	8.8	0.78			108			34			38	30	
	Unloaded		65	17	21.5	0.58	0.77	11.8	0.75			101			37			35	26	
	Unloaded		66	16	22.7	0.58	0.71	10.8	0.82			108			34			37	30	
	Unloaded	120/72	67	17	16.3	0.43	0.57	8.5	0.75	7.43	25	103	85	17	37	38	1	35	26	0.31
0.5	20		73	16	24.1	0.65	0.81	11.1	0.80			105			36			35	28	
1.0	20		76	14	20.4	0.69	0.78	10.3	0.88			103			37			28	25	
1.5	40		77	13	22.2	0.66	0.88	11.4	0.75			97			40			32	24	
2.0	40	129/72	84	20	22.1	0.65	0.88	10.5	0.74	7.42	25	97	81	18	41	40	-1	31	23	0.29
2.5	60		89	15	30.4	0.90	1.15	12.9	0.78			98			40			32	25	
3.0	60		91	13	23.3	0.74	0.95	10.4	0.78			91			44			30	23	
3.5	80		93	17	32.1	1.02	1.23	13.2	0.83			102			40			30	25	
4.0	80	150/75	98	21	37.7	1.16	1.34	13.7	0.87	7.39	24	101	77	27	41	41	0	31	27	0.30
4.5	100		103	18	39.4	1.26	1.41	13.7	0.89			102			41			30	27	
5.0	100		105	21	47.8	1.48	1.55	14.8	0.95			107			39			31	30	
5.5	120		106	20	47.2	1.53	1.58	14.9	0.97			107			40			30	29	
6.0	120	174/75	114	25	47.9	1.56	1.61	14.1	0.97	7.38	24	104	73	35	42	41	-1	29	28	0.27
6.5	140		124	27	61.6	1.92	1.83	14.8	1.05			110			33			31	32	
7.0	140		126	29	70.1	2.18	2.04	16.2	1.07			109			41			31	33	
7.5	160		132	31	75.6	2.25	2.01	15.2	1.12			115			36			32	36	
8.0	160	204/78	138	34	83.6	2.43	2.14	15.5	1.14	7.37	22	116	74	42	36	38	2	33	38	0.31
8.5	180		145	34	88.6	2.63	2.23	15.4	1.18			116			36			33	38	
9.0	180	213/84	149	10	97.6	2.86	2.37	15.9	1.21	7.36	20	119	72	47	37	36	-1	34	41	0.29
	Recovery		141	35	91.4	2.67	2.11	15.0	1.27			120			35			33	42	
	Recovery		122	35	84.5	2.26	1.59	13.0	1.42			124			33			36	51	
	Recovery		111	29	68.1	1.74	1.20	10.8	1.45			125			32			38	55	
	Recovery	213/72	106	23	51.2	1.32	0.96	9.1	1.38	7.33	18	123	99	24	32	34	2	37	51	0.31

maximum work rate is normal, certain measurements become abnormal during exercise, indicating that the patient has ventilation-perfusion mismatching (branchpoint 2.3). These include mild arterial hypoxemia and a significant progressive increase in $P(A-a)_{O_2}$ as work rate is increased. Moreover, $P(a-ET)_{CO_2}$ is increased at the maximum $\dot{V}O_2$, and VD/VT is borderline normal.

CONCLUSION

Ventilation-perfusion mismatching during exercise in an asymptomatic, 48-year-old man, with maximum exercise performance at the lower limit of normal. Putting this together with the history of a pleural effusion 12 years previously, pleural plaques, and pulmonary fibrosis evident on chest x-ray studies, the strong possibility exists that this patient is evidencing early features of pulmonary asbestosis. The persistent cigarette smoking (high level of blood carboxyhemoglobin) in this asbestos-exposed worker provides a major neoplastic threat. It also makes him a high-risk candidate for heart disease and emphysema.

CASE 47 *Asbestosis, mild*

CLINICAL FINDINGS

This 55-year-old male shipyard worker with a long history of asbestos and former cigarette exposure complained of shortness of breath only after climbing three to four flights of stairs and a daily cough productive of scant, yellow-tinged sputum. He denied any other symptoms or illnesses. No rales were noted on examination. Chest roentgenograms revealed minimal, but definite, fibrosis, typical of asbestosis. Exercise testing was requested to ascertain whether physiologic abnormalities were associated with the asbestosis.

EXERCISE FINDINGS

The patient performed exercise on a cycle ergometer. He pedalled at 60 rpm without an added load for 3 minutes. The work rate was then increased 10 W per minute to tolerance. Arterial blood was sampled every second minute, and intra-arterial pressure was recorded from a percutaneously placed brachial artery catheter. The patient stopped exercise because of shortness of breath. The ECG showed nonspecific T-wave abnormalities and occasional ventricular premature contractions at rest and during exercise.

TABLE 47-1. *Selected Respiratory Function Data*

MEASUREMENT	PREDICTED	MEASURED
Age, yr		55
Sex		Male
Height, cm		181
Weight, kg	82	84
Hematocrit, %		45
VC, L	4.24	3.50
IC, L	2.83	2.26
TLC, L	6.32	5.15
FEV$_1$, L	3.35	2.94
FEV$_1$/VC, %	79	84
MVV, L/min	135	107
D$_{LCO}$, ml/mm Hg/min	27.3	22.7

TABLE 47-2. *Selected Exercise Data*

MEASUREMENT	PREDICTED	MEASURED
Maximum $\dot{V}O_2$, L/min	2.50	2.03
Maximum HR, beats/min	165	154
Maximum O$_2$ pulse, ml/beat	15.1	13.2
$\Delta \dot{V}O_2/\Delta WR$, ml/min/W	10.3	8.7
AT, L/min	> 1.08	1.3
Blood pressure, mm Hg (rest, max)		156/90,216/99
Maximum $\dot{V}E$, L/min		93
Exercise breathing reserve, L/min	> 15	14
Pa$_{O_2}$, mm Hg (rest, max ex)		88,99
P(A − a)$_{O_2}$ mm Hg (rest, max ex)		14,21
P(a − ET)$_{CO_2}$, mm Hg (rest, max ex)		3, −2
V$_D$/V$_T$ (rest, max ex)		0.37,0.30
HCO$_3^-$, mEq/L (rest, 2-min recov)		25,20

TABLE 47-3.

Time min	Work rate watts	BP mm Hg	HR min⁻¹	f min⁻¹	$\dot{V}_E$ L/min BTPS	$\dot{V}_{CO_2}$ L/min STPD	$\dot{V}_{O_2}$ L/min STPD	$\frac{\dot{V}_{O_2}}{HR}$ ml/beat	R	pH	HCO₃ meq/L	PO2, mm Hg ET	a	(A-a)	PCO2, mm Hg ET	a	(a-ET)	$\frac{\dot{V}_E}{\dot{V}_{CO_2}}$	$\frac{\dot{V}_E}{\dot{V}_{O_2}}$	VD VT
	Rest	156/90								7.43	25		79			38				
	Rest		81	21	12.3	0.24	0.32	4.0	0.75			106			35			44	33	
	Rest		83	23	11.8	0.23	0.31	3.7	0.74			106			35			43	32	
	Rest		88	21	11.9	0.23	0.30	3.4	0.77			108			34			44	34	
	Rest	162/96	80	22	11.2	0.23	0.31	3.9	0.74	7.42	24	105	88	14	35	38	3	41	30	0.37
	Rest		84	18	11.4	0.23	0.31	3.7	0.74			104			36			43	32	
	Rest		86	20	12.2	0.25	0.32	3.7	0.78			106			36			42	33	
	Unloaded		97	21	16.3	0.40	0.50	5.2	0.80			105			37			36	29	
	Unloaded		93	33	21.8	0.48	0.66	7.1	0.73			102			37			40	29	
	Unloaded		93	32	23.8	0.52	0.64	6.9	0.81			109			34			41	33	
	Unloaded		95	30	22.7	0.53	0.69	7.3	0.77			104			37			38	29	
	Unloaded		94	36	22.3	0.51	0.67	7.1	0.76			100			38			38	29	
	Unloaded	192/96	96	35	29.2	0.65	0.75	7.8	0.87	7.43	25	108	91	16	34	38	4	40	35	0.39
0.5	20		97	36	26.6	0.62	0.78	8.0	0.79			105			36			38	30	
1.0	20		98	39	28.3	0.62	0.78	8.0	0.79			108			35			40	32	
1.5	40		95	41	28.7	0.62	0.80	8.4	0.78			204			37			41	32	
2.0	40	192/90	103	26	27.7	0.75	0.98	9.5	0.77	7.43	25	101	87	16	38	38	0	34	26	0.31
2.5	60		104	31	28.3	0.73	0.91	8.8	0.80			104			37			35	28	
3.0	60		110	35	40.2	1.02	1.16	10.5	0.88			110			35			36	32	
3.5	80		113	36	39.6	1.06	1.29	11.4	0.82			104			38			34	28	
4.0	80	198/93	120	28	35.4	1.07	1.41	11.8	0.76	7.41	25	97	89	11	42	40	-2	31	23	0.28
4.5	100		128	37	47.4	1.26	1.39	10.9	0.91			110			37			35	32	
5.0	100		130	52	55.2	1.36	1.44	11.1	0.94			113			35			37	35	
5.5	120		130	49	60.6	1.50	1.50	11.5	1.00			113			35			38	38	
6.0	120	201/93	131	58	66.8	1.64	1.67	12.7	0.98	7.43	23	114	98	16	34	35	1	38	37	0.32
6.5	140		138	50	68.0	1.73	1.72	12.5	1.01			114			35			37	37	
7.0	140		140	50	73.4	1.87	1.78	12.7	1.05			115			35			37	39	
7.5	160		148	60	87.0	2.09	1.93	13.0	1.08			119			32			39	42	
8.0	160	198/99	149	59	92.9	2.24	2.03	13.6	1.10	7.43	22	119	99	20	32	33	1	39	43	0.32
8.5	180	216/99	154	55	89.3	2.21	2.02	13.1	1.09	7.42	20	117	99	21	34	32	-2	38	42	0.28
	Recovery		146	32	61.5	1.73	1.64	11.2	1.05			115			35			34	36	
	Recovery		132	32	53.4	1.37	1.14	8.6	1.20			118			35			37	44	
	Recovery		128	28	37.8	0.96	0.76	5.9	1.26			121			33			37	47	
	Recovery	189/93	125	27	30.1	0.75	0.63	5.0	1.19	7.39	20	119	114	7	34	33	-1	37	44	0.27

Interpretation

COMMENTS

Resting pulmonary function studies showed a mild restrictive defect with parallel loss of pulmonary capillary bed.

ANALYSIS

In flow chart 1, maximum $\dot{V}_{O_2}$ is decreased, but the anaerobic threshold is normal. See flow chart 3. At branchpoint 3.1, the breathing reserve is borderline low. The VD/VT is borderline normal, but the $P(A-a)_{O_2}$ and $P(a-ET)_{CO_2}$ are normal. At branchpoint 3.2, the patient has a high breathing frequency, typical of restrictive lung disease. If we had used flow chart 2, we would have arrived (through branchpoints 2.1 and 2.3) at the diagnosis of lung disease.

CONCLUSION

This patient with asbestosis shows mild abnormalities both at rest and with exercise. There is evidence of mild restrictive lung disease at rest. Exercise testing reveals a slightly low maximum $\dot{V}_{O_2}$. The high breathing frequency suggests ventilatory limitation; however, the disease at the time of testing has resulted in minimal physiologic impairments.

FIG. 47-A.

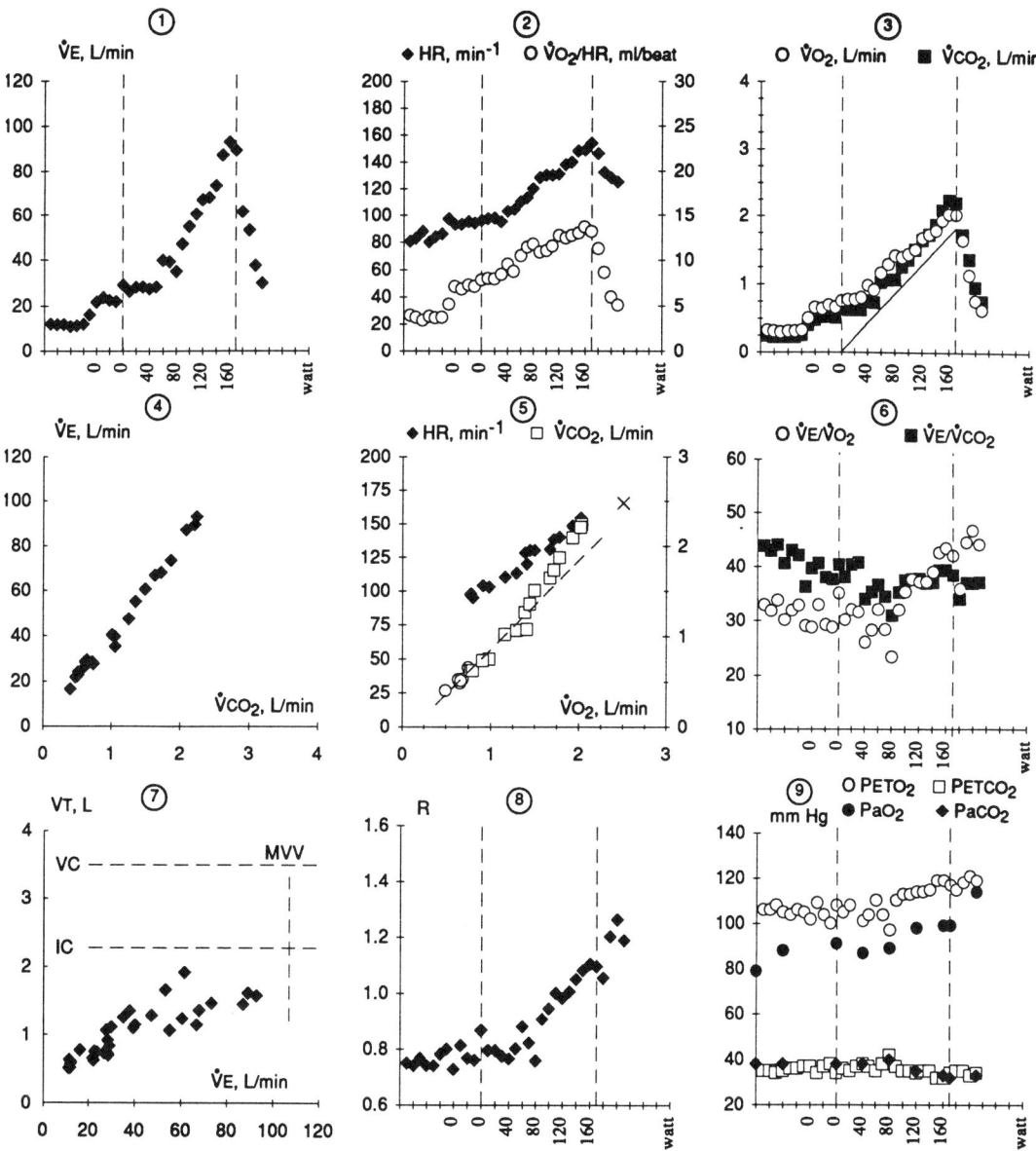

1. Vertical dashed lines in panels 1 to 3 and 6, 8, and 9 indicate the beginning and the end of increasing work period.

2. Unloaded cycling is performed for 3 minutes before the left vertical dashed line.

3. In panel 3, the diagonal line shows the increase of $\dot{V}O_2$ at a slope of 10 ml/min/W.

4. In panel 5, the diagonal dashed line has a slope of 1; the "x" in the upper right is the predicted maximum heart rate and $\dot{V}O_2$ for the subject.

Case 48   *Asbestosis*

Clinical Findings

This 67-year-old woman was referred for exercise testing. She had been exposed to asbestos for 3 years while working in a shipyard, approximately 40 years earlier. She had never smoked. Three years prior to this evaluation she noted fatigability, clubbing of fingernails, and shortness of breath. She was unable to climb a flight of stairs or walk rapidly on the level. A transbronchial lung biopsy at that time was reported as showing "fibrosis." Her symptoms improved markedly on 80 mg prednisone, but this medication was stopped after 1 year because of concern for its side effects. Five months prior to this evaluation she was started on oxygen therapy but corticosteroids were not reintroduced. Examination revealed a thin woman with fine inspiratory rales in the lateral and inferior lung fields that did not clear with coughing. There was dramatic digital clubbing. Chest roentgenograms showed extensive pulmonary infiltrates, compatible with interstitial pulmonary fibrosis. There was also a small patch of pleural calcification on the left. Resting ECG was normal.

Exercise Findings

The patient performed exercise on a cycle ergometer. She pedalled at 60 rpm without added load for 3 minutes. The work rate was then increased 5 W per minute to her symptom-limited maximum. Arterial blood was sampled every second minute, and intra-arterial blood pressure was recorded from a percutaneously placed brachial artery catheter. The patient stopped exercising because of dyspnea. She developed some premature atrial contractions during exercise but ECG otherwise was not remarkable.

TABLE 48-1. *Selected Respiratory Function Data*

MEASUREMENT	PREDICTED	MEASURED
Age, yr		67
Sex		Female
Height, cm		163
Weight, kg	63	48
Hematocrit, %		38
VC, L	2.77	1.51
IC, L	1.85	0.70
TLC, L	4.82	2.65
FEV_1, L	2.19	1.24
FEV_1/VC, %	79	82
MVV, L/min	82	33
D_{LCO}, ml/mm Hg/min	22.3	6.4

TABLE 48-2. *Selected Exercise Data*

MEASUREMENT	PREDICTED	MEASURED
Maximum $\dot{V}O_2$, L/min	1.12	0.42
Maximum HR, beat/min	153	108
Maximum O_2 pulse, ml/beat	7.3	4.1
AT, L/min	> 0.56	indeterminate
Blood pressure, mm Hg (rest, max)		122/74,140/80
Maximum $\dot{V}E$, L/min		29
Exercise breathing reserve, L/min	> 15	4
Pa_{O_2}, mm Hg (rest, max ex)		58,46
$P(A-a)_{O_2}$, mm Hg (rest, max ex)		41,64
$P(a-ET)_{CO_2}$, mm Hg (rest, max ex)		8,10
V_D/V_T (rest, heavy ex)		0.56,0.55
HCO_3^-, mEq/L (rest, 2-min recov)		25,24

Fig. 48-A.

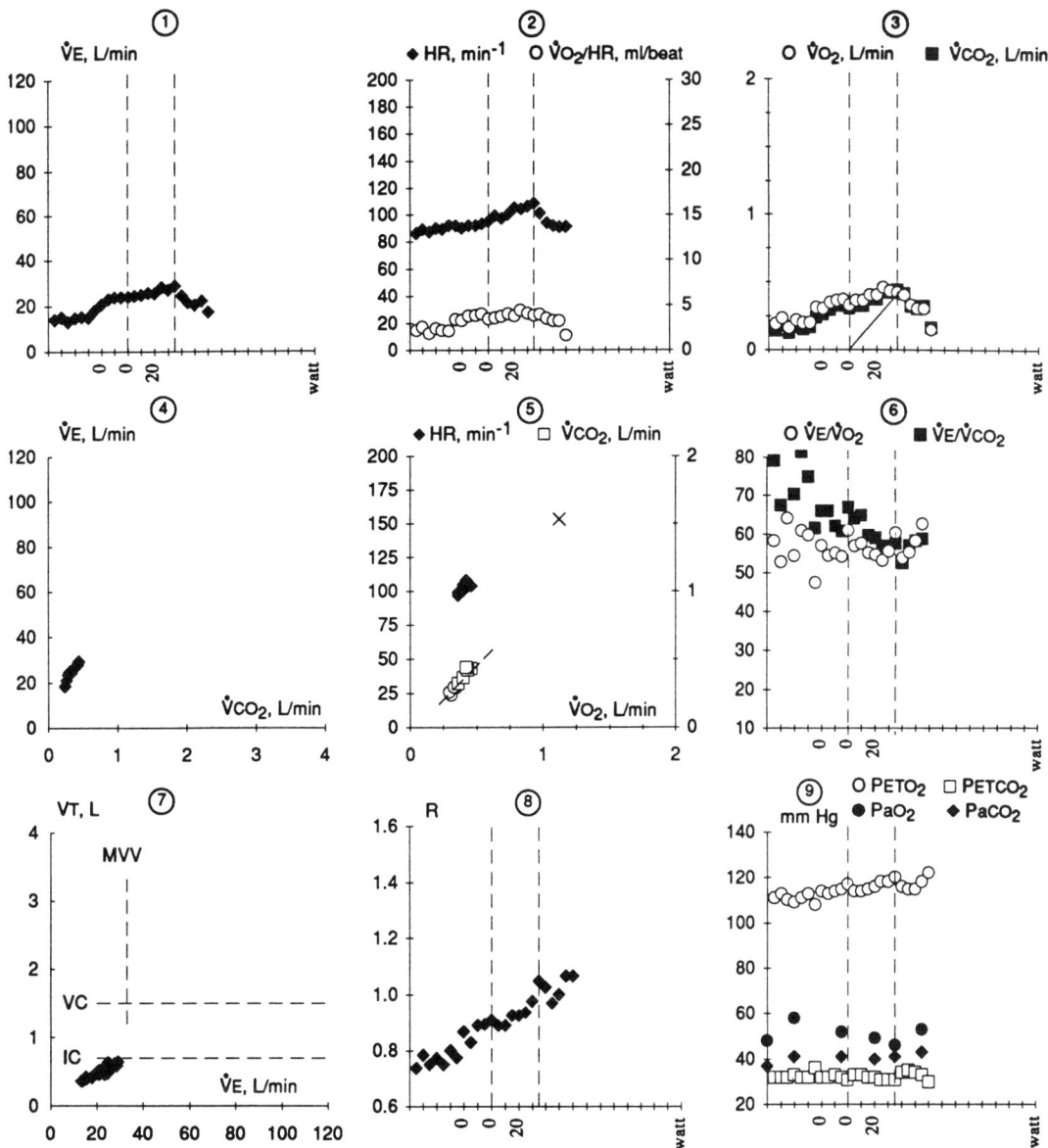

1. Vertical dashed lines in panels 1 to 3 and 6, 8, and 9 indicate the beginning and the end of increasing work period.

2. Unloaded cycling is performed for 3 minutes before the left vertical dashed line.

3. In panel 3, the diagonal line shows the increase of $\dot{V}O_2$ at a slope of 10 ml/min/W.

4. In panel 5, the diagonal dashed line has a slope of 1; the "x" in the upper right is the predicted maximum heart rate and $\dot{V}O_2$ for the subject.

TABLE 48-3.

Time min	Work rate watts	BP mm Hg	HR min⁻¹	f min⁻¹	$\dot{V}E$ L/min BTPS	$\dot{V}CO_2$ L/min STPD	$\dot{V}O_2$ L/min STPD	$\dfrac{\dot{V}O_2}{HR}$ ml/beat	R	pH	HCO₃ meq/L	PO2 ET	PO2 a	PO2 (A-a)	PCO2 ET	PCO2 a	PCO2 (a-ET)	$\dfrac{\dot{V}E}{\dot{V}CO_2}$	$\dfrac{\dot{V}E}{\dot{V}O_2}$	VD/VT
	Rest	122/74								7.44	25	111	48			37				
	Rest		86	38	14.3	0.14	0.19	2.2	0.74			113			32			79	58	
	Rest		89	36	15.2	0.18	0.23	2.6	0.78			113			32			67	53	
	Rest		87	37	13.4	0.12	0.16	1.8	0.75			110			32			85	64	
	Rest	119/71	90	36	15.0	0.17	0.22	2.4	0.77	7.40	25	109	58	41	33	41	8	70	54	0.56
	Rest		89	39	15.5	0.15	0.20	2.2	0.75			111			32			81	61	
	Rest		92	37	15.1	0.16	0.20	2.2	0.80			113			32			75	60	
	Unloaded		92	42	18.3	0.24	0.31	3.4	0.77			108			36			61	48	
	Unloaded		90	46	21.0	0.26	0.30	3.3	0.87			114			32			66	57	
	Unloaded		92	51	23.4	0.29	0.35	3.8	0.83			113			32			66	54	
	Unloaded		92	49	24.0	0.32	0.36	3.9	0.89			114			33			62	55	
	Unloaded	126/71	93	48	24.1	0.33	0.37	4.0	0.89	7.41	26	115	52	53	32	41	9	61	54	0.54
	Unloaded		95	50	24.3	0.30	0.33	3.5	0.91			117			31			67	61	
0.5	10		99	50	24.7	0.32	0.36	3.6	0.89			114			33			64	57	
1.0	10		97	51	25.0	0.32	0.36	3.7	0.89			114			33			65	57	
1.5	20		100	47	26.0	0.37	0.40	4.0	0.93			115			32			59	55	
2.0	20	137/74	105	47	25.8	0.37	0.40	3.8	0.93	7.41	25	116	49	58	32	40	8	59	55	0.54
2.5	30		104	49	28.6	0.43	0.46	4.4	0.93			118			31			57	53	
3.0	30		106	45	27.6	0.42	0.43	4.1	0.98			118			31			57	55	
3.5	40	140/80	108	45	29.1	0.44	0.42	3.9	1.05	7.39	24	120	46	64	31	41	10	57	60	0.55
	Recovery		101	39	24.8	0.41	0.40	4.0	1.03			116			34			52	54	
	Recovery		94	41	21.7	0.32	0.33	3.5	0.97			115			35			57	55	
	Recovery		92	40	20.8	0.30	0.30	3.3	1.00			115			34			58	58	
	Recovery	134/68	91	43	22.4	0.32	0.30	3.3	1.07	7.36	24	118	53	56	33	43	10	59	62	0.55
	Recovery		91	43	17.8	0.16	0.15	1.6	1.07			122			30			88	94	

Interpretation

COMMENTS

Results of the respiratory function studies indicate that this patient has a moderately severe restrictive defect with a marked reduction in diffusing capacity (Table 48-1). The ECG is normal.

ANALYSIS

In flow chart 1, the maximum $\dot{V}O_2$ is markedly reduced and the anaerobic threshold is indeterminate (Table 48-2). See flow chart 5: VD/VT, $P(a-\text{ET})_{CO_2}$, and $P(A-a)_{O_2}$ during exercise are markedly abnormal (branchpoint 5.1). The breathing reserve is low (branchpoint 5.3). The breathing frequency is high at rest and is maintained at a high level of approximately 50 breaths per minute through the incremental exercise period. The max-

imum ventilation achieved is approximately the patient's maximum ability to breathe (branchpoint 5.7). The foregoing findings lead to the diagnosis of restrictive lung disease. Supporting this diagnosis is the progressive decrease in Pa_{O_2} and increase in $P(A-a)_{O_2}$ at each work rate performed (Table 48-3 and panel 9, Fig. 48-A). An additional measurement consistent with restrictive lung disease is the high tidal volume/inspiratory capacity ratio (panel 7, Fig. 48-A). An O_2 flow limitation is demonstrated by the small rise in $\dot{V}O_2$ and the failure of O_2 pulse to rise (panels 3 and 2, respectively, in Fig. 48-A) as work rate is increased.

CONCLUSION

Exercise tolerance is limited by restrictive lung disease.

CASE 49 *Idiopathic interstitial lung disease*

CLINICAL FINDINGS

This 45-year-old woman had developed dyspnea, diffuse pulmonary infiltrates, and hypoxemia 6 months previously and was treated with oral corticosteroids without lung biopsy or specific diagnosis. She was no longer receiving medication but still had dyspnea after walking three blocks. She had never smoked and had no known exposure to known toxins except that she worked in a pet shop and sprayed bleach on cages to clean them. She had no other significant illnesses. She was evaluated to determine the pathophysiology of her dyspnea.

EXERCISE FINDINGS

The patient performed exercise on a cycle ergometer. She pedalled at 60 rpm without an added load for 3 minutes. The work rate was then increased 5 W per minute to her symptom-limited maximum. Arterial blood was sampled every second minute, and intra-arterial blood pressure was recorded from a percutaneously placed brachial artery catheter. Resting and exercise ECGs were normal. The patient stopped exercise because of leg fatigue. By ear oximetry, the baseline O_2 saturation was 96% at rest and 93% at peak exercise.

TABLE 49-1. *Selected Respiratory Function Data*

MEASUREMENT	PREDICTED	MEASURED
Age, yr		45
Sex		Female
Height, cm		152
Weight, kg	56	51
Hematocrit, %		49
VC, L	2.92	1.81
IC, L	1.95	1.23
TLC, L	4.29	3.62
FEV_1, L	2.41	1.42
FEV_1/VC, %	83	78
MVV, L/min	92	56
D_{LCO}, ml/mm Hg/min	22.7	4.3

TABLE 49-2. *Selected Exercise Data*

MEASUREMENT	PREDICTED	MEASURED
Maximum $\dot{V}_{O_2}$, L/min	1.44	0.88
Maximum HR, beats/min	174	174
Maximum O_2 pulse, ml/beat	8.3	5.1
$\Delta\dot{V}_{O_2}/\Delta$WR, ml/min/W	10.3	8.7
AT, L/min	> 0.69	0.65
Blood pressure, mm Hg (rest, max ex)		150/90,183/99
Maximum $\dot{V}_E$, L/min		56
Exercise breathing reserve, L/min	> 15	0
Pa_{O_2}, mm Hg (rest, max ex)		93,74
$P(A-a)_{O_2}$ mm Hg (rest, max ex)		24,50
$P(a-ET)_{CO_2}$, mm Hg (rest, max ex)		1,5
V_D/V_T (rest, max ex)		0.31,0.38
HCO_3^-, mEq/L (rest, recov)		23,17

TABLE 49-3.

Time min	Work rate watts	BP mm Hg	HR min⁻¹	f min⁻¹	$\dot{V}E$ L/min BTPS	$\dot{V}CO_2$ L/min STPD	$\dot{V}O_2$ L/min STPD	$\dfrac{\dot{V}O_2}{HR}$ ml/beat	R	pH	HCO3 meq/L	PO2, mm Hg ET	a	(A-a)	PCO2, mm Hg ET	a	(a-ET)	$\dfrac{\dot{V}E}{\dot{V}CO_2}$	$\dfrac{\dot{V}E}{\dot{V}O_2}$	$\dfrac{VD}{VT}$
	Rest	150/84								7.42	23		80			36				
	Rest		82	20	9.8	0.22	0.29	3.5	0.76			105			35			37	28	
	Rest		83	22	8.5	0.16	0.18	2.2	0.89			107			35			41	37	
	Rest		82	22	11.3	0.26	0.31	3.8	0.84			109			34			36	30	
	Rest	150/90	86	23	11.6	0.23	0.23	2.7	1.00	7.45	23	116	93	24	32	33	1	42	42	0.31
	Rest		88	21	11.4	0.24	0.23	2.6	1.04			117			31			40	42	
	Rest		93	25	11.5	0.22	0.23	2.5	0.96			112			34			43	41	
	Unloaded		105	25	15.7	0.33	0.31	3.0	1.06			119			30			41	44	
	Unloaded		111	28	14.9	0.34	0.38	3.4	0.89			107			36			37	33	
	Unloaded		114	28	17.2	0.42	0.48	4.2	0.88			109			35			35	31	
	Unloaded		114	26	18.7	0.45	0.47	4.1	0.96			112			34			37	35	
	Unloaded		117	26	20.7	0.50	0.52	4.4	0.96			113			33			37	36	
	Unloaded	177/96	118	27	19.3	0.47	0.51	4.3	0.92	7.41	22	113	75	37	34	36	2	36	33	0.30
0.5	5		117	25	20.4	0.50	0.52	4.4	0.96			112			33			37	35	
1.0	5		120	27	21.3	0.51	0.53	4.4	0.96			114			33			37	36	
1.5	10		121	27	22.6	0.55	0.57	4.7	0.96			113			33			37	36	
2.0	10	177/96	124	29	22.5	0.53	0.55	4.4	0.96	7.41	21	114	75	40	32	34	2	38	36	0.29
2.5	15		128	29	24.1	0.58	0.59	4.6	0.98			116			32			37	37	
3.0	15		130	30	23.8	0.58	0.57	4.4	1.02			104			37			37	37	
3.5	20		139	28	24.6	0.64	0.65	4.7	0.98			110			36			35	34	
4.0	20	180/99	142	28	22.8	0.63	0.68	4.8	0.93	7.39	21	110	80	32	37	36	-1	32	30	0.23
4.5	25		145	36	33.0	0.80	0.74	5.1	1.08			113			36			37	40	
5.0	25		148	37	35.8	0.83	0.78	5.3	1.06			118			32			39	42	
5.5	30		151	36	32.8	0.79	0.71	4.7	1.11			118			33			38	42	
6.0	30	180/96	158	44	40.0	0.87	0.74	4.7	1.18	7.39	20	122	77	43	30	34	4	42	49	0.35
6.5	35		159	47	43.6	0.91	0.77	4.8	1.18			123			29			44	51	
7.0	35		165	46	43.8	0.90	0.77	4.7	1.17			123			28			44	52	
7.5	40		165	48	42.1	0.89	0.79	4.8	1.13			122			29			43	48	
8.0	40	180/96	168	48	46.6	0.95	0.82	4.9	1.16	7.39	19	123	74	47	28	32	4	45	52	0.36
8.5	45		171	49	49.0	0.98	0.83	4.9	1.18			124			28			46	54	
9.0	45	183/99	174	55	56.0	1.08	0.88	5.1	1.23	7.38	18	127	74	50	26	31	5	48	58	0.38
	Recovery		169	40	43.2	0.92	0.79	4.7	1.16			128			28			43	50	
	Recovery		163	41	40.9	0.82	0.64	3.9	1.28			126			27			46	58	
	Recovery		153	30	23.4	0.61	0.53	3.5	1.15			121			30			34	39	
	Recovery	165/90	146	28	24.6	0.53	0.46	3.2	1.15	7.35	17	122	98	24	29	31	2	42	48	0.30

Interpretation

COMMENTS

This case is presented to show the effects of severe pulmonary vascular disease accompanying interstitial lung disease. The resting respiratory studies show extremely severe DL_{CO} reduction despite only mild to moderate restriction and normal resting Pa_{O_2}.

ANALYSIS

In flow chart 1, the patient had a low maximum $\dot{V}O_2$ and anaerobic threshold (Table 49-2). In flow chart 4, the patient had a negligible breathing reserve (branchpoint 4.1) and a high VD/VT (branchpoint 4.2) leading to a tentative diagnosis of "lung disease with impaired peripheral oxygenation." She had confirmatory findings of a high VT/IC, low oximeter saturation, high breathing frequency, positive $P(a-ET)_{CO_2}$, and wide and increasing $P(A-a)_{O_2}$, and a steep HR versus $\dot{V}O_2$ relationship. The $\Delta\dot{V}O_2/\Delta WR$ is within normal limits, but the low and unchanging O_2 pulse is striking (panels 2 and 5 of Fig. 49-A). The decrease in O_2 saturation is not abrupt (branchpoint 4.5), which excludes a significant right to left shunt.

CONCLUSION

Although the patient has ventilatory limitation, she also has evidence of severe pulmonary vascular disease with decreased pulmonary blood flow because of decreased stroke volume. The cardiac output is so limited that, even at peak exercise, there apparently is adequate time for reasonable equilibration of the end-capillary red cells with alveolar Po_2.

Fɪɢ. 49-A.

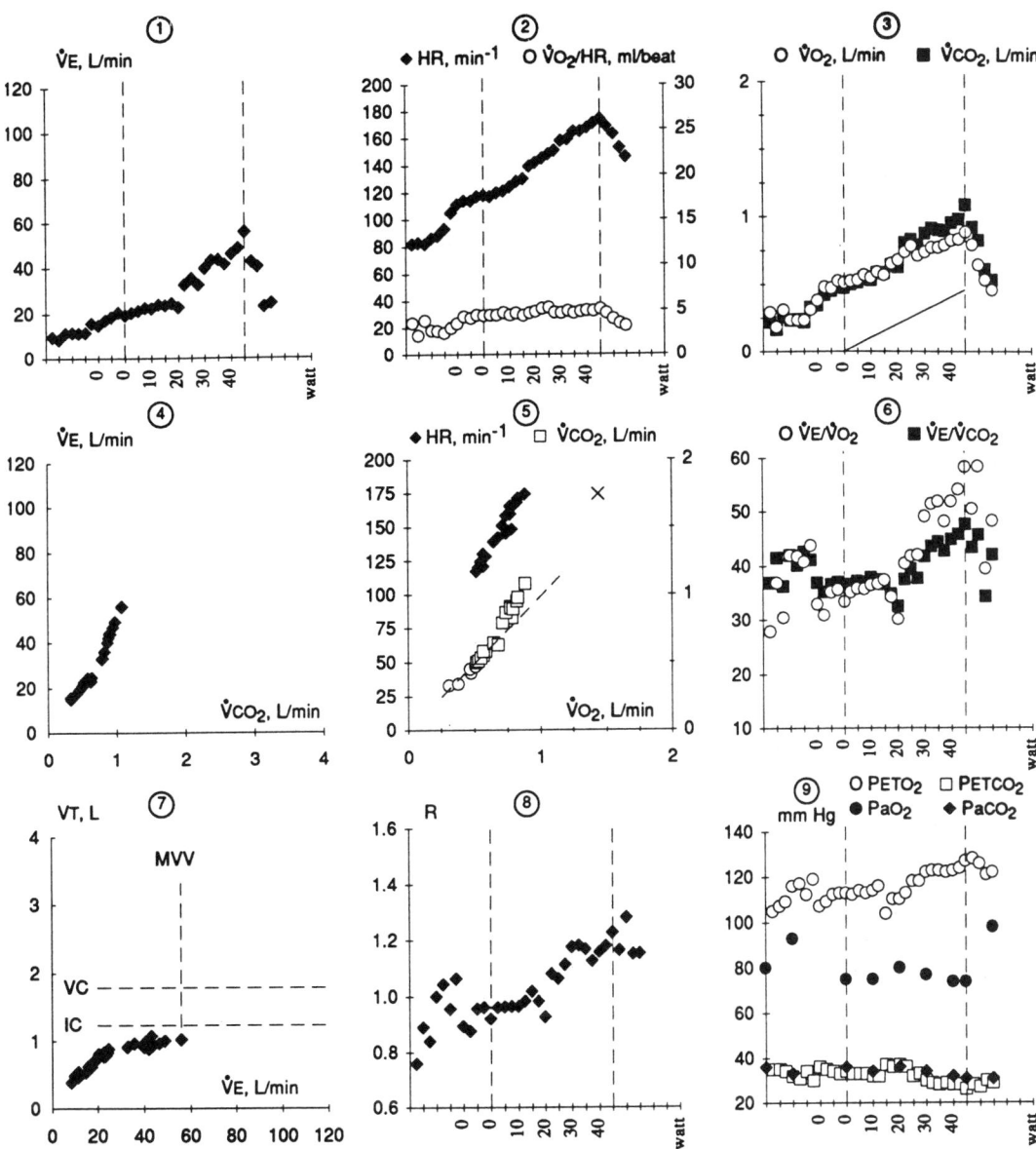

1. Vertical dashed lines in panels 1 to 3 and 6, 8, and 9 indicate the beginning and the end of increasing work period.

2. Unloaded cycling is performed for 3 minutes before the left vertical dashed line.

3. In panel 3, the diagonal line shows the increase of $\dot{V}O_2$ at a slope of 10 ml/min/W.

4. In panel 5, the diagonal dashed line has a slope of 1; the "x" in the upper right is the predicted maximum heart rate and $\dot{V}O_2$ for the subject.

CASE 50 *Mixed connective tissue disease with interstitial and pulmonary vascular disease*

CLINICAL FINDINGS

This 38-year-old man with known mixed connective tissue disease and restrictive lung disease of 3 years' duration was referred for evaluation to determine his level of disability. He had had a productive cough for 3 years and had been dyspneic for over 2 years. He had never smoked, but had been exposed to multiple chemical agents in a rubber factory. His current medications were prednisone, theophylline, and cimetidine.

EXERCISE FINDINGS

The patient performed exercise on a cycle ergometer. He pedalled at 60 rpm without an added load for 3 minutes. The work rate was then increased 15 W per minute to his symptom-limited maximum. Arterial blood was sampled every second minute and intra-arterial blood pressure was recorded from a percutaneously passed brachial artery catheter. Resting ECG was normal except for occasional premature ectopic beats. The frequency of these increased during exercise to a maximum of 12 per minute. No ST or T wave abnormalities occurred. Exercise was stopped because the patient seemed unsteady and indicated that he was lightheaded. These symptoms cleared in a few minutes. He also indicated that he was out of breath, but did not identify this as the cause of stopping.

TABLE 50-1. *Selected Respiratory Function Data*

MEASUREMENT	PREDICTED	MEASURED
Age, yr		38
Sex		Male
Height, cm		188
Weight, kg	88	88
Hematocrit, %		43
VC, L	5.09	2.28
IC, L	3.39	1.36
TLC, L	7.14	3.43
FEV_1, L	4.09	1.99
FEV_1/VC, %	81	87
MVV, L/min		
direct	163	107
indirect	164	80
D_{LCO}, ml/mm Hg/min	32.7	10.7

TABLE 50-2. *Selected Exercise Data*

MEASUREMENT	PREDICTED	MEASURED
Maximum $\dot{V}_{O_2}$, L/min	3.21	1.07
Maximum HR, beats/min	182	128
Maximum O_2 pulse, ml/beat	17.6	8.4
$\Delta\dot{V}_{O_2}/\Delta WR$, ml/min/W	10.3	7.3
AT, L/min	> 1.35	< 0.9
Blood pressure, mm Hg (rest, max ex)		141/90,222/102
Maximum $\dot{V}_E$, L/min		76
Exercise breathing reserve, L/min		
using direct MVV	> 15	31
using indirect MVV	> 15	4
Pa_{O_2}, mm Hg (rest, max ex)		79,63
$P(A-a)_{O_2}$, mm Hg (rest, max ex)		16,58
$P(a-ET)_{CO_2}$, mm Hg (rest, max ex)		5,9
V_D/V_T (rest, max ex)		0.46,0.48
HCO_3^-, mEq/L (rest, recov)		25,20

Fɪɢ. 50-A.

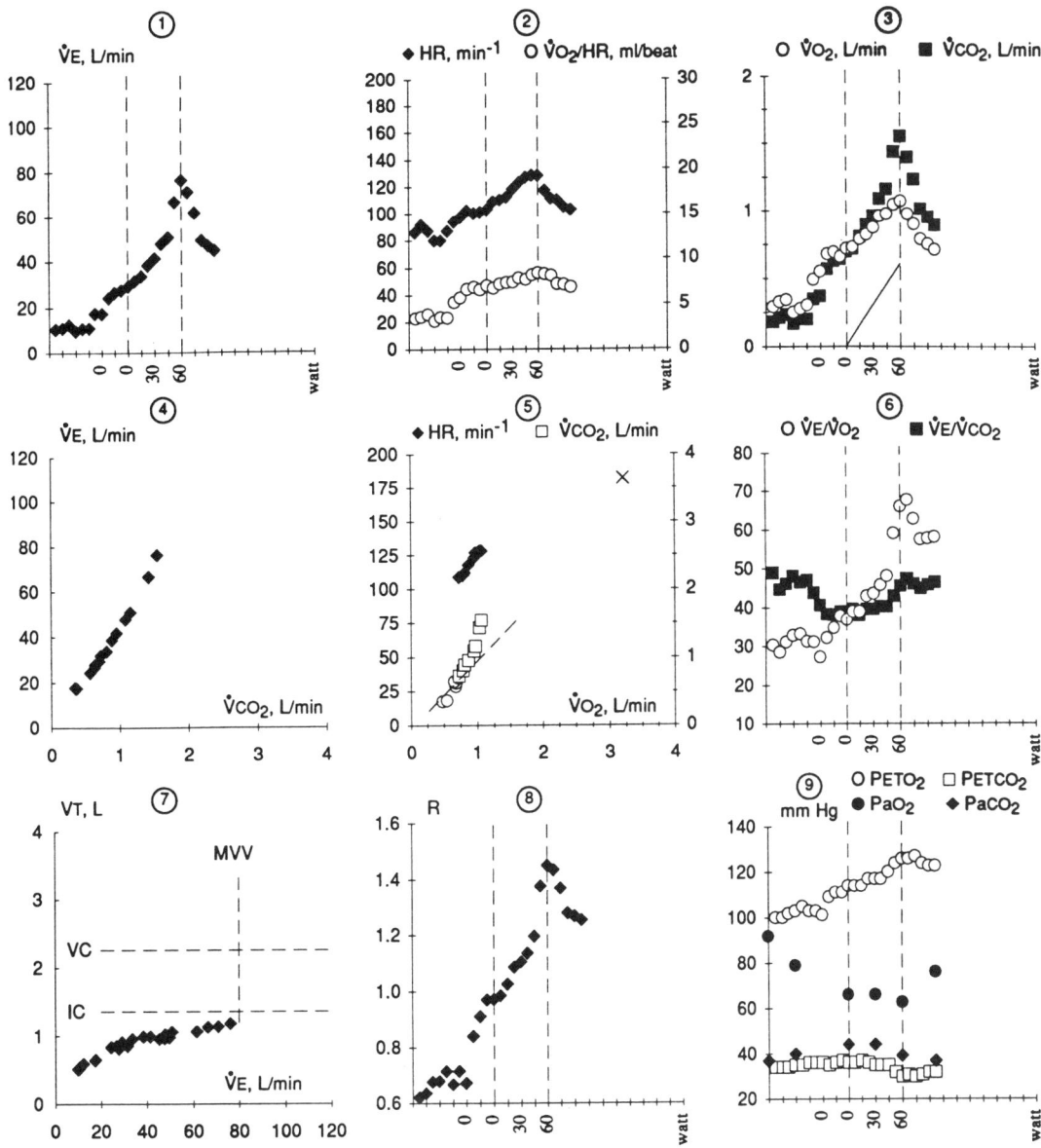

1. Vertical dashed lines in panels 1 to 3 and 6, 8, and 9 indicate the beginning and the end of increasing work period.

2. Unloaded cycling is performed for 3 minutes before the left vertical dashed line.

3. In panel 3, the diagonal line shows the increase of $\dot{V}O_2$ at a slope of 10 ml/min/W.

4. In panel 5, the diagonal dashed line has a slope of 1; the "x" in the upper right is the predicted maximum heart rate and $\dot{V}O_2$ for the subject.

TABLE 50-3.

Time min	Work rate watts	BP mm Hg	HR min⁻¹	f min⁻¹	V̇E L/min BTPS	V̇CO2 L/min STPD	V̇O2 L/min STPD	V̇O2/HR ml/beat	R	pH	HCO3 meq/L	PO2, mm Hg ET	a	(A-a)	PCO2, mm Hg ET	a	(a-ET)	V̇E/VCO2	V̇E/VO2	VD/VT
	Rest	141/90								7.45	25		92			37				
	Rest		86	20	10.5	0.18	0.29	3.4	0.62			100			34			49	30	
	Rest		92	20	11.1	0.21	0.33	3.6	0.64			100			34			45	28	
	Rest		87	21	12.4	0.23	0.34	3.9	0.68			102			34			46	31	
	Rest	156/96	80	19	9.8	0.17	0.25	3.1	0.68	7.41	25	103	79	16	35	40	5	48	33	0.46
	Rest		80	20	11.0	0.20	0.28	3.5	0.71			105			35			47	33	
	Rest		87	20	11.1	0.20	0.30	3.4	0.67			103			36			47	31	
	Unloaded		94	27	17.6	0.35	0.49	5.2	0.71			103			36			44	31	
	Unloaded		97	27	17.3	0.37	0.55	5.7	0.67			101			36			41	27	
	Unloaded		102	29	24.3	0.57	0.68	6.7	0.84			109			35			38	32	
	Unloaded		100	31	26.6	0.63	0.69	6.9	0.91			111			36			38	35	
	Unloaded		101	34	27.8	0.64	0.66	6.5	0.97			111			37			39	38	
	Unloaded	192/99	103	32	29.2	0.70	0.72	7.0	0.97	7.38	26	114	66	39	36	44	8	38	37	0.44
0.5	15		109	37	31.6	0.72	0.73	6.7	0.99			114			36			40	39	
1.0	15		110	35	33.7	0.81	0.79	7.2	1.03			114			37			38	39	
1.5	30		112	39	38.5	0.89	0.82	7.3	1.09			117			36			40	43	
2.0	30	204/102	118	42	41.5	0.96	0.87	7.4	1.10	7.38	26	117	66	43	35	44	9	40	44	0.46
2.5	45		123	47	47.8	1.09	0.96	7.8	1.14			117			35			40	46	
3.0	45		127	48	50.8	1.16	0.97	7.6	1.20			120			35			40	48	
3.5	60		128	59	66.5	1.43	1.04	8.1	1.38			124			32			43	59	
4.0	60	222/102	128	64	76.1	1.55	1.07	8.4	1.45	7.38	23	126	63	58	30	39	9	46	66	0.48
	Recovery		117	62	70.9	1.39	0.97	8.3	1.43			126			31			47	68	
	Recovery		111	58	61.5	1.23	0.90	8.1	1.37			127			30			46	63	
	Recovery		110	51	49.7	1.01	0.79	7.2	1.28			124			31			45	57	
	Recovery		105	49	47.5	0.95	0.75	7.1	1.27			123			32			46	58	
	Recovery	180/88	103	47	45.2	0.89	0.71	6.9	1.25	7.35	20	123	76	43	32	37	5	46	58	0.45

Interpretation

COMMENTS

This patient shows the effect of severe interstitial lung disease on cardiac output, presumably because of increased pulmonary vascular resistance. The resting respiratory function studies show severe restriction with severe loss of available pulmonary capillary bed and mild hypoxemia.

ANALYSIS

In flow chart 1, the patient had a low maximum $\dot{V}O_2$ and an extremely low anaerobic threshold (Table 50-2). In flow chart 4, the patient had a low breathing reserve using the indirect MVV (branchpoint 4.1). At branchpoint 4.2 we are directed to "lung disease with impaired peripheral oxygenation" by the finding of a high VD/VT. Confirmatory findings of ventilatory limitation to exercise are the high breathing frequency (64) and high VT/IC. Especially impressive are the small increases in $\dot{V}O_2$ and O_2 pulse, the arrhythmia, and

the lightheadedness, all indicating difficulty in perfusion and/or oxygenation of the myocardium and brain as peak exercise is reached. (If we had decided that the breathing reserve were normal (branchpoint 4.1) we would also have been directed through branchpoint 4.3 with high ventilatory equivalents to "abnormal pulmonary circulation" and from there through branchpoint 4.5 to pulmonary vascular disease without clear evidence of a right to left shunt.)

CONCLUSION

This patient demonstrates significant gas exchange, ventilatory, and cardiovascular defects, all because of his severe interstitial lung disease. Although he has no evidence of intrinsic heart disease, he has severe impairment in increasing his cardiac output. The increased CO_2 production secondary to his metabolic acidosis and the high ventilatory requirement because of his increased VD/VT combine to create an unusually large ventilatory requirement in a patient with reduced ventilatory capacity.

Case 51 *Interstitial lung disease*

Clinical Findings

This 20-year-old man with a history of exposure to crop dusting was found after extensive work-up and open lung biopsy to have an interstitial pneumonitis with mica deposits. The patient noted severe dyspnea with walking one block or climbing two flights of stairs. He denies cough, wheezing, orthopnea, chest pain, syncope, peripheral edema, or cyanosis. He was being re-evaluated following institution of daily prednisone.

Exercise Findings

The patient performed exercise on a cycle ergometer. He pedalled at 60 rpm without an added load for 3 minutes. The work rate was then increased 10 W per minute to tolerance. Arterial blood was sampled every second minute and intra-arterial pressure was recorded from a percutaneously placed brachial artery catheter. The patient was well motivated and cooperative and stopped exercise because of fatigue and shortness of breath. No ECG abnormalities occurred at rest or during exercise, but the patient developed a significant pulsus paradoxus (blood pressure variations with breathing).

TABLE 51-1. *Selected Respiratory Function Data*

MEASUREMENT	PREDICTED	MEASURED
Age, yr		20
Sex		Male
Height, cm		160
Weight, kg	66	48
Hematocrit, %		51
VC, L	3.52	1.25
IC, L	2.37	0.74
FEV$_1$, L	2.99	1.21
FEV$_1$/VC, %	85	97
MVV, L/min	125	51

TABLE 51-2. *Selected Exercise Data*

MEASUREMENT	PREDICTED	MEASURED
Maximum $\dot{V}O_2$, L/min	2.46	0.74
Maximum HR, beats/min	200	182
Maximum O_2 pulse, ml/beat	12.3	4.1
$\Delta\dot{V}O_2/\Delta WR$, ml/min/W	10.3	4.2
AT, L/min	> 0.98	< 0.55
Blood pressure, mm Hg (rest, max ex)		118/81,165–126/102–63
Maximum $\dot{V}E$, L/min		47
Exercise breathing reserve, L/min	> 15	4
Pa$_{O_2}$, mm Hg (rest, max ex)		73,85
P(a−a)$_{O_2}$ mm Hg (rest, max ex)		15,36
P(a−ET)$_{CO_2}$, mm Hg (rest, max ex)		3,4
V$_D$/V$_T$ (rest, max ex)		0.37,0.36
HCO$_3^-$, mEq/L (rest, 2-min recov)		28,14

Table 51-3.

Time min	Work rate watts	BP mm Hg	HR min⁻¹	f min⁻¹	V̇E L/min BTPS	V̇CO2 L/min STPD	V̇O2 L/min STPD	V̇O2/HR ml/beat	R	pH	HCO3 meq/L	PO2 ET	PO2 a	PO2 (A-a)	PCO2 ET	PCO2 a	PCO2 (a-ET)	V̇E/V̇CO2	V̇E/V̇O2	VD/VT
	Rest	96/68								7.40	27	77			45					
	Rest		96	24	8.9	0.19	0.30	3.1	0.63			89			45			36	23	
	Rest		93	23	9.0	0.20	0.29	3.1	0.69			93			45			35	24	
	Rest		91	21	8.7	0.20	0.29	3.2	0.69			95			43			35	24	
	Rest	118/81	90	23	9.3	0.21	0.30	3.3	0.70	7.40	28	97	73	15	43	46	3	35	24	0.37
	Rest		89	22	8.9	0.20	0.27	3.0	0.74			97			43			35	26	
	Rest		91	24	9.5	0.20	0.28	3.1	0.71			96			43			37	27	
	Unloaded		112	27	12.8	0.33	0.48	4.3	0.69			90			46			32	22	
	Unloaded		115	33	16.8	0.44	0.53	4.6	0.83			100			44			32	26	
	Unloaded		123	34	18.2	0.50	0.54	4.4	0.93			100			47			31	28	
	Unloaded		130	33	19.0	0.54	0.54	4.2	1.00			103			47			30	30	
	Unloaded		134	35	20.2	0.58	0.55	4.1	1.05			105			47			30	31	
	Unloaded	147/93	135	34	19.9	0.58	0.53	3.9	1.09	7.35	27	108	77	27	46	49	3	29	32	0.34
0.5	10		139	46	20.7	0.56	0.51	3.7	1.10			100			51			30	33	
1.0	10		146	42	25.1	0.71	0.60	4.1	1.18			112			44			30	36	
1.5	20		150	40	24.4	0.67	0.55	3.7	1.22			112			44			31	38	
2.0	20	156/96	157	43	26.5	0.72	0.59	3.8	1.22	7.33	25	113	79	30	43	48	5	32	39	0.37
2.5	30		156	46	29.6	0.81	0.67	4.3	1.21			110			45			32	38	
3.0	30		168	48	31.5	0.86	0.65	3.9	1.32			116			43			32	42	
3.5	40		174	50	32.9	0.89	0.67	3.9	1.33			116			43			32	43	
4.0	40	156/90	177	54	37.1	0.98	0.68	3.8	1.44	7.28	22	119	81	33	42	47	5	33	48	0.39
4.5	50		178	52	36.3	1.00	0.68	3.8	1.47			120			42			32	47	
5.0	50		180	55	40.9	1.07	0.69	3.8	1.55			121			41			34	53	
5.5	60	65-126/102-6	182	61	47.3	1.23	0.74	4.1	1.66	7.23	17	124	85	36	38	42	4	34	57	0.36
	Recovery		180	61	45.9	1.16	0.71	3.9	1.63			124			38			35	57	
	Recovery		180	55	38.4	0.94	0.63	3.5	1.49			122			39			36	54	
	Recovery		176	56	38.4	0.90	0.62	3.5	1.45			123			38			37	54	
	Recovery		172	54	35.4	0.79	0.58	3.4	1.36			123			36			39	53	
	Recovery	136/69	164	54	31.5	0.68	0.55	3.4	1.24	7.15	14	121	92	23	36	41	5	40	49	0.40
	Recovery		160	47	27.7	0.58	0.46	2.9	1.26			123			35			41	52	

Interpretation

COMMENTS

Resting respiratory function studies showed severe restrictive lung disease. Arterial blood gases revealed a chronic, compensated respiratory acidosis with mild hypoxemia.

ANALYSIS

In flow chart 1, maximum V̇O2 and the anaerobic threshold are both markedly reduced. Proceeding to flow chart 4 through branchpoints 4.1 and 4.2, we come to lung disease with impaired peripheral oxygenation, but we are also instructed to look at the box with abnormal pulmonary circulation. The high breathing frequency, high ratio of tidal volume to inspiratory capacity (panel 7 of Fig 51-A), and the breathing reserve are all typical of severe restrictive lung disease. The elevated VD/VT and positive P(a − ET)$_{CO_2}$ indicate inadequate perfusion of ventilated airspaces. The lack of severe hypoxemia is at first puzzling; the extremely low O2 pulse and low anaerobic threshold tell us that stroke volume must be extremely low. On reflection, it seems likely that the right ventricle has not hypertrophied in response to the increased pulmonary vascular resistance caused by the underlying lung disease. Thus, the cardiac output is relatively fixed, as indicated by the failure of V̇O2 to increase despite the increasing work rate. Because cardiac output does not increase, residence time in the pulmonary capillary remains unchanged. This allows satisfactory equilibration of

FIG. 51-A.

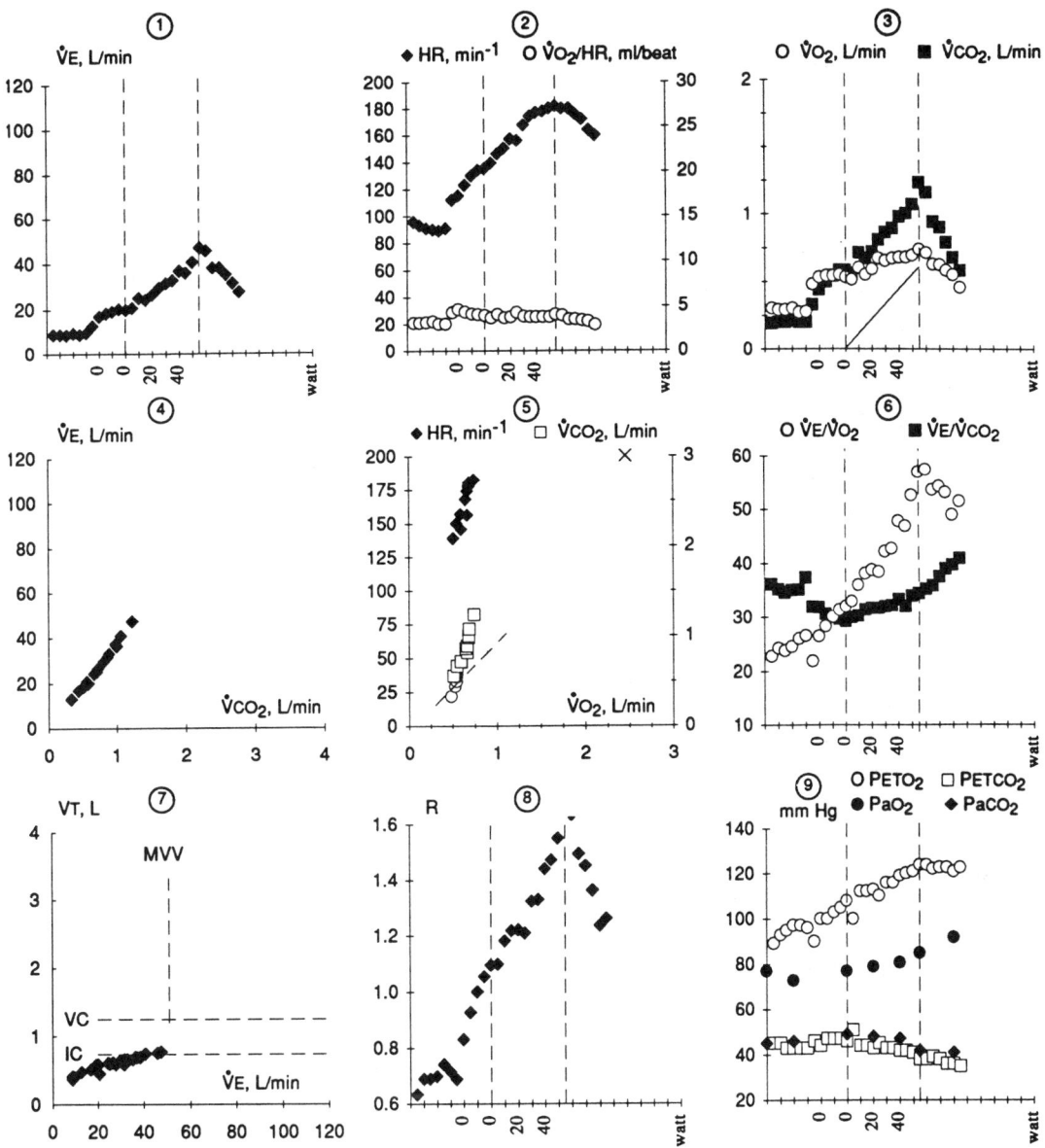

1. Vertical dashed lines in panels 1 to 3 and 6, 8, and 9 indicate the beginning and the end of increasing work period.

2. Unloaded cycling is performed for 3 minutes before the left vertical dashed line.

3. In panel 3, the diagonal line shows the increase of $\dot{V}O_2$ at a slope of 10 ml/min/W.

4. In panel 5, the diagonal dashed line has a slope of 1; the "x" in the upper right is the predicted maximum heart rate and $\dot{V}O_2$ for the subject.

the end-capillary red cells with the alveolar gas O_2. The striking increase in $\dot{V}CO_2$ is in contrast to $\dot{V}O_2$. This is explained by the severe metabolic (lactic) acidosis that the patient develops as a result of the failure of cardiac output to increase in response to exercise (arterial HCO_3^- decreases 14 mEq/L in 8 minutes).

CONCLUSION

This is an unusual patient with extremely severe restrictive lung disease and secondary pulmonary vascular disease with high dead space ventilation, extremely low stroke volume and cardiac output, but without significant hypoxemia.

CASE 52 *Sarcoidosis*

CLINICAL FINDINGS

This 39-year-old woman was referred for follow-up exercise testing with complaints of mild shortness of breath of 1 year's duration and diminished exercise tolerance of 18 months' duration. One year previously, following an episode of hepatitis of undetermined origin, she was found to have an enlarging right lower lung field cystic lesion. Noninvasive preoperative exercise testing at that time suggested cardiovascular limitation. During thoracic surgery, pulmonary artery pressure was normal. The resected lesion contained non-caseating granulomata compatible with sarcoidosis. No organisms were seen or cultured. The patient had never smoked cigarettes and took no medications. Her exercise test was repeated with an intra-arterial catheter.

EXERCISE FINDINGS

The patient performed exercise on a cycle ergometer. She pedalled at 60 rpm without an added load for 3 minutes. The work rate was then increased 15 W per minute to tolerance. Arterial blood was sampled every second minute, and intra-arterial pressure was recorded from a percutaneously placed brachial artery catheter. The patient stopped exercise because of lightheadedness and shortness of breath. No ECG abnormalities occurred at rest or during exercise.

TABLE 52-1. *Selected Respiratory Function Data*

MEASUREMENT	PREDICTED	MEASURED
Age, yr		39
Sex		Female
Height, cm		162
Weight, kg	63	68
Hematocrit, %		41
VC, L	3.38	2.89
IC, L	2.25	1.80
TLC, L	5.84	4.34
FEV_1, L	2.75	2.40
FEV_1/VC, %	81	88
MVV, L/min	105	98
DL_{CO}, ml/mm Hg/min	24.2	17.9

TABLE 52-2. *Selected Exercise Data*

MEASUREMENT	PREDICTED	MEASURED
Maximum $\dot{V}O_2$, L/min	1.70	1.12
Maximum HR, beats/min	181	173
Maximum O_2 pulse, ml/beat	9.4	6.5
$\Delta \dot{V}O_2/\Delta WR$, ml/min/W	10.3	7.3
AT, L/min	> 0.81	< 0.65
Blood pressure, mm Hg (rest, max)		146/88,189/105
Maximum $\dot{V}E$, L/min		55
Exercise breathing reserve, L/min	> 15	43
Pa_{O_2}, mm Hg (rest, max ex)		104,119
$P(A-a)_{O_2}$, mm Hg (rest, max ex)		7,7
$P(a-ET)_{CO_2}$, mm Hg (rest, max ex)		0, −4
VD/VT (rest, max ex)		0.30,0.19
HCO_3^-, mEq/L (rest, 2-min recov)		22,13

Fig. 52-A.

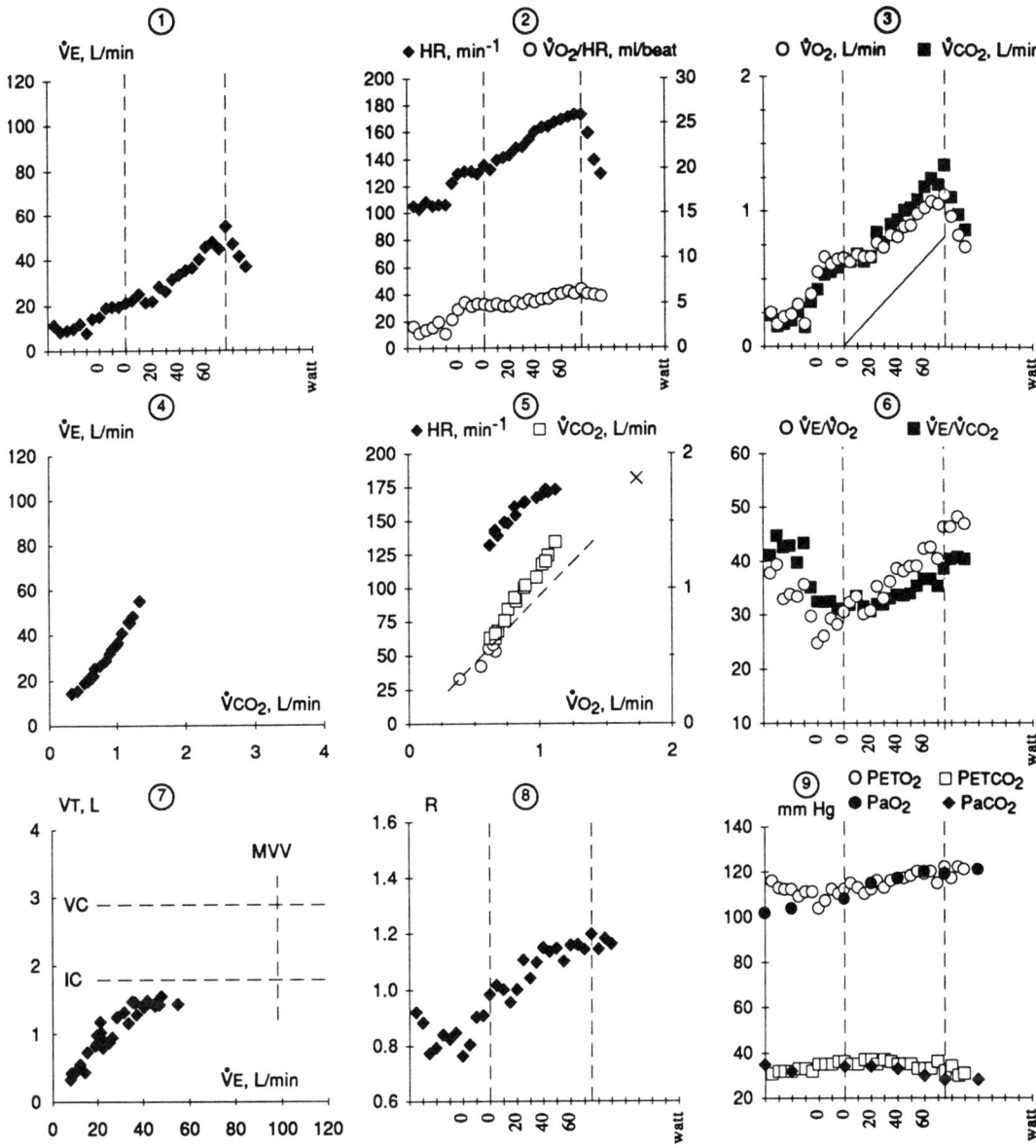

1. Vertical dashed lines in panels 1 to 3 and 6, 8, and 9 indicate the beginning and the end of increasing work period.

2. Unloaded cycling is performed for 3 minutes before the left vertical dashed line.

3. In panel 3, the diagonal line shows the increase of $\dot{V}O_2$ at a slope of 10 ml/min/W.

4. In panel 5, the diagonal dashed line has a slope of 1; the "x" in the upper right is the predicted maximum heart rate and $\dot{V}O_2$ for the subject.

Table 52-3.

Time min	Work rate watts	BP mm Hg	HR min⁻¹	f min⁻¹	V̇E L/min BTPS	V̇CO₂ L/min STPD	V̇O₂ L/min STPD	V̇O₂/HR ml/beat	R	pH	HCO₃ meq/L	PO₂ ET	PO₂ a	PO₂ (A-a)	PCO₂ ET	PCO₂ a	PCO₂ (a-ET)	V̇E/V̇CO₂	V̇E/V̇O₂	VD/VT
	Rest	156/90								7.41	22	102			35					
	Rest		105	23	11.4	0.23	0.25	2.4	0.92			116			31			41	38	
	Rest		103	20	8.4	0.15	0.17	1.7	0.88			113			32			45	39	
	Rest		108	23	9.2	0.17	0.22	2.0	0.77			112			32			43	33	
	Rest	146/88	105	23	10.1	0.19	0.24	2.3	0.79	7.43	21	112	104	7	32	32	0	43	34	0.30
	Rest		106	22	12.2	0.26	0.31	2.9	0.84			109			33			40	33	
	Rest		106	24	8.1	0.14	0.17	1.6	0.82			111			33			43	36	
	Unloaded		122	33	14.4	0.33	0.39	3.2	0.85			111			32			35	30	
	Unloaded		129	21	15.4	0.42	0.55	4.3	0.76			104			35			32	25	
	Unloaded		131	23	19.1	0.53	0.66	5.0	0.80			107			35			32	26	
	Unloaded		131	23	19.8	0.55	0.61	4.7	0.90			112			35			32	29	
	Unloaded		129	20	19.7	0.58	0.64	5.0	0.91			110			36			31	28	
	Unloaded	165/99	135	18	21.3	0.64	0.65	4.8	0.98	7.39	20	112	108	8	36	34	-2	31	30	0.17
0.5	10		132	28	22.4	0.63	0.62	4.7	1.02			115			35			32	32	
1.0	10		139	29	25.2	0.68	0.68	4.9	1.00			113			35			33	33	
1.5	20		141	21	21.6	0.63	0.66	4.7	0.95			110			37			31	30	
2.0	20	168/97	143	24	22.2	0.66	0.66	4.6	1.00	7.38	20	112	115	1	37	34	-3	31	31	0.15
2.5	30		148	23	28.7	0.84	0.76	5.1	1.11			116			35			32	35	
3.0	30		149	28	26.5	0.76	0.73	4.9	1.04			113			37			32	33	
3.5	40		154	24	31.7	0.90	0.82	5.3	1.10			116			36			33	36	
4.0	40	189/105	160	29	33.7	0.93	0.81	5.1	1.15	7.37	19	117	117	3	35	33	-2	34	39	0.21
4.5	50		163	24	35.6	1.00	0.88	5.4	1.14			117			35			34	38	
5.0	50		164	25	36.7	1.02	0.89	5.4	1.15			118			35			34	39	
5.5	60		167	29	40.7	1.08	0.98	5.9	1.10			120			33			35	39	
6.0	60	189/105	169	31	45.8	1.18	1.02	6.0	1.16	7.35	16	119	120	3	33	30	-3	37	42	0.20
6.5	70		171	31	48.1	1.24	1.07	6.3	1.16			120			33			37	42	
7.0	70		173	32	45.2	1.20	1.05	6.1	1.14			115			36			35	40	
7.5	80	189/105	173	38	55.0	1.34	1.12	6.5	1.20	7.32	14	122	119	7	32	28	-4	39	46	0.19
	Recovery		159	33	47.2	1.10	0.96	6.0	1.15			117			34			40	46	
	Recovery	118/60	139	28	41.8	0.97	0.82	5.9	1.18			122			30			41	48	
	Recovery		129	29	37.2	0.86	0.74	5.7	1.16			121			31			40	47	
										7.27	13	121			28					

Interpretation

COMMENTS

The resting respiratory function studies were similar to her pre-lung resection values and showed mild restrictive lung disease. The resting blood gases reveal a mild compensated respiratory alkalosis or metabolic acidosis.

ANALYSIS

In flow chart 1, maximum $\dot{V}O_2$ and the anaerobic threshold are both decreased, sending us through branchpoint 1.3 to flow chart 4. The breathing reserve is high (branchpoint 4.1). The mildly elevated ventilatory equivalents can be accounted for by the low Pa_{CO_2}. The normal VD/VT and $P(A-a)_{O_2}$ (branchpoint 4.3) indicate uniform ventilation-perfusion ratios. The hematocrit is normal (branchpoint 4.4). The maximum O_2 pulse is extremely low and increases slowly as work rate is increased. The patient had no leg pain or electrocardiographic abnormality; the heart rate reserve was low. These findings are compatible with a cardiomyopathy or peripheral muscle dysfunction secondary to sarcoidosis at either or both sites.

CONCLUSION

The patient exercised maximally and developed a significant lactic acidosis. Pulmonary disease does not explain her low $\dot{V}O_2$max. Sarcoidosis of either the myocardium or a defect in electron transport in the peripheral musculature could explain this patient's findings.

CASE 53 *Sarcoidosis, severe: Air and oxygen breathing*

CLINICAL FINDINGS

This 29-year-old man with a 6-year history of sarcoidosis was referred for evaluation of the pathophysiology of his worsening dyspnea. He was on continuous O_2 supplementation and beclomethasone diproprionate (Vanceril) inhaler, but he was not currently taking systemic corticosteroids. His weight was stable. He had smoked cigarettes for only 1 year.

EXERCISE FINDINGS

The patient performed exercise on a cycle ergometer while he breathed room air. The test was repeated while he was breathing 100% O_2. On both occasions, he pedalled at 60 rpm without an added load for 3 minutes. The work rate was then increased 10 W per minute to tolerance. Arterial blood was sampled every second minute, and intra-arterial pressure was recorded from a percuta-neously placed brachial artery catheter. The patient stopped exercise because of shortness of breath while breathing room air and because of leg fatigue while breathing O_2. The resting ECG showed right axis deviation and inverted T waves anteriorly. The T waves became upright during exercise. No arrhythmias were noted.

TABLE 53-1. *Selected Respiratory Function Data*

MEASUREMENT	PREDICTED	MEASURED
Age, yr		29
Sex		Male
Height, cm		171
Weight, kg	73	58
Hematocrit, %		45
VC, L	4.28	3.11
IC, L	2.85	1.59
TLC, L	5.82	4.78
FEV_1, L	3.46	2.27
FEV_1/VC, %	81	73
MVV, L/min, indirect	138	91
DL_{CO}, ml/mm Hg/min	29.9	6.9

TABLE 53-2. *Selected Exercise Data*

		MEASURED	
MEASUREMENT	PREDICTED	AIR	100% O_2
Maximum work rate, W		40	70
Maximum $\dot{V}O_2$, L/min	2.64	0.8	
Maximum HR, beats/min	191	149	150
Maximum O_2 pulse, ml/beat	13.6	5.7	
AT, L/min	> 1.08	0.7	
Blood pressure, mm Hg (rest, max ex)		114/72,135/78	111/69,141/87
Maximum $\dot{V}E$, L/min		64	70
Exercise breathing reserve, L/min	> 15	27	21
PA_{O_2}, mm Hg (rest, max ex)		42,35	585,605
$P(A-a)_{O_2}$ mm Hg (rest, max ex)		52,74	84,57
$P(a-ET)_{CO_2}$, mm Hg (rest, max ex)		16,22	19,28
VD/VT (rest, max ex)		0.57,0.67	0.63,0.71
HCO_3^-, mEq/L (rest, 2-min recov)		27,24	25,24

FIG. 53-A. *Air breathing.*

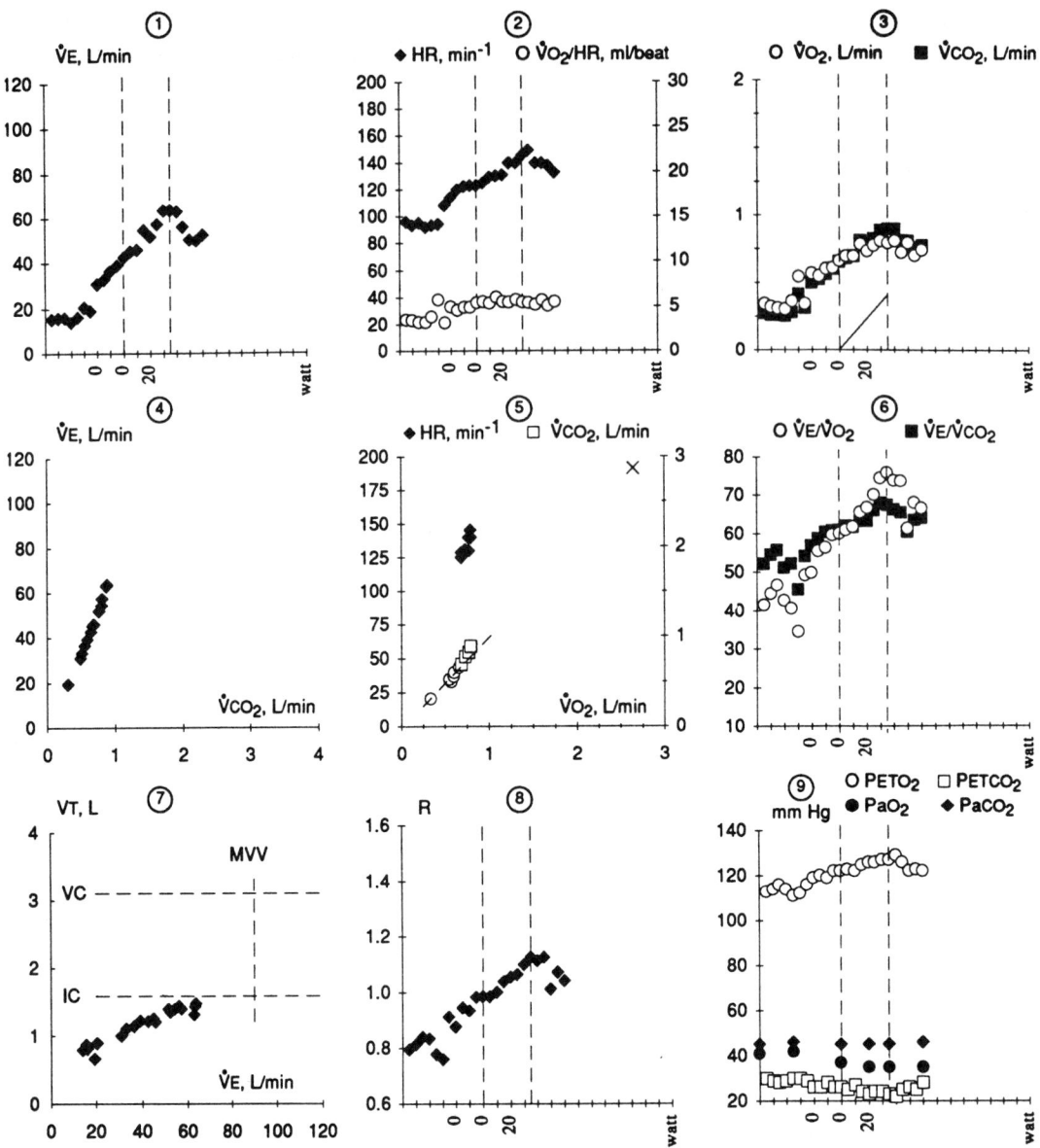

1. Vertical dashed lines in panels 1 to 3 and 6, 8, and 9 indicate the beginning and the end of increasing work period.

2. Unloaded cycling is performed for 3 minutes before the left vertical dashed line.

3. In panel 3, the diagonal line shows the increase of $\dot{V}O_2$ at a slope of 10 ml/min/W.

4. In panel 5, the diagonal dashed line has a slope of 1; the "x" in the upper right is the predicted maximum heart rate and $\dot{V}O_2$ for the subject.

FIG. 53-B. *Oxygen breathing.*

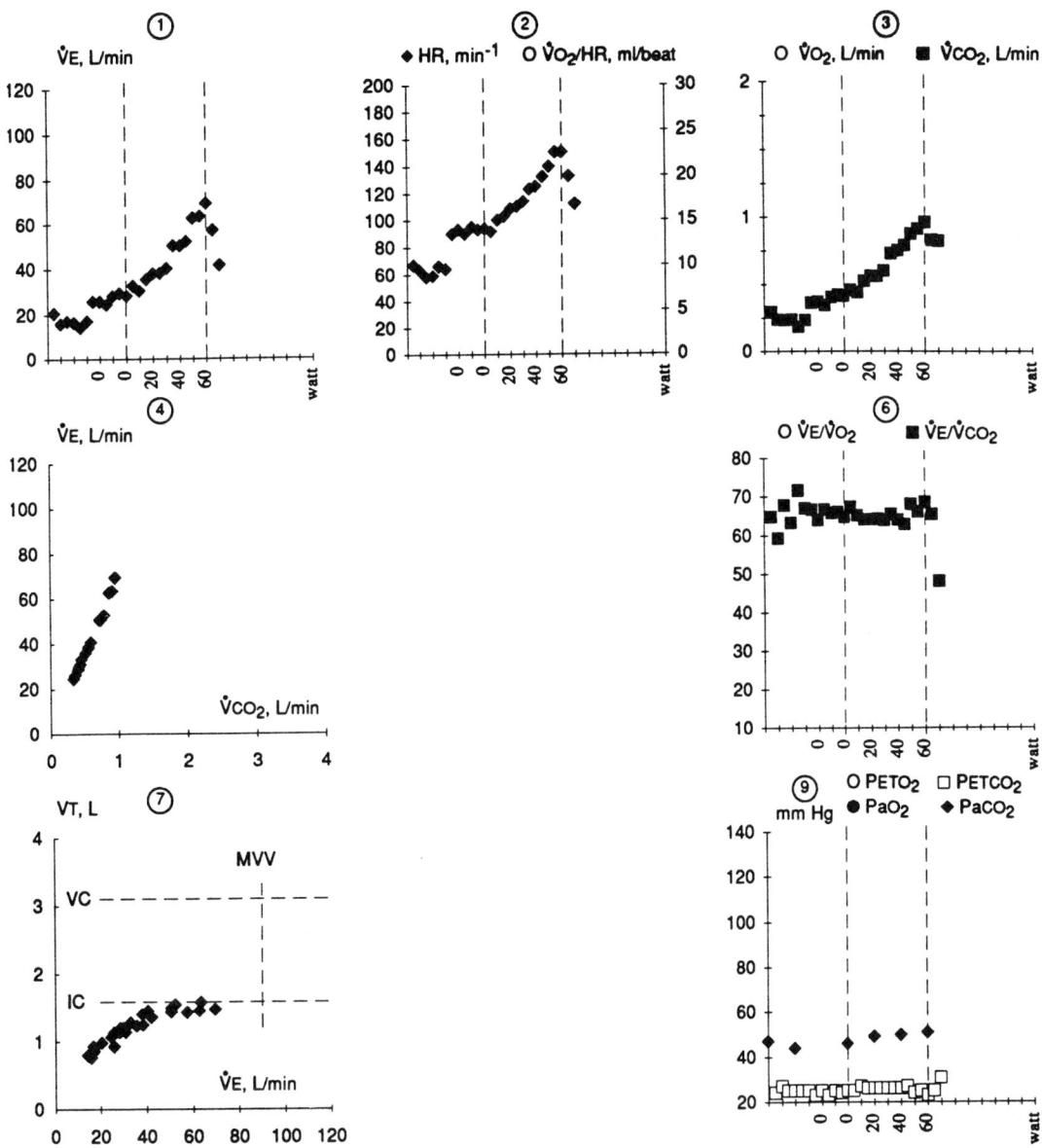

1. Vertical dashed lines in panels 1 to 3 and 6 and 9 indicate the beginning and the end of increasing work period.
2. Unloaded cycling is performed for 3 minutes before the left vertical dashed line.

TABLE 53-3. *Air breathing.*

Time min	Work rate watts	BP mm Hg	HR min⁻¹	f min⁻¹	$\dot{V}_E$ L/min BTPS	$\dot{V}_{CO_2}$ L/min STPD	$\dot{V}_{O_2}$ L/min STPD	$\dfrac{\dot{V}_{O_2}}{HR}$ ml/beat	R	pH	HCO₃ meq/L	PO₂ ET	PO₂ a	PO₂ (A-a)	PCO₂ ET	PCO₂ a	PCO₂ (a-ET)	$\dfrac{\dot{V}_E}{\dot{V}_{CO_2}}$	$\dfrac{\dot{V}_E}{\dot{V}_{O_2}}$	$\dfrac{V_D}{V_T}$
	Rest	111/66								7.39	27		41			45				
	Rest		96	18	15.6	0.27	0.34	3.5	0.79			113			30			52	41	
	Rest		93	19	15.8	0.26	0.32	3.4	0.81			114			29			55	44	
	Rest		95	19	16.1	0.26	0.31	3.3	0.84			116			28			56	47	
	Rest		92	18	14.3	0.25	0.30	3.3	0.83			114			29			51	43	
	Rest	114/72	93	20	16.3	0.28	0.36	3.9	0.78	7.38	27	111	42	52	30	46	16	52	41	0.57
	Rest		94	23	20.6	0.41	0.54	5.7	0.76			112			30			45	35	
	Unloaded		108	29	19.2	0.31	0.34	3.1	0.91			116			29			54	49	
	Unloaded		114	31	31.0	0.50	0.57	5.0	0.88			119			26			57	50	
	Unloaded		120	30	33.0	0.52	0.55	4.6	0.95			120			26			59	55	
	Unloaded		122	32	36.5	0.56	0.60	4.9	0.93			119			28			60	56	
	Unloaded		123	32	39.1	0.60	0.61	5.0	0.98			122			26			61	60	
	Unloaded	116/72	123	35	42.5	0.65	0.66	5.4	0.98	7.38	26	122	37	67	26	45	19	61	60	0.64
0.5	10		125	36	45.1	0.68	0.69	5.5	0.99			123			25			62	61	
1.0	10		129	38	45.8	0.69	0.69	5.3	1.00			122			27			62	62	
1.5	20		130	39	54.4	0.81	0.78	6.0	1.04			125			24			63	65	
2.0	20	129/78	131	37	51.7	0.77	0.73	5.6	1.05	7.37	26	126	35	72	23	45	22	63	67	0.65
2.5	30		140	41	57.4	0.82	0.77	5.5	1.06			126			24			66	70	
3.0	30		140	44	63.3	0.88	0.80	5.7	1.10			127			24			68	74	
3.5	40	135/78	145	43	63.6	0.89	0.79	5.4	1.13	7.35	24	127	35	74	23	45	22	67	76	0.67
	Recovery		149	48	63.0	0.89	0.80	5.4	1.11			129			22			66	74	
	Recovery		140	39	56.3	0.81	0.72	5.1	1.13			126			25			65	74	
	Recovery		140	36	50.5	0.80	0.79	5.6	1.01			122			26			59	60	
	Recovery		138	34	50.1	0.75	0.70	5.1	1.07			123			25			63	67	
	Recovery	114/69	133	39	52.5	0.77	0.74	5.6	1.04	7.33	24	122	35	70	28	46	18	64	66	0.66

TABLE 53-4. *Oxygen breathing.*

Time min	Work rate watts	BP mm Hg	HR min⁻¹	f min⁻¹	$\dot{V}_E$ L/min BTPS	$\dot{V}_{CO_2}$ L/min STPD	$\dot{V}_{O_2}$ L/min STPD	$\dfrac{\dot{V}_{O_2}}{HR}$ ml/beat	R	pH	HCO₃ meq/L	PO₂ ET	PO₂ a	PO₂ (A-a)	PCO₂ ET	PCO₂ a	PCO₂ (a-ET)	$\dfrac{\dot{V}_E}{\dot{V}_{CO_2}}$	$\dfrac{\dot{V}_E}{\dot{V}_{O_2}}$	$\dfrac{V_D}{V_T}$
	Rest									7.34	25	519				47				
	Rest		67	21	20.6	0.29									24			65		
	Rest		63	21	16.0	0.24									27			59		
	Rest		58	19	17.2	0.23									25			68		
	Rest	111/69	59	18	16.7	0.24				7.36	24	585	84		25	44	19	63		0.63
	Rest		66	18	14.4	0.18									25			72		
	Rest		64	20	17.1	0.23									25			67		
	Unloaded		90	23	25.9	0.36									23			67		
	Unloaded		93	28	26.0	0.37									25			64		
	Unloaded		90	23	24.6	0.34									23			67		
	Unloaded		95	25	28.4	0.40									25			66		
	Unloaded		93	25	29.8	0.42									24			66		
	Unloaded	116/75	94	24	28.6	0.41				7.35	25	615	52		25	46	21	65		0.66
0.5	10		92	26	33.1	0.46									25			67		
1.0	10		100	27	30.9	0.44									27			65		
1.5	20		103	29	35.8	0.52									26			64		
2.0	20	120/78	108	27	38.1	0.56				7.33	25	620	44		26	49	23	64		0.68
2.5	30		110	31	38.6	0.56									26			64		
3.0	30		114	28	40.6	0.60									26			64		
3.5	40		123	35	50.6	0.73									26			65		
4.0	40	132/81	125	34	50.8	0.75				7.31	25	612	51		26	50	24	64		0.69
4.5	50		132	34	52.5	0.79									27			63		
5.0	50		140	43	62.8	0.87									24			68		
5.5	60		150	40	63.5	0.91									25			66		
6.0	60	141/87	150	47	69.6	0.96				7.28	24	605	57		23	51	28	68		0.71
	Recovery		133	40	57.6	0.83									25			65		
	Recovery		112	31	42.1	0.82									31			48		

Interpretation

COMMENTS

Resting respiratory function studies showed mild to moderate restrictive and obstructive components in ventilatory mechanics, an extremely low $D_{L_{CO}}$, and severe arterial hypoxemia.

ANALYSIS

In flow chart 1, both the maximum $\dot{V}_{O_2}$ and anaerobic threshold are severely reduced. Proceeding to flow chart 4 through branchpoint 4.1, the breathing reserve is normal, but the high $\dot{V}_E/\dot{V}_{CO_2}$ (branchpoint 4.3) and high V_D/V_T (branchpoint 4.2) direct us to the boxes with lung disease with impaired oxygenation and abnormal pulmonary circulation. The findings support these diagnoses with high dead space ventilation increasing the ventilatory requirements at rest and all work levels. With O_2 breathing, there is no evidence of a right to left shunt, but ventilatory drive is reduced and the patient is able to tolerate a considerably higher work rate.

CONCLUSION

This patient with sarcoidosis with some disturbance in ventilatory mechanics has severe gas exchange abnormality due to the accompanying marked pulmonary vascular destruction. He has severe hypoxemia at rest and during exercise without supplemental oxygen; his ability to perform work is increased with oxygen. From sequential exercise testing it became evident that his pulmonary microcirculation was disappearing (increasing V_D/V_T and $\dot{V}_E/\dot{V}_{O_2}$ and worsening hypoxemia) despite stable ventilatory mechanics. The patient was treated with unilateral lung transplantation.

CASE 54 *Interstitial pneumonitis: Pre- and post-corticosteroid therapy*

CLINICAL FINDINGS

This 37-year-old housewife developed progressive shortness of breath. She was found to have the pattern of interstitial lung disease on chest x-ray studies and was referred for exercise testing.

EXERCISE FINDINGS

The patient performed exercise on a cycle ergometer. She pedalled at 60 rpm without added load for 3 minutes. The work rate was then increased 15 W per minute to her symptom-limited maximum. Arterial blood was sampled every second minute, and intra-arterial blood pressure was recorded from a percutaneously placed brachial artery catheter. Her resting and exercise ECGs were normal. In the initial study she stopped exercise because

of shortness of breath. After the first exercise test she was treated with prednisone. Her exercise test was repeated 6 months later, at which time she was taking 30 mg prednisone daily. She was asymptomatic at the time of the second test.

TABLE 54-1. *Selected Respiratory Function Data*

MEASUREMENT	PREDICTED	BEFORE TREATMENT	AFTER TREATMENT
Age, yr		37	
Sex		Female	
Height, cm		168	
Weight, kg	66	57	
Hematocrit, %		42	
VC, L	3.76	1.71	3.85
IC, L	2.50	1.31	2.25
FEV_1, L	3.08	1.52	3.10
FEV_1/VC, %	82	89	81
MVV, L/min	120	66	130
D_{LCO}, ml/mm Hg/min	28.5	16.2	

TABLE 54-2. *Selected Exercise Data*

MEASUREMENT	PREDICTED	BEFORE TREATMENT	AFTER TREATMENT
Maximum $\dot{V}_{O_2}$, L/min	1.72	1.35	2.01
Maximum HR, beats/min	183	149	174
Maximum O_2 pulse, ml/beat	9.4	9.1	11.6
$\Delta\dot{V}_{O_2}/\Delta WR$, ml/min/W	10.3	9.5	9.8
AT, L/min	> 0.79	0.80	1.0
Blood pressure, mm Hg (rest, max)		119/68,190/81	125/75,181/88
Maximum $\dot{V}_E$, L/min		58	86
Exercise breathing reserve, L/min	> 15	8	44
Pa_{O_2}, mm Hg (rest, max ex)		65,51	117,98
$P(A-a)_{O_2}$, mm Hg (rest, max ex)		43,65	−1,26
$P(a-ET)_{CO_2}$, mm Hg (rest, max ex)		3,3	−3,−2
V_D/V_T (rest, heavy ex)		0.40,0.32	0.22,0.15
HCO_3^-, mEq/L (rest, 2-min recov)		25,21	24,15

FIG. 54-A. *Before treatment.*

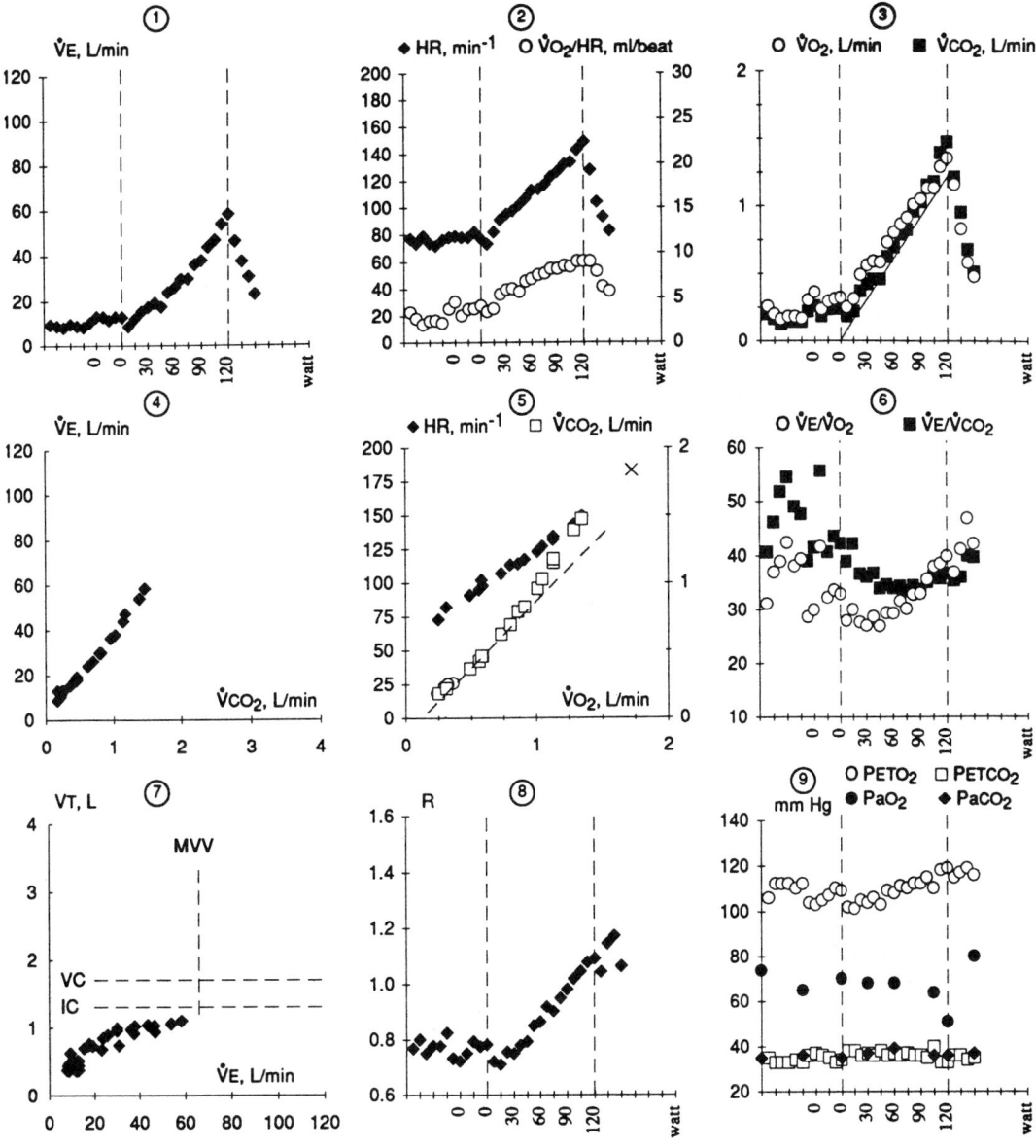

1. Vertical dashed lines in panels 1 to 3 and 6, 8, and 9 indicate the beginning and the end of increasing work period.

2. Unloaded cycling is performed for 3 minutes before the left vertical dashed line.

3. In panel 3, the diagonal line shows the increase of $\dot{V}O_2$ at a slope of 10 ml/min/W.

4. In panel 5, the diagonal dashed line has a slope of 1; the "x" in the upper right is the predicted maximum heart rate and $\dot{V}O_2$ for the subject.

Fig. 54-B. *After treatment.*

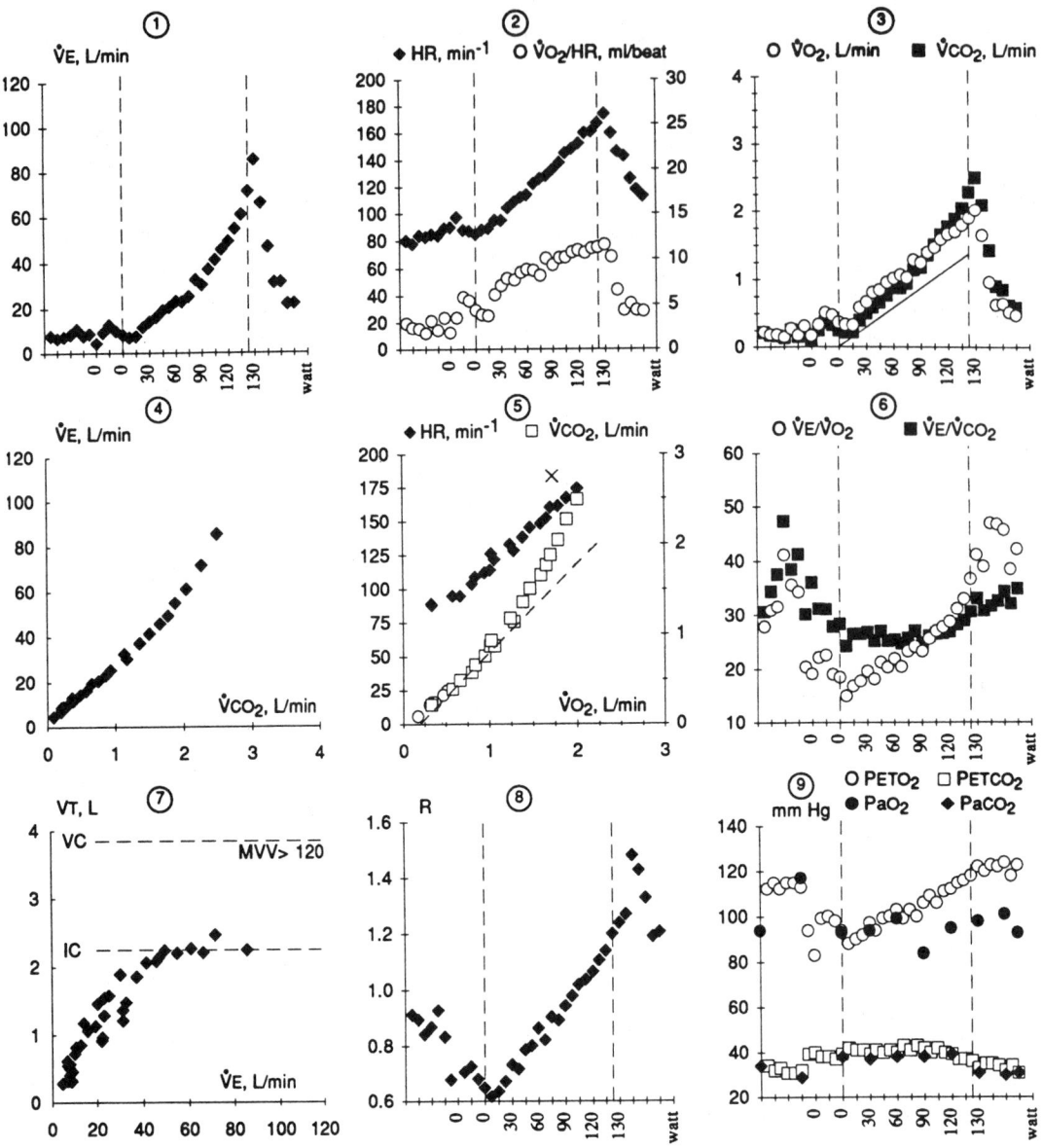

1. Vertical dashed lines in panels 1 to 3 and 6, 8, and 9 indicate the beginning and the end of increasing work period.

2. Unloaded cycling is performed for 3 minutes before the left vertical dashed line.

3. In panel 3, the diagonal line shows the increase of $\dot{V}O_2$ at a slope of 10 ml/min/W.

4. In panel 5, the diagonal dashed line has a slope of 1; the "x" in the upper right is the predicted maximum heart rate and $\dot{V}O_2$ for the subject.

TABLE 54-3. *Before treatment.*

Time min	Work rate watts	BP mm Hg	HR min⁻¹	f min⁻¹	$\dot{V}_E$ L/min BTPS	$\dot{V}_{CO_2}$ L/min STPD	$\dot{V}_{O_2}$ L/min STPD	$\frac{\dot{V}_{O_2}}{HR}$ ml/beat	R	pH	HCO₃ meq/L	PO2, mm Hg ET	a	(A-a)	PCO2, mm Hg ET	a	(a-ET)	$\frac{\dot{V}_E}{\dot{V}_{CO_2}}$	$\frac{\dot{V}_E}{\dot{V}_{O_2}}$	$\frac{V_D}{V_T}$
	Rest									7.47	25	74			35					
	Rest		77	15	9.4	0.20	0.26	3.4	0.77			106			35			41	31	
	Rest		74	19	9.0	0.16	0.20	2.7	0.80			112			33			46	37	
	Rest		79	21	8.0	0.12	0.16	2.0	0.75			112			33			52	39	
	Rest		74	22	9.5	0.14	0.18	2.4	0.78			112			33			55	42	
	Rest		72	24	8.9	0.14	0.18	2.5	0.78			110			34			49	38	
	Rest	119/68	76	19	8.3	0.14	0.17	2.2	0.82	7.45	25	112	65	43	33	36	3	48	39	0.40
	Unloaded		78	20	10.3	0.22	0.30	3.8	0.73			104			36			39	29	
	Unloaded		79	25	12.9	0.26	0.36	4.6	0.72			103			37			41	30	
	Unloaded		78	34	12.9	0.18	0.24	3.1	0.75			105			36			56	42	
	Unloaded		78	23	11.3	0.23	0.29	3.7	0.79			107			35			41	32	
	Unloaded		82	29	12.9	0.24	0.31	3.8	0.77			110			33			43	34	
	Unloaded	125/68	77	24	12.6	0.25	0.32	4.2	0.78	7.44	23	109	70	37	34	35	1	42	33	0.35
0.5	15		73	20	8.7	0.18	0.25	3.4	0.72			102			38			39	28	
1.0	15		82	32	12.0	0.22	0.31	3.8	0.71			101			38			42	30	
1.5	30		91	22	15.4	0.37	0.49	5.4	0.76			105			36			37	28	
2.0	30	131/68	95	23	17.1	0.42	0.56	5.9	0.75	7.44	25	104	68	35	37	37	0	36	27	0.31
2.5	45		98	26	19.1	0.46	0.59	6.0	0.78			106			36			37	29	
3.0	45		102	23	17.6	0.46	0.58	5.7	0.79			103			38			34	27	
3.5	60		107	28	23.8	0.62	0.73	6.8	0.85			109			36			35	29	
4.0	60	146/75	113	29	25.9	0.69	0.80	7.1	0.86	7.43	25	108	68	38	37	39	2	34	29	0.32
4.5	75		114	31	29.8	0.79	0.86	7.5	0.92			111			36			34	32	
5.0	75		117	30	29.9	0.82	0.91	7.8	0.90			110			37			33	30	
5.5	90		123	37	36.2	0.96	1.01	8.2	0.95			112			36			34	33	
6.0	90		127	37	37.8	1.03	1.05	8.3	0.98			112			36			34	33	
6.5	105		132	42	43.8	1.15	1.13	8.6	1.02			115			35			35	36	
7.0	105	190/78	134	50	47.0	1.18	1.13	8.4	1.04	7.42	23	110	64	51	40	36	-4	36	38	0.31
7.5	120		143	51	54.0	1.39	1.29	9.0	1.08			118			33			36	39	
8.0	120	190/81	149	53	58.4	1.47	1.35	9.1	1.09	7.41	22	119	51	65	33	36	3	37	40	0.32
	Recovery		128	45	46.6	1.21	1.16	9.1	1.04			115			36			35	37	
	Recovery		104	41	37.6	0.95	0.83	8.0	1.14			117			36			36	41	
	Recovery		93	41	30.7	0.68	0.58	6.2	1.17			119			34			40	47	
	Recovery	190/81	83	34	23.1	0.51	0.48	5.8	1.06	7.36	21	116	80	35	35	37	2	40	42	0.36

Interpretation

COMMENTS

The resting respiratory function studies indicate that this patient had severe restrictive lung disease before therapy, which improved markedly after therapy (Table 54-1). The resting ECG is normal. The "after-treatment" exercise test was performed 6 months after the first test.

ANALYSIS

In flowchart 1, the maximum $\dot{V}_{O_2}$ and the anaerobic threshold are abnormal (Table 54-2). See flow chart 4: The patient's breathing reserve is low (branchpoint 4.1). V_D/V_T is high (branchpoint 4.2). This leads to the diagnosis of lung disease with an O_2 flow problem. Characteristically, this is a restrictive lung disease. Confirming restrictive lung disease as the major pathophysiologic disorder are a high V_T/IC ratio (panel 7, Figure 54-A), breathing frequency exceeding 50 breaths per minute at the patient's maximum work rate (Table 54-3), $P(A-a)_{O_2}$ increasing and Pa_{O_2} decreasing systematically with work rate, and increased values of $P(a-ET)_{CO_2}$ and V_D/V_T (Table 54-3).

After treatment, the maximum $\dot{V}_{O_2}$ improved significantly and exceeded the predicted value. Arterial hypoxemia with exercise is no longer present and $P(a-ET)_{CO_2}$ and V_D/V_T are normal, suggesting that the ventilation-perfusion abnormality observed before treatment was corrected. Moreover, the strikingly abnormal breathing pattern observed during pre-treatment exercise resolves after treatment (compare panels 7 of Figs. 54-A and 54-B).

CONCLUSION

Restrictive lung disease has limited exercise performance. Therapy reverses these abnormalities.

TABLE 54-4. *After treatment.*

Time min	Work rate watts	BP mm Hg	HR min^{-1}	f min^{-1}	$\dot{V}E$ L/min BTPS	$\dot{V}CO_2$ L/min STPD	$\dot{V}O_2$ L/min STPD	$\frac{\dot{V}O_2}{HR}$ ml/beat	R	pH	HCO$_3$ meq/L	PO2, mm Hg ET	a	(A-a)	PCO2, mm Hg ET	a	(a-ET)	$\frac{\dot{V}E}{\dot{V}CO_2}$	$\frac{\dot{V}E}{\dot{V}O_2}$	VD/VT
	Rest	125/75								7.45	23		94			34				
	Rest		80	15	7.7	0.21	0.23	2.9	0.91			112			34			31	28	
	Rest		78	11	6.8	0.17	0.19	2.4	0.89			115			32			35	31	
	Rest		84	13	7.1	0.16	0.19	2.3	0.84			112			33			37	32	
	Rest		83	24	8.2	0.13	0.15	1.8	0.87			115			31			47	41	
	Rest		85	13	10.7	0.25	0.27	3.2	0.93			115			31			38	36	
	Rest	119/75	84	19	7.8	0.15	0.18	2.1	0.83	7.50	22	113	117	-1	32	29	-3	41	34	0.22
	Unloaded		89	28	8.7	0.21	0.31	3.5	0.68			94			39			30	20	
	Unloaded		90	16	4.6	0.09	0.17	1.9	0.53			83			40			36	19	
	Unloaded		97	20	9.2	0.24	0.34	3.5	0.71			99			38			31	22	
	Unloaded		88	15	12.8	0.37	0.51	5.8	0.73			100			38			31	23	
	Unloaded		87	14	10.1	0.32	0.47	5.4	0.68			98			37			28	19	
	Unloaded	125/75	85	14	8.0	0.24	0.37	4.4	0.65	7.43	25	94	93	3	39	38	-1	28	18	0.17
0.5	15		88	21	6.9	0.21	0.34	3.9	0.62			88			42			24	15	
1.0	15		89	23	7.5	0.21	0.33	3.7	0.64			90			41			26	17	
1.5	30		95	14	11.5	0.39	0.58	6.1	0.67			92			41			26	18	
2.0	30	125/69	95	12	14.1	0.49	0.67	7.1	0.73	7.44	25	97	94	8	39	37	-2	27	20	0.12
2.5	45		104	15	15.9	0.58	0.81	7.8	0.72			94			41			25	18	
3.0	45		109	17	19.2	0.66	0.84	7.7	0.79			99			40			27	21	
3.5	60		112	14	20.4	0.76	0.95	8.5	0.80			100			41			25	20	
4.0	60	144/75	114	15	23.3	0.87	1.01	8.9	0.86	7.43	25	103	99	8	40	38	-2	25	22	0.10
4.5	75		122	18	23.1	0.87	1.06	8.7	0.82			99			43			25	20	
5.0	75		126	16	25.3	0.93	1.03	8.2	0.90			103			41			26	23	
5.5	90		128	22	32.6	1.14	1.28	10.0	0.89			100			43			27	24	
6.0	90	156/75	133	16	30.3	1.17	1.24	9.3	0.94	7.42	24	106	84	26	42	38	-4	25	23	0.08
6.5	105		138	20	37.2	1.36	1.39	10.1	0.98			109			40			26	26	
7.0	105		145	20	41.4	1.50	1.47	10.1	1.02			106			42			26	27	
7.5	120		148	22	45.8	1.65	1.59	10.7	1.04			111			40			27	28	
8.0	120	181/81	152	22	49.4	1.77	1.66	10.9	1.07	7.40	24	112	95	18	39	39	0	27	29	0.17
8.5	135		160	25	55.0	1.88	1.70	10.6	1.11			115			37			28	31	
9.0	135		161	27	61.2	2.04	1.79	11.1	1.14			116			37			29	33	
9.5	130		167	29	71.7	2.27	1.89	11.3	1.20			118			36			31	37	
10.0	130	181/88	174	38	85.6	2.49	2.01	11.6	1.24	7.40	19	122	98	26	33	31	-2	33	41	0.15
	Recovery		160	30	66.5	2.08	1.64	10.3	1.27			120			35			31	39	
	Recovery		146	22	46.9	1.42	0.96	6.6	1.48			123			35			32	47	
	Recovery		143	23	31.3	0.90	0.63	4.4	1.43			122			34			33	47	
	Recovery	181/81	126	26	31.4	0.85	0.64	5.1	1.33	7.36	17	124	101	25	32	30	-2	34	46	0.15
	Recovery		118	24	22.0	0.62	0.52	4.4	1.19			118			34			32	38	
	Recovery	175/75	113	23	22.2	0.58	0.48	4.2	1.21	7.36	17	123	93	30	31	31	0	35	42	0.18

CASE 55 *Interstitial pulmonary fibrosis: Air and oxygen breathing*

CLINICAL FINDINGS

This 47-year-old man had developed dyspnea 12 years previously. A histologic diagnosis of pulmonary alveolar proteinosis was then made by open lung biopsy. Following lung lavage he became asymptomatic until 10 months prior to evaluation when progressive dyspnea first became evident when he was skiing at high altitudes. Although previously active in sports, he was unable to walk more than 30 yards on flat ground at a normal pace. He coughed with exercise and sometimes produced clear sputum. He denied smoking, wheezing, or edema. The results of his examination were normal except for digital clubbing and infrequent fine inspiratory rales at the lung bases. Chest roentgenogram showed increased interstitial markings with honeycombing.

EXERCISE FINDINGS

The patient performed exercise on a cycle ergometer breathing room air, and, after a 30 minute rest, breathing 100% oxygen. He pedalled at 60 rpm without added load for 3 minutes. The work rate was increased 15 W every minute to his symptom-limited maximum. Arterial blood was sampled every second minute, and intra-arterial blood pressure was recorded from a percutaneously placed brachial artery catheter. When breathing room air, he stopped exercise because of fatigue and lightheadedness. When breathing oxygen he stopped because of leg pain and general fatigue. Resting and exercise ECGs were normal.

TABLE 55-1. *Selected Respiratory Function Data*

MEASUREMENT	PREDICTED	MEASURED
Age, yr		47
Sex		Male
Height, cm		174
Weight, kg	77	85
Hematocrit, %		41
VC, L	4.49	2.20
IC, L	2.99	1.14
TLC, L	6.48	3.17
FEV$_1$, L	3.58	2.01
FEV$_1$/VC, %	80	91
MVV, L/min, direct	151	112
MVV, L/min, indirect	143	80
D$_{LCO}$, ml/mm Hg/min	30.7	13.9

TABLE 55-2. *Selected Exercise Data*

MEASUREMENT	PREDICTED	ROOM AIR	OXYGEN
Maximum V̇$_{O_2}$, L/min	2.60	1.23	
Maximum HR, beats/min	173	150	154
Maximum O$_2$ pulse, ml/beat	15.0	8.2	
ΔV̇$_{O_2}$/ΔWR, ml/min/W	10.3	8.6	
AT, L/min	> 1.12	0.85	
Blood pressure, mm Hg (rest, max)		120/75,175/84*	138/87,195/90*
Maximum V̇$_E$, L/min		72	56
Exercise breathing reserve, L/min	> 15	8	32
Pa$_{O_2}$, mm Hg (rest, max ex)		62,37	568,284
P(A−a)$_{O_2}$, mm Hg (rest, max ex)		30,73	102,365
P(a−ET)$_{CO_2}$, mm Hg (rest, max ex)		6,10	4,12
V$_D$/V$_T$ (rest, heavy ex)		0.54,0.54	0.51,0.56
HCO$_3^-$, mEq/L (rest, 2-min recov)		23,20	26,22

* Systolic pulsus paradoxus of 70 mm Hg.

FIG. 55-A. *Air breathing.*

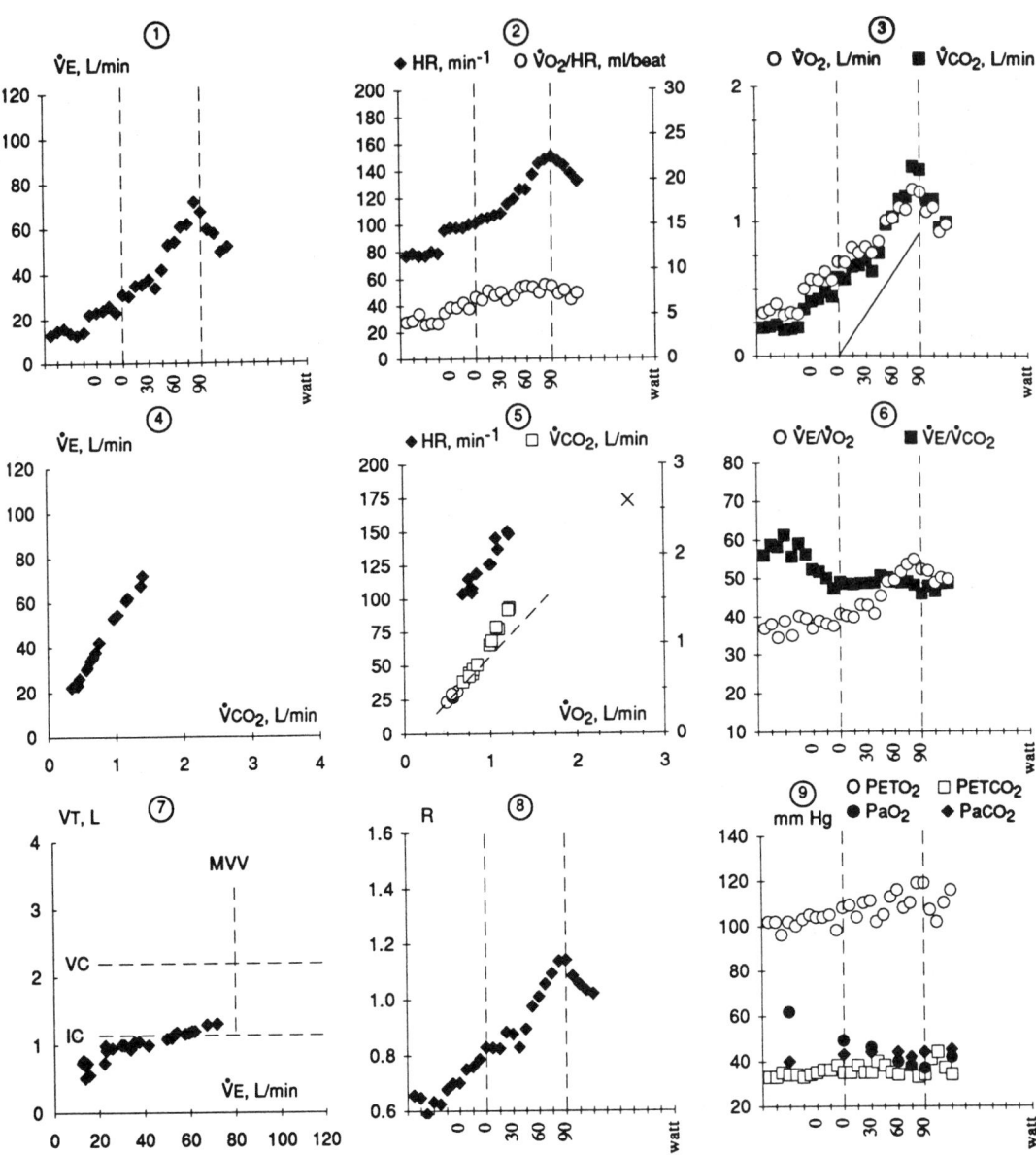

1. Vertical dashed lines in panels 1 to 3 and 6, 8, and 9 indicate the beginning and the end of increasing work period.

2. Unloaded cycling is performed for 3 minutes before the left vertical dashed line.

3. In panel 3, the diagonal line shows the increase of $\dot{V}O_2$ at a slope of 10 ml/min/W.

4. In panel 5, the diagonal dashed line has a slope of 1; the "x" in the upper right is the predicted maximum heart rate and $\dot{V}O_2$ for the subject.

FIG. 55-B. *Oxygen breathing.*

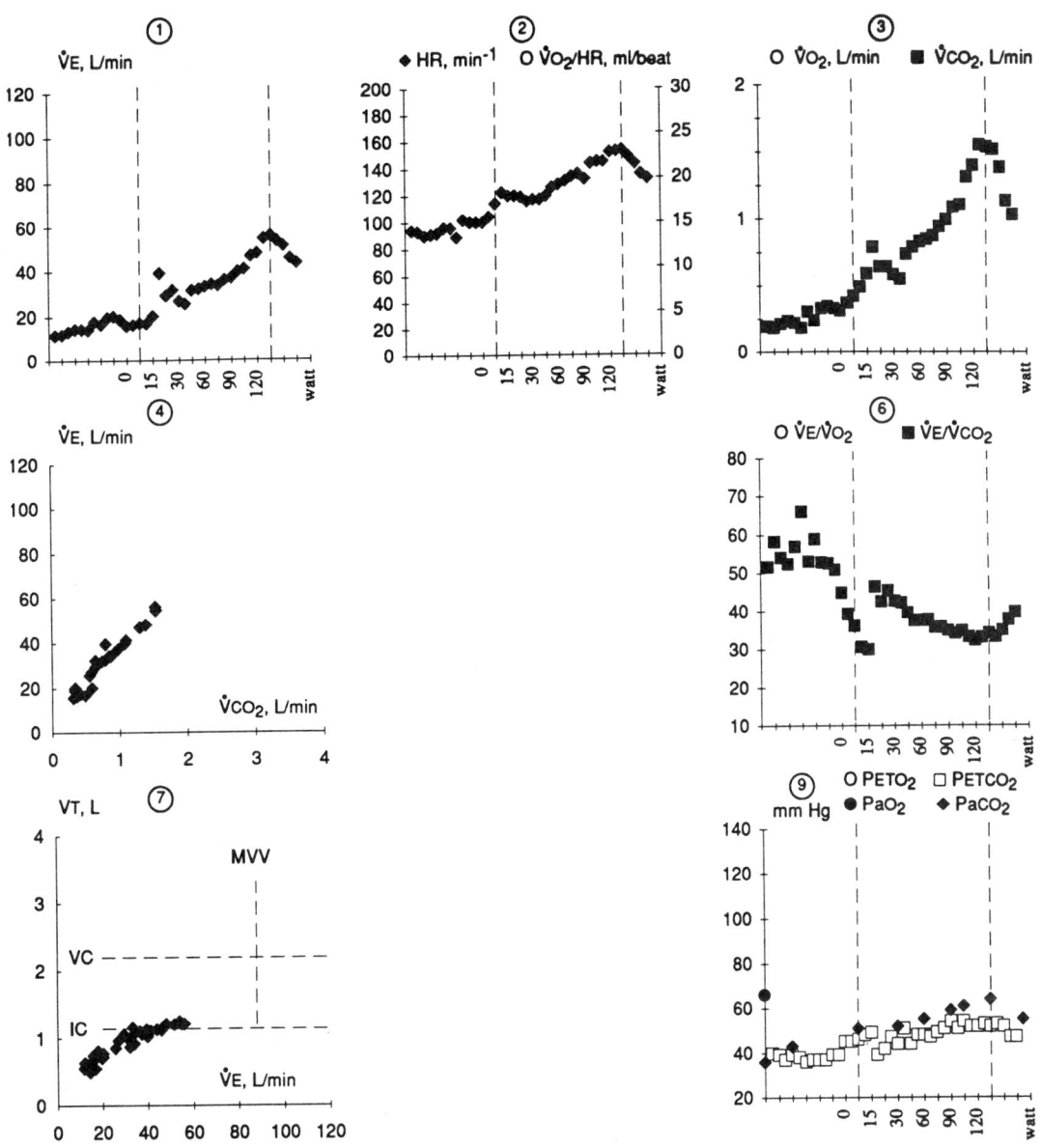

1. Vertical dashed lines in panels 1 to 3 and 6 and 9 indicate the beginning and the end of increasing work period.
2. Unloaded cycling is performed for 3 minutes before the left vertical dashed line.

Interpretation

COMMENTS

This case of severe interstitial lung disease is presented to illustrate two major points: (1) The impaired peripheral oxygenation that may be caused by pulmonary fibrosis; and (2) the presence of a major increasing contribution of the carotid bodies to breathing, in association with arterial hypoxemia.

The results of the resting respiratory function studies indicate that this patient has a severe restrictive disorder, with no evidence of airflow obstruction (Table 55-1). The resting ECG is normal.

ANALYSIS

In flow chart 1, the maximum $\dot{V}O_2$ and anaerobic threshold are reduced (Table 55-2). See flow chart 4: The breathing reserve is borderline normal

TABLE 55-3. *Air breathing.*

Time min	Work rate watts	BP mm Hg	HR min⁻¹	f min⁻¹	V̇E L/min BTPS	V̇CO2 L/min STPD	V̇O2 L/min STPD	V̇O2/HR ml/beat	R	pH	HCO3 meq/L	PO2 ET	PO2 a	PO2 (A-a)	PCO2 ET	PCO2 a	PCO2 (a-ET)	V̇E/V̇CO2	V̇E/V̇O2	VD/VT
	Rest		77	17	13.2	0.21	0.32	4.2	0.66			102			33			56	37	
	Rest		79	20	14.6	0.22	0.34	4.3	0.65			102			33			59	38	
	Rest		77	28	15.8	0.23	0.39	5.1	0.59			96			35			58	34	
	Rest	120/75	77	27	13.9	0.19	0.30	3.9	0.63	7.37	23	102	62	30	34	40	6	61	39	0.54
	Rest		80	17	12.6	0.20	0.32	4.0	0.63			100			34			56	35	
	Rest		79	20	14.1	0.21	0.31	3.9	0.68			103			33			59	40	
	Unloaded		96	30	22.2	0.35	0.50	5.2	0.70			105			34			56	39	
	Unloaded		98	25	23.0	0.40	0.57	5.8	0.70			104			35			52	37	
	Unloaded		98	25	23.8	0.42	0.56	5.7	0.75			104			36			52	39	
	Unloaded		98	27	25.8	0.47	0.62	6.3	0.76			105			36			50	38	
	Unloaded		100	23	22.8	0.44	0.56	5.6	0.79			98			38			47	37	
	Unloaded	153/81	101	31	31.0	0.58	0.70	6.9	0.83	7.35	23	108	49	51	35	43	8	49	41	0.54
0.5	15		104	30	30.1	0.57	0.69	6.6	0.83			109			35			48	40	
1.0	15		105	35	34.8	0.66	0.80	7.6	0.83			104			38			48	40	
1.5	30		107	34	35.5	0.67	0.76	7.1	0.88			110			35			49	43	
2.0	30	159/75	108	36	37.6	0.71	0.81	7.5	0.88	7.34	23	111	46	55	35	44	9	49	43	0.55
2.5	45		115	36	33.8	0.63	0.76	6.6	0.83			102			40			49	40	
3.0	45		119	42	41.9	0.76	0.85	7.1	0.89			105			38			50	45	
3.5	60		126	46	52.8	0.98	1.00	7.9	0.98			113			35			50	49	
4.0	60	177/90	126	46	54.3	1.03	1.02	8.1	1.01	7.33	23	116	40	66	34	44	10	49	49	0.56
4.5	75		137	51	60.9	1.16	1.10	8.0	1.05			108			39			49	51	
5.0	75	186/90	145	52	62.1	1.18	1.08	7.4	1.09	7.33	22	110	38	73	38	42	4	49	53	0.54
5.5	90		148	55	72.0	1.40	1.23	8.3	1.14			119			33			48	55	
6.0	90	186/93	150	52	67.5	1.38	1.21	8.1	1.14	7.31	22	119	37	73	34	44	10	46	52	0.53
	Recovery		147	51	59.7	1.16	1.07	7.3	1.08			107			41			48	52	
	Recovery		144	50	57.9	1.16	1.10	7.6	1.05			102			44			46	49	
	Recovery		138	46	49.9	0.95	0.92	6.7	1.03			110			37			48	50	
	Recovery	174/90	132	47	52.1	0.99	0.97	7.3	1.02	7.27	20	116	42	64	34	45	11	49	50	0.56

(branchpoint 4.1). Taking the right branchpoint, the V̇E/V̇CO2 at the anaerobic threshold is markedly elevated (branchpoint 4.3). This leads the interpreter to the diagnosis of "abnormal pulmonary circulation." However, branchpoint 4.3 states that if the vital capacity is low, as it is in this patient, one should go to the low breathing reserve branch of branchpoint 4.1. The reason for this is that patients with restrictive lung disease can have an unusually high MVV when measured directly. One can conclude, therefore, that the breathing reserve for the patient is high. If the MVV were calculated from the FEV₁ (2.01 × 40), the MVV would be 80.4 L/min in this patient, and the breathing reserve would then, in fact, be low. Thus, this branchpoint 4.3 instruction is designed to detect patients who have abnormal pulmonary circulation secondary to restrictive lung disease.

Following the low breathing reserve branch of branchpoint 4.1, we consider branchpoint 4.2 and the high VD/VT. From this, we conclude that this patient has restrictive lung disease with an O_2 flow problem. Findings confirming this diagnosis are: (1) the high VT/IC ratio (panel 7, Fig. 55-A), (2) the low and progressively decreasing Pa_{O_2} as work rate is increased (panel 9, Fig. 55-A), (3) a breathing frequency greater than 50 at the maximum V̇O2 (Table 55-3), (4) an increased $P(a - ET)_{CO_2}$ (panel 9, Fig. 55-A), (5) a steep heart rate response to the increasing oxygen uptake (panel 5, Fig. 55-A), (6) a low O_2 pulse with a flat contour as the work rate is increased (panel 2, Fig. 55-A), (7) a reduced $\Delta\dot{V}_{O_2}/\Delta WR$ (Table 55-2 and panel 3, Fig. 55-A), and (8) $P(A - a)_{O_2}$ increasing with increasing work rate (Table 55-3). Note that all these confirmatory findings are characteristic of restrictive lung disease.

O_2 breathing allows the patient to increase his maximum work rate from 90 to 135 W (Table 55-4 and Fig. 55-B). This was accomplished primarily by decreasing ventilatory drive. In contrast to regulating arterial P_{CO_2} around 40 as the patient did

TABLE 55-4. *Oxygen breathing.*

Time min	Work rate watts	BP mm Hg	HR min⁻¹	f min⁻¹	V̇E L/min BTPS	V̇CO2 L/min STPD	V̇O2 L/min STPD	V̇O2/HR ml/beat	R	pH	HCO3 meq/L	PO2 ET	PO2 a	PO2 (A-a)	PCO2 ET	PCO2 a	PCO2 (a-ET)	V̇E/V̇CO2	V̇E/V̇O2	VD/VT
	Rest	132/84								7.44	24	66				36				
	Rest		94	21	11.6		0.19								40			52		
	Rest		93	19	12.1		0.18								39			58		
	Rest		90	23	13.3		0.21								37			54		
	Rest	138/87	91	29	14.5		0.23			7.39	26	568	102		39	43	4	52		0.51
	Rest		92	23	14.5		0.22								38			57		
	Rest		96	25	14.0		0.18								36			66		
	Rest		96	22	17.8		0.30								37			53		
	Rest		89	30	16.7		0.24								37			59		
	Unloaded		102	28	19.8		0.33								37			53		
	Unloaded		100	26	20.1		0.34								39			53		
	Unloaded		100	25	18.9		0.33								39			51		
	Unloaded		100	21	15.7		0.31								45			45		
	Unloaded		104	22	16.4		0.37								45			39		
	Unloaded	192/108	114	24	17.2		0.42			7.33	26	540	122		46	51	5	36		0.47
0.5	15		122	22	16.9		0.49								48			31		
1.0	15		120	28	20.1		0.59								49			30		
1.5	15		120	35	39.6		0.79								39			46		
2.0	15		119	28	29.5		0.64								42			42		
2.5	30		116	37	32.2		0.64								47			45		
3.0	30	186/96	117	28	27.1		0.58			7.31	26	505	156		44	52	8	43		0.56
3.5	45		117	30	25.7		0.55								51			42		
4.0	45		120	32	32.0		0.74								44			40		
4.5	60		126	34	32.4		0.79								48			37		
5.0	60	192/99	128	29	33.5		0.83			7.28	25	467	191		48	55	7	37		0.54
5.5	75		131	32	34.6		0.85								47			38		
6.0	75		134	37	34.2		0.87								49			36		
6.5	90		136	33	36.5		0.94								51			36		
7.0	90	196/102	132	35	37.5		0.99			7.25	25	409	245		54	59	5	35		0.53
7.5	105		144	39	40.1		1.08								51			34		
8.0	105	207/102	145	37	41.3		1.10			7.23	25	350	302		54	61	7	35		0.55
8.5	120		145	40	47.0		1.31								52			33		
9.0	120		152	40	48.3		1.39								52			32		
9.5	135		153	45	54.7		1.54								53			33		
10.0	135	210/102	154	46	56.1		1.53			7.20	25	284	365		52	64	12	34		0.56
	Recovery		149	43	53.9		1.51								53			33		
	Recovery		144	43	51.7		1.38								52			35		
	Recovery		136	41	46.1		1.13								47			38		
	Recovery		133	39	44.1		1.03								47			40		
		192/102								7.22	22		475			55				

with breathing air, 100% O_2 breathing attenuated ventilatory drive (carotid body inhibition) causing Pa_{CO_2} to increase to 64 at the maximum work rate achieved. At each work rate during O_2 breathing, the breathing frequency (f) is decreased (compare Table 55-3 with Table 55-4). O_2 breathing allows the patient to breathe less and to be less breathless. The breathing frequency is only 35 ($\dot{V}E$ = 37.5) at 90 W when breathing O_2 as compared to 52 ($\dot{V}E$ = 67.5) during air breathing, at the same work rate. The heart rate is considerably more rapid during air breathing (150) than during O_2 breathing (132) at 90 W.

CONCLUSION

The patient has severe interstitial lung disease, with an important O_2 flow problem probably created by a combination of arterial hypoxemia and pulmonary vascular disease. O_2 breathing attenuates ventilatory drive and provides relief of dyspnea.

CASE 56 *Pulmonary alveolar proteinosis: Air and oxygen breathing*

CLINICAL FINDINGS

This 19-year-old man was hospitalized because of increasing shortness of breath, productive cough, and fatigue of 6 weeks' duration. He denied fever, sweats, chest pain, or exposure to infectious or toxic agents other than automobile paint fumes, tobacco, and occasional marijuana. He was thin, afebrile, tachycardic, and tachypneic with diffuse coarse rales bilaterally. Chest roentgenograms revealed a diffuse alveolar infiltrate, and blood gases showed hypoxemia and hypercapnia. An open lung biopsy showed pulmonary alveolar proteinosis. Exercise tests were performed while the patient was breathing room air and then 100% O_2 prior to bilateral lung lavage.

EXERCISE FINDINGS

The patient performed exercise on a cycle ergometer twice in the same morning with a 40-minute rest period between tests. On both occasions, arterial blood was sampled every second minute, and intra-arterial pressure was recorded from a percutaneously placed brachial artery catheter. He pedalled at 60 rpm without an added load for 3 minutes. The work rate was then increased 15 W per minute to tolerance. The patient was well motivated and cooperative and stopped exercise on both occasions because of dyspnea and chest tightness. No ECG abnormalities were noted.

TABLE 56-1. *Selected Respiratory Function Data*

MEASUREMENT	PREDICTED	MEASURED
Age, yr		19
Sex		Male
Height, cm		180
Weight, kg	82	68
Hematocrit, %		49
VC, L	4.46	2.46
IC, L	2.98	1.50
TLC, L	6.7	3.40
FEV$_1$, L	3.79	2.20
FEV$_1$/VC, %	85	89
MVV, L/min		
direct	134	101
indirect	152	88
D$_{LCO}$, ml/mm Hg/min	36.5	8.4

TABLE 56-2. *Selected Exercise Data*

MEASUREMENT	PREDICTED	ROOM AIR	OXYGEN
Maximum V̇$_{O_2}$, L/min	3.26	1.42	
Maximum HR, beats/min	201	150	150
Maximum O$_2$ pulse, ml/beat	16.2	9.5	
ΔV̇$_{O_2}$/ΔWR, ml/min/W	10.3	11.9	
AT, L/min	> 1.31	1.4	
Work rate, max, W		75	120
Blood pressure, mm Hg (rest, max ex)		102/57,144/72	114/62,132/72
Maximum V̇$_E$, L/min		84	73
Exercise breathing reserve, L/min			
using direct MVV	> 15	17	28
using indirect MVV	> 15	4	15
Pa$_{O_2}$, mm Hg (rest, max ex)		52,38	306,164
P(A−a)$_{O_2}$, mm Hg (rest, max ex)		57,76	371,506
P(a−ET)$_{CO_2}$, mm Hg (rest, max ex)		−1,5	1,5
V$_D$/V$_T$ (rest, max ex)		0.42,0.59	0.49,0.48
HCO$_3^-$, mEq/L (rest, recov)		23,21	23,20

FIG. 56-A. *Air breathing.*

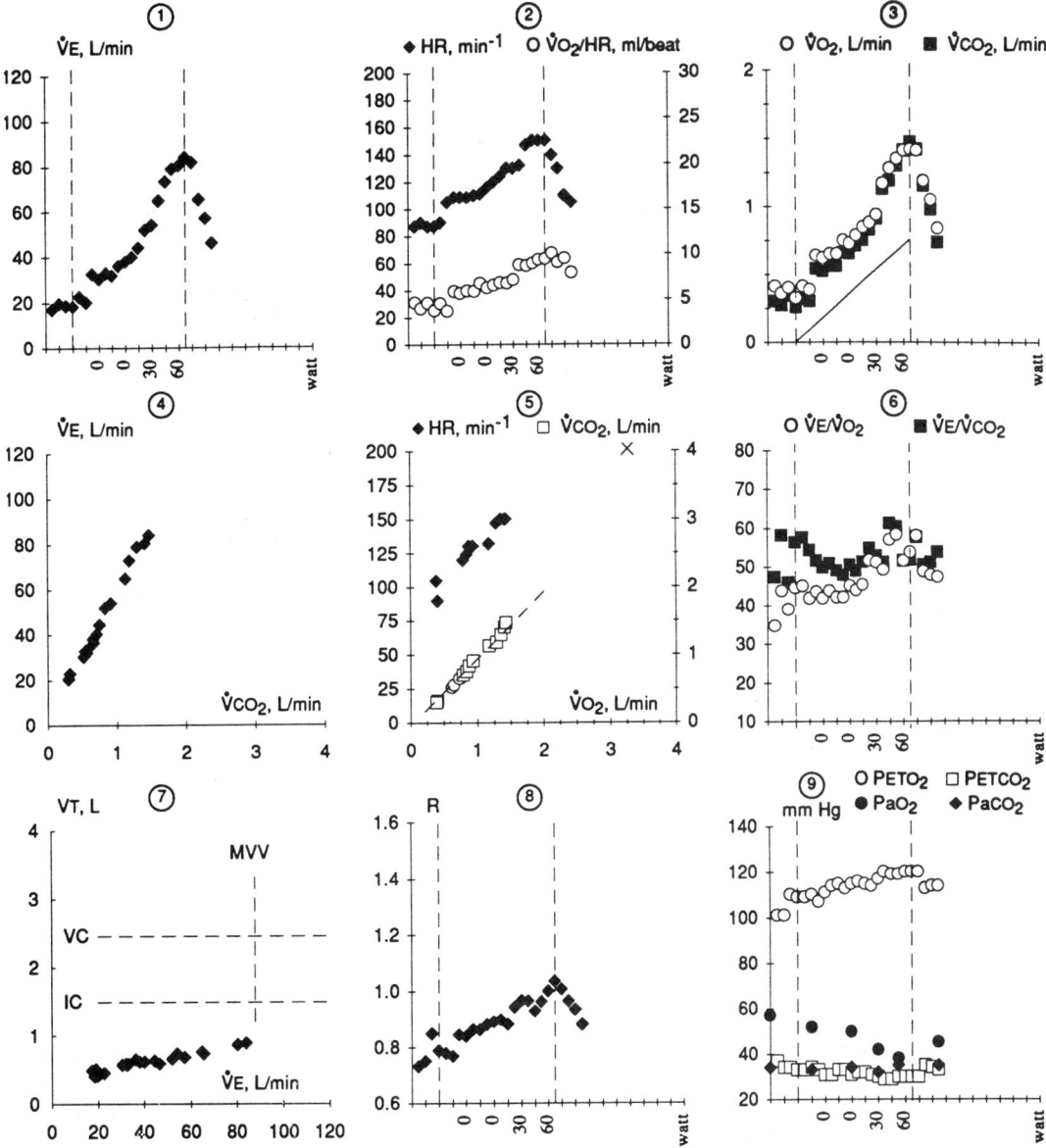

1. Vertical dashed lines in panels 1 to 3 and 6, 8, and 9 indicate the beginning and the end of increasing work period.

2. Unloaded cycling is performed for 3 minutes before the left vertical dashed line.

3. In panel 3, the diagonal line shows the increase of $\dot{V}_{O_2}$ at a slope of 10 ml/min/W.

4. In panel 5, the diagonal dashed line has a slope of 1; the "x" in the upper right is the predicted maximum heart rate and $\dot{V}_{O_2}$ for the subject.

Fig. 56-B. *Oxygen breathing.*

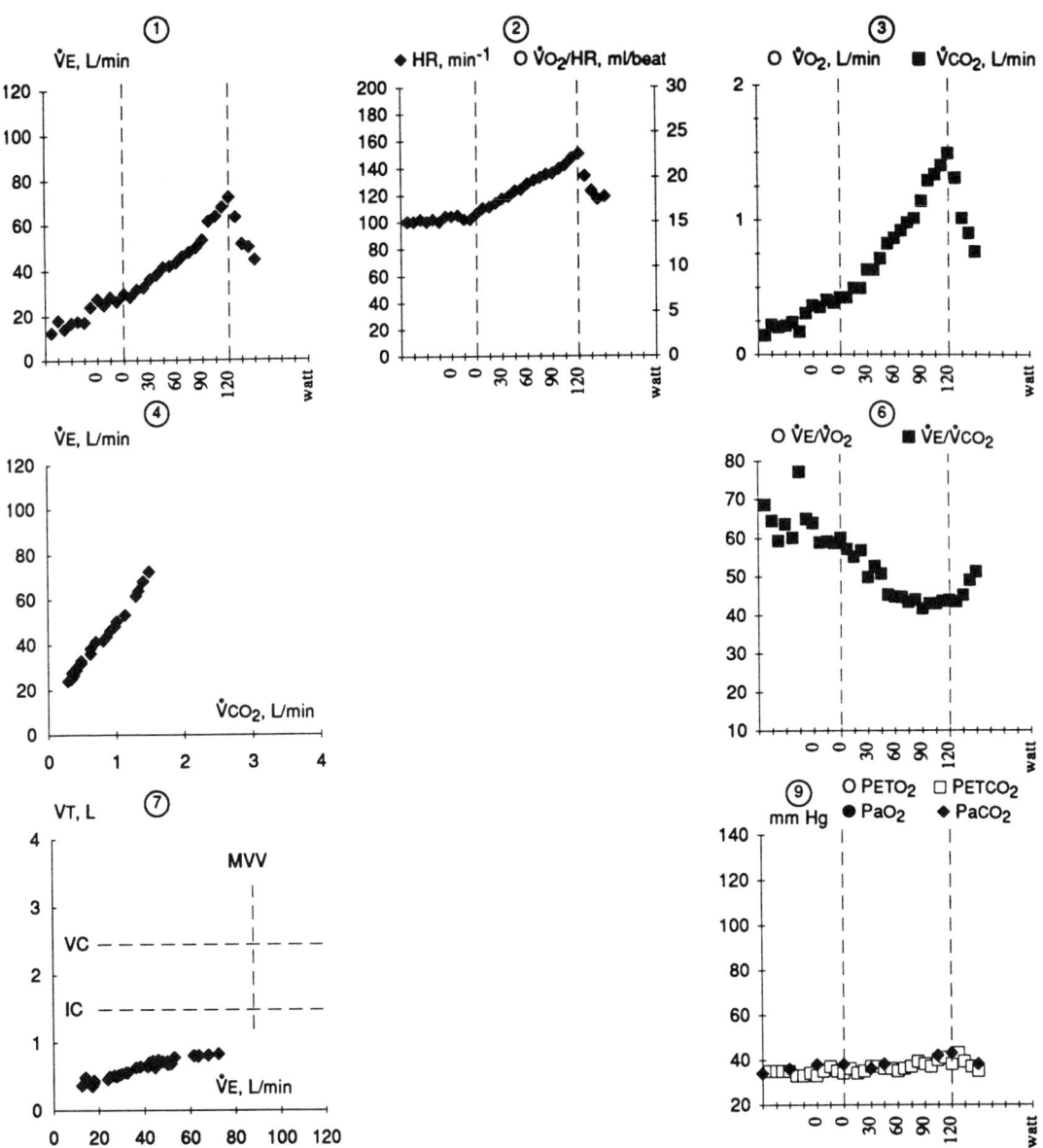

1. Vertical dashed lines in panels 1 to 3 and 6 and 9 indicate the beginning and the end of increasing work period.
2. Unloaded cycling is performed for 3 minutes before the left vertical dashed line.

TABLE 56-3. *Air breathing.*

Time min	Work rate watts	BP mm Hg	HR min⁻¹	f min⁻¹	V̇E L/min BTPS	V̇CO2 L/min STPD	V̇O2 L/min STPD	V̇O2/HR ml/beat	R	pH	HCO3 meq/L	PO2 ET	PO2 a	PO2 (A-a)	PCO2 ET	PCO2 a	PCO2 (a-ET)	V̇E/V̇CO2	V̇E/V̇O2	VD/VT
	Rest	102/57								7.45	23		57			34				
	Rest		87	35	17.2	0.30	0.41	4.7	0.73			101			37			47	35	
	Rest		90	48	19.8	0.27	0.36	4.0	0.75			101			34			58	44	
	Rest		87	37	18.8	0.34	0.40	4.6	0.85			110			34			46	39	
	Rest		87	45	18.5	0.26	0.33	3.8	0.79			109			33			56	44	
0.5			90	50	22.7	0.32	0.41	4.6	0.78			109			33			58	45	
1.0		99/60	105	47	20.3	0.30	0.39	3.7	0.77	7.45	23	110	52	57	34	33	-1	54	42	0.42
1.5	Unloaded		109	57	32.7	0.54	0.64	5.9	0.84			107			33			52	44	
2.0	Unloaded		109	53	30.4	0.52	0.62	5.7	0.84			111			31			50	42	
2.5	Unloaded		109	57	33.3	0.56	0.65	6.0	0.86			114			31			51	44	
3.0	Unloaded		110	55	32.1	0.56	0.65	5.9	0.86			115			33			49	42	
3.5	Unloaded		111	56	36.4	0.66	0.75	6.8	0.88			113			33			48	42	
4.0	Unloaded	123/69	116	62	38.1	0.65	0.73	6.3	0.89	7.45	23	115	50	63	31	34	3	51	45	0.43
4.5	15		120	65	40.2	0.71	0.79	6.6	0.90			116			32			49	44	
5.0	15		124	70	44.4	0.75	0.85	6.9	0.88			115			32			51	45	
5.5	30		130	79	52.1	0.83	0.88	6.8	0.94			114			31			55	52	
6.0	30	126/72	130	73	54.2	0.91	0.94	7.2	0.97	7.46	22	117	42	75	30	32	2	53	51	0.43
6.5	45		132	85	64.9	1.13	1.17	8.9	0.97			120			29			51	49	
7.0	45		147	5	73.2	1.19	1.28	8.7	0.93			119			29			61	57	
7.5	60	144/72	150	3	78.8	1.30	1.35	9.0	0.96	7.43	23	119	38	76	30	35	5	60	58	0.59
8.0	60		150	93	80.4	1.41	1.41	9.4	1.00			120			30			51	51	
8.5	75		150	94	84.2	1.47	1.42	9.5	1.04			120			30			52	54	
	Recovery		140	2	81.8	1.42	1.41	10.1	1.01			120			30			57	58	
	Recovery		130	89	65.6	1.15	1.19	9.2	0.97			113			35			50	49	
	Recovery		110	84	57.3	0.98	1.05	9.5	0.93			114			34			51	48	
	Recovery	144/72	105	79	46.5	0.74	0.84	8.0	0.88	7.39	21	114	45	66	33	35	2	54	47	0.46

Interpretation

COMMENTS

This case is presented to show the effects of O_2 breathing on work capacity in a patient with hypoxemia and restrictive lung disease and the differences between direct and indirect MVV measures in such patients. Resting respiratory function studies showed severe restrictive disease with low DL_{CO}, indicating loss of effective alveolar capillary bed, moderate hypoxemia, and mild hypocapnia.

ANALYSIS

In flow chart 1, in the room air study the maximum $\dot{V}O_2$ was low, but the anaerobic threshold was within normal limits (Table 56-2). This leads us to flow chart 3 and the category of lung disease through branchpoint 3.1 because of the borderline normal breathing reserve using the direct MVV. If we had used the indirect MVV, the breathing reserve would have been clearly low (abnormal). Confirmatory findings are high VD/VT, positive $P(a-ET)_{CO_2}$, and wide $P(A-a)_{O_2}$. Restrictive lung disease is confirmed because of the high breathing frequency of over 90 per minute (branchpoint 3.2). In the O_2 study, the patient exercised to a considerably higher work rate with a lower $\dot{V}E_{max}$, confirming that the patient did indeed have ventilatory limitation during the room air study. The low O_2 pulse while the patient was breathing room air is predominantly due to the low arterial O_2 content (Sa_{O_2} approximated 75% during late exercise) and the resultant reduced maximal arteriovenous O_2 content difference at maximal exercise, rather than a reduced stroke volume such as is found with primary cardiac defects. The patient developed a mild metabolic acidosis on both studies and some respiratory acidosis during O_2 breathing. The latter study demonstrates a large right to left shunt-like effect typical of this disorder.[1]

CONCLUSION

This is a typical case of pulmonary alveolar proteinosis with restriction and severe gas exchange

TABLE 56-4. *Oxygen breathing.*

Time min	Work rate watts	BP mm Hg	HR min⁻¹	f min⁻¹	$\dot{V}E$ L/min BTPS	$\dot{V}CO_2$ L/min STPD	$\dot{V}O_2$ L/min STPD	$\dfrac{\dot{V}O_2}{HR}$ ml/beat	R	pH	HCO₃ meq/L	PO2, mm Hg ET	a	(A-a)	PCO2, mm Hg ET	a	(a-ET)	$\dfrac{\dot{V}E}{\dot{V}CO_2}$	$\dfrac{\dot{V}E}{\dot{V}O_2}$	$\dfrac{VD}{VT}$
	Rest	114/62								7.44	23	359				34				
	Rest		100	34	12.5	0.14									35			69		
	Rest		100	44	17.9	0.22									35			64		
	Rest		102	29	14.3	0.20									35			59		
	Rest	99/63	100	43	17.0	0.21				7.41	22	306	371		35	36	1	64		0.49
	Rest		102	40	17.8	0.24									33			60		
	Rest		100	48	17.2	0.17									33			77		
	Unloaded		104	52	23.9	0.30									34			65		
	Unloaded	102/63	104	56	27.7	0.36				7.40	23	221	454		33	38	5	64		0.53
	Unloaded		105	50	24.8	0.35									35			59		
	Unloaded		102	55	28.3	0.40									37			59		
	Unloaded		102	51	26.6	0.38									35			59		
	Unloaded	102/69	106	56	29.9	0.42				7.40	23	227	448		34	38	4	60		0.52
0.5	15		110	54	28.6	0.42									36			57		
1.0	15		111	56	31.7	0.49									34			55		
1.5	30		114	58	32.7	0.49									35			57		
2.0	30	102/60	117	57	36.1	0.63				7.39	21	189	488		37	36	-1	50		0.45
2.5	45		119	59	38.2	0.63									37			53		
3.0	45	108/60	123	64	41.4	0.71				7.39	23	163	512		36	38	2	51		0.48
3.5	60		124	59	42.0	0.82									36			45		
4.0	60		128	60	43.5	0.86									35			45		
4.5	75		131	62	46.2	0.92									36			44		
5.0	75		133	66	48.0	0.98									37			43		
5.5	90		135	69	50.1	1.01									39			44		
6.0	90		136	68	53.3	1.14									38			42		
6.5	105		139	76	61.8	1.29									37			43		
7.0	105	126/66	142	79	63.9	1.33				7.34	22	157	514		40	42	2	43		0.47
7.5	120		147	83	68.1	1.40									41			44		
8.0	120	132/72	150	87	72.5	1.49				7.32	22	164	506		38	43	5	44		0.49
	Recovery		134	80	63.6	1.31									43			43		
	Recovery		123	75	51.8	1.01									39			45		
	Recovery		117	74	50.3	0.90									37			49		
	Recovery	117/60	119	70	44.8	0.76				7.33	20	185	490		35	38	3	51		0.48

abnormalities. The patient was limited both by his ventilatory ability and by hypoxemia. Young patients with interstitial lung disease often develop strong ventilatory muscles that allow them to exercise at a higher rate than might otherwise be expected. The directly measured MVV, performed at a high breathing frequency, was 101 L/min, whereas the indirect MVV, calculated as 40 times the FEV₁ was 88 L/min. Bilateral lung lavage performed after this study was helpful in improving the patient's exercise tolerance.

Reference

1. Selecky, P.A., Wasserman, K., Benfield, J.R., and Lippman, M.: The clinical and physiological effect of whole-lung lavage in pulmonary alveolar proteinosis: a ten-year experience. Ann. Thorac. Surg., 24:451–461, 1977.

CASE 57 *Alveolar proteinosis: Pre- and post-whole lung lavage*

CLINICAL FINDINGS

This 25-year-old graduate student was found to have alveolar proteinosis, proved by transbronchial lung biopsy, several years previously. He had had whole lung lavage twice previously, at yearly intervals, with improvement on both occasions. Despite the dyspnea associated with this illness, he was very physically active, running an average of 70 miles per week. He returned because of increasing dyspnea. Examination revealed a thin, muscular man who was not cyanotic. Chest roentgenograms showed bilateral infiltrates typical of alveolar proteinosis.

EXERCISE FINDINGS

The patient performed exercise on a cycle ergometer with similar protocols before and shortly after separate lavages of the right and left lungs. He pedalled at 60 rpm without added load for 3 minutes. The work rate was then increased 25 or 30 W per minute to his symptom-limited maximum. Arterial blood was sampled every second minute, and intra-arterial blood pressure was recorded from a percutaneously placed brachial artery catheter. Resting 12-lead and exercise single-lead ECG were normal. On both tests, the patient stopped exercise because of leg fatigue.

TABLE 57-1. *Selected Respiratory Function Data*

MEASUREMENT	PREDICTED	PRE-LAVAGE	POST-LAVAGE
Age, yr		25	
Sex		Male	
Height, cm		165	
Weight, kg	70	52	
Hematocrit, %		48	47
VC, L	4.46	2.06	2.98
IC, L	2.98	1.36	1.60
TLC, L	5.93	3.28	4.10
FEV_1, L	3.63	1.67	2.44
FEV_1/VC, %	81	81	82
MVV, L/min	163	97	121
D_{LCO}, ml/mm Hg/min	29.5	20.0	28.7

TABLE 57-2. *Selected Exercise Data*

MEASUREMENT	PREDICTED	PRE-LAVAGE	POST-LAVAGE
Maximum $\dot{V}_{O_2}$, L/min	2.52	2.70	3.07
Maximum HR, beats/min	195	165	175
Maximum O_2 pulse, ml/beat	12.9	16.4	17.5
$\Delta\dot{V}_{O_2}/\Delta WR$, ml/min/W	10.3	9.2	9.1
AT, L/min	> 1.02	2.1	2.1
Maximum $\dot{V}_E$, L/min		125	133
Exercise breathing reserve, L/min	> 15	−28	−12
Pa_{O_2}, mm Hg (rest, max ex)		82,53	93,64
$P(A-a)_{O_2}$, mm Hg (rest, max ex)		16,64	12,55
$P(a-ET)_{CO_2}$, mm Hg (rest, max ex)		−1,6	−1,−5
V_D/V_T (rest, heavy ex)		0.20,0.36	0.25,0.21
HCO_3^-, mEq/L (rest, heavy ex)		26,21	24,15

FIG. 57-A. *Pre-whole lung lavage.*

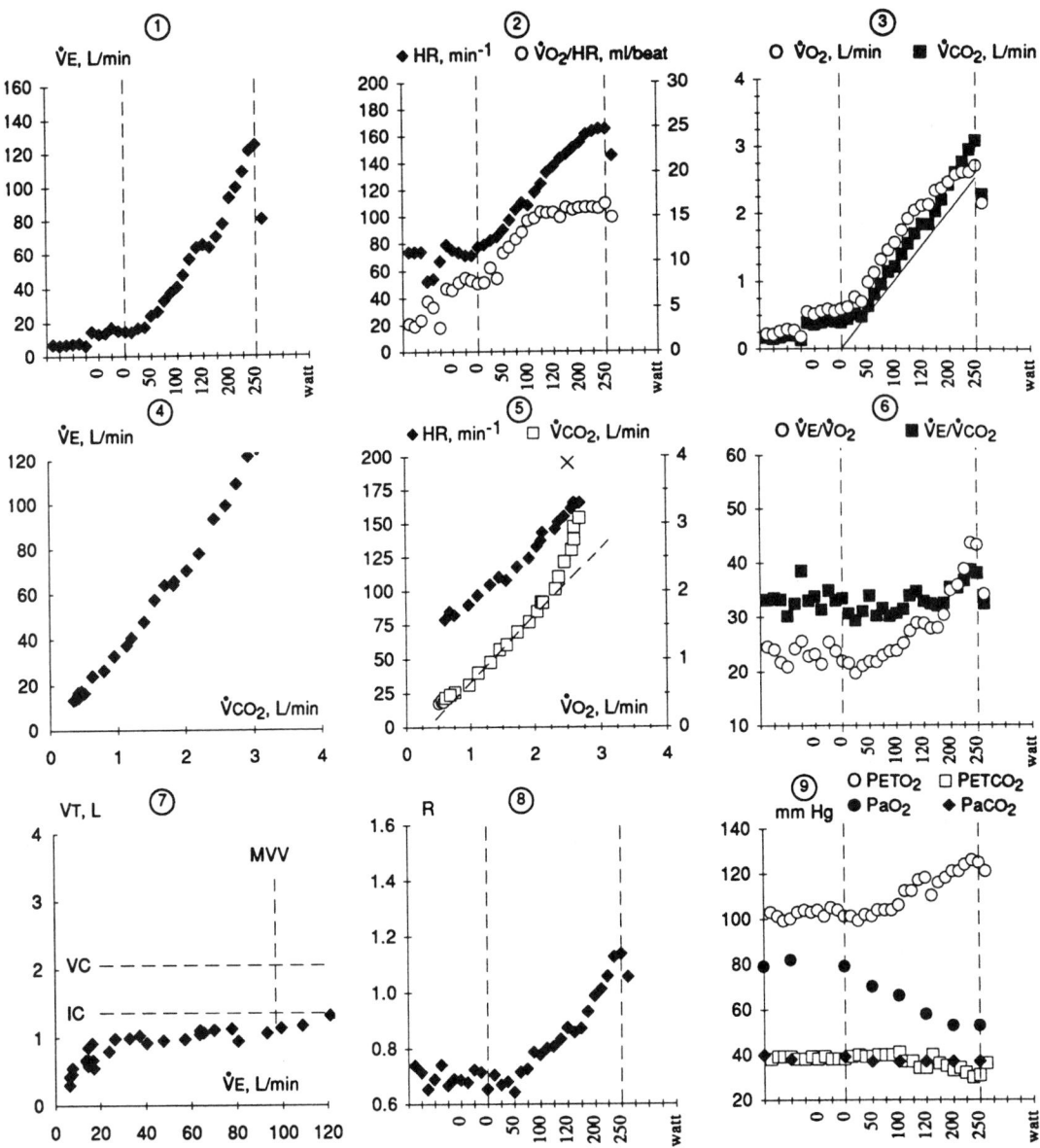

1. Vertical dashed lines in panels 1 to 3 and 6, 8, and 9 indicate the beginning and the end of increasing work period.
2. Unloaded cycling is performed for 3 minutes before the left vertical dashed line.
3. In panel 3, the diagonal line shows the increase of $\dot{V}O_2$ at a slope of 10 ml/min/W.
4. In panel 5, the diagonal dashed line has a slope of 1; the "x" in the upper right is the predicted maximum heart rate and $\dot{V}O_2$ for the subject.

FIG. 57-B. *Post-whole lung lavage.*

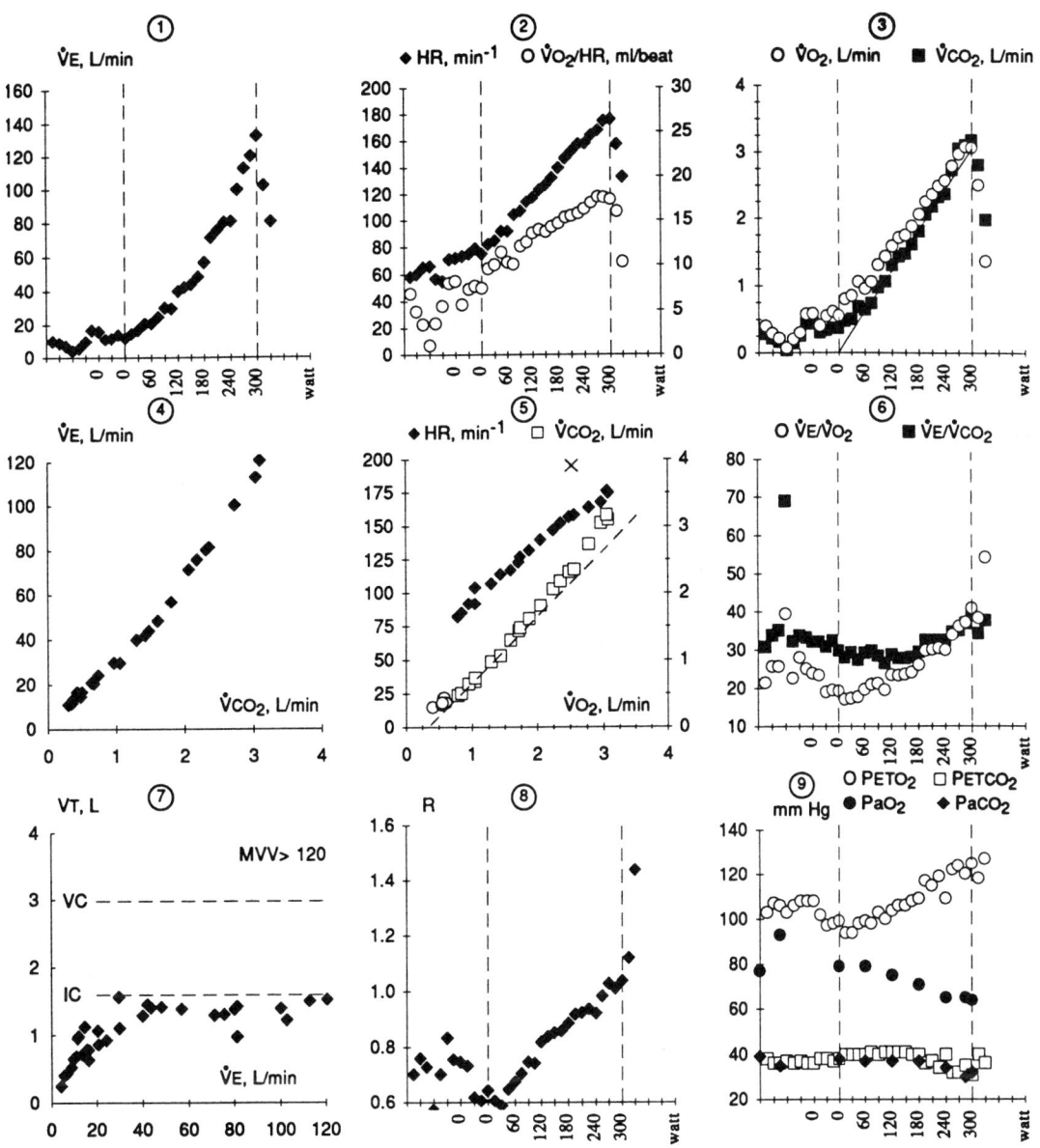

1. Vertical dashed lines in panels 1 to 3 and 6, 8, and 9 indicate the beginning and the end of increasing work period.

2. Unloaded cycling is performed for 3 minutes before the left vertical dashed line.

3. In panel 3, the diagonal line shows the increase of $\dot{V}O_2$ at a slope of 10 ml/min/W.

4. In panel 5, the diagonal dashed line has a slope of 1; the "x" in the upper right is the predicted maximum heart rate and $\dot{V}O_2$ for the subject.

TABLE 57-3. *Pre-whole lung lavage.*

Time min	Work rate watts	BP mm Hg	HR min⁻¹	f min⁻¹	$\dot{V}E$ L/min BTPS	$\dot{V}CO_2$ L/min STPD	$\dot{V}O_2$ L/min STPD	$\dfrac{\dot{V}O_2}{HR}$ ml/beat	R	pH	HCO₃ meq/L	PO2 mm Hg ET	a	(A-a)	PCO2 mm Hg ET	a	(a-ET)	$\dfrac{\dot{V}E}{\dot{V}CO_2}$	$\dfrac{\dot{V}E}{\dot{V}O_2}$	$\dfrac{VD}{VT}$
	Rest									7.43	26		79			40				
	Rest		74	16	7.0	0.17	0.23	3.1	0.74			103			38			33	25	
	Rest		74	15	6.3	0.15	0.21	2.8	0.71			101			39			34	24	
	Rest		74	16	7.0	0.17	0.26	3.5	0.65			99			39			33	22	
	Rest		52	16	7.4	0.20	0.29	5.6	0.69	7.44	25	100	82	16	39	38	-1	30	21	0.20
	Rest		54	14	7.7	0.20	0.27	5.0	0.74			103			38			33	24	
	Rest		67	21	6.4	0.12	0.18	2.7	0.67			104			38			38	26	
	Unloaded		79	25	14.7	0.38	0.55	7.0	0.69			103			39			33	23	
	Unloaded		75	20	13.5	0.35	0.51	6.8	0.69			104			38			34	23	
	Unloaded		73	21	13.7	0.38	0.56	7.7	0.68			101			39			31	21	
	Unloaded		71	25	16.8	0.42	0.58	8.2	0.72			105			38			35	25	
	Unloaded		71	23	15.2	0.40	0.56	7.9	0.71			104			38			33	24	
	Unloaded		77	24	14.7	0.38	0.58	7.5	0.66	7.43	25	101	79	16	38	39	1	33	22	0.29
0.5	25		79	17	14.6	0.43	0.61	7.7	0.70			101			39			31	22	
1.0	25		82	18	16.5	0.51	0.76	9.3	0.67			99			40			29	20	
1.5	50		85	31	17.2	0.47	0.69	8.1	0.68			102			39			31	21	
2.0	50		90	30	23.9	0.63	0.98	10.9	0.64	7.43	24	101	70	27	39	37	-2	34	22	0.28
2.5	75		97	27	26.5	0.80	1.12	11.5	0.71			104			40			30	22	
3.0	75		105	33	32.8	0.95	1.31	12.5	0.73			104			40			32	23	
3.5	100		110	36	37.3	1.14	1.45	13.2	0.79			104			40			30	24	
4.0	100		108	44	40.7	1.21	1.56	14.4	0.78	7.44	25	106	66	39	41	37	-4	31	24	0.21
4.5	125		118	50	47.8	1.39	1.74	14.7	0.80			112			37			31	25	
5.0	125		124	59	57.4	1.55	1.92	15.5	0.81			112			37			34	27	
5.5	120		133	61	63.9	1.70	2.04	15.3	0.83			117			34			35	29	
6.0	120		137	61	65.6	1.84	2.11	15.4	0.87	7.43	24	118	58	51	34	37	3	33	29	0.27
6.5	175		143	58	64.1	1.83	2.13	14.9	0.86			110			40			32	28	
7.0	175		146	63	70.2	2.03	2.33	16.0	0.87			116			36			32	28	
7.5	200		151	69	77.8	2.21	2.37	15.7	0.93			118			35			33	30	
8.0	200		155	87	93.3	2.43	2.46	15.9	0.99	7.41	23	121	53	60	33	37	4	35	35	0.31
8.5	225		161	87	99.4	2.60	2.57	16.0	1.01			121			34			35	36	
9.0	225		163	93	108.9	2.76	2.61	16.0	1.06			124			32			37	39	
9.5	250		165	92	121.4	2.94	2.61	15.8	1.13			126			30			39	44	
10.0	250		165	96	124.9	3.07	2.70	16.4	1.14	7.36	21	125	53	64	31	37	6	38	43	0.36
	Recovery		145	85	80.6	2.27	2.15	14.8	1.06			121			36			32	34	

Interpretation

COMMENTS

Respiratory function studies indicate moderately severe restrictive lung disease that improves after lung lavage (Table 57-1). The resting ECG is normal. The post-lavage exercise study was done 7 days after completion of whole lung lavage and 11 days after the pre-lavage study.

ANALYSIS

In flow chart 1, because this patient is so exceptionally well trained, his maximum $\dot{V}O_2$ and anaerobic threshold are substantially greater than predicted. Nevertheless, the rate of rise in $\dot{V}O_2$ decreases above the anaerobic threshold before lavage (panel 3, Fig. 57-A). The maximum $\dot{V}O_2$, even before lavage, is significantly above predicted (Table 57-2). See flow chart 2: The O_2 pulse is supra-normal and his ECG is normal at maximum $\dot{V}O_2$. His blood gases, however, while normal at rest, become abnormal during exercise, with Pa_{O_2} progressively decreasing and $P(A-a)_{O_2}$ progressively increasing with work rate (Table 57-3) (branchpoint 2.1). The VD/VT is abnormal (branchpoint 2.3). At the maximum work rate performed, the patient has a marked tachypnea (Table 57-3). The tidal volume remains constant at the level of the inspiratory capacity from a relatively light work rate to the maximum (panel 7, Fig. 57-A), with the increase in minute ventilation

Table 57-4. *Post-whole lung lavage.*

Time min	Work rate watts	BP mm Hg	HR min⁻¹	f min⁻¹	V̇E L/min BTPS	V̇CO2 L/min STPD	V̇O2 L/min STPD	V̇O2/HR ml/beat	R	pH	HCO3 meq/L	PO2, mm Hg ET	a	(A-a)	PCO2, mm Hg ET	a	(a-ET)	V̇E/V̇CO2	V̇E/V̇O2	VD/VT
	Rest									7.40	24	77			39					
	Rest		58	15	9.9	0.28	0.40	6.9	0.70			103			38			31	22	
	Rest		60	17	8.9	0.22	0.29	4.8	0.76			107			36			34	26	
	Rest		65	16	7.0	0.16	0.22	3.4	0.73	7.43	23	106	93	12	36	35	-1	35	26	0.24
	Rest		66	17	4.2	0.04	0.07	1.1	0.57			103			37			69	39	
	Rest		57	14	5.7	0.14	0.20	3.5	0.70			106			36			32	23	
	Rest		55	15	9.7	0.25	0.30	5.5	0.83			108			37			34	28	
	Unloaded		71	26	16.5	0.43	0.57	8.0	0.75			108			36			33	25	
	Unloaded		72	20	15.8	0.44	0.59	8.2	0.75			108			36			32	24	
	Unloaded		73	16	11.0	0.30	0.41	5.6	0.73			102			38			32	24	
	Unloaded		75	12	11.5	0.34	0.55	7.3	0.62			97			38			31	19	
	Unloaded		79	19	13.6	0.37	0.61	7.7	0.61			98			37			32	20	
	Unloaded		75	12	11.8	0.36	0.56	7.5	0.64	7.41	24	99	79	16	38	38	0	30	19	0.22
0.5	30		82	13	14.6	0.48	0.79	9.6	0.61			94			40			28	17	
1.0	30		85	21	16.5	0.50	0.85	10.0	0.59			94			40			29	17	
1.5	60		92	19	20.3	0.68	1.05	11.4	0.65			98			40			27	18	
2.0	60		92	24	20.8	0.64	0.95	10.3	0.67	7.41	23	99	79	20	40	37	-3	29	20	0.18
2.5	90		104	26	24.2	0.74	1.05	10.1	0.70			98			41			30	21	
3.0	90		107	27	29.8	0.97	1.30	12.1	0.75			103			40			28	21	
3.5	120		114	19	29.7	1.06	1.43	12.5	0.74			100			41			26	20	
4.0	120		117	31	40.0	1.30	1.59	13.6	0.82	7.40	23	104	75	31	41	37	-4	29	24	0.18
4.5	150		123	29	42.1	1.43	1.71	13.9	0.84			106			41			28	23	
5.0	150		127	31	43.7	1.48	1.74	13.7	0.85			106			41			28	24	
5.5	180		132	34	48.2	1.61	1.88	14.2	0.86			108			40			28	24	
6.0	180		140	41	56.8	1.81	2.05	14.6	0.88	7.40	23	109	71	38	40	37	-3	29	26	0.20
6.5	210		147	55	71.4	2.06	2.25	15.3	0.92			117			36			32	30	
7.0	210		152	58	75.8	2.18	2.36	15.5	0.92			115			37			33	30	
7.5	240		157	58	80.2	2.32	2.48	15.8	0.94			119			34			32	30	
8.0	240		158	57	81.3	2.36	2.56	16.2	0.92	7.40	21	109	65	49	40	34	-6	32	30	0.20
8.5	270		164	72	100.3	2.73	2.78	17.0	0.98			122			32			34	34	
9.0	270		168	75	113.0	3.04	2.96	17.6	1.03			124			32			35	36	
9.5	300		175	79	120.7	3.10	3.07	17.5	1.01	7.35	16	120	65	55	35	30	-5	37	37	0.21
10.0	300		176	96	132.8	3.17	3.06	17.4	1.04	7.30	15	125	64	55	31	32	1	39	41	0.29
	Recovery		157	84	102.9	2.80	2.50	15.9	1.12			118			40			34	38	
	Recovery		133	83	81.2	1.97	1.37	10.3	1.44			127			36			38	54	

achieved, almost solely, by increasing breathing frequency. This exercise response is consistent with restrictive lung disease, despite a supra-normal maximum V̇O2.

Although the patient exceeds the predicted V̇O2max value for sedentary males of his size, he clearly has physiologic abnormalities that limit his exercise performance, as evidenced by his improved exercise performance following bilateral whole lung lavage (Table 57-2, and contrasting data in Tables 57-3 and 57-4). Because of the mechanical limitation to lung expansion imposed by the alveolar filling disorder, and perhaps some pulmonary fibrosis, the patient has to increase minute ventilation during exercise primarily by increasing breathing frequency. The minute ventilation at maximum exercise exceeds his MVV (negative breathing reserve), reflecting his high motivation and possibly some exercise bronchodilatation. In the second study the ventilatory pattern of restrictive disease persists but is more mild. The degree of arterial hypoxemia and the increase in $P(A-a)_{O_2}$ are also considerably reduced following whole lung lavage (compare Table 57-3 with Table 57-4), whereas the upper portion of the V̇CO2 versus V̇O2 plot is shallower and O2 pulse is higher at higher work rates (compare panels 5 and 2 of Fig. 57-A and B).

Conclusion

The patient has restrictive lung disease that improved following therapy.

CASE 58 *Pulmonary microlithiasis: Air and oxygen breathing*

CLINICAL FINDINGS

This 63-year-old Iranian man had previously been diagnosed by lung biopsy as having pulmonary microlithiasis. He had never smoked. He had had slowly progressive dyspnea over 30 years until he was limited to walking a few steps. He occasionally had hemoptysis. He had been treated with corticosteroids and bronchodilators without apparent benefit. Exercise testing was requested to obtain optimal assessment of his cardiorespiratory function prior to lung lavage or other therapeutic intervention. Resting ECG showed nonspecific ST-T wave changes.

EXERCISE FINDINGS

Exercise tests recorded while the patient was breathing room air and then 100% O_2 were performed on the same day on a cycle ergometer with an intermediate rest period. On both occasions, arterial blood was sampled every second minute, and intra-arterial pressure was recorded from a percutaneously placed brachial artery catheter. The patient pedalled at 60 rpm without an added load for 3 minutes. The work rate was then increased 5 W per minute to tolerance. The patient was well motivated and cooperative and stopped exercise on both occasions because of dyspnea. No further ECG abnormalities were noted during or after exercise.

TABLE 58-1. *Selected Respiratory Function Data*

MEASUREMENT	PREDICTED	MEASURED
Age, yr		63
Sex		Male
Height, cm		164
Weight, kg	69	55
Hematocrit, %		51
VC, L	3.36	1.37
IC, L	2.24	0.73
TLC, L	5.28	2.70
FEV$_1$, L	2.61	1.31
FEV$_1$/VC, %	78	92
MVV, L/min		
direct	117	62
indirect	104	52
D$_{LCO}$, ml/mm Hg/min	23.9	6.0

TABLE 58-2. *Selected Exercise Data*

MEASUREMENT	PREDICTED	ROOM AIR	OXYGEN
Maximum V̇$_{O_2}$, L/min	1.69	0.60	
Maximum HR, beats/min	151	110	138
Maximum O$_2$ pulse, ml/beat	11.2	5.6	
ΔV̇$_{O_2}$/ΔWR, ml/min/W	10.3	10.3	
AT, L/min	> 0.75	< 0.55	
Work rate, max, W		15	40
Blood pressure, mm Hg (rest, max ex)		147/84,186/87	135/81,153/99
Maximum V̇$_E$, L/min		63	54
Exercise breathing reserve, L/min			
using direct MVV	> 15	−1	8
using indirect MVV	> 15	−11	−2
Pa$_{O_2}$, mm Hg (rest, max ex)		40,34	364,344
P(A−a)$_{O_2}$ mm Hg (rest, max ex)		48,88	292,304
P(a−ET)$_{CO_2}$, mm Hg (rest, max ex)		16,17	21,22
V$_D$/V$_T$ (rest, max ex)		0.65,0.64	0.68,0.71
HCO$_3^-$, mEq/L (rest, recov)		31,27	29,28

Fig. 58-A. *Air breathing.*

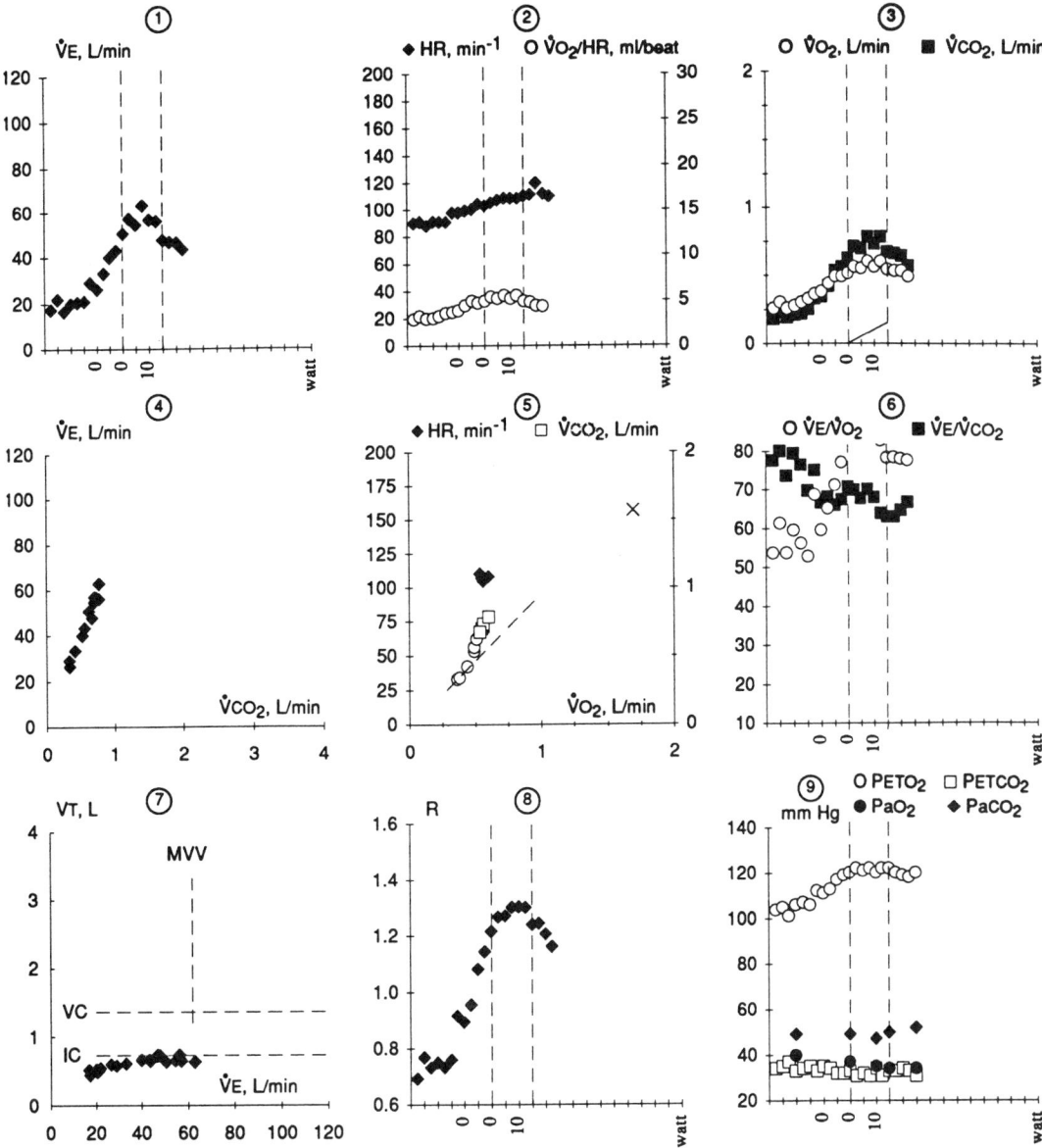

1. Vertical dashed lines in panels 1 to 3 and 6, 8, and 9 indicate the beginning and the end of increasing work period.
2. Unloaded cycling is performed for 3 minutes before the left vertical dashed line.
3. In panel 3, the diagonal line shows the increase of $\dot{V}O_2$ at a slope of 10 ml/min/W.
4. In panel 5, the diagonal dashed line has a slope of 1; the "x" in the upper right is the predicted maximum heart rate and $\dot{V}O_2$ for the subject.

FIG. 58-B. *Oxygen breathing.*

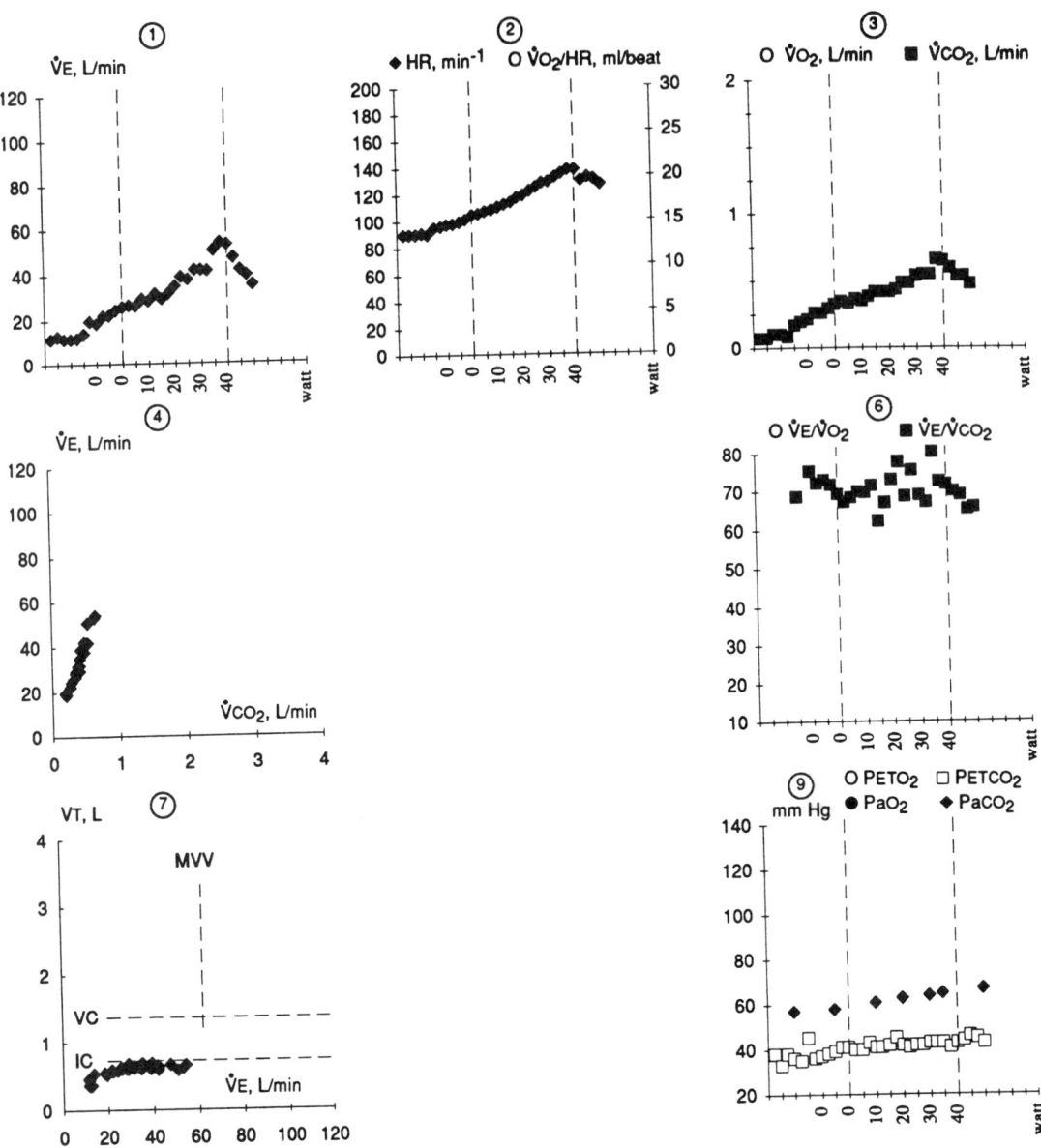

1. Vertical dashed lines in panels 1 to 3 and 6 and 9 indicate the beginning and the end of increasing work period.
2. Unloaded cycling is performed for 3 minutes before the left vertical dashed line.

TABLE 58-3. *Air breathing.*

Time min	Work rate watts	BP mm Hg	HR min⁻¹	f min⁻¹	$\dot V_E$ L/min BTPS	$\dot V_{CO_2}$ L/min STPD	$\dot V_{O_2}$ L/min STPD	$\dfrac{\dot V_{O_2}}{HR}$ ml/beat	R	pH	HCO₃ meq/L	PO2, mm Hg ET	a	(A-a)	PCO2, mm Hg ET	a	(a-ET)	$\dfrac{\dot V_E}{\dot V_{CO_2}}$	$\dfrac{\dot V_E}{\dot V_{O_2}}$	$\dfrac{V_D}{V_T}$
	Rest	147/84	90	39	17.3	0.18	0.26	2.9	0.69			104			34			78	54	
	Rest		91	40	21.8	0.23	0.30	3.3	0.77			105			35			80	61	
	Rest		88	32	16.7	0.19	0.26	3.0	0.73			101			37			74	54	
	Rest	147/84	91	38	19.9	0.21	0.28	3.1	0.75	7.41	31	106	40	48	33	49	16	79	60	0.65
	Rest		91	42	20.4	0.22	0.30	3.3	0.73			107			34			77	56	
	Rest		91	42	21.0	0.25	0.33	3.6	0.76			106			35			70	53	
	Unloaded		98	50	29.0	0.33	0.36	3.7	0.92			112			33			75	69	
	Unloaded		98	44	26.4	0.34	0.38	3.9	0.89			111			35			67	60	
	Unloaded		99	55	33.3	0.42	0.44	4.4	0.95			113			34			68	65	
	Unloaded		100	61	40.1	0.53	0.49	4.9	1.08			117			32			66	71	
	Unloaded		104	65	43.3	0.56	0.49	4.7	1.14			119			32			67	77	
	Unloaded	174/84	103	80	50.6	0.62	0.51	5.0	1.22	7.40	30	120	37	71	33	49	16	71	86	0.65
0.5	5		105	89	57.1	0.71	0.56	5.3	1.27			122			31			70	88	
1.0	5		107	84	54.5	0.70	0.55	5.1	1.27			121			32			68	86	
1.5	10		108	99	63.0	0.78	0.60	5.6	1.30			122			31			70	91	
2.0	10	186/90	108	83	56.7	0.73	0.56	5.2	1.30	7.39	28	120	35	77	34	47	13	68	89	0.64
2.5	15		108	77	56.2	0.78	0.60	5.6	1.30			122			31			64	83	
3.0	15	186/87	110	66	47.8	0.67	0.54	4.9	1.24	7.36	28	122	34	74	33	50	17	63	78	0.64
	Recovery		111	64	47.0	0.66	0.53	4.8	1.25			120			33			63	78	
	Recovery		120	65	46.8	0.64	0.53	4.4	1.21			119			34			64	78	
	Recovery		112	68	43.8	0.57	0.49	4.4	1.16			118			33			67	78	
	Recovery		110								7.33	27	120	34		31	52	21			

Interpretation

COMMENTS

This case shows the effects of oxygen breathing on exercise capacity and blood gases in a patient severely disabled with interstitial lung disease. Resting respiratory function studies showed severe restrictive disease with low $D_{L_{CO}}$, severe hypoxemia, and moderate hypercapnia.

ANALYSIS

In flow chart 1, in the room air study the maximum $\dot V_{O_2}$ and the anaerobic threshold were reduced (Table 58-2). This leads us through branchpoints 1.1, 1.2, and 1.3 to flow chart 4. We arrive at the diagnosis of "lung disease with impaired peripheral oxygenation" through branchpoint 4.1 (low breathing reserve) and branchpoint 4.2 (high V_D/V_T). The patient filled all the requirements in both this box and the "abnormal pulmonary circulation" box. With O_2 breathing, a large shunt was not found. The high breathing frequency, negative breathing reserve, and high tidal volume to inspiratory capacity ratio all indicate severe ventilatory limitation. The gas exchange abnormalities (hypoxemia, positive $P(a-ET)_{CO_2}$, and high V_D/V_T) were striking and reflect lung units with abnormally high and abnormally low ventilation-perfusion ratios. With O_2 breathing, exercise capacity was significantly increased, as arterial O_2 saturation and content increased. As a consequence of carotid body suppression with O_2, the ventilatory response was decreased compared to air breathing, and a more severe respiratory acidosis developed. In addition, note the extremely low O_2 pulse while the patient was breathing air. Arterial O_2 capacity was 21.3 ml/100 ml, and air breathing O_2 content was approximately 15 ml/100 ml. Thus, a major part of the reduction in O_2 pulse is due to hypoxemia, with some reduction likely due to a low stroke volume.

CONCLUSION

This patient demonstrates the gas exchange and ventilatory defects found in severe interstitial lung disease and demonstrates the improvement from O_2 supplementation.

TABLE 58-4. *Oxygen breathing.*

Time min	Work rate watts	BP mm Hg	HR min⁻¹	f min⁻¹	$\dot{V}_E$ L/min BTPS	$\dot{V}CO_2$ L/min STPD	$\dot{V}O_2$ L/min STPD	$\dfrac{\dot{V}O_2}{HR}$ ml/beat	R	pH	HCO₃ meq/L	PO2, mm Hg ET	a	(A-a)	PCO2, mm Hg ET	a	(a-ET)	$\dfrac{\dot{V}_E}{\dot{V}CO_2}$	$\dfrac{\dot{V}_E}{\dot{V}O_2}$	$\dfrac{V_D}{V_T}$
	Rest	120/78	90	31	11.6	0.07									38			128		
	Rest		90	35	12.8	0.07									33			140		
	Rest		90	25	11.5	0.10									38			94		
	Rest	135/81	91	26	11.6	0.10				7.32	29		364	292	36	57	21	94		0.68
	Rest		90	31	12.1	0.08									35			118		
	Rest		95	26	13.9	0.17									45			69		
	Unloaded		96	37	19.6	0.19									36			87		
	Unloaded		97	34	18.7	0.21									37			75		
	Unloaded		98	37	21.9	0.26									38			72		
	Unloaded	147/90	99	39	22.3	0.26				7.32	29		437	218	39	58	19	73		0.68
	Unloaded		101	42	24.4	0.29									41			72		
	Unloaded		104	41	25.7	0.32									41			69		
0.5	5		105	43	26.5	0.34									40			67		
1.0	5		107	43	26.2	0.33									40			68		
1.5	10		108	48	29.3	0.36									43			70		
2.0	10	147/90	110	47	28.4	0.35				7.29	29		423	229	41	61	20	70		0.68
2.5	15		112	51	31.5	0.38									41			71		
3.0	15		114	43	29.2	0.41									42			62		
3.5	20		117	49	31.6	0.41									45			67		
4.0	20	141/84	119	57	34.8	0.41				7.28	29		387	263	42	63	21	73		0.70
4.5	25		122	64	38.9	0.43									41			78		
5.0	25		125	58	37.9	0.48									42			69		
5.5	30		128	70	42.2	0.48									42			76		
6.0	30	153/99	129	66	42.1	0.53				7.26	28		361	288	43	64	21	69		0.70
6.5	35		132	64	41.7	0.54									43			67		
7.0	35		135	86	50.7	0.54				7.25	28		344	304	43	65	22	80		0.71
7.5	40		138	81	54.1	0.65									41			73		
8.0	40		138	84	53.1	0.64									43			72		
	Recovery		130	70	47.3	0.59									44			70		
	Recovery		132	65	42.0	0.53									46			69		
	Recovery		131	57	39.4	0.53									45			65		
	Recovery	151/102	127	51	35.2	0.47				7.23	28		380	266	43	67	24	66		0.70

CASE 59 *Pulmonary vascular disease, thromboembolic*

CLINICAL FINDINGS

This 50-year-old shipyard worker had felt well until one year prior to evaluation when he noted the insidious but progressive development of dyspnea and easy fatigability. Six months later, he had had the abrupt onset of severe substernal chest pain and dyspnea, which resulted in hospitalization and treatment for a suspected myocardial infarction. Following discharge from the hospital, he had lost 25 to 30 pounds by watching his diet but remained somewhat dyspneic. There was no personal or family history of hypertension or diabetes mellitus. He had smoked 3 to 4 cigarettes daily until 2 years earlier. Physical examination was normal. Chest roentgenograms showed minimal pleural thickening bilaterally. Resting ECG showed normal QRS complexes and negative T waves in V1 to V3, suggesting right ventricular strain.

EXERCISE FINDINGS

The patient performed exercise on a cycle ergometer. He pedalled at 60 rpm without added load for 3 minutes. The work rate was then increased 15 W per minute. Arterial blood was sampled every second minute, and intra-arterial blood pressure was recorded from a percutaneously placed brachial artery catheter. At 105 W work rate the pedal came off the cycle ergometer. After 30 minutes rest, the study was restarted with an increase of 20 W every minute. The patient stopped exercise because of overall fatigue and exhaustion; he denied having chest pain or dyspnea. There was a 0.5-mm ST segment depression in leads II, V5, and V6 that disappeared at 3 minutes of recovery.

TABLE 59-1. *Selected Respiratory Function Data*

MEASUREMENT	PREDICTED	MEASURED
Age, yr		50
Sex		Male
Height, cm		185
Weight, kg	86	92
Hematocrit, %		46
VC, L	5.10	4.68
IC, L	3.40	2.94
TLC, L	7.45	5.94
FEV_1, L	4.06	3.62
FEV_1/VC, %	80	77
MVV, L/min	161	152
D_{LCO}, ml/mm Hg/min	32.3	21.2

TABLE 59-2. *Selected Exercise Data*

MEASUREMENT	PREDICTED	MEASURED
Maximum $\dot{V}_{O_2}$, L/min	2.78	1.92
Maximum HR, beats/min	170	164
Maximum O_2 pulse, ml/beat	16.4	11.7
$\Delta\dot{V}_{O_2}/\Delta WR$, ml/min/W	10.3	8.9
AT, L/min	> 1.20	1.4
Blood pressure, mm Hg (rest, max)		125/80,161/92
Maximum $\dot{V}_E$, L/min		104
Exercise breathing reserve, L/min	> 15	48
Pa_{O_2}, mm Hg (rest, max ex)		83,56
$P(A-a)_{O_2}$, mm Hg (rest, max ex)		26,63
$P(a-ET)_{CO_2}$, mm Hg (rest, max ex)		5,9
V_D/V_T (rest, heavy ex)		0.40,0.45
HCO_3^-, mEq/L (rest, 2-min recov)		22,19

TABLE 59-3.

Time min	Work rate watts	BP mm Hg	HR min⁻¹	f min⁻¹	V̇E L/min BTPS	V̇CO₂ L/min STPD	V̇O₂ L/min STPD	V̇O₂/HR ml/beat	R	pH	HCO₃ meq/L	PO₂, mm Hg			PCO₂, mm Hg			V̇E/V̇CO₂	V̇E/V̇O₂	VD/VT
												ET	a	(A-a)	ET	a	(a-ET)			
	Rest	125/80								7.41	21		73			34				
	Rest		82	24	12.9	0.22	0.25	3.0	0.88			116			28			49	43	
	Rest		82	22	14.7	0.28	0.35	4.3	0.80			112			29			46	37	
	Rest		81	21	14.8	0.28	0.35	4.3	0.80			110			30			46	37	
	Rest	119/83	81	16	12.0	0.23	0.29	3.6	0.79	7.42	22	112	83	26	29	34	5	46	37	0.40
	Unloaded		94	23	26.8	0.56	0.66	7.0	0.85			109			30			44	38	
	Unloaded	140/86	92	26	26.1	0.55	0.63	6.8	0.87	7.42	22	116	69	42	28	35	7	43	38	0.40
0.5	20		100	25	28.9	0.64	0.77	7.7	0.83			113			29			42	35	
1.0	20		100	22	32.8	0.72	0.86	8.6	0.84			115			28			43	36	
1.5	40		104	20	34.2	0.77	0.91	8.8	0.85			115			28			42	36	
2.0	40		108	22	37.1	0.84	0.99	9.2	0.85			115			28			42	36	
2.5	60		111	25	45.2	0.97	1.10	9.9	0.88			118			27			44	39	
3.0	60	146/86	115	25	47.2	1.02	1.16	10.1	0.88	7.42	22	116	64	47	28	35	7	44	39	0.42
3.5	80		121	27	52.5	1.16	1.31	10.8	0.89			116			28			43	38	
4.0	80		125	29	56.5	1.21	1.31	10.5	0.92			120			25			45	41	
4.5	100		132	27	60.8	1.32	1.41	10.7	0.94			120			26			44	41	
5.0	100	155/89	137	28	63.9	1.39	1.47	10.7	0.95	7.43	22	121	60	55	25	33	8	44	42	0.39
5.5	120		143	27	69.1	1.52	1.58	11.0	0.96			122			25			44	42	
6.0	120		147	28	72.8	1.62	1.66	11.3	0.98			123			25			43	42	
6.5	140		152	33	87.8	1.80	1.74	11.4	1.03			124			24			47	49	
7.0	140	161/92	156	31	89.7	1.88	1.79	11.5	1.05	7.40	20	124	58	60	24	33	9	46	49	0.42
7.5	160		160	34	94.8	1.97	1.88	11.8	1.05			125			24			47	49	
8.0	160	155/86	164	37	104.5	2.07	1.92	11.7	1.08	7.40	20	126	56	63	24	33	9	49	53	0.45
	Recovery		144	29	85.2	1.86	1.80	12.5	1.03			123			25			44	46	
	Recovery		127	27	73.4	1.62	1.52	12.0	1.07			122			26			44	47	
	Recovery		116	23	54.5	1.23	1.14	9.8	1.08			122			27			43	46	
	Recovery	152/86	109	20	35.7	0.84	0.79	7.2	1.06	7.37	19	119	73	45	30	34	4	40	43	0.36

Interpretation

COMMENTS

This case is presented because it illustrates the use of exercise testing for detecting significant pulmonary vascular disease and correcting an erroneous diagnosis. The patient's physician assumed that symptoms of chest pain, dyspnea, and easy fatigability had been due to a myocardial infarction. That diagnosis could not be supported by myocardial enzyme concentrations or specific ECG changes. Radionuclide ventilation-perfusion scans confirmed the presence of many perfusion without ventilation defects, characteristic of pulmonary thromboembolic disease.

The results of the resting respiratory function studies indicate that this patient had normal lung mechanics. He had a significant reduction in diffusing capacity, however (Table 59-1). The ECG was suggestive of right ventricular strain.

ANALYSIS

In flow chart 1, the maximum V̇O₂ is reduced while the anaerobic threshold is normal (Table 59-2). See flow chart 3: The breathing reserve is normal, which directs us to branchpoint 3.3, where the ECG is within normal limits. The criteria for "poor effort, musculoskeletal disorder, or myocardial ischemia" are not met, so we retrace our path to branchpoint 3.1. Although the breathing reserve is not low, we note the unusually high V̇E/V̇CO₂, (panel 6, Fig. 59-A) despite the normal Pa_{CO_2}, indicating a high fraction of wasted ventilation. We also note the abnormally high VD/VT, $P(A-a)_{O_2}$, and $P(a-ET)_{CO_2}$, all evidence of lung disease with ventilation-perfusion mismatching. The patient's findings are not explained by the uncomplicated obstructive or restrictive lung disease suggested in flow chart 3. Recognizing that the patient also has a persistently low maximum O₂ pulse (panel

FIG. 59-A.

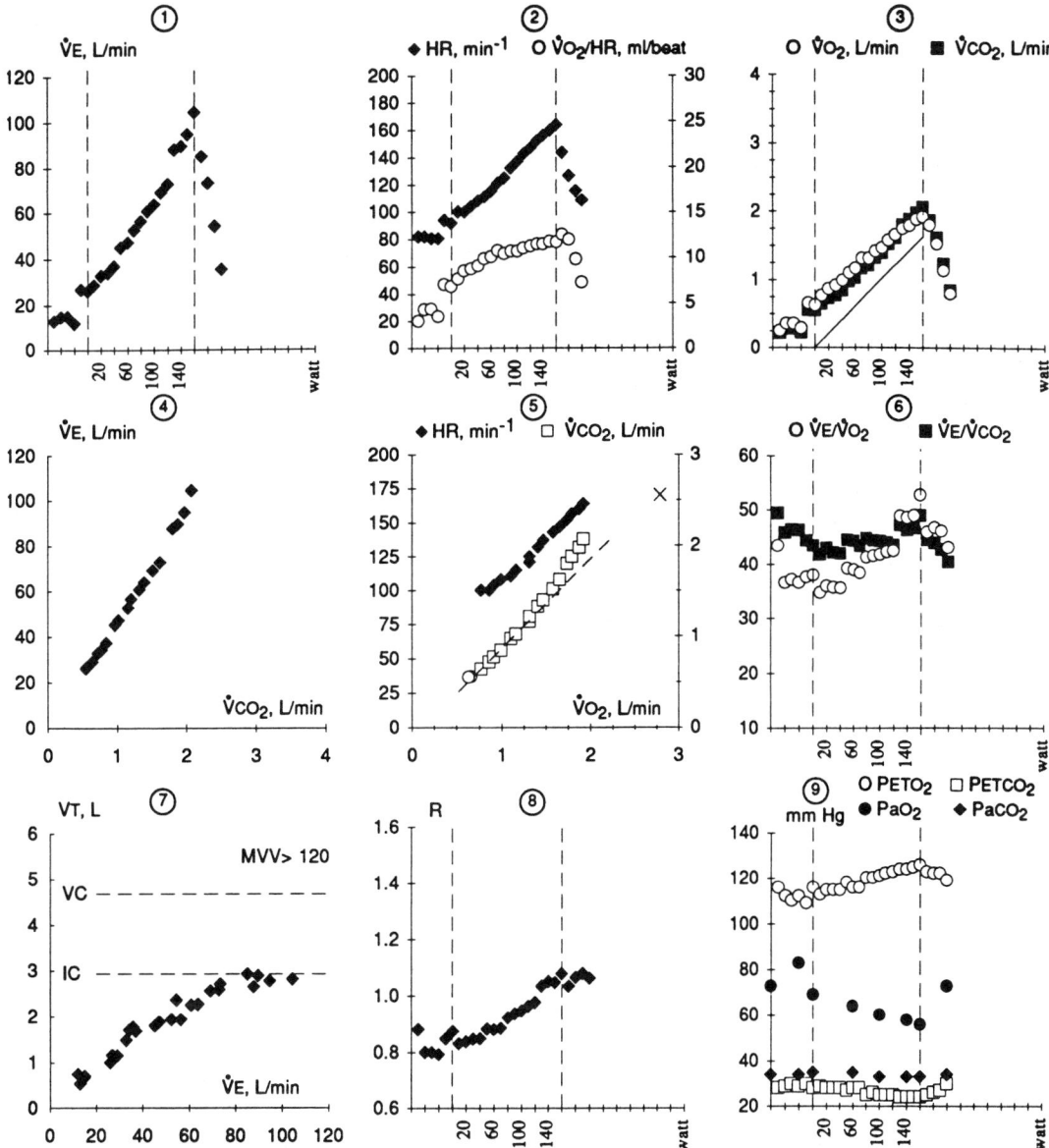

1. Vertical dashed lines in panels 1 to 3 and 6, 8, and 9 indicate the beginning and the end of increasing work period.

2. Unloaded cycling is performed for 3 minutes before the left vertical dashed line.

3. In panel 3, the diagonal line shows the increase of $\dot{V}_{O_2}$ at a slope of 10 ml/min/W.

4. In panel 5, the diagonal dashed line has a slope of 1; the "x" in the upper right is the predicted maximum heart rate and $\dot{V}_{O_2}$ for the subject.

2, Fig. 59-A), we consider flow chart 5. The abnormal gas exchange (branchpoint 5.1), normal breathing reserve (branchpoint 5.3) and decreasing Pa_{O_2} (branchpoint 5.6) direct us to "pulmonary vascular disease." Here the first five criteria for this diagnosis are well satisfied. The patient was not tested with 100% O_2, but the lack of an abrupt decrease in Pa_{O_2} during exercise suggests that a right to left shunt through a potentially patent foramen ovale does not occur.

CONCLUSION

This patient had pulmonary vascular disease, previously unrecognized, probably of thromboembolic origin. The patient eventually died of thromboembolic disease.

CASE 60 *Pulmonary vasculitis: Air and oxygen breathing*

CLINICAL FINDINGS

This 54-year-old executive had apparently been in good health until 11 years previously, when he had had a documented acute myocardial infarction. Coronary arteriogram had been normal 1 year later. Five years ago he had developed fatigue, jaundice, Raynaud's phenomenon, renal failure, and peripheral neuropathy with a histologic diagnosis of membranoproliferative glomerulonephritis secondary to vasculitis. Diffuse cerebritis with panhypopituitarism had followed; this had responded well to corticosteroids, cyclophosphamide, and endocrine replacement therapy. Three years ago, progressive exertional dyspnea had begun without cough, pleurisy, or wheezing. A pulmonary nodule had developed and was biopsied. Histologic examination had showed an organizing exudate, hemorrhage, and severe arteriolar wall thickening. The patient had never smoked or abused drugs or alcohol. Physical examination revealed acrocyanosis without clubbing, clear lungs, and normal heart sounds. Exercise testing was performed to evaluate the possible efficacy of supplemental oxygen.

EXERCISE FINDINGS

The patient performed exercise tests on the cycle ergometer. On both occasions he pedalled at 60 rpm without added load for 3 minutes. The work rate was then increased 15 W every minute.

The first test was done during air breathing, and the second was done while breathing 100% oxygen. Arterial blood was sampled every second minute, and intra-arterial blood pressure recorded from a percutaneously inserted brachial artery catheter.

During air breathing, the patient stopped because of leg fatigue and complained of shortness of breath. While breathing 100% O_2, the patient complained of leg fatigue only. Resting ECG showed a rightward axis, poor R wave progression in the precordial leads and T wave inversion in V4. There was no ectopy or abnormality of ST segments, although the T wave inversion increased during exercise.

TABLE 60-1. *Selected Respiratory Function Data*

MEASUREMENT	PREDICTED	MEASURED
Age, yr		54
Sex		Male
Height, cm		170
Weight, kg	74	64
Hematocrit, %		38
VC, L	4.03	4.07
IC, L	2.68	3.16
FEV$_1$, L	3.18	3.38
FEV$_1$/VC, %	79	83
MVV, L/min	137	143
D$_{LCO}$, ml/mm Hg/min	26.5	8.0

TABLE 60-2. *Selected Exercise Data*

MEASUREMENT	PREDICTED	ROOM AIR	OXYGEN
Maximum work rate, W	160	90	90
Maximum V̇O$_2$, L/min	2.11	0.96	
Maximum HR, beats/min	166	132	131
Maximum O$_2$ pulse, ml/beat	12.7	7.3	
ΔV̇O$_2$/ΔWR, ml/min/W	10.3	8.8	
AT, L/min	> 0.91	< 0.75	
Blood pressure, mm Hg (rest, max)		129/69,204/84	126/75,201/87
Maximum V̇E, L/min		117	89
Exercise breathing reserve, L/min	> 15	26	54
Pa$_{O_2}$, mm Hg (rest, max ex)		114,90	692,678
P(A − a)$_{O_2}$, mm Hg (rest, max ex)		10,41	−8,4
P(a − ET)$_{CO_2}$, mm Hg (rest, max ex)		7,9	10,12
V$_D$/V$_T$ (rest, heavy ex)		0.44,0.52	0.52,0.57
HCO$_3^-$, mEq/L (rest, 2-min recov)		18,12	18,15

FIG. 60-A. *Air breathing.*

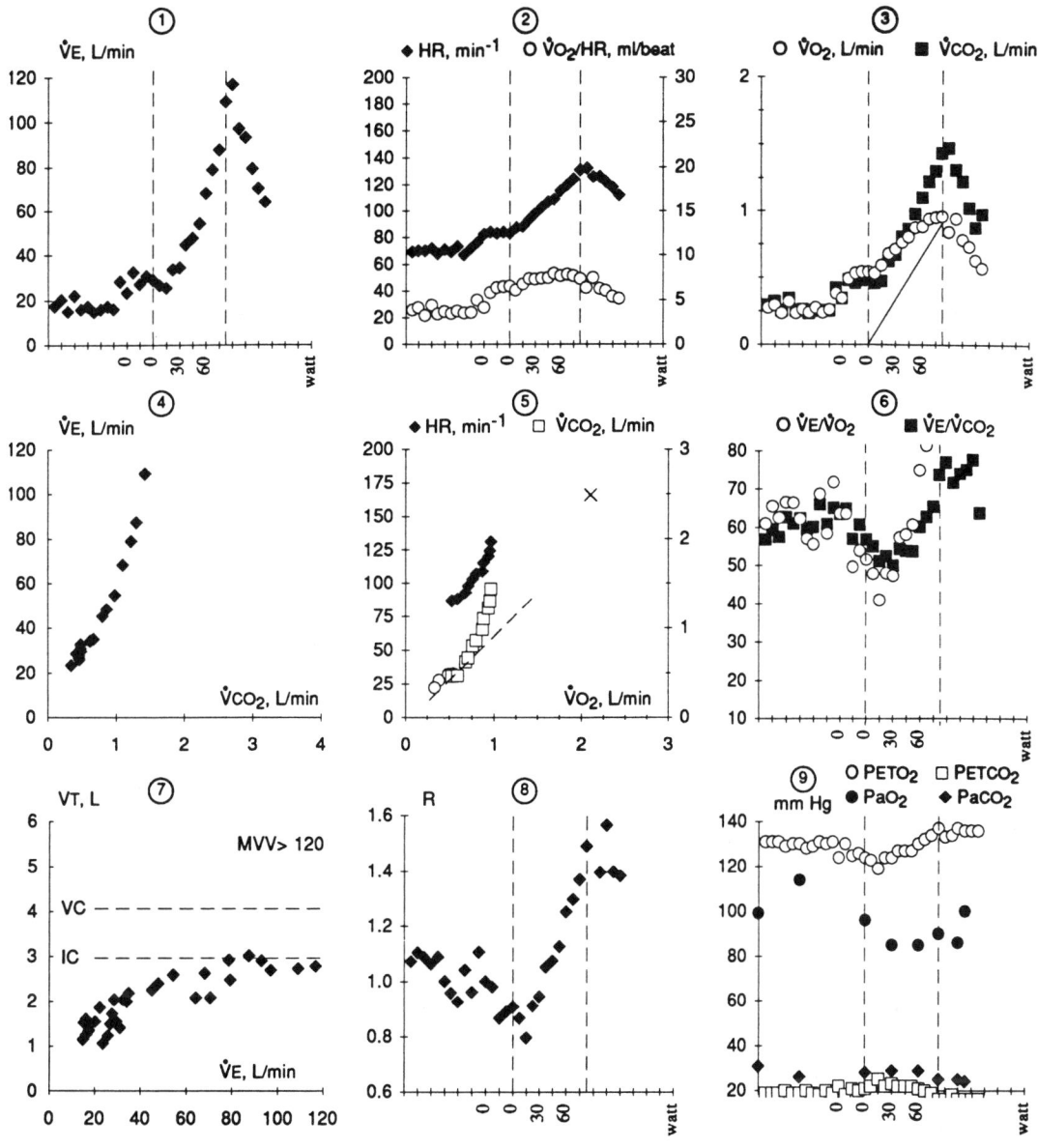

1. Vertical dashed lines in panels 1 to 3 and 6, 8, and 9 indicate the beginning and the end of increasing work period.

2. Unloaded cycling is performed for 3 minutes before the left vertical dashed line.

3. In panel 3, the diagonal line shows the increase of $\dot{V}O_2$ at a slope of 10 ml/min/W.

4. In panel 5, the diagonal dashed line has a slope of 1; the "x" in the upper right is the predicted maximum heart rate and $\dot{V}O_2$ for the subject.

FIG. 60-B. *Oxygen breathing.*

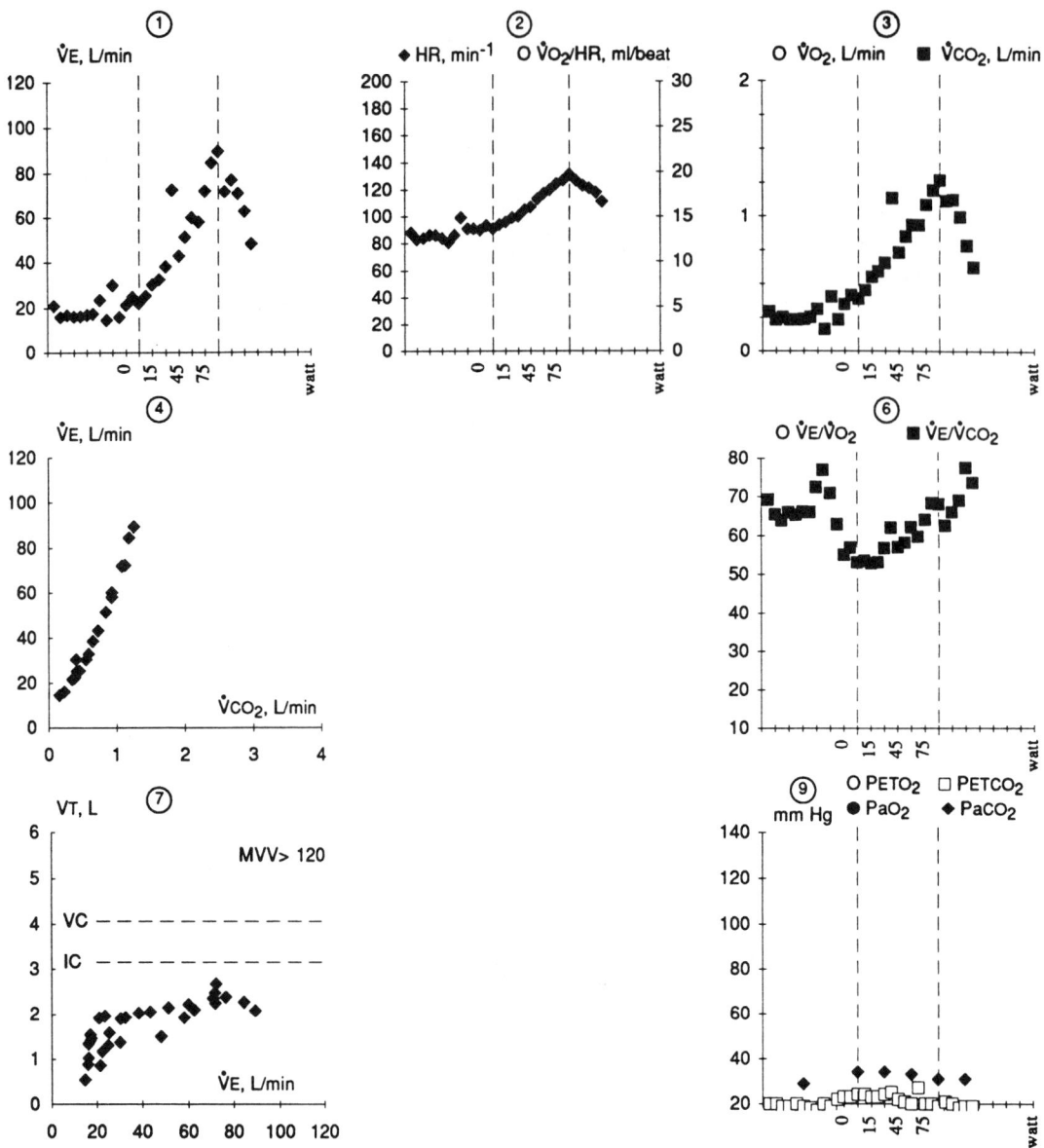

1. Vertical dashed lines in panels 1 to 3 and 6 and 9 indicate the beginning and the end of increasing work period.
2. Unloaded cycling is performed for 3 minutes before the left vertical dashed line.

TABLE 60-3. *Air breathing.*

Time min	Work rate watts	BP mm Hg	HR min⁻¹	f min⁻¹	V̇E L/min BTPS	V̇CO2 L/min STPD	V̇O2 L/min STPD	V̇O2/HR ml/beat	R	pH	HCO3 meq/L	PO2 ET	PO2 a	PO2 (A-a)	PCO2 ET	PCO2 a	PCO2 (a-ET)	V̇E/V̇CO2	V̇E/V̇O2	VD/VT
	Rest	129/69								7.38	18		99			31				
	Rest		69	12	17.5	0.29	0.27	3.9	1.07			131			19			57	61	
	Rest		70	13	20.1	0.32	0.29	4.1	1.10			131			19			59	66	
	Rest		70	10	15.2	0.25	0.23	3.3	1.09			131			19			57	62	
	Rest		72	12	22.3	0.34	0.32	4.4	1.06			129			20			63	67	
	Rest		68	10	16.1	0.25	0.23	3.4	1.09			130			19			61	66	
	Rest	126/69	71	13	17.3	0.26	0.26	3.7	1.00	7.44	17	130	114	10	19	26	7	62	62	0.44
	Rest		69	13	14.8	0.23	0.24	3.5	0.96			128			20			60	57	
	Rest		73	13	16.1	0.25	0.27	3.7	0.93			129			19			60	56	
	Rest		67	13	17.6	0.25	0.24	3.6	1.04			131			18			66	69	
	Rest		72	13	16.3	0.25	0.26	3.6	0.96			130			20			61	58	
	Unloaded		76	14	28.5	0.42	0.38	5.0	1.11			131			19			65	72	
	Unloaded		82	22	23.5	0.34	0.34	4.1	1.00			124			22			64	64	
	Unloaded		84	16	32.5	0.48	0.49	5.8	0.98			130			18			65	64	
	Unloaded		83	16	27.6	0.46	0.53	6.4	0.87			125			21			57	50	
	Unloaded		84	22	31.0	0.48	0.54	6.4	0.89			126			20			61	54	
	Unloaded	147/75	83	19	29.4	0.49	0.54	6.5	0.91	7.41	17	124	96	24	21	28	7	57	51	0.43
0.5	15		87	18	26.8	0.46	0.53	6.1	0.87			123			22			55	48	
1.0	15		88	21	25.8	0.47	0.59	6.7	0.80			119			25			51	41	
1.5	30		93	17	34.0	0.62	0.68	7.3	0.91			124			22			53	48	
2.0	30	156/78	98	16	34.9	0.67	0.71	7.2	0.94	7.39	17	124	85	35	23	29	6	50	47	0.39
2.5	45		103	20	45.2	0.80	0.76	7.4	1.05			127			22			54	57	
3.0	45		107	20	48.1	0.86	0.80	7.5	1.08			127			22			54	58	
3.5	60		109	21	54.5	0.98	0.87	8.0	1.13			127			22			54	61	
4.0	60	183/84	115	26	68.3	1.10	0.88	7.7	1.25	7.38	17	130	85	41	21	29	8	60	75	0.49
4.5	75		120	27	78.9	1.22	0.94	7.8	1.30			132			20			63	81	
5.0	75		124	29	87.6	1.30	0.95	7.7	1.37			134			19			65	90	
5.5	90	204/84	131	40	109.1	1.43	0.96	7.3	1.49	7.38	15	137	90	41	16	25	9	74	110	0.52
	Recovery		132	42	116.9	1.47	0.84	6.4	1.75			133			16			77	135	
	Recovery		126	36	97.1	1.31	0.94	7.5	1.39			134			18			72	100	
	Recovery	198/87	126	32	93.1	1.22	0.78	6.2	1.56	7.37	14	137	86	46	16	25	9	74	116	0.52
	Recovery	192/78	122	32	79.4	1.02	0.73	6.0	1.40	7.33	12	136	100	31	16	24	8	75	105	0.50
	Recovery		118	34	70.6	0.87	0.63	5.3	1.38			136			16			78	107	
	Recovery		112	31	64.4	0.97	0.57	5.1	1.70			136			16			64	108	

Interpretation

COMMENTS

Except for the very low diffusing capacity, the results of this patient's respiratory function studies are normal (Table 60-1).

ANALYSIS

In flow chart 1, during air breathing, the maximum V̇O2 and the anaerobic threshold are significantly reduced (Table 60-2). See flow chart 4. The breathing reserve is normal (branchpoint 4.1). The ventilatory equivalent is significantly increased, but part of this increase is due to chronic and acute hyperventilation (Table 60-3) (branchpoint 4.3); however, the patient has a high VD/VT and abnormal $P(a - ET)_{CO_2}$ and $P(A - a)_{O_2}$ at the maximum work rate performed, providing confirmatory evidence of marked ventilation-perfusion mismatching. In view of the patient's normal respiratory mechanics, the ventilation-perfusion abnormality is probably due to pulmonary vascular disease. Further support that pulmonary vascular disease is limiting the cardiac output increase is provided by the confirmatory findings listed in the abnormal pulmonary circulation diagnostic box in flow chart 4: (1) a steep and steepening heart rate in-

TABLE 60-4. *Oxygen breathing.*

Time min	Work rate watts	BP mm Hg	HR min⁻¹	f min⁻¹	$\dot{V}E$ L/min BTPS	$\dot{V}CO_2$ L/min STPD	$\dot{V}O_2$ L/min STPD	$\frac{\dot{V}O_2}{HR}$ ml/beat	R	pH	HCO₃ meq/L	PO2, mm Hg ET	a	(A-a)	PCO2, mm Hg ET	a	(a-ET)	$\frac{\dot{V}E}{\dot{V}CO_2}$	$\frac{\dot{V}E}{\dot{V}O_2}$	$\frac{VD}{VT}$
	Rest		88	11	21.0	0.29									20			69		
	Rest		83	12	16.1	0.23									20			66		
	Rest		84	11	16.9	0.25									19			64		
	Rest		86	12	16.2	0.23									19			66		
	Rest		86	16	16.4	0.23									20			65		
	Rest	120/72	84	12	16.9	0.24				7.40	18	692	-8		19	29	10	66			0.52
	Rest		81	12	17.5	0.25									18			66		
	Rest		86	12	23.5	0.31									17			73		
	Unloaded		99	27	14.6	0.16									20			77		
	Unloaded		91	22	30.2	0.40									19			71		
	Unloaded		91	18	16.0	0.23									22			63		
	Unloaded		90	25	21.4	0.35									23			55		
	Unloaded		93	19	24.9	0.41									23			57		
	Unloaded	132/72	91	19	22.3	0.39				7.36	19	678	1		24	34	10	53			0.48
0.5	15		94	16	25.4	0.45									24			53		
1.0	15		96	16	30.4	0.55									23			53		
1.5	30		99	17	32.7	0.59									23			53		
2.0	30	156/75	100	19	38.4	0.65				7.35	18	645	34		24	34	10	57			0.53
2.5	45		105	27	72.3	1.13									25			62		
3.0	45		107	21	43.3	0.73									22			57		
3.5	60		113	24	51.4	0.85									21			58		
4.0	60	189/81	117	27	60.1	0.93				7.35	18	683	-3		20	33	13	62			0.56
4.5	75		120	30	58.1	0.93									27			60		
5.0	75		124	32	72.0	1.08									20			64		
5.5	90		127	37	84.3	1.19									20			68		
6.0	90	201/87	131	43	89.4	1.26				7.34	16	678	4		19	31	12	68			0.57
	Recovery		127	29	71.7	1.11									21			62		
	Recovery		123	32	76.5	1.12									20			66		
	Recovery		121	30	70.8	0.99									18			69		
	Recovery	186/78	118	30	62.9	0.78				7.31	15	682	0		19	31	12	77			0.61
	Recovery		111	32	48.3	0.62									19			74		

crease with increasing $\dot{V}O_2$ (panel 5, Fig. 60-A), (2) a low O_2 pulse that fails to increase as work rate is increased (panel 2, Fig. 60-A), and (3) a low $\Delta\dot{V}O_2/\Delta WR$ that decreases with increasing work rate (panel 3, Fig. 60-A).

Pa_{O_2} decreases during exercise but remains within the normal range (panel 9, Fig. 60-A). The high Pa_{O_2} measured during exercise with the patient breathing 100% O_2 confirms the absence of the development of a right to left shunt (usually through the foramen ovale). This might be contrasted with Case 61, a patient with pulmonary vascular disease in whom a right to left shunt through the foramen ovale did develop during exercise.

100% O_2 breathing had little effect on this patient's exercise performance. This suggests that this patient has little pulmonary vasodilatation in response to high O_2 breathing. Ventilation, however, is considerably reduced with O_2 breathing demonstrating a suppression of ventilatory drive during exercise. Despite this reduction in ventilation and dyspnea, there was no improvement in exercise performance. This suggests that the patient is not ventilatory limited.

Resting arterial bicarbonate is low, demonstrating a compensated metabolic acidosis at rest. The metabolic acidosis worsens with exercise (Table 60-2).

CONCLUSION

Severe pulmonary vascular disease has limited exercise performance.

CASE 61 *Pulmonary hypertension with patent foramen ovale*

CLINICAL FINDINGS

This 61-year-old woman had first noted mild exertional dyspnea 3 years prior to evaluation. Four months prior to evaluation she had "caught the flu" and soon thereafter developed recurring episodes of depression and confusion. Medical evaluation revealed hypoxemia. With oxygen therapy her mental status returned to normal. She also admitted to squeezing substernal chest pain, usually associated with exercise, but this symptom was not prominent. There was no history of cigarette smoking, exposure to environmental toxins, pulmonary emboli, or thrombophlebitis. She was given alprazolam for her mental symptoms and propranolol for systemic hypertension. On referral, examination revealed mild obesity, hypertension, and a prominent S4. Chest roentgenogram showed enlarged pulmonary arteries. Resting ECG revealed right axis deviation, an R much greater than S in V1, and negative T waves in leads V1 to V4.

EXERCISE FINDINGS

The patient performed exercise on a cycle ergometer. She pedalled at 60 rpm without added load for 3 minutes. The work rate was then increased 5 W per minute to her symptom-limited maximum. Arterial blood was sampled every second minute, and intra-arterial blood pressure was recorded from a percutaneously placed brachial artery catheter. She stopped exercise because of shortness of breath. There were no arrhythmias, ST segment, or T wave changes with exercise. Following a rest period of 30 minutes, the exercise study was repeated while the patient was breathing 100% oxygen.

TABLE 61-1. *Selected Respiratory Function Data*

MEASUREMENT	PREDICTED	MEASURED
Age, yr		61
Sex		Female
Height, cm		147
Weight, kg	53	61
Hematocrit, %		37
VC, L	2.33	2.31
IC, L	1.56	1.59
TLC, L	3.66	4.53
FEV$_1$, L	1.90	1.59
FEV$_1$/VC, %	81	69
MVV, L/min	73	59
D$_{LCO}$, ml/mm Hg/min	17.6	17.3

TABLE 61-2. *Selected Exercise Data*

MEASUREMENT	PREDICTED	ROOM AIR	OXYGEN
Maximum work rate, W		20	25
Maximum V̇$_{O_2}$, L/min	1.23	0.62	
Maximum HR, beats/min	159	87	85
Maximum O$_2$ pulse, ml/beat	7.8	7.1	
AT, L/min	> 0.61	indeterminate	
Blood pressure, mm Hg (rest, max)		186/90,204/90	172/84,210/102
Maximum V̇$_E$, L/min		38	42
Exercise breathing reserve, L/min	> 15	21	17
Pa$_{O_2}$, mm Hg (rest, max ex)		71,40	550,70
P(A−a)$_{O_2}$, mm Hg (rest, max ex)		42,79	138,612
P(a−ET)$_{CO_2}$, mm Hg (rest, max ex)		5,12	4,9
V$_D$/V$_T$ (rest, heavy ex)		0.31,0.47	0.34,0.47
HCO$_3^-$, mEq/L (rest, 2-min recov)		22,20	22,18

FIG. 61-A. *Air breathing.*

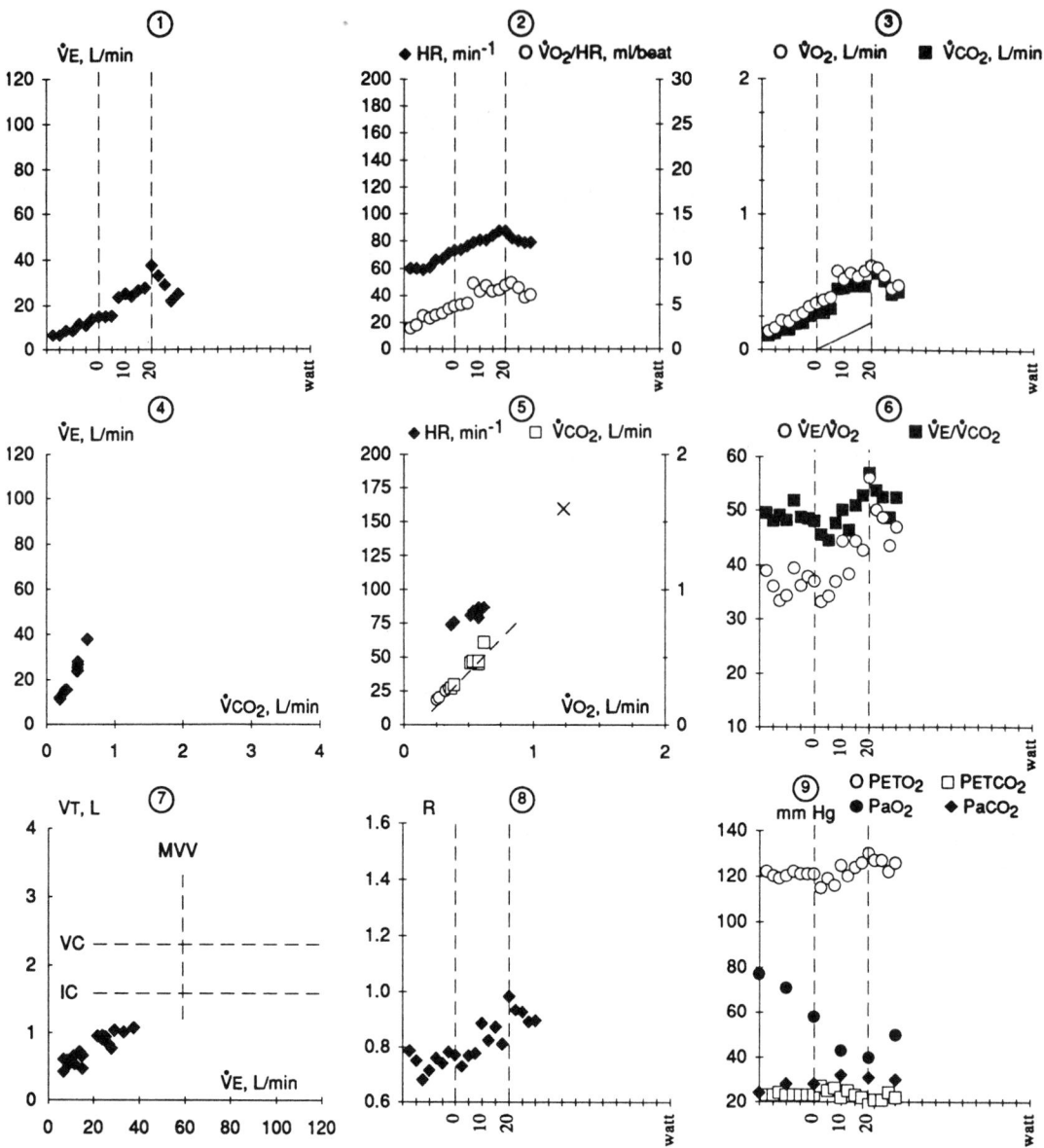

1. Vertical dashed lines in panels 1 to 3 and 6, 8, and 9 indicate the beginning and the end of increasing work period.

2. Unloaded cycling is performed for 3 minutes before the left vertical dashed line.

3. In panel 3, the diagonal line shows the increase of $\dot{V}O_2$ at a slope of 10 ml/min/W.

4. In panel 5, the diagonal dashed line has a slope of 1; the "x" in the upper right is the predicted maximum heart rate and $\dot{V}O_2$ for the subject.

FIG. 61-B. *Oxygen breathing.*

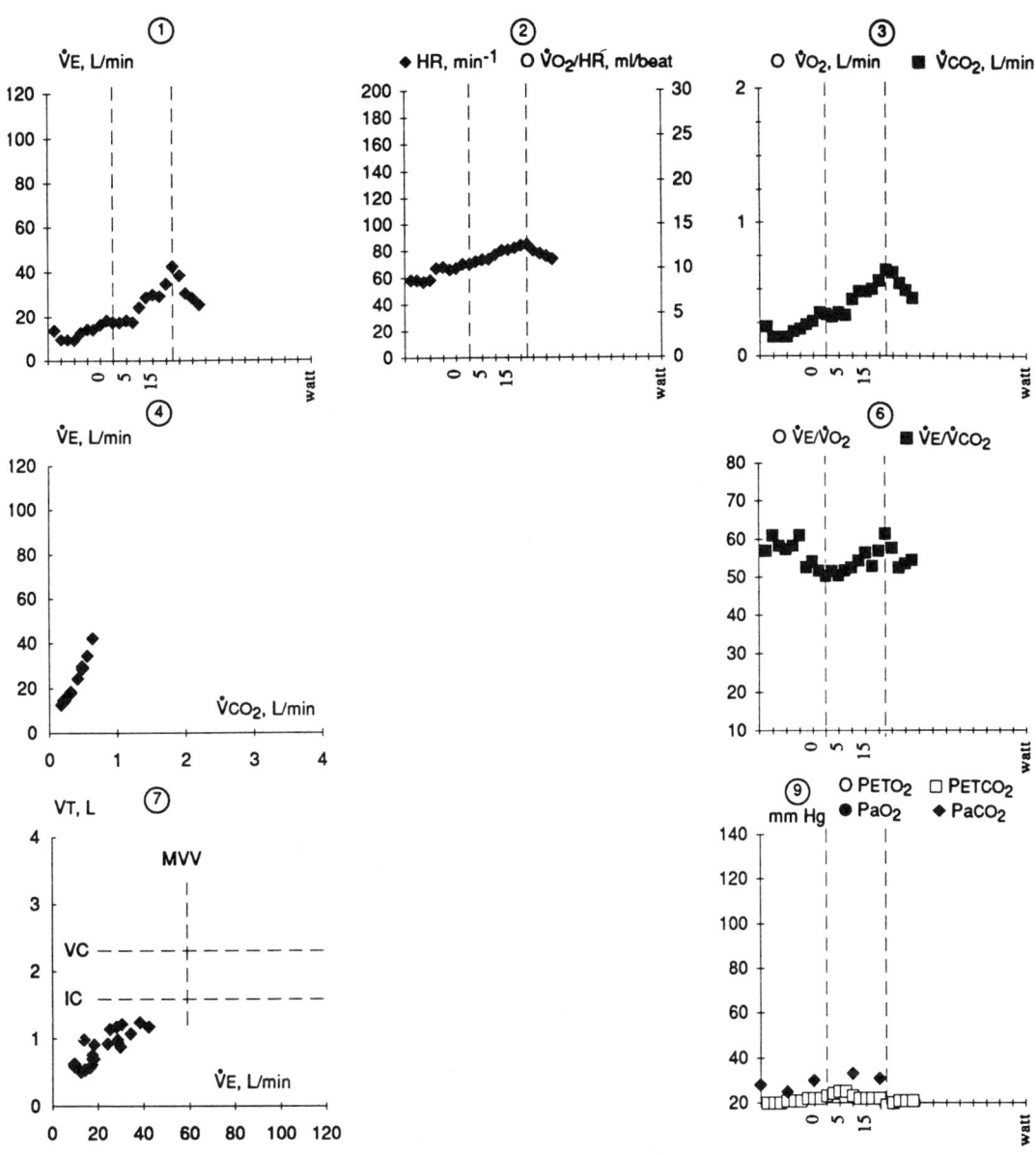

1. Vertical dashed lines in panels 1 to 3 and 6 and 9 indicate the beginning and the end of increasing work period.
2. Unloaded cycling is performed for 3 minutes before the left vertical dashed line.

TABLE 61-3. *Air breathing.*

Time min	Work rate watts	BP mm Hg	HR min⁻¹	f min⁻¹	$\dot{V}E$ L/min BTPS	$\dot{V}CO_2$ L/min STPD	$\dot{V}O_2$ L/min STPD	$\dfrac{\dot{V}O_2}{HR}$ ml/beat	R	pH	HCO₃ meq/L	PO₂, mm Hg ET	a	(A-a)	PCO₂, mm Hg ET	a	(a-ET)	$\dfrac{\dot{V}E}{\dot{V}CO_2}$	$\dfrac{\dot{V}E}{\dot{V}O_2}$	$\dfrac{VD}{VT}$
	Rest	186/90								7.56	21		77			24				
	Rest		60	16	6.8	0.11	0.14	2.3	0.79			122			23			49	39	
	Rest		60	11	6.7	0.12	0.16	2.7	0.75			120			23			48	36	
	Rest		59	17	8.8	0.15	0.22	3.7	0.68			119			24			49	33	
	Rest	206/114	61	14	8.4	0.15	0.21	3.4	0.71	7.52	22	120	71	42	23	28	5	48	34	0.31
	Unloaded		66	22	11.7	0.19	0.25	3.8	0.76			122			23			52	39	
	Unloaded		67	17	11.2	0.20	0.27	4.0	0.74			121			23			49	36	
	Unloaded		71	19	13.7	0.25	0.32	4.5	0.78			121			23			48	38	
	Unloaded	191/94	73	23	14.9	0.27	0.35	4.8	0.77	7.50	21	121	58	57	23	28	5	48	37	0.31
0.5	5		74	32	15.0	0.27	0.37	5.0	0.73			115			27			45	33	
1.0	5		76	23	15.3	0.30	0.39	5.1	0.77			119			25			44	34	
1.5	10		79	26	23.6	0.45	0.58	7.3	0.78			116			26			48	37	
2.0	10	202/96	81	27	25.3	0.46	0.52	6.4	0.88	7.47	23	125	43	72	22	32	10	50	44	0.42
2.5	15		81	25	23.9	0.47	0.57	7.0	0.82			120			25			46	38	
3.0	15		84	32	26.6	0.47	0.54	6.4	0.87			124			23			51	44	
3.5	20		87	36	27.8	0.47	0.58	6.7	0.81			126			22			53	43	
4.0	20	204/90	87	35	37.7	0.61	0.62	7.1	0.98	7.45	21	130	40	79	19	31	12	57	56	0.47
	Recovery		82	33	33.3	0.57	0.61	7.4	0.93			127			21			54	50	
	Recovery		80	28	29.1	0.51	0.55	6.9	0.93			127			21			52	49	
	Recovery		79	23	21.9	0.41	0.46	5.8	0.89			122			24			49	43	
	Recovery	198/87	79	27	24.8	0.43	0.48	6.1	0.90	7.45	20	126	50	67	22	30	8	52	47	0.41

TABLE 61-4. *Oxygen breathing.*

Time min	Work rate watts	BP mm Hg	HR min⁻¹	f min⁻¹	$\dot{V}E$ L/min BTPS	$\dot{V}CO_2$ L/min STPD	$\dot{V}O_2$ L/min STPD	$\dfrac{\dot{V}O_2}{HR}$ ml/beat	R	pH	HCO₃ meq/L	PO₂, mm Hg ET	a	(A-a)	PCO₂, mm Hg ET	a	(a-ET)	$\dfrac{\dot{V}E}{\dot{V}CO_2}$	$\dfrac{\dot{V}E}{\dot{V}O_2}$	$\dfrac{VD}{VT}$
	Rest	171/78								7.50	21		67			28				
	Rest		58	14	13.7	0.22									20			57		
	Rest		58	16	9.9	0.14									20			61		
	Rest		57	16	9.5	0.14									20			58		
	Rest	172/84	58	15	9.3	0.14				7.53	21		550	138	21	25	4	57		0.34
	Unloaded		67	25	12.6	0.18									21			58		
	Unloaded		68	27	14.5	0.20									21			61		
	Unloaded		66	26	14.3	0.23									22			53		
	Unloaded	180/87	67	29	16.5	0.26				7.48	22		386	297	22	30	8	54		0.40
	Unloaded		70	20	18.2	0.32									22			52		
	Unloaded		70	23	17.5	0.31									23			50		
0.5	5		72	28	17.3	0.29									24			51		
1.0	5		73	26	18.3	0.32									25			50		
1.5	10		74	25	17.6	0.30									25			52		
2.0	10	180/84	77	26	24.2	0.42				7.44	22		100	580	23	33	10	52		0.45
2.5	15		80	29	28.5	0.48									22			54		
3.0	15		81	34	29.9	0.48									22			56		
3.5	20		82	31	29.0	0.50									22			53		
4.0	20	210/102	84	32	34.5	0.56				7.45	21		70	612	22	31	9	57		0.47
4.5	25		85	36	42.3	0.64									19			61		
	Recovery		80	31	38.4	0.62									20			58		
	Recovery		78	25	30.5	0.54									21			53		
	Recovery		76	24	28.2	0.49									21			53		
	Recovery	198/92	74	22	25.2	0.43									21			54		

Interpretation

COMMENTS

The results of this patient's resting respiratory function tests show mild airway obstruction (Table 61-1). The ECG is compatible with right ventricular hypertrophy. The exercise test was repeated with the subject breathing 100% oxygen to evaluate the possible development of a right to left shunt through a foramen ovale when exercise-induced right atrial pressure exceeds left atrial pressure—a possible cause of activity-induced hypoxemia, which might contribute to this patient's symptoms.

ANALYSIS

In flow chart 1, the maximum oxygen uptake is reduced while the anaerobic threshold is indeterminate, but probably low. (Table 61-2). See flow chart 4: The breathing reserve is normal (branchpoint 4.1). The $\dot{V}_E/\dot{V}_{CO_2}$ during exercise is high (branchpoint 4.3). The patient is hyperventilating, however, and the arterial CO_2 must be taken into account (see Fig. 3-14), or the indices of ventilation-perfusion mismatching (V_D/V_T, $P(_A-a)_{O_2}$ and $P(a-_{ET})_{CO_2}$) must be directly measured. Because they were measured and, in fact, are high (Table 61-3), the diagnosis of an abnormal pulmonary circulation is made. The abnormal measurements listed under this diagnosis provide confirmation.

At the lowest work rate, Pa_{O_2} abruptly decreases and continues to decrease as the work rate is increased. Moreover, $P(a-_{ET})_{CO_2}$ continues to increase as work rate is increased and the abnormalities in V_D/V_T become progressively more severe (Table 61-3). The changes in Pa_{O_2}, P_{CO_2} and V_D/V_T suggest the development of a right to left shunt during exercise. Clearly, the patient is also oxygen-flow limited in that $\dot{V}_{O_2}$ and oxygen pulse fail to increase with increasing work rate (panels 3 and 2, respectively, Fig. 61-A).

To document that a right to left shunt develops with exercise, Pa_{O_2} was measured at rest and during exercise while the patient was breathing 100% oxygen. At rest, Pa_{O_2} is normal (550 mm Hg); with mild exercise, it drops to 70 mm Hg. This can only be explained by the development of a right to left shunt with exercise (in contrast with Case 60).

Subsequently, the patient had right heart catheterization. Pulmonary artery pressures were confirmed to be at systemic pressure levels; the catheter slipped easily through the foramen ovale into the left atrium.

CONCLUSION

This patient has a pulmonary hypertension with an exercise-induced right to left shunt through the foramen ovale.

CASE 62 *Mild pulmonary vascular disease and systemic hypertension*

CLINICAL FINDINGS

This 66-year-old shipyard worker stated that he was in excellent health. Two weeks prior to evaluation he had had an episode of severe shortness of breath, awakening him from his sleep at a Colorado camp site at 11,000 feet of altitude. He had driven there from Los Angeles in the previous 24 hours. He had had no relief until he was driven down to an altitude of 7000 feet. He had a 40 pack year history of cigarette smoking with a nonproductive cough. He denied other symptoms. The physical examination was normal except for mild obesity. Chest roentgenograms revealed moderate nodular pleural plaques with evidence of minimal pulmonary fibrosis. Resting ECG showed left anterior superior hemiblock.

EXERCISE FINDINGS

The patient performed exercise on a cycle ergometer. He pedalled at 60 rpm without added load for 3 minutes. The work rate was then increased 20 W per minute to his symptom-limited maximum. Arterial blood was sampled every second minute, and intra-arterial blood pressure was recorded from a percutaneously placed brachial artery catheter. The patient stopped exercising because of leg fatigue and shortness of breath. Exercise ECGs were normal except for the appearance of infrequent premature ventricular contractions during the last two work rates.

TABLE 62-1. *Selected Respiratory Function Data*

MEASUREMENT	PREDICTED	MEASURED
Age, yr		66
Sex		Male
Height, cm		178
Weight, kg	80	84
Hematocrit, %		41
VC, L	4.18	3.48
IC, L	2.79	2.96
TLC, L	6.56	5.95
FEV$_1$, L	3.26	2.76
FEV$_1$/VC, %	78	79
MVV, L/min	132	93
D$_{LCO}$, ml/mm Hg/min	25.6	22.7

TABLE 62-2. *Selected Exercise Data*

MEASUREMENT	PREDICTED	MEASURED
Maximum V̇O$_2$, L/min	2.12	1.58
Maximum HR, beats/min	154	141
Maximum O$_2$ pulse, ml/beat	13.7	11.6
ΔV̇O$_2$/ΔWR, ml/min/W	10.3	7.7
AT, L/min	> 0.95	1.1
Blood pressure, mm Hg (rest, max)		167/86,241/104
Maximum V̇E, L/min		70
Exercise breathing reserve, L/min	> 15	23
Pa$_{O_2}$, mm Hg (rest, max ex)		87,90
P(A−a)$_{O_2}$, mm Hg (rest, max ex)		19,23
P(a−ET)$_{CO_2}$, mm Hg (rest, max ex)		−2,3
V$_D$/V$_T$ (rest, heavy ex)		0.38,0.33
HCO$_3^-$, mEq/L (rest, 2-min recov)		24,17

FIG. 62-A.

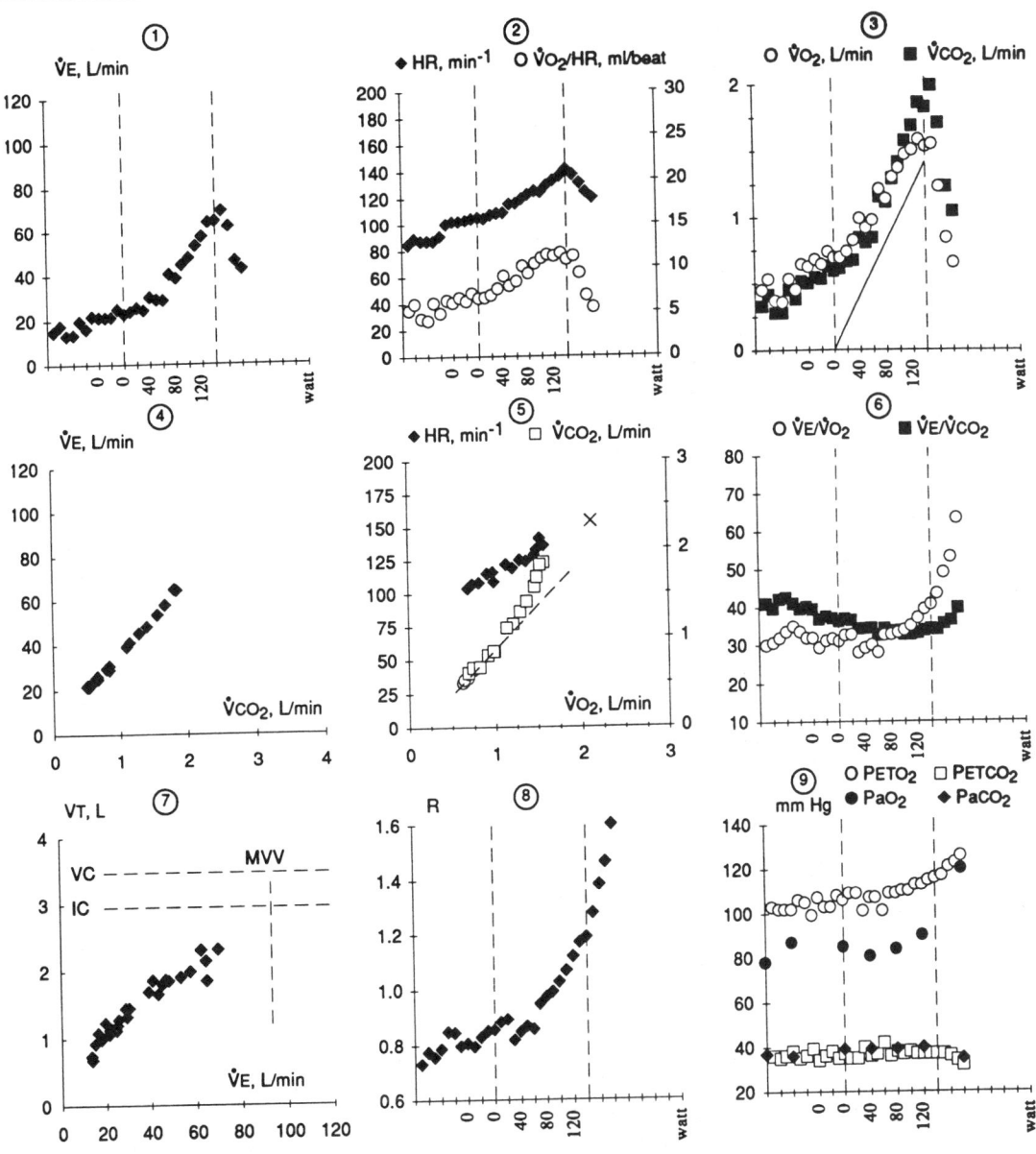

1. Vertical dashed lines in panels 1 to 3 and 6, 8, and 9 indicate the beginning and the end of increasing work period.

2. Unloaded cycling is performed for 3 minutes before the left vertical dashed line.

3. In panel 3, the diagonal line shows the increase of $\dot{V}O_2$ at a slope of 10 ml/min/W.

4. In panel 5, the diagonal dashed line has a slope of 1; the "x" in the upper right is the predicted maximum heart rate and $\dot{V}O_2$ for the subject.

Interpretation

COMMENTS

Results of the resting respiratory function studies show the vital capacity to be at the low end of the normal range (Table 62-1). The resting ECG is slightly abnormal, as noted in "Clinical Findings."

ANALYSIS

In flow chart 1, the maximum $\dot{V}O_2$ is reduced and the anaerobic threshold is normal (Table 62-2). See flow chart 3. The breathing reserve is normal (branchpoint 3.1), and infrequent ventricular premature contractions appear during late exercise (branchpoint 3.3). This gives preference to the di-

TABLE 62-3.

Time min	Work rate watts	BP mm Hg	HR min⁻¹	f min⁻¹	$\dot{V}E$ L/min BTPS	$\dot{V}CO_2$ L/min STPD	$\dot{V}O_2$ L/min STPD	$\dfrac{\dot{V}O_2}{HR}$ ml/beat	R	pH	HCO3 meq/L	PO2, mm Hg ET	a	(A-a)	PCO2, mm Hg ET	a	(a-ET)	$\dfrac{\dot{V}E}{\dot{V}CO_2}$	$\dfrac{\dot{V}E}{\dot{V}O_2}$	$\dfrac{VD}{VT}$
	Rest	167/86								7.42	24	78			37					
	Rest		85	16	14.9	0.33	0.45	5.3	0.73			103			36			41	30	
	Rest		89	18	17.8	0.41	0.53	6.0	0.77			102			35			40	31	
	Rest		87	18	13.3	0.28	0.37	4.3	0.76			102			36			42	32	
	Rest	161/89	87	20	13.6	0.28	0.36	4.1	0.79	7.41	22	102	87	19	38	36	-2	43	33	0.38
	Rest		87	16	19.8	0.45	0.53	6.1	0.85			106			35			41	35	
	Rest		91	15	16.3	0.38	0.45	4.9	0.84			105			36			40	33	
	Unloaded		100	19	22.0	0.51	0.64	6.4	0.80			99			39			40	32	
	Unloaded		102	20	21.4	0.50	0.62	6.1	0.81			107			34			39	32	
	Unloaded		102	19	21.4	0.54	0.68	6.7	0.79			103			36			37	29	
	Unloaded		103	20	21.5	0.53	0.64	6.2	0.83			103			38			37	31	
	Unloaded		104	21	25.1	0.63	0.74	7.1	0.85			108			35			37	32	
	Unloaded	191/95	105	20	23.0	0.59	0.69	6.6	0.86	7.39	23	106	85	21	37	39	2	36	31	0.36
0.5	20		104	21	24.2	0.61	0.69	6.6	0.88			109			35			37	32	
1.0	20		107	20	25.8	0.66	0.74	6.9	0.89			109			35			37	33	
1.5	40		108	22	24.7	0.67	0.82	7.6	0.82			101			40			34	28	
2.0	40	194/92	109	21	30.5	0.84	0.99	9.1	0.85	7.39	23	107	81	24	36	39	3	34	29	0.33
2.5	60		115	22	29.4	0.80	0.92	8.0	0.87			107			37			34	30	
3.0	60		116	20	29.0	0.84	0.98	8.4	0.86			101			42			33	28	
3.5	80		119	22	41.1	1.15	1.21	10.2	0.95			109			36			34	32	
4.0	80	218/98	122	23	39.1	1.11	1.14	9.3	0.97	7.37	22	109	84	26	38	39	1	33	33	0.32
4.5	100		125	25	45.2	1.29	1.30	10.4	0.99			110			37			33	33	
5.0	100		124	26	48.3	1.41	1.37	11.0	1.03			110			38			33	34	
5.5	120		129	28	53.6	1.57	1.47	11.4	1.07			113			37			33	35	
6.0	120	239/98	133	29	57.8	1.68	1.50	11.3	1.12	7.34	21	113	90	23	37	40	3	33	37	0.33
6.5	140		136	30	64.5	1.85	1.58	11.6	1.17			115			37			33	39	
7.0	140	241/104	141	35	65.0	1.82	1.53	10.9	1.19			116			37			34	41	
	Recovery		137	30	69.7	1.98	1.55	11.3	1.28			117			37			34	43	
	Recovery		131	27	62.4	1.70	1.23	9.4	1.38			121			36			35	49	
	Recovery		124	25	46.8	1.23	0.84	6.8	1.46			123			34			36	53	
	Recovery	200/80	120	26	43.3	1.04	0.65	5.4	1.60	7.29	17	126	120	5	32	35	3	40	63	0.36

agnostic box of "myocardial ischemia," rather than "poor effort," especially because the reduced $\Delta\dot{V}O_2/\Delta WR$ strongly suggests a circulatory limitation. Because the VD/VT and $P(a-ET)CO_2$ are elevated, we proceed to flow chart 5, although the $P(A-a)O_2$ is within normal limits (branchpoint 5.1). Taking the abnormal branch, the breathing reserve is found to be normal (branchpoint 5.3). PaO_2 does not decrease with increasing work rate (branchpoint 5.6). The results of these findings are compatible with a circulatory limitation. The ECG is normal except for infrequent premature ventricular contractions. The patient does not have a chronic metabolic acidosis but does develop an acute metabolic acidosis at the highest work rate

performed (Table 62-3). $\Delta\dot{V}O_2/\Delta WR$ is low (Table 62-2), and $\dot{V}O_2$ and O_2 pulse fail to increase as the subject approaches his symptom-limited maximum work rate, confirmatory evidence of a circulatory limitation. The abnormalities in gas exchange at the lung are compatible with pulmonary vascular disease; however, systemic hypertension and peripheral vascular disease might also contribute to the impaired O_2 utilization.

CONCLUSION

This patient has circulatory limitation, mild pulmonary vascular disease possibly secondary to fibrosing alveolitis, and systemic hypertension.

CASE 63 *Pulmonary vascular disease, secondary to interstitial and obstructive lung disease*

CLINICAL FINDINGS

This 70-year-old retired shipyard worker complained of shortness of breath after climbing a flight of stairs. He had a 50 pack year smoking history but had stopped 3 months prior to the evaluation. He took triamterene, hydrochlorothiazide, and methyldopa for hypertension but denied any history of heart or lung disease. The physical examination was not remarkable. Resting ECG showed left axis deviation, left atrial enlargement, and left ventricular hypertrophy. Chest roentgenograms showed moderate pleural thickening with some calcification plus moderate interstitial fibrosis.

EXERCISE FINDINGS

The patient performed exercise on a cycle ergometer. He pedalled at 60 rpm without added load for 3 minutes. The work rate was then increased 15 W per minute to his symptom-limited maximum. Arterial blood was sampled every second minute, and intra-arterial blood pressure was recorded from a percutaneously placed brachial artery catheter. Except for an increase in rate, the ECG pattern remained unchanged during exercise. The patient stopped exercise because of shortness of breath and a dry mouth.

TABLE 63-1. *Selected Respiratory Function Data*

MEASUREMENT	PREDICTED	MEASURED
Age, yr		70
Sex		Male
Height, cm		187
Weight, kg	87	76
Hematocrit, %		47
VC, L	4.69	3.64
IC, L	3.13	2.28
TLC, L	7.39	6.02
FEV_1, L	3.65	2.19
FEV_1/VC, %	78	60
MVV, L/min	140	90
D_{LCO}, ml/mm Hg/min	29.4	10.8

TABLE 63-2. *Selected Exercise Data*

MEASUREMENT	PREDICTED	MEASURED
Maximum $\dot{V}_{O_2}$, L/min	2.01	1.32
Maximum HR, beats/min	150	152
Maximum O_2 pulse, ml/beat	13.4	8.7
$\Delta\dot{V}_{O_2}/\Delta WR$, ml/min/W	10.3	7.4
AT, L/min	> 0.91	0.95
Blood pressure, mm Hg (rest, max)		176/86,227/89
Maximum $\dot{V}_E$, L/min		88
Exercise breathing reserve, L/min	> 15	2
Pa_{O_2}, mm Hg (rest, max ex)		64,52
$P(A-a)_{O_2}$, mm Hg (rest, max ex)		43,68
$P(a-ET)_{CO_2}$, mm Hg (rest, max ex)		6,4
V_D/V_T (rest, heavy ex)		0.45,0.48
HCO_3^-, mEq/L (rest, 2-min recov)		27,19

TABLE 63-3.

Time min	Work rate watts	BP mm Hg	HR min⁻¹	f min⁻¹	V̇E L/min BTPS	V̇CO2 L/min STPD	V̇O2 L/min STPD	V̇O2/HR ml/beat	R	pH	HCO3 meq/L	PO2, mm Hg ET	a	(A-a)	PCO2, mm Hg ET	a	(a-ET)	V̇E/V̇CO2	V̇E/V̇O2	VD/VT
	Rest									7.45	27	59			39					
	Rest	176/86	89	22	18.5	0.35	0.38	4.3	0.92			115			31			48	44	
	Rest		89	22	18.8	0.34	0.37	4.2	0.92			116			30			50	46	
	Rest		88	20	17.0	0.33	0.36	4.1	0.92			115			31			46	43	
	Rest		89	20	16.0	0.30	0.33	3.7	0.91			114			31			48	43	
	Rest		86	20	15.9	0.29	0.31	3.6	0.94			115			31			49	46	
	Rest		88	19	15.2	0.30	0.32	3.6	0.94			115			31			45	42	
	Rest	185/89	90	17	16.7	0.36	0.39	4.3	0.92	7.43	26	111	64	43	34	40	6	42	39	0.45
	Rest		89	22	17.8	0.33	0.35	3.9	0.94			116			30			48	46	
	Unloaded		93	38	30.0	0.49	0.51	5.5	0.96			117			30			55	52	
	Unloaded		95	28	23.1	0.42	0.45	4.7	0.93			115			31			49	46	
	Unloaded		97	30	27.4	0.52	0.57	5.9	0.91			115			30			48	44	
	Unloaded		98	34	31.2	0.57	0.59	6.0	0.97			117			30			50	48	
	Unloaded		98	35	33.5	0.62	0.63	6.4	0.98			117			31			49	48	
	Unloaded	197/89	101	31	32.4	0.65	0.65	6.4	1.00	7.43	26	116	62	48	31	40	9	46	46	0.49
0.5	15		103	38	36.5	0.67	0.65	6.3	1.03			118			30			50	51	
1.0	15		102	33	37.6	0.76	0.74	7.3	1.03			119			30			46	47	
1.5	30		106	44	40.9	0.75	0.73	6.9	1.03			119			30			50	51	
2.0	30	206/86	107	36	41.8	0.85	0.82	7.7	1.04	7.42	24	117	60	53	31	38	7	46	47	0.46
2.5	45		109	42	46.8	0.91	0.90	8.3	1.01			119			30			48	48	
3.0	45		113	53	53.3	0.96	0.92	8.1	1.04			121			28			51	53	
3.5	60		116	52	58.4	1.08	1.01	8.7	1.07			119			29			50	53	
4.0	60	209.86	120	55	66.6	1.24	1.11	9.3	1.12	7.42	25	123	57	57	27	39	12	50	56	0.52
4.5	75		122	55	68.4	1.28	1.13	9.3	1.13			123			28			50	56	
5.0	75		134	53	72.1	1.40	1.21	9.0	1.16			123			28			48	56	
5.5	90		131	57	79.9	1.51	1.25	9.5	1.21			125			27			50	60	
6.0	90	221/92	134	54	72.4	1.45	1.22	9.1	1.19	7.40	23	121	53	65	30	37	7	47	56	0.47
6.5	105		143	60	84.7	1.64	1.33	9.3	1.23			125			27			49	60	
7.0	105	227/89	152	60	87.5	1.68	1.32	8.7	1.27	7.38	21	125	52	68	32	36	4	49	62	0.48
	Recovery		136	45	72.4	1.57	1.24	9.1	1.27			123			30			44	55	
	Recovery		131	39	64.1	1.39	1.08	8.2	1.29			123			30			44	56	
	Recovery		126	37	56.0	1.18	0.89	7.1	1.33			125			29			45	59	
	Recovery	233/98	122	34	48.1	1.03	0.76	6.2	1.36	7.34	19	121	74	47	34	36	2	44	59	0.43

Interpretation

COMMENTS

This case is presented because of its mixed pathophysiologic features. Despite the patient's denial of a history of lung disease, the results of his respiratory function studies indicate that he has mild to moderate obstructive as well as mild restrictive lung disease as evidenced by the reduced FEV_1/VC, total lung capacity, and vital capacity. Accompanying these changes is a marked reduction in diffusing capacity (Table 63-1). The resting ECG reflects changes associated with long-standing systemic hypertension, for which he is being treated.

ANALYSIS

In flow chart 1, the maximum $\dot{V}O_2$ is reduced and the anaerobic threshold is borderline normal (Table 63-2). See flow chart 3. The breathing reserve is low (branchpoint 3.1), whereas the findings of a high VD/VT, $P(a-ET)_{CO_2}$, and $P(A-a)_{O_2}$ support the diagnosis of "lung disease." The heart rate reserve is negative, not high, however. The high breathing frequency during most of the exercise period (branchpoint 3.2) is more typical of re-

FIG. 63-A.

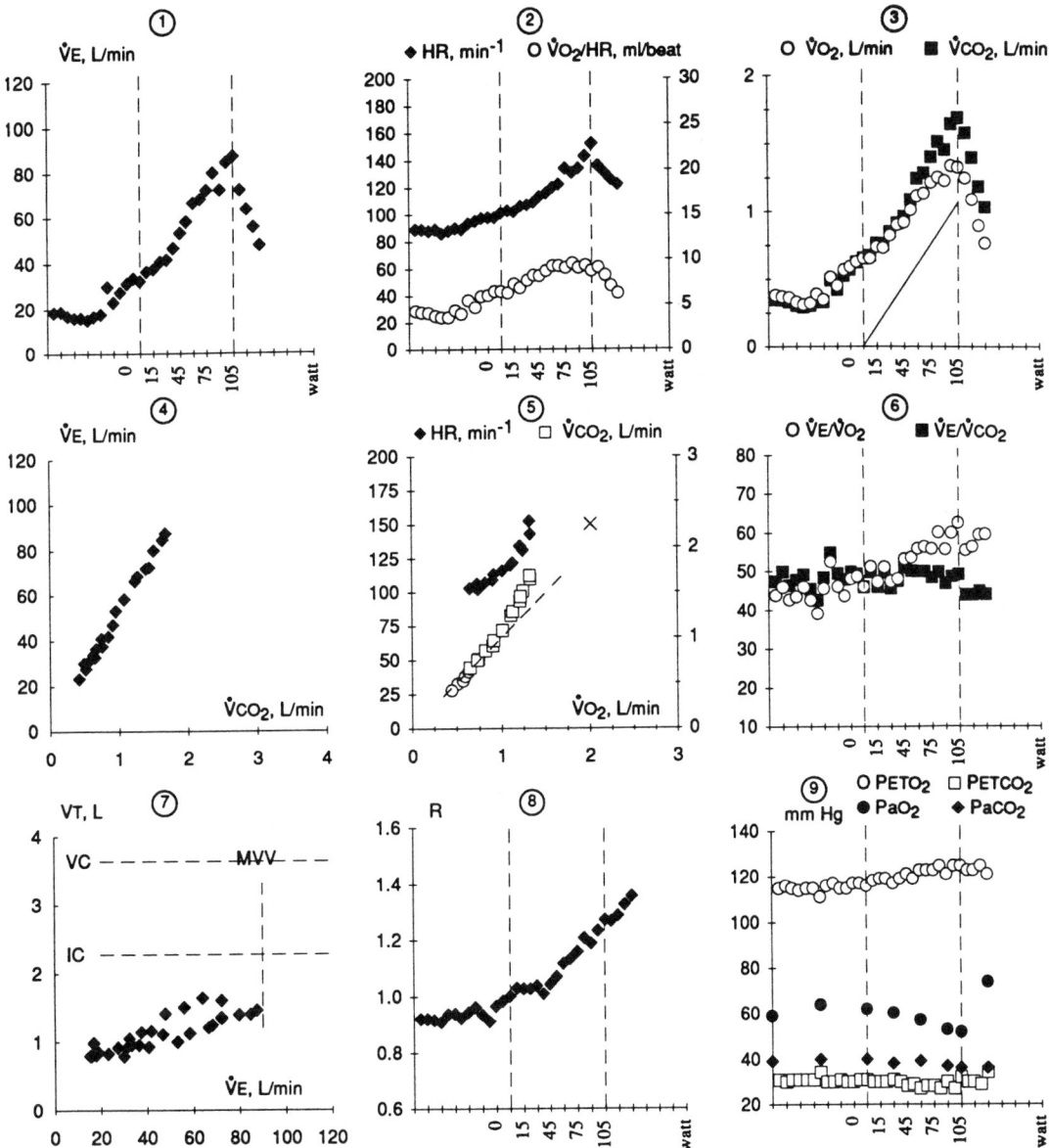

1. Vertical dashed lines in panels 1 to 3 and 6, 8, and 9 indicate the beginning and the end of increasing work period.
2. Unloaded cycling is performed for 3 minutes before the left vertical dashed line.
3. In panel 3, the diagonal line shows the increase of $\dot{V}O_2$ at a slope of 10 ml/min/W.
4. In panel 5, the diagonal dashed line has a slope of 1; the "x" in the upper right is the predicted maximum heart rate and $\dot{V}O_2$ for the subject.

strictive than obstructive lung disease, although the patient manifests both disorders at rest. We must also consider the patient's other exercise findings. The plateau in $\dot{V}O_2$ and O_2 pulse as well as the low $\Delta\dot{V}O_2/\Delta WR$, low heart rate reserve, and progressive hypoxemia are all characteristic of pulmonary vascular disease secondary to interstitial lung disease (see flow chart 4 (abnormal pulmonary circulation) or flow chart 5 (pulmonary vascular disease) for details).

CONCLUSION

Pulmonary vascular disease has limited exercise performance, probably secondary to interstitial lung disease.

CASE 64 *Pulmonary arterio-venous fistulae*

CLINICAL FINDINGS

This 26-year-old man with multiple pulmonary arterio-venous malformations and recurrent brain abscesses was referred for exercise testing to assess his pathophysiologic status before undergoing embolization therapy. He denied shortness of breath and until recently had worked as an aerobics instructor. The patient was well developed muscularly, without rales or murmurs, but with marked clubbing and cyanosis. A recent study while the patient was at rest breathing oxygen showed a calculated right to left shunt of 53%.

EXERCISE FINDINGS

The patient performed exercise on a cycle ergometer. He pedalled at 60 rpm without an added load for 3 minutes. The work rate was then increased continuously at a rate of 20 W per minute to tolerance. Blood was sampled every second minute, and intra-arterial pressure was recorded from a percutaneously placed brachial artery catheter. Heart rate and rhythm were continuously monitored; 12-lead ECGs were obtained during rest, exercise, and recovery. The patient appeared to give an excellent effort and stopped exercise because of general and leg fatigue, without dyspnea or chest pain. No arrhythmias or ischemic changes were noted on ECGs.

TABLE 64-1. *Selected Respiratory Function Data*

MEASUREMENT	PREDICTED	MEASURED
Age, yr		26
Sex		Male
Height, cm		189
Weight, kg	87	64
Hemoglobin, g/100 ml		21.8
VC, L	5.55	4.18
IC, L	3.70	2.94
FEV$_1$, L	4.50	3.95
FEV$_1$/VC, %	81	94
MVV, L/min		
direct	183	169
indirect	180	158

TABLE 64-2. *Selected Exercise Data*

MEASUREMENT	PREDICTED	MEASURED
Maximum $\dot{V}O_2$, L/min	3.12	2.19
Maximum HR, beats/min	194	160
Maximum O_2 pulse, ml/beat	16.1	13.7
$\Delta \dot{V}O_2/\Delta WR$, ml/min/W	10.3	9.9
AT, L/min	> 1.28	1.5
Blood pressure, mm Hg (rest, max)		144/84,180/90
Maximum $\dot{V}E$, L/min		123
Exercise breathing reserve, L/min	> 15	35
Sa_{O_2}, % (rest, max ex)		76,64
Pa_{O_2}, mm Hg (rest, max ex)		39,39
$P(A-a)_{O_2}$, mm Hg (rest, max ex)		74,76
$P(a-ET)_{CO_2}$, mm Hg (rest, max ex)		9,15
V_D/V_T (rest, max ex)		0.42,0.52
HCO_3^-, mEq/L (rest, 2-min recov)		22,16

TABLE 64-3.

Time min	Work rate watts	BP mm Hg	HR min⁻¹	f min⁻¹	$\dot{V}E$ L/min BTPS	$\dot{V}CO_2$ L/min STPD	$\dot{V}O_2$ L/min STPD	$\dfrac{\dot{V}O_2}{HR}$ ml/beat	R	pH	HCO₃ meq/L	PO2, mm Hg ET	a	(A-a)	PCO2, mm Hg ET	a	(a-ET)	$\dfrac{\dot{V}E}{\dot{V}CO_2}$	$\dfrac{\dot{V}E}{\dot{V}O_2}$	$\dfrac{VD}{VT}$
	Rest									7.43	22		51			33				
	Rest		92	21	22.8	0.38	0.43	4.7	0.88			124	;		22			55	49	
	Rest		92	21	22.8	0.38	0.43	4.7	0.88			121			22			55	49	
	Rest		92	21	22.8	0.38	0.43	4.7	0.88			124			22			55	49	
	Rest		78	28	18.5	0.31	0.37	4.7	0.84	7.45	22	121	39	74	23	32	9	52	44	0.42
	Rest		83	21	18.6	0.31	0.35	4.2	0.89			123			22			54	48	
	Rest		87	23	17.0	0.27	0.31	3.6	0.87			120			24			56	49	
	Unloaded		88	23	19.1	0.31	0.35	4.0	0.89			124			21			55	49	
	Unloaded		104	29	23.8	0.46	0.61	5.9	0.75			118			24			46	35	
	Unloaded		90	31	30.1	0.59	0.76	8.4	0.78			118			25			47	36	
	Unloaded		86	30	31.3	0.61	0.73	8.5	0.84			120			25			47	39	
	Unloaded		90	30	36.0	0.68	0.80	8.9	0.85			120			25			49	42	
	Unloaded	144/84	91	26	29.9	0.61	0.73	8.0	0.84	7.43	22	118	38	73	30	34	4	45	38	0.41
0.5	10		91	31	38.8	0.74	0.88	9.7	0.84			120			25			49	41	
1.0	20		92	27	32.4	0.66	0.78	8.5	0.85			119			25			46	39	
1.5	30		94	29	36.1	0.72	0.84	8.9	0.86			120			26			47	40	
2.0	40	150/90	96	27	37.2	0.81	0.95	9.9	0.85	7.42	22	118	39	72	25	34	9	43	37	0.39
2.5	50		97	30	40.4	0.85	0.98	10.1	0.87			121			24			45	39	
3.0	60		100	33	40.2	0.90	1.03	10.3	0.87			119			25			42	36	
3.5	70		103	32	40.6	0.94	1.06	10.3	0.89			120			26			40	36	
4.0	80	162/90	102	34	46.2	0.95	1.09	10.7	0.87	7.42	22	121	39	73	25	34	9	46	40	0.42
4.5	90		111	32	58.2	1.16	1.24	11.2	0.94			119			26			48	45	
5.0	100		111	36	63.6	1.25	1.28	11.5	0.98			123			24			48	47	
5.5	110		115	35	63.7	1.30	1.35	11.7	0.96			119			27			47	45	
6.0	120	174/96	122	38	69.0	1.42	1.44	11.8	0.99	7.38	20	124	39	76	24	35	11	46	46	0.45
6.5	130		127	39	73.7	1.54	1.53	12.0	1.01			124			25			46	46	
7.0	140		136	44	90.2	1.78	1.70	12.5	1.05			126			23			49	51	
7.5	150		161	43	92.9	1.90	1.80	11.2	1.06			126			24			47	50	
8.0	160	180/90	149	41	91.5	1.93	1.84	12.3	1.05	7.36	20	121	39	76	27	36	9	46	48	0.46
8.5	170		154	53	115.0	2.23	2.03	13.2	1.10			125			24			50	54	
9.0	180	180/96	160	53	123.3	2.42	2.19	13.7	1.11	7.31	19	127	39	76	23	38	15	49	54	0.52
	Recovery		162	49	115.0	2.12	1.84	11.4	1.15			129			28			52	60	
	Recovery		140	45	106.9	1.75	1.37	9.8	1.28			132			20			59	75	
	Recovery		125	41	86.4	1.32	0.99	7.9	1.33			134			18			63	84	
	Recovery	156/84	124	41	73.7	1.15	0.88	7.1	1.31	7.30	16	134	43	79	19	34	15	61	80	0.56

Fig. 64-A.

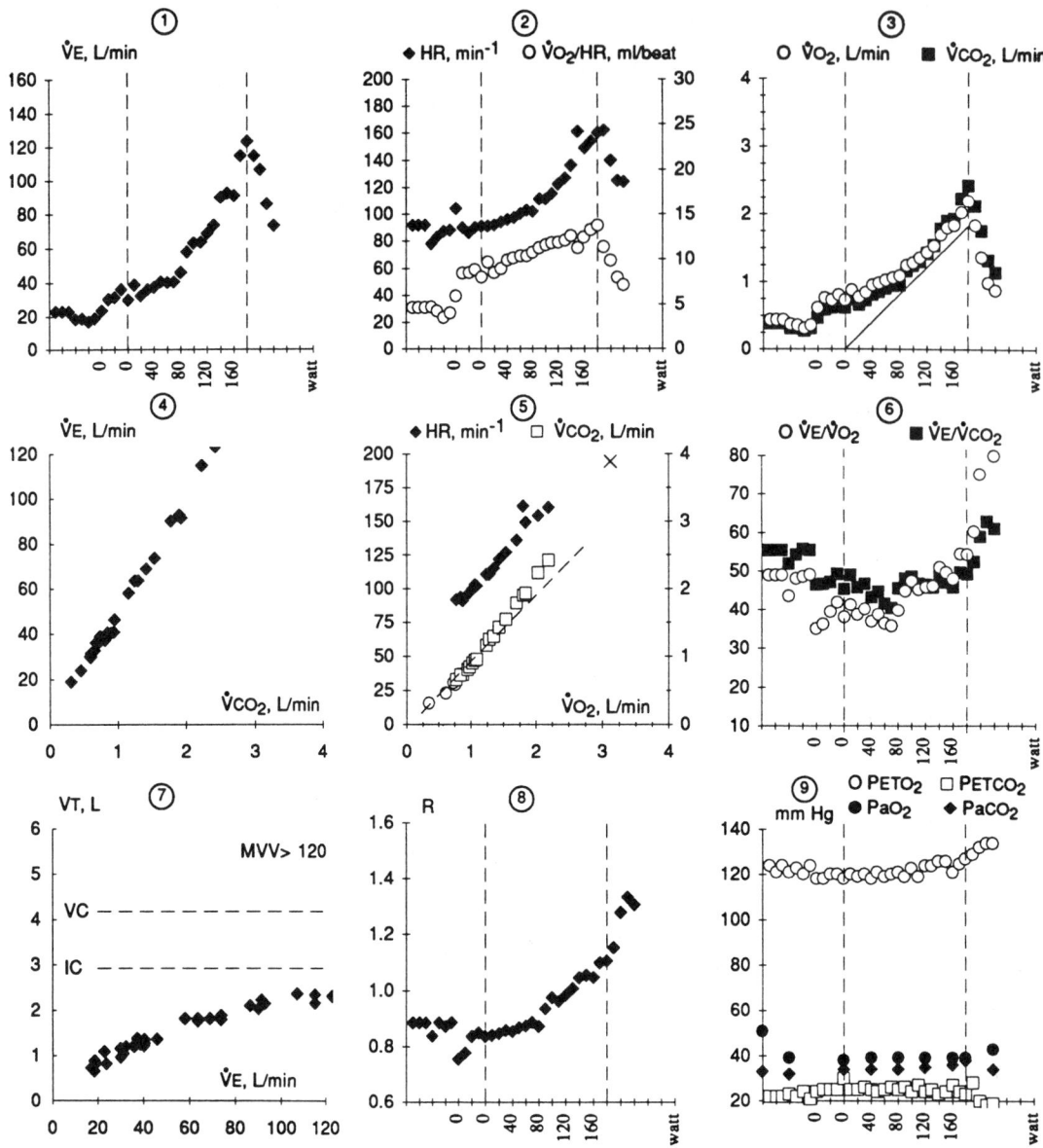

1. Vertical dashed lines in panels 1 to 3 and 6, 8, and 9 indicate the beginning and the end of increasing work period.

2. Unloaded cycling is performed for 3 minutes before the left vertical dashed line.

3. In panel 3, the diagonal line shows the increase of $\dot{V}O_2$ at a slope of 10 ml/min/W.

4. In panel 5, the diagonal dashed line has a slope of 1; the "x" in the upper right is the predicted maximum heart rate and $\dot{V}O_2$ for the subject.

Interpretation

COMMENTS

Resting respiratory function studies showed restrictive lung disease with good ventilatory ability. The patient was thin, cyanotic, and polycythemic. Resting arterial blood analysis showed hypoxemia and a chronic respiratory alkalosis.

ANALYSIS

In flow chart 1, the maximum $\dot{V}O_2$ is low, but the anaerobic threshold is normal (Table 64-2). Also striking are the severe hypoxemia, low P_{ETCO_2}, and high V_D/V_T. We are directed through branchpoints 1.1 1.2, and 1.3 to flow chart 3, which leads us through branchpoints 3.1 and 3.3 to "poor effort or musculo-skeletal disorder," which does not fit well with the patient's known findings. Using flow chart 4, the normal breathing reserve (branchpoint 4.1) and the high $\dot{V}E/\dot{V}CO_2$ (branchpoint 4.3) lead us to "abnormal pulmonary circulation," where the patient meets most of the criteria. If we had used flow chart 5, we would have arrived through branchpoints 5.1 and 5.3 at branchpoint 5.6 at "pulmonary vascular disease." The low O_2 saturation during persistent exercise confirms a large right to left shunt.

The finding of a lower than predicted O_2 pulse is of interest, especially in view of the high O_2 capacity (30.8 ml/100 ml versus the normal 21 ml/100 ml). Because of the low arterial saturation, arterial content is only approximately 20 ml/100 ml.

Likely, mixed venous O_2 saturation is normal, resulting in a higher than normal content (because of the polycythemia). Thus, the patient has no evidence of reduced ventricular stroke volume or reduced cardiac output. Clearly, much of the right ventricular output bypasses the aerated alveoli. Therefore, the blood that goes through the pulmonary capillaries must be exposed to alveoli with low P_{CO_2} values for the systemic arterial values that receive venous blood to have Pa_{CO_2} as low as 33 or 35 mm Hg. Thus, the P_{ACO_2} and P_{ETCO_2} values are extremely low, and the V_D/V_T values are extremely high. In this patient, these findings indicate an abnormal pulmonary circulation, not necessarily pulmonary hypertension. Finally, the high exercise breathing frequency and V_T/IC are typical of restrictive lung disease.

CONCLUSION

The patient has a large right to left shunt at rest and at exercise because of pulmonary arterio-venous malformations. The high V_D/V_T values and positive $P(a - ET)_{CO_2}$ indicate that ventilation is relatively ineffective in removing CO_2 from the blood, consistent with a high fraction of right ventricular output bypassing the alveolar capillaries. In this patient, the wide $P(A - a)_{O_2}$, positive $P(a - ET)_{CO_2}$, and high V_D/V_T, which increase with exercise, indicate a large shunt rather than the ordinary maldistribution of ventilation found in many others with lung diseases.

CASE 65 *Poor effort*

CLINICAL FINDINGS

This 37-year-old male electrician was referred for evaluation because of his 5-year exposure to asbestos while working in a shipyard. He stated that he had had a daily productive cough for a year and that he could only climb 6 or 7 steps before he had to stop to catch his breath. He stated that he had smoked approximately half a package of cigarettes daily for the last 13 years. He denied other problems and took no medications. Physical and chest roentgenographic examinations were normal.

EXERCISE FINDINGS

The patient performed exercise on a cycle ergometer. He pedalled at 60 rpm without an added load for 3 minutes. The work rate was then increased 25 W per minute to his symptom-limited maximum. Blood was sampled every second minute, and intra-arterial blood pressure was recorded from a percutaneously passed brachial artery catheter. The patient was apprehensive and was unhappy about having a test performed. He breathed rapidly and shallowly on the mouthpiece despite reassurance and encouragement. He slowed his pedalling frequency after 2 minutes of incremental work and stopped pedalling at a work rate of 100 W, complaining of generalized fatigue, tingling in the hands, and lightheadedness. These symptoms resolved within 5 minutes. After an hour of rest, explanation, and encouragement to breathe at a slower rate, the test was repeated using an increment of 20 W/min. This time, the patient began to hyperventilate as soon as exercise began. He stopped cycling at a work rate of 60 W with a heart rate of 99. Complete data from the first test and selected data from the second test are presented. Resting and exercise ECGs were normal.

TABLE 65-1. *Selected Respiratory Function Data*

MEASUREMENT	PREDICTED	MEASURED
Age, yr		37
Sex		Male
Height, cm		170
Weight, kg	80	87
Hematocrit, %		46
VC, L	4.52	4.20
IC, L	3.01	3.07
TLC, L	6.29	5.29
FEV$_1$, L	3.64	3.66
FEV$_1$/VC, %	81	87
MVV, L/min	152	129
D$_{LCO}$, ml/mm Hg/min	29.9	24.7

TABLE 65-2. *Selected Exercise Data*

MEASUREMENT	PREDICTED	MEASURED
Maximum $\dot{V}O_2$, L/min	3.00	1.43
Maximum HR, beats/min	183	112
Maximum O_2 pulse, ml/beat	16.4	12.8
$\Delta\dot{V}O_2/\Delta WR$, ml/min/W	10.3	10.1
AT, L/min	> 1.26	indeterminate
Blood pressure, mm Hg (rest, max ex)		146/93,174/105
Maximum $\dot{V}E$, L/min		64
Exercise breathing reserve, L/min	> 15	65
Pa$_{O_2}$, mm Hg (rest, max ex)		89,117
P(a−a)$_{O_2}$ mm Hg (rest, max ex)		6,7
P(a−ET)$_{CO_2}$, mm Hg (rest, max ex)		0,−3
V$_D$/V$_T$ (rest, max ex)		0.37,0.19
HCO$_3^-$, mEq/L (rest, recov)		23,20
Carboxyhemoglobin, rest, %		6.5

TABLE 65-3.

Time min	Work rate watts	BP mm Hg	HR min⁻¹	f min⁻¹	V̇E L/min BTPS	V̇CO2 L/min STPD	V̇O2 L/min STPD	V̇O2/HR ml/beat	R	pH	HCO3 meq/L	PO2, mm Hg ET	a	(A-a)	PCO2, mm Hg ET	a	(a-ET)	V̇E/V̇CO2	V̇E/V̇O2	VD/VT
	Rest	146/93								7.42	23		95			36				
	Rest		72	37	20.9	0.41	0.39	5.4	1.05			117			33			43	46	
	Rest		73	31	15.1	0.29	0.32	4.4	0.91			109			36			43	39	
	Rest		73	32	9.8	0.16	0.21	2.9	0.76			104			38			44	34	
	Rest	153/102	73	29	11.3	0.20	0.32	4.4	0.63	7.41	23	97	89	6	37	37	0	44	28	0.37
	Rest		74	26	12.8	0.27	0.40	5.4	0.68			95			38			39	26	
	Rest		77	31	15.8	0.33	0.46	6.0	0.72			96			38			40	29	
	Unloaded		82	33	30.3	0.72	0.69	8.4	1.04			115			32			38	40	
	Unloaded		88	42	33.3	0.71	0.61	6.9	1.16			122			30			42	49	
	Unloaded		90	49	45.5	0.90	0.68	7.6	1.32			127			28			46	61	
	Unloaded		85	50	45.7	0.88	0.67	7.9	1.31			127			27			47	62	
	Unloaded		85	57	39.6	0.68	0.51	6.0	1.33			129			25			51	68	
	Unloaded		85	50	33.0	0.58	0.49	5.8	1.18			126			25			50	59	
	Unloaded	168/105	85	53	38.7	0.66	0.54	6.4	1.22	7.52	21	128	122	6	24	26	2	52	63	0.32
	Unloaded		83	54	45.6	0.79	0.65	7.8	1.22			129			23			52	63	
0.5	25		88	54	47.2	0.79	0.65	7.4	1.22			128			23			54	66	
1.0	25		89	56	60.6	0.99	0.79	8.9	1.25			127			24			56	71	
1.5	50		94	59	62.8	1.06	0.92	9.8	1.15			130			21			55	63	
2.0	50	168/102	94	54	54.7	0.97	0.95	10.1	1.02	7.56	19	126	123	5	23	22	-1	52	53	0.22
2.5	75		103	51	61.9	1.13	1.09	10.6	1.04			123			25			51	53	
3.0	75		103	51	62.9	1.19	1.15	11.2	1.03			126			23			49	51	
3.5	100		110	46	53.2	1.13	1.21	11.0	0.93			114			30			44	41	
4.0	100	174/105	112	46	64.0	1.39	1.43	12.8	0.97	7.52	20	120	117	7	28	25	-3	43	42	0.19
	Recovery		96	47	52.5	1.13	1.20	12.5	0.94			119			28			43	40	
	Recovery		86	46	45.4	0.91	0.90	10.5	1.01			122			27			46	46	
	Recovery		79	52	46.6	0.77	0.61	7.7	1.26			130			22			55	69	
	Recovery	168/108	78	43	34.9	0.55	0.45	5.8	1.22	7.54	20	130	126	3	22	24	2	57	69	0.33

TABLE 65-4. *Selected Measures Early in Second Study*

TIME (min)	WORK RATE	f (/min)	V̇E (L/min)	R	pH	Paco2 (mm Hg)	HCO3⁻ (mEq/L)
0					7.42	34	22
0.5	rest	32	26.6	1.08			
1	rest	29	16.6	1.00			
1.5	rest	22	17.7	0.97			
2	rest	22	12.2	0.77	7.45	29	20
2.5	rest	23	12.3	0.71			
3	rest	25	18.3	0.80			
3.5	unloaded	35	30.9	0.93			
4	unloaded	39	34.9	1.07			
4.5	unloaded	37	32.6	0.95			
5	unloaded	46	44.5	1.08			
5.5	unloaded	51	55.7	1.18			
6	unloaded	49	51.0	1.14	7.57	21	19

Interpretation

COMMENTS

Resting respiratory function was normal; the normal inspiratory capacity and low expiratory reserve volume are typical of obesity rather than intrinsic restrictive lung disease.

ANALYSIS

In flow chart 1, the maximum V̇O2 was low, and the anaerobic threshold was indeterminate (Table 65-2). This leads us to flow chart 5, where we note that gas exchange was normal (branchpoint 5.1), the heart rate reserve was high (branchpoint 5.2), and the breathing reserve was high (branchpoint 5.5). The ΔV̇O2/ΔWR was normal (branchpoint 5.8), leading to the diagnosis of poor effort. The normal ECG, minimal decline in HCO3⁻, and R < 1.0 at exercise cessation all signify the absence of cardiac ischemia or significant metabolic acidosis. Thus, we can safely conclude that the evaluee gave a poor effort. We were unable to encourage him to improve his performance when tested an hour later. The abrupt hyperventilation and respiratory alkalosis early in the second study (Table 65-4) are typical of patients with anxiety or voluntary hyperventilation. An irregular breathing pat-

FIG. 65-A.

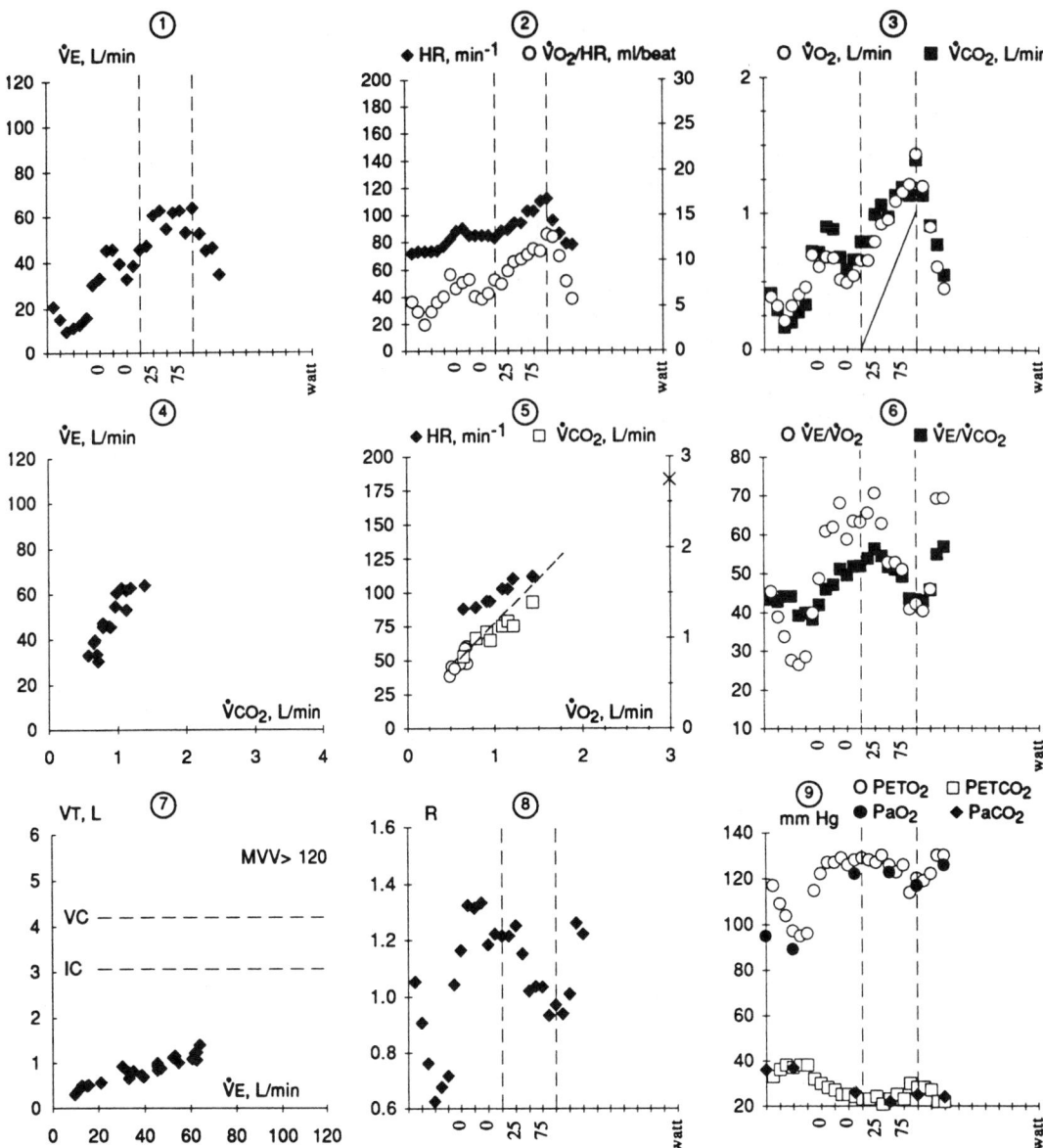

1. Vertical dashed lines in panels 1 to 3 and 6, 8, and 9 indicate the beginning and the end of increasing work period.

2. Unloaded cycling is performed for 3 minutes before the left vertical dashed line.

3. In panel 3, the diagonal line shows the increase of $\dot{V}O_2$ at a slope of 10 ml/min/W.

4. In panel 5, the diagonal dashed line has a slope of 1; the "x" in the upper right is the predicted maximum heart rate and $\dot{V}O_2$ for the subject.

tern is more consistent with volitional lack of cooperation.

CONCLUSION

This case study shows poor effort on the part of the patient. No evidence indicated abnormal gas exchange, ventilatory limitation, metabolic acidosis or cardiovascular limitation. The symptoms and findings are typical of acute respiratory alkalosis of variable degree. Because of the high ventilatory equivalents that might suggest a gas exchange abnormality, blood gas analysis is helpful in excluding ventilation-perfusion mismatching.

CASE 66 *Poor effort*

CLINICAL FINDINGS

This 59-year-old shipyard worker had been made aware of an abnormality in his chest x-ray 1 year prior to evaluation. Retrospectively, he felt that he had had some shortness of breath for 2 years when jogging or climbing stairs. He had smoked cigarettes for 20 years, until age 35. Results of physical, laboratory, and roentgenographic examinations were normal except for prostatic enlargement and extensive pleural calcification.

EXERCISE FINDINGS

The patient performed exercise on a cycle ergometer. He pedalled at 60 rpm without added load for 3 minutes. The work rate was then increased 20 W per minute to his symptom-limited maximum. Arterial blood was sampled every second minute, and intra-arterial blood pressure was recorded from a percutaneously placed brachial artery catheter. The patient pedalled irregularly during the test. He stopped pedalling, complaining of shortness of breath and leg fatigue, and stated he could go no further. Resting and exercise ECG were normal.

TABLE 66-1. *Selected Respiratory Function Data*

MEASUREMENT	PREDICTED	MEASURED
Age, yr		59
Sex		Male
Height, cm		173
Weight, kg	76	72
Hematocrit, %		44
VC, L	3.65	3.05
IC, L	2.44	2.44
TLC, L	5.57	4.93
FEV$_1$, L	2.87	2.49
FEV$_1$/VC, %	79	82
MVV, L/min	121	110
D$_{LCO}$, ml/mm Hg/min	22.6	24.6

TABLE 66-2. *Selected Exercise Data*

MEASUREMENT	PREDICTED	MEASURED
Maximum V̇$_{O_2}$, L/min	2.13	1.08
Maximum HR, beats/min	161	110
Maximum O$_2$ pulse, ml/beat	13.2	9.8
AT, L/min	> 0.94	indeterminate
Blood pressure, mm Hg (rest, max)		135/78,144/78
Maximum V̇$_E$, L/min		30
Exercise breathing reserve, L/min	> 15	80
Pa$_{O_2}$, mm Hg (rest, max ex)		98,96
P(A − a)$_{O_2}$, mm Hg (rest, max ex)		0,10
P(a − ET)$_{CO_2}$, mm Hg (rest, max ex)		0, −3
V$_D$/V$_T$ (rest, heavy ex)		0.35,0.36
HCO$_3^-$, mEq/L (rest, 2-min recov)		25,24

TABLE 66-3.

Time min	Work rate watts	BP mm Hg	HR min⁻¹	f min⁻¹	$\dot{V}E$ L/min BTPS	$\dot{V}CO_2$ L/min STPD	$\dot{V}O_2$ L/min STPD	$\frac{\dot{V}O_2}{HR}$ ml/beat	R	pH	HCO₃ meq/L	PO2, mm Hg ET	a	(A-a)	PCO2, mm Hg ET	a	(a-ET)	$\frac{\dot{V}E}{\dot{V}CO_2}$	$\frac{\dot{V}E}{\dot{V}O_2}$	VD VT
	Rest	135/78								7.51	24	118			30					
	Rest		73	19	8.2	0.17	0.23	3.2	0.74			97			39			39	29	
	Rest		76	14	4.9	0.11	0.15	2.0	0.73			96			39			34	25	
	Rest		76	19	8.7	0.19	0.26	3.4	0.73			97			40			37	27	
	Rest	132/78	78	20	11.2	0.26	0.36	4.6	0.72	7.41	25	95	98	0	40	40	0	37	26	0.35
	Rest		78	19	9.0	0.18	0.24	3.1	0.75			101			39			41	31	
	Rest		83	18	12.3	0.32	0.41	4.9	0.78			99			39			34	26	
	Unloaded		89	26	14.5	0.37	0.47	5.3	0.79			97			41			33	26	
	Unloaded		90	29	17.6	0.42	0.57	6.3	0.74			100			39			36	27	
	Unloaded		92	27	18.6	0.47	0.55	6.0	0.85			106			38			35	30	
	Unloaded		90	32	21.9	0.49	0.53	5.9	0.92			112			40			39	36	
	Unloaded		87	37	23.1	0.51	0.50	5.7	1.02			112			36			39	40	
	Unloaded	144/78	87	26	23.5	0.55	0.50	5.7	1.10	7.43	23	115	104	13	35	36	1	39	43	0.34
0.5	20		89	29	17.2	0.44	0.49	5.5	0.90			102			40			33	30	
1.0	20		95	20	14.3	0.41	0.50	5.3	0.82			95			40			31	25	
1.5	40		100	23	17.4	0.52	0.67	6.7	0.78			92			44			30	23	
2.0	40	144/78	101	36	25.0	0.58	0.68	6.7	0.85	7.41	24	98	96	10	42	39	-3	38	32	0.36
2.5	60		110	25	29.7	0.89	1.08	9.8	0.82			91			44			31	26	
	Recovery	150/78	97	25	26.2	0.67	0.65	6.7	1.03	7.41	23	110	102	12	37	37	0	36	37	0.32
	Recovery		93	31	18.6	0.46	0.46	4.9	1.00			107			40			35	35	
	Recovery		88	38	16.0	0.32	0.33	3.8	0.97			105			40			40	39	
	Recovery		81	28	18.5	0.37	0.35	4.3	1.06			115			34			44	46	
	Recovery		84	30	14.5	0.27	0.28	3.3	0.96			110			37			44	43	
	Recovery	132/84	82	30	15.4	0.28	0.30	3.7	0.93	7.41	24	113	94	16	34	38	4	46	43	0.42
	Recovery		88	16	11.0	0.25	0.27	3.1	0.93			113			35			39	36	

Interpretation

COMMENTS

Resting respiratory function (Table 66-1) is within normal limits.

ANALYSIS

In flow chart 1, the maximum $\dot{V}O_2$ is significantly reduced and the anaerobic threshold is indeterminate (Table 66-2). See flow chart 5. The resting VD/VT is normal, but it does not decrease appropriately during exercise. Only light exercise was performed, however, and the lack of a decrease might be spurious owing to the low tidal volume, tachypnea, and low work rate performed (Table 66-3). Because $P(a-ET)CO_2$ and $P(A-a)O_2$ are normal (branchpoint 5.1), we conclude that the indices of ventilation relative to perfusion are normal. Heart rate reserve (branchpoint 5.2) is high and the breathing reserve (branchpoint 5.5) is also high (Table 66-3). The $\Delta\dot{V}O_2/\Delta WR$ (branchpoint 5.8) cannot be measured because of the brevity of exercise. There is no exercise hypertension. These findings place the patient in the diagnostic category of poor effort. The following findings are consistent with this diagnosis: (1) the normal exercise ECG; (2) R of only 0.82 at the maximum $\dot{V}O_2$; (3) minimal decline in HCO_3^- induced by the exercise (Table 66-3); and the previously mentioned high heart rate reserve, high breathing reserve, normal blood gases, and normal indices of ventilation-perfusion mismatching.

CONCLUSION

This patient has made a poor effort.

Fig. 66-A.

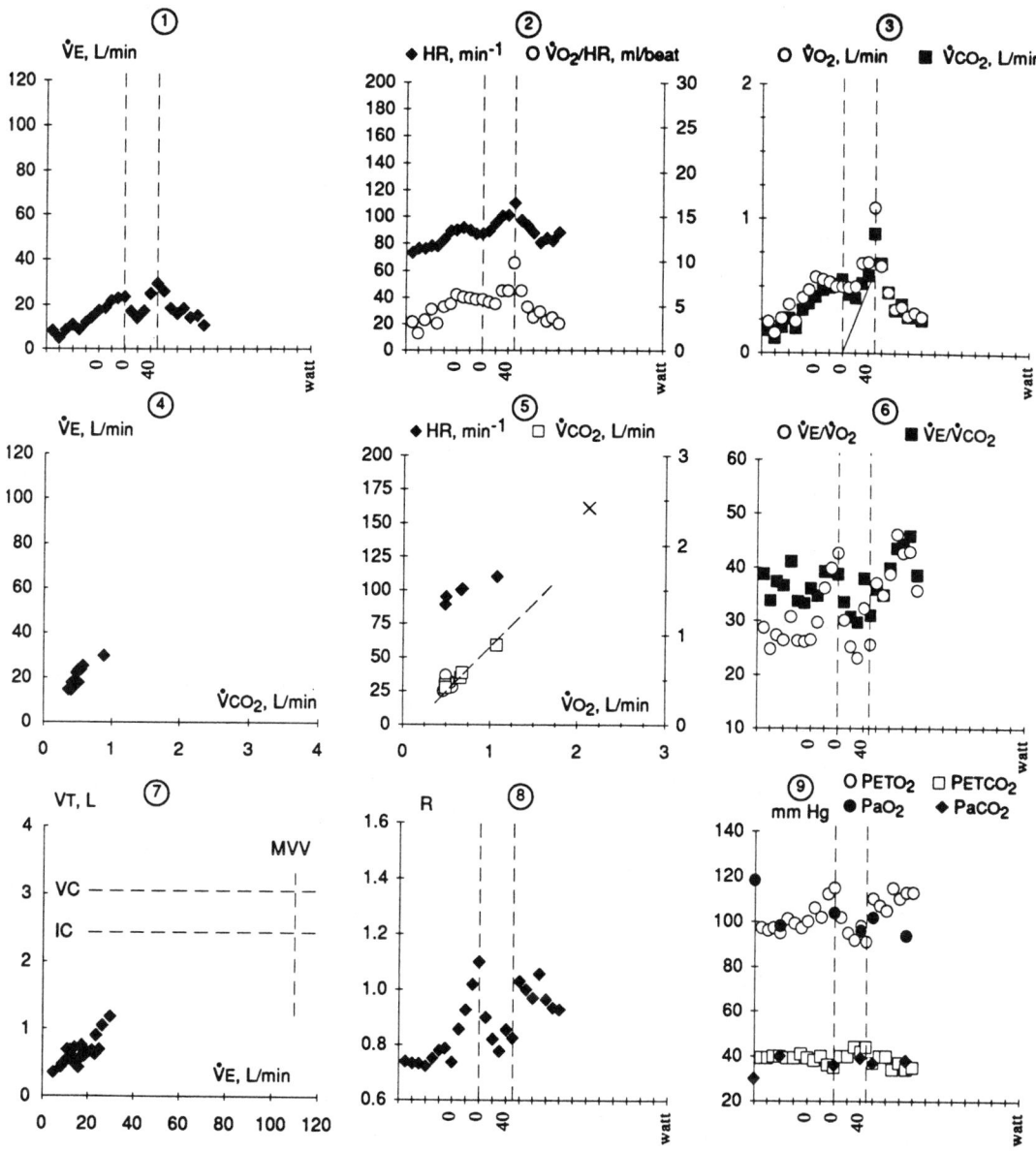

1. Vertical dashed lines in panels 1 to 3 and 6, 8, and 9 indicate the beginning and the end of increasing work period.

2. Unloaded cycling is performed for 3 minutes before the left vertical dashed line.

3. In panel 3, the diagonal line shows the increase of $\dot{V}O_2$ at a slope of 10 ml/min/W.

4. In panel 5, the diagonal dashed line has a slope of 1; the "x" in the upper right is the predicted maximum heart rate and $\dot{V}O_2$ for the subject.

CASE 67 *Poor effort with acute hyperventilation and anxiety in a moderately obese man*

CLINICAL FINDINGS

This 56-year-old shipyard worker complained of progressive dyspnea on exertion, evident when climbing two flights of stairs. He had also noted anterior chest pain with exertion, relieved by rest, associated with dyspnea and diaphoresis but not with palpitations, lightheadedness, syncope, or numbness. He had stopped smoking 20 years previously after 20 pack years. He took no medications but had been told that he had hypertension several years ago. Physical examination and resting ECG were normal. Chest x-ray showed mild pleural thickening bilaterally.

EXERCISE FINDINGS

After percutaneous insertion of a brachial artery catheter, while being positioned on the cycle ergometer, the patient became lightheaded and syncopal. The patient was placed on a guerney in the reverse Trendelenburg position. Continuous monitoring revealed a transient sinus bradycardia as low as 25 with normal blood pressure. The bradycardia lasted only a few minutes. After 15 minutes he felt well and was able to exercise. He pedalled at 60 rpm without added load for 3 minutes. The work rate was then increased 15 W every minute. Arterial blood was sampled every second minute, and intra-arterial blood pressure was recorded from the brachial artery catheter. Mild chest pain began at 45 W; exercise was stopped at 90 W because of the patient's continuing and increasing chest pain, which was typical of his usual symptom. There were no ST abnormalities nor was there arrhythmia during or after exercise.

TABLE 67-1. *Selected Respiratory Function Data*

MEASUREMENT	PREDICTED	MEASURED
Age, yr		56
Sex		Male
Height, cm		172
Weight, kg	75	98
Hematocrit, %		46
VC, L	4.10	3.16
IC, L	2.74	2.55
TLC, L	6.17	4.77
FEV$_1$, L	3.23	2.78
FEV$_1$/VC, %	79	88
MVV, L/min	137	98
D$_{LCO}$, ml/mm Hg/min	26.3	20.9

TABLE 67-2. *Selected Exercise Data*

MEASUREMENT	PREDICTED	MEASURED
Maximum V̇$_{O_2}$, L/min	2.38	1.51
Maximum HR, beats/min	164	130
Maximum O$_2$ pulse, ml/beat	14.5	11.6
ΔV̇$_{O_2}$/ΔWR, ml/min/W	10.3	9.3
AT, L/min	> 1.05	1.4
Blood pressure, mm Hg (rest, max)		168/96,228/111
Maximum V̇$_E$, L/min		79
Exercise breathing reserve, L/min	> 15	19
Pa$_{O_2}$, mm Hg (rest, max ex)		112,100
P(A−a)$_{O_2}$, mm Hg (rest, max ex)		21,25
P(a−ET)$_{CO_2}$, mm Hg (rest, max ex)		2,0
V$_D$/V$_T$ (rest, heavy ex)		0.30,0.24
HCO$_3^-$, mEq/L (rest, 2-min recov)		24,20

FIG. 67-A.

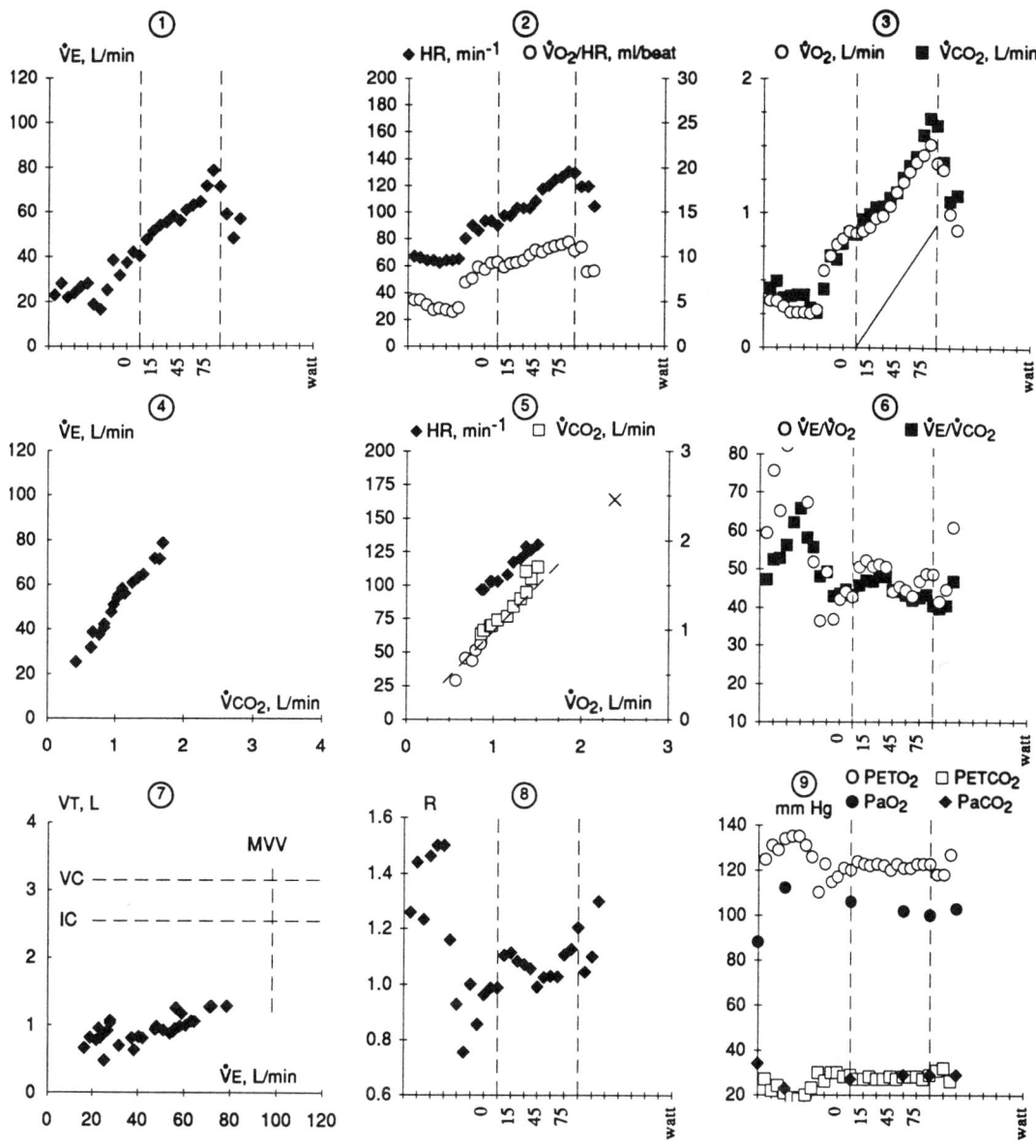

1. Vertical dashed lines in panels 1 to 3 and 6, 8, and 9 indicate the beginning and the end of increasing work period.

2. Unloaded cycling is performed for 3 minutes before the left vertical dashed line.

3. In panel 3, the diagonal line shows the increase of $\dot{V}O_2$ at a slope of 10 ml/min/W.

4. In panel 5, the diagonal dashed line has a slope of 1; the "x" in the upper right is the predicted maximum heart rate and $\dot{V}O_2$ for the subject.

Interpretation

COMMENTS

Resting respiratory function studies reveal the patient to have a mild restrictive defect of the type generally seen with obesity (normal inspiratory capacity, but reduced expiratory reserve volume)

(Table 67-1). The patient is, in fact, 23 kg overweight. Resting ECG is normal. As the patient was getting ready to cycle, he became lightheaded and hypotensive. His blood pressure decreased and he developed a marked bradycardia consistent with a vasovagal reaction. When placed in a supine position, the patient's pulse and blood pres-

TABLE 67-3.

Time min	Work rate watts	BP mm Hg	HR min⁻¹	f min⁻¹	V̇E L/min BTPS	V̇CO2 L/min STPD	V̇O2 L/min STPD	V̇O2/HR ml/beat	R	pH	HCO3 meq/L	PO2, mm Hg ET	a	(A-a)	PCO2, mm Hg ET	a	(a-ET)	V̇E/V̇CO2	V̇E/V̇O2	VD/VT
	Rest	168/96								7.47	24	88			34					
	Rest		67	24	22.8	0.44	0.35	5.2	1.26			125			27			47	59	
	Rest		66	26	27.9	0.49	0.34	5.2	1.44			131			22			52	76	
	Rest		64	28	21.9	0.37	0.30	4.7	1.23			129			24			53	65	
	Rest	156/87	64	29	23.8	0.38	0.26	4.1	1.46	7.59	22	134	112	21	21	23	2	56	82	0.30
	Rest		62	29	26.7	0.39	0.26	4.2	1.50			135			19			62	93	
	Rest		64	27	27.9	0.39	0.26	4.1	1.50			135			18			66	98	
	Rest		64	23	18.8	0.29	0.25	3.9	1.16			131			20			58	67	
	Rest		65	25	16.6	0.26	0.28	4.3	0.93			126			23			56	52	
	Unloaded		80	53	25.2	0.43	0.57	7.1	0.75			110			30			48	36	
	Unloaded		90	61	38.6	0.68	0.68	7.6	1.00			123			26			49	49	
	Unloaded		86	45	31.7	0.65	0.76	8.8	0.86			115			30			43	37	
	Unloaded		93	46	37.5	0.77	0.80	8.6	0.96			117			30			44	42	
	Unloaded		93	52	42.2	0.85	0.86	9.2	0.99			121			28			44	44	
	Unloaded	207/108	90	49	40.4	0.84	0.85	9.4	0.99	7.52	22	120	106	17	29	27	-2	43	43	0.23
0.5	15		97	51	47.7	0.95	0.86	8.9	1.10			124			27			46	50	
1.0	15		97	55	51.1	0.99	0.89	9.2	1.11			123			27			47	52	
1.5	30		103	61	53.9	1.04	0.96	9.3	1.08			122			28			47	51	
2.0	30		103	61	55.4	1.05	0.98	9.5	1.07			123			27			48	51	
2.5	45		103	59	58.1	1.11	1.05	10.2	1.06			122			27			48	51	
3.0	45		108	59	56.0	1.15	1.16	10.7	0.99			120			28			44	44	
3.5	60		117	61	61.0	1.26	1.23	10.5	1.02			123			27			44	45	
4.0	60	216/108	120	59	63.2	1.35	1.31	10.9	1.03	7.49	22	121	102	20	28	29	1	43	44	0.28
4.5	75		124	61	64.5	1.42	1.38	11.1	1.03			121			28			42	43	
5.0	75		126	56	71.8	1.58	1.43	11.3	1.10			123			28			42	47	
5.5	90		130	61	78.7	1.70	1.51	11.6	1.13			123			27			43	49	
6.0	90	228/111	129	56	71.3	1.65	1.37	10.6	1.20	7.46	20	123	100	25	29	29	0	40	49	0.24
	Recovery		119	50	58.9	1.38	1.32	11.1	1.05			118			31			40	41	
	Recovery		119	49	48.2	1.09	0.99	8.3	1.10			118			32			40	44	
	Recovery		104	45	56.7	1.13	0.87	8.4	1.30			127			26			47	61	
										7.45	20		103			29				

sure became normal and he resumed his position on the cycle ergometer for testing; however, he acutely hyperventilated at rest, demonstrating a marked respiratory alkalosis in his arterial blood (Table 67-3).

ANALYSIS

In flow chart 1, the maximum V̇O2 is reduced while the anaerobic threshold is normal (Table 67-2), which directs us through branchpoints 1.1, 1.2, and 1.3 to flow chart 3. The breathing reserve (branchpoint 3.1) and ECG (branchpoint 3.3) are normal, directing us to "poor effort or musculoskeletal disorder." The V̇D/V̇T, $P(A-a)_{O_2}$, and $P(a-ET)_{CO_2}$ are normal and the heart rate reserve is high. The change in bicarbonate from rest to recovery is only 4 mEq/L, which is less than expected for a normal maximal exercise effort. These findings, indicate that the patient's maximum V̇O2

is due to poor effort, possibly secondary to apprehension. He does have significant obesity and hypertension however. Re-evaluation is in order when the patient is less anxious.

CONCLUSION

This study shows poor effort with acute resting hyperventilation and anxiety in a moderately obese man. The combination of high heart rate reserve and normal breathing reserve without objective evidence of either myocardial, pulmonary vascular, peripheral vascular, or underlying lung disease suggests that this patient's reduced maximum oxygen uptake, and perhaps symptom of dyspnea, is psychogenic. The pre-exercise vasovagal reaction and the acute hyperventilation in the anticipation of exercise are consistent with this interpretation.

CASE 68 *Skeletal disease limiting exercise*

CLINICAL FINDINGS

This 60-year-old former shipyard worker had enjoyed apparent good health except for arthritis of the right hip of many years' duration and hypertension, which had not been treated. He had smoked cigarettes for a short period of time 3 decades previously. Chest roentgenograms showed fibrotic changes at both bases, but no rales were heard on physical examination.

EXERCISE FINDINGS

The patient felt more comfortable walking on the treadmill than pedalling the cycle ergometer. After insertion of a brachial artery catheter he walked at 1.6 mph on the level followed by increments in grade of 2% per minute. He stopped exercise after 11 minutes because of pain in the right hip. He had no shortness of breath or palpitations. The ECG remained normal.

TABLE 68-1. *Selected Respiratory Function Data*

MEASUREMENT	PREDICTED	MEASURED
Age, yr		60
Sex		Male
Height, cm		175
Weight, kg	78	97
Hematocrit, %		44
VC, L	3.77	4.09
IC, L	2.52	3.01
TLC, L	5.77	5.72
FEV_1, L	2.96	3.21
FEV_1/VC, %	78	78
MVV, L/min	122	94
$D_{L_{CO}}$, ml/min Hg/min	25.0	23.9

TABLE 68-2. *Selected Exercise Data*

MEASUREMENT	PREDICTED	MEASURED
Maximum $\dot{V}_{O_2}$, L/min	2.57	1.62
Maximum HR, beats/min	160	123
Maximum O_2 pulse, ml/beat	16.1	14.0
AT, L/min	> 1.13	1.45
Blood pressure, mm Hg (rest, max)		186/117,213/123
Maximum $\dot{V}_E$, L/min		52
Exercise breathing reserve, L/min	> 15	42
Pa_{O_2}, mm Hg (rest, max ex)		90,80
$P(A-a)_{O_2}$, mm Hg (rest, max ex)		10,32
$P(a-ET)_{CO_2}$, mm Hg (rest, max ex)		1,−3
V_D/V_T (rest, heavy ex)		0.39,0.25
HCO_3^-, mEq/L (rest, 2-min recov)		24,23

TABLE 68-3.

Time min	Treadmill grade, %	BP mm Hg	HR min⁻¹	f min⁻¹	V̇E L/min BTPS	V̇CO2 L/min STPD	V̇O2 L/min STPD	V̇O2/HR ml/beat	R	pH	HCO3 meq/L	PO2 ET	PO2 a	PO2 (A-a)	PCO2 ET	PCO2 a	PCO2 (a-ET)	V̇E/V̇CO2	V̇E/V̇O2	VD/VT
	Rest	186/117								7.44	23		100			34				
	Rest		86	19	14.1	0.35	0.46	5.3	0.76			103			37			36	27	
	Rest		85	20	13.7	0.30	0.37	4.4	0.81			110			35			40	32	
	Rest		83	25	12.5	0.23	0.30	3.6	0.77			100			39			45	35	
	Rest	192/126	84	20	11.1	0.23	0.31	3.7	0.74	7.41	24	102	90	10	38	39	1	41	30	0.39
	Rest		86	21	12.5	0.30	0.40	4.7	0.75			97			41			36	27	
	Rest		90	20	13.4	0.29	0.34	3.8	0.85			111			35			40	34	
	0		103	24	31.1	0.81	0.81	7.9	1.00			114			34			36	36	
	0		95	24	27.7	0.70	0.76	8.0	0.92			110			36			37	34	
	0		101	23	21.6	0.58	0.77	7.6	0.75			97			39			34	26	
	0	216/129	103	29	22.4	0.64	0.91	8.8	0.70	7.41	22	93	74	28	41	36	-5	31	22	0.21
	0		109	23	22.5	0.66	0.95	8.7	0.69			91			41			31	22	
	0		111	22	28.6	0.84	1.17	10.5	0.72			90			41			32	23	
0.5	2		105	24	30.1	0.85	1.07	10.2	0.79			103			38			33	26	
1.0	2		105	26	33.0	0.90	1.18	11.2	0.76			100			39			34	26	
1.5	4		106	28	34.6	0.93	1.16	10.9	0.80			104			39			35	28	
2.0	4	216/126	106	33	31.9	0.88	1.06	10.0	0.83	7.41	23	103	80	27	39	37	-2	33	27	0.27
2.5	6		107	32	30.9	0.85	1.07	10.0	0.79			100			40			33	26	
3.0	6		107	38	29.4	0.80	1.06	9.9	0.75			97			40			33	25	
3.5	8		108	31	35.0	0.98	1.16	10.7	0.84			106			38			33	28	
4.0	8	210/123	109	25	35.8	1.02	1.20	11.0	0.85	7.41	23	106	81	27	38	37	-1	33	28	0.28
4.5	10		112	30	37.8	1.08	1.32	11.8	0.82			99			41			33	27	
5.0	10		111	28	36.8	1.07	1.31	11.8	0.82			102			40			32	26	
5.5	12		114	28	37.4	1.10	1.30	11.4	0.85			102			41			32	27	
6.0	12	216/123	114	33	44.3	1.23	1.42	12.5	0.87	7.40	23	106	81	26	39	38	-1	34	29	0.31
6.5	14		121	30	41.1	1.21	1.43	11.8	0.85			101			41			32	27	
7.0	14		119	30	48.3	1.41	1.55	13.0	0.91			106			40			32	30	
7.5	16		122	33	51.5	1.47	1.60	13.1	0.92			107			39			33	30	
8.0	16	213/123	123	32	49.9	1.44	1.56	12.7	0.92	7.40	22	107	80	32	39	36	-3	33	30	0.25
	Recovery		116	34	52.2	1.49	1.62	14.0	0.92			108			39			33	30	
	Recovery		112	27	40.4	1.21	1.34	12.0	0.90			107			40			31	28	
	Recovery		101	28	28.7	0.77	0.84	8.3	0.92			107			39			34	31	
	Recovery	192/126	97	38	21.7	0.50	0.61	6.3	0.82	7.39	23	100	90	14	42	39	-3	37	30	0.34

Interpretation

COMMENTS

The results of the respiratory function studies are within normal limits (Table 68-1). The patient had significant systemic hypertension at the time of the study (Table 68-3). Because of arthritis of the right hip, treadmill walking was used for exercise testing. The rate of walking was slow (1.6 mph) to avoid discomfort to the patient and also so the arterial pressure could be closely monitored.

ANALYSIS

In flow chart 1, the maximum V̇O2 is significantly reduced but the anaerobic threshold is normal (Table 68-2). See flow chart 3. The breathing reserve at maximum exercise is high (branchpoint 3.1). The ECG is normal (branchpoint 3.3). The diagnosis at this point reveals either poor effort or that the patient has a musculoskeletal disorder. The normal V_D/V_T, borderline $P(A-a)_{O_2}$, normal $P(a-ET)_{CO_2}$, high heart rate reserve, and only 1 mEq/L decrease in bicarbonate 2 minutes after the start of recovery support either of these diagnoses. From the patient's history, musculoskeletal disorder seems most likely.

CONCLUSION

Musculoskeletal disorder has limited exercise performance.

Fɪɢ. 68-A.

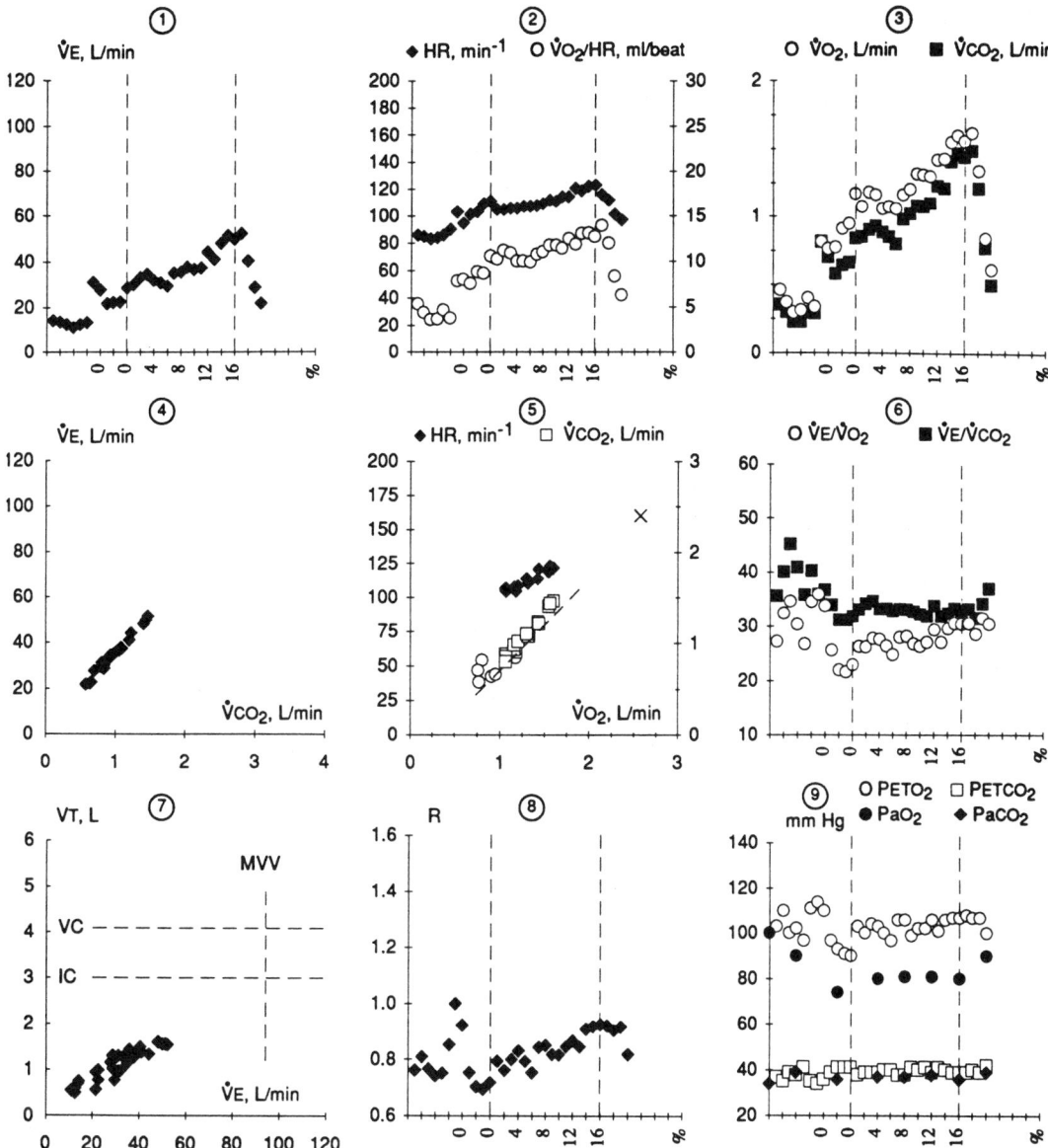

1. Vertical dashed lines in panels 1 to 3 and 6, 8, and 9 indicate the beginning and the end of increasing work period.

2. Zero grade walking is performed for 3 minutes before the left vertical dashed line.

3. In panel 5, the diagonal dashed line has a slope of 1; the "x" in the upper right is the predicted maximum heart rate and $\dot{V}O_2$ for the subject.

CASE 69 *Ankylosing spondylitis*

CLINICAL FINDINGS

This 51-year-old airline employee had first developed symptoms of ankylosing spondylitis, primarily involving the neck and thoracic spine, approximately 6 years prior to evaluation. He had received some relief of pain with indomethacin. He had stopped smoking over 10 years previously. On the basis of pleural changes at the apices, he had been treated for tuberculosis several years ago although the tuberculin skin test was negative. To maintain fitness, he had begun running approximately 3 miles a day. In recent months he had felt as if he "could not get enough air into his lungs" and found himself taking gasping breaths. Physical examination revealed reduced neck movement and thoracic expansion. Chest roentgenograms revealed apical pleural thickening. ECG was normal.

EXERCISE FINDINGS

The patient performed exercise on a cycle ergometer. He pedalled at 60 rpm without added load for 3 minutes. The work rate was then increased 20 W per minute to his symptom-limited maximum. He stopped exercise because of shortness of breath. Exercise ECGs were normal except for a single interpolated ventricular premature contraction.

TABLE 69-1. *Selected Respiratory Function Data*

MEASUREMENT	PREDICTED	MEASURED
Age, yr		51
Sex		Male
Height, cm		178
Weight, kg	80	79
Hematocrit, %		39
VC, L	4.62	3.61
IC, L	3.08	2.60
FEV$_1$, L	3.67	2.76
FEV$_1$/VC, %	79	76
MVV, L/min, direct	151	132 at f = 80/min
MVV, L/min, indirect	147	110

TABLE 69-2. *Selected Exercise Data*

MEASUREMENT	PREDICTED	MEASURED
Maximum $\dot{V}O_2$, L/min	2.52	2.54
Maximum HR, beats/min	169	170
Maximum O$_2$ pulse, ml/beat	14.9	14.9
$\Delta\dot{V}O_2/\Delta WR$, ml/min/W	10.3	9.4
AT, L/min	> 1.08	1.4
Blood pressure, mm Hg (rest, max)		126/86, 206/84
Maximum $\dot{V}E$, L/min		108
Exercise breathing reserve, L/min	> 15	2

Fig. 69-A.

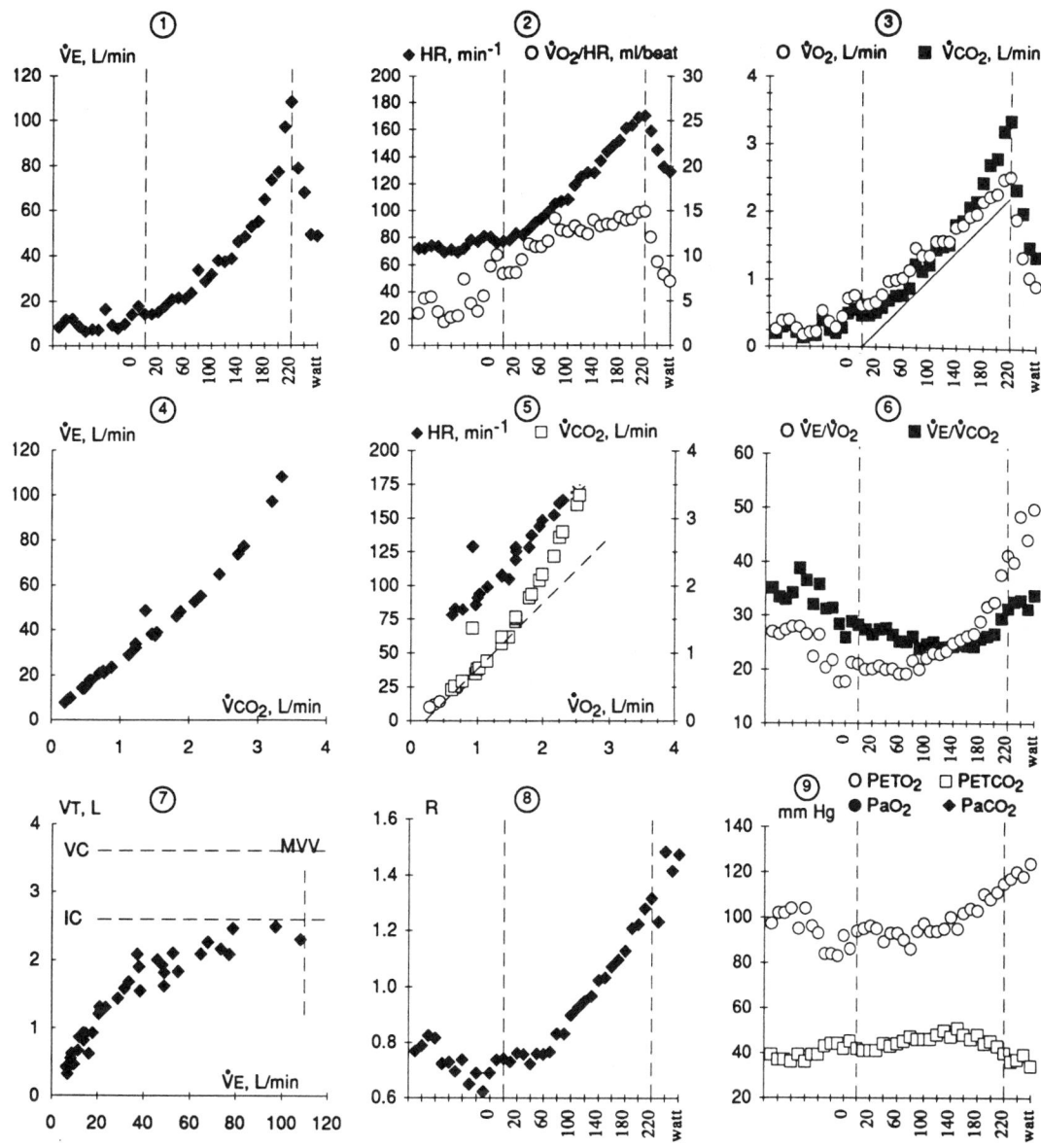

1. Vertical dashed lines in panels 1 to 3 and 6, 8, and 9 indicate the beginning and the end of increasing work period.

2. Unloaded cycling is performed for 3 minutes before the left vertical dashed line.

3. In panel 3, the diagonal line shows the increase of $\dot{V}O_2$ at a slope of 10 ml/min/W.

4. In panel 5, the diagonal dashed line has a slope of 1; the "x" in the upper right is the predicted maximum heart rate and $\dot{V}O_2$ for the subject.

Interpretation

COMMENTS

The results of spirometry and total lung capacity measurement suggest that the patient has mild restrictive disease (Table 69-1) consequent to his ankylosing spondylitis. This is reflected in part by a reduction in the inspiratory capacity (loss of his ability to expand his chest wall). The resting ECG is normal.

ANALYSIS

In flow chart 1, the maximum $\dot{V}O_2$ and the anaerobic threshold are normal (Table 69-2). See flow chart 2. The ECG and O_2 pulse at maximum $\dot{V}O_2$

TABLE 69-3.

Time min	Work rate watts	BP mm Hg	HR min⁻¹	f min⁻¹	$\dot{V}E$ L/min BTPS	$\dot{V}CO_2$ L/min STPD	$\dot{V}O_2$ L/min STPD	$\dfrac{\dot{V}O_2}{HR}$ ml/beat	R	pH	HCO₃ meq/L	PO2, mm Hg ET	a	(A-a)	PCO2, mm Hg ET	a	(a-ET)	$\dfrac{\dot{V}E}{\dot{V}CO_2}$	$\dfrac{\dot{V}E}{\dot{V}O_2}$	VD VT
	Rest		72	15	8.3	0.20	0.26	3.6	0.77			97			39			35	27	
	Rest		72	17	11.5	0.30	0.38	5.3	0.79			102			37			34	26	
	Rest		74	14	12.1	0.33	0.40	5.4	0.83			102			37			33	27	
	Rest		73	14	8.7	0.22	0.27	3.7	0.81			104			36			34	28	
	Rest		69	15	6.3	0.13	0.18	2.6	0.72			95			39			39	28	
	Rest	126/86	71	16	7.2	0.16	0.22	3.1	0.73			104			36			37	27	
	Rest		69	22	7.0	0.16	0.23	3.3	0.70			96			39			32	22	
	Rest		72	26	16.2	0.39	0.53	7.4	0.74			93			39			36	26	
	Unloaded		78	19	9.1	0.24	0.37	4.7	0.65			84			43			31	20	
	Unloaded		77	18	7.8	0.20	0.29	3.8	0.69			84			44			31	22	
	Unloaded		81	21	9.7	0.28	0.45	5.6	0.62			83			44			28	18	
	Unloaded		80	15	13.9	0.49	0.71	8.9	0.69			92			42			26	18	
	Unloaded		76	19	17.7	0.56	0.76	10.0	0.74			86			45			29	21	
	Unloaded		77	16	14.3	0.46	0.62	8.1	0.74			94			42			28	21	
0.5	20		78	17	14.0	0.46	0.63	8.1	0.73			95			41			27	20	
1.0	20	158/86	83	16	14.8	0.51	0.67	8.1	0.76			96			41			26	20	
1.5	40		82	19	17.7	0.59	0.78	9.5	0.76			95			41			27	21	
2.0	40	174/84	86	17	20.7	0.70	0.97	11.3	0.72			89			44			28	20	
2.5	60		91	17	21.4	0.76	1.00	11.0	0.76			93			43			26	20	
3.0	60		94	16	21.0	0.78	1.03	11.0	0.76			93			44			25	19	
3.5	80		99	18	23.5	0.88	1.15	11.6	0.77			90			45			25	19	
4.0	80	178/78	105	20	33.6	1.23	1.48	14.1	0.83			86			47			26	22	
4.5	100		107	20	28.9	1.14	1.37	12.8	0.83			94			46			24	20	
5.0	100		108	20	31.8	1.23	1.37	12.7	0.90			97			46			24	22	
5.5	120		119	20	38.0	1.46	1.58	13.3	0.92			94			46			25	23	
6.0	120	190/86	125	18	37.5	1.51	1.59	12.7	0.95			94			48			24	23	
6.5	140		128	25	38.8	1.53	1.58	12.3	0.97			95			50			24	23	
7.0	140		128	23	46.1	1.82	1.78	13.9	1.02			100			47			24	25	
7.5	160		137	25	48.3	1.88	1.82	13.3	1.03			95			51			25	25	
8.0	160	206/84	144	25	52.7	2.08	1.94	13.5	1.07			102			48			24	26	
8.5	180		148	30	55.1	2.17	1.98	13.4	1.10			104			46			24	27	
9.0	180		152	31	64.8	2.44	2.16	14.2	1.13			103			48			25	29	
9.5	200		161	34	73.6	2.71	2.24	13.9	1.21			110			44			26	32	
10.0	200		163	37	77.2	2.80	2.29	14.0	1.22			108			45			26	32	
10.5	220		169	39	97.2	3.20	2.50	14.8	1.28			111			43			29	38	
11.0	220		170	47	108.3	3.34	2.54	14.9	1.31			115			40			31	41	
	Recovery		159	32	78.9	2.35	1.91	12.0	1.23			117			36			32	40	
	Recovery		145	30	67.9	2.00	1.35	9.3	1.48			120			37			33	48	
	Recovery	160/78	133	27	49.1	1.50	1.06	8.0	1.42			118			39			31	44	
	Recovery		129	30	48.8	1.37	0.93	7.2	1.47			124			34			34	50	

are normal (branchpoint 2.1). The subject is not obese (branchpoint 2.2). The normal ventilatory equivalent for CO_2 at the anaerobic threshold suggests that ventilation-perfusion matching is normal. The observation that tidal volume reaches the inspiratory capacity (panel 7, Figure 69-A) reflects the changes that would be expected from restrictive pulmonary or chest wall disease. Note that the indirect MVV is close to the maximum exercise ventilation resulting in virtually no breathing reserve. This is further evidence of ventilatory limitation.

CONCLUSION

Exertional dyspnea, developing secondary to restrictive changes in the chest wall, is consequent to ankylosing spondylitis.

CASE 70 *Myasthenia gravis*

CLINICAL FINDINGS

This 62-year-old retired shipyard worker had been found to have myasthenia gravis 21 years earlier. He had taken 30 mg of pyridostigmine bromide with benefit for many years. He had a 20 pack year history of smoking cigarettes but had stopped 21 years ago. He had a daily minimally productive cough. He took digoxin for an arrhythmia and reserpine for hypertension. He complained of gradually increasing shortness of breath in the last 3 years, evident when walking 2 to 3 blocks slowly or climbing a flight of stairs. There was no evidence of pulmonary or cardiovascular disease on physical examination. Chest roentgenogram was normal except for old granulomatous disease. Resting ECG showed sinus bradycardia and ST segment depression in V5 and V6 consistent with digitalis effect.

EXERCISE FINDINGS

The patient performed exercise on a cycle ergometer. He pedalled at 60 rpm without added load for 3 minutes. The work rate was then increased 15 W per minute to his symptom-limited maximum. Arterial blood was sampled every second minute, and intra-arterial blood pressure was recorded from a percutaneously placed brachial artery catheter. He stopped exercise complaining of leg pain and generalized fatigue. A single premature ventricular contraction occurred at 60 W.

TABLE 70-1. *Selected Respiratory Function Data*

MEASUREMENT	PREDICTED	MEASURED
Age, yr		62
Sex		Male
Height, cm		178
Weight, kg	80	80
Hematocrit, %		39
VC, L	3.87	2.96
IC, L	2.58	2.08
TLC, L	5.95	4.64
FEV_1, L	3.03	2.42
FEV_1/VC, %	78	82
MVV, L/min	123	56
D_{LCO}, ml/min Hg/min	24.7	25.6

TABLE 70-2. *Selected Exercise Data*

MEASUREMENT	PREDICTED	MEASURED
Maximum $\dot{V}_{O_2}$, L/min	2.21	1.09
Maximum HR, beats/min	158	102
Maximum O_2 pulse, ml/beat	14.0	10.8
$\Delta\dot{V}_{O_2}/\Delta$WR, ml/min/W	10.3	10.5
AT, L/min	> 0.97	> 1.1
Blood pressure, mm Hg (rest, max)		153/84,210/84
Maximum $\dot{V}_E$, L/min		37
Exercise breathing reserve, L/min	> 15	19
Pa_{O_2}, mm Hg (rest, max ex)		95,86
$P(A-a)_{O_2}$, mm Hg (rest, max ex)		8,21
$P(a-ET)_{CO_2}$, mm Hg (rest, max ex)		3,1
V_D/V_T (rest, heavy ex)		0.39,0.31
HCO_3^-, mEq/L (rest, 2-min recov)		25,23

TABLE 70-3.

Time min	Work rate watts	BP mm Hg	HR min⁻¹	f min⁻¹	$\dot{V}E$ L/min BTPS	$\dot{V}CO_2$ L/min STPD	$\dot{V}O_2$ L/min STPD	$\dfrac{\dot{V}O_2}{HR}$ ml/beat	R	pH	HCO₃ meq/L	PO2, mm Hg ET	a	(A-a)	PCO2, mm Hg ET	a	(a-ET)	$\dfrac{\dot{V}E}{\dot{V}CO_2}$	$\dfrac{\dot{V}E}{\dot{V}O_2}$	VD/VT
	Rest	153/84								7.42	24		97			38				
	Rest		77	23	16.8	0.38	0.39	5.1	0.97			114			34			39	38	
	Rest		74	32	13.6	0.27	0.30	4.1	0.90			112			34			40	36	
	Rest		74	24	10.4	0.18	0.21	2.8	0.86			111			34			46	40	
	Rest	138/78	77	23	10.6	0.20	0.26	3.4	0.77	7.43	25	107	95	8	35	38	3	43	33	0.39
	Unloaded		76	27	14.9	0.35	0.48	6.3	0.73			101			38			36	26	
	Unloaded		80	25	15.2	0.39	0.55	6.9	0.71			96			39			34	24	
	Unloaded		82	20	19.0	0.55	0.73	8.9	0.75			95			41			31	24	
	Unloaded		80	24	14.8	0.37	0.47	5.9	0.79			99			41			34	27	
	Unloaded		80	31	17.4	0.44	0.56	7.0	0.79			101			39			34	26	
	Unloaded	165/81	80	27	15.8	0.42	0.53	6.6	0.79	7.41	26	101	86	15	40	41	1	32	25	0.30
0.5	15		81	27	17.9	0.46	0.53	6.5	0.87			105			39			34	29	
1.0	15		82	26	28.1	0.76	0.78	9.5	0.97			103			39			34	33	
1.5	30		83	28	18.0	0.43	0.50	6.0	0.86			102			40			36	31	
2.0	30	162/78	90	27	24.2	0.69	0.84	9.3	0.82			101			39			32	26	
2.5	45		91	33	27.0	0.74	0.84	9.2	0.88			102			41			33	29	
3.0	45		93	39	28.0	0.77	0.84	9.0	0.92			106			40			32	29	
3.5	60		98	26	26.2	0.84	0.96	9.8	0.88			103			42			29	25	
4.0	60	192/81	101	32	35.3	1.05	1.09	10.8	0.96	7.38	24	104	86	21	41	42	1	31	30	0.31
4.5	75		102	35	32.8	1.00	1.06	10.4	0.94			107			40			30	28	
	Recovery		99	36	37.4	1.05	0.98	9.9	1.07	7.38	24	108	92	19	41	41	0	33	35	0.33
	Recovery		94	36	32.8	0.87	0.78	8.3	1.12			115			36			34	38	
	Recovery		84	33	22.3	0.61	0.59	7.0	1.03			109			40			32	33	
	Recovery		85	28	22.0	0.61	0.59	6.9	1.03			111			39			32	33	
	Recovery	174/84	82	30	21.8	0.54	0.46	5.6	1.17	7.38	23	117	94	22	36	39	3	36	42	0.33

Interpretation

COMMENTS

This patient appears to have mild restrictive lung or chest wall disease (Table 70-1). Because the diffusing capacity is within normal limits and the MVV is significantly reduced, the latter is more likely. The resting ECG is normal except for the digitalis effect.

ANALYSIS

In flow chart 1, the maximum oxygen uptake is reduced but the anaerobic threshold is normal (Table 70-2). See flow chart 3. The breathing reserve at the maximum work rate is normal (branchpoint 3.1). The ECG remained normal except for the digitalis effect (branchpoint 3.3). This suggests that the patient either made poor effort or had a musculoskeletal disorder. The indices of ventilation-perfusion mismatching are normal, supporting the concept that this patient does not have significant pulmonary disease. (Note VD/VT of 0.31 to 0.33 is considered to be normal in view of the low level of exercise performed.) The high heart rate reserve and small decrease in bicarbonate support the observation that the cardiovascular system was not highly stressed. The reduced maximum $\dot{V}O_2$, with the strikingly reduced MVV, suggests that this patient is limited by a musculoskeletal defect.

CONCLUSION

Exercise limitation without cardiovascular or ventilatory impairment. Limitation is most likely secondary to myasthenia gravis.

Fig. 70-A.

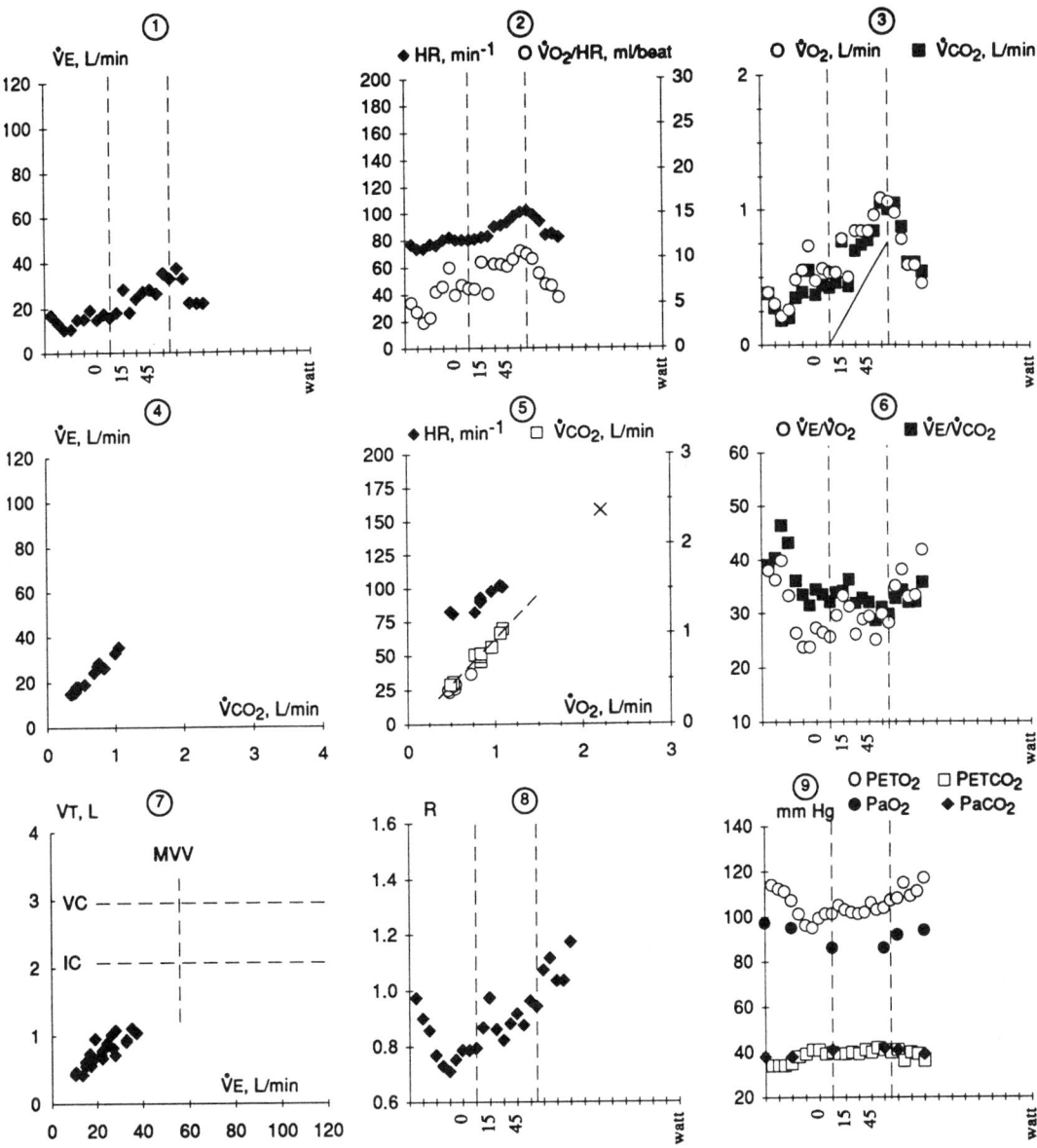

1. Vertical dashed lines in panels 1 to 3 and 6, 8, and 9 indicate the beginning and the end of increasing work period.
2. Unloaded cycling is performed for 3 minutes before the left vertical dashed line.
3. In panel 3, the diagonal line shows the increase of $\dot{V}O_2$ at a slope of 10 ml/min/W.
4. In panel 5, the diagonal dashed line has a slope of 1; the "x" in the upper right is the predicted maximum heart rate and $\dot{V}O_2$ for the subject.

CASE 71 *Aortic and mitral stenosis and obstructive airway disease*

CLINICAL FINDINGS

This 43-year-old man developed dyspnea and precordial pain at rest and on exertion 3 weeks prior to study. He had a history of "passing out" with or without prior feelings of lightheadedness. He also noted cough and sputum production with exertion. He was a welder and an extremely heavy smoker, but he stated that he had reduced his smoking to several cigarettes daily. Evaluation, including cardiac catheterization, revealed severe aortic stenosis (1.4 cm² valvular area) and moderate mitral stenosis (1.6 cm²), normal coronary arteries, and an elevated pulmonary artery pressure of 50/25 mm Hg and wedge pressure of 16 mm Hg. Medications included a systemic β-blocker, theophylline, and a β-agonist inhaler. Physical examination was consistent with aortic stenosis and mitral valve disease, but the patient had no pulmonary rales or wheezes.

EXERCISE FINDINGS

The patient performed exercise on a cycle ergometer. He pedalled at 60 rpm without an added load for 3 minutes. The work rate was then increased 15 W per minute to tolerance. Blood was sampled every second minute, and intra-arterial blood pressure was recorded from a percutaneously placed brachial artery catheter. The resting ECG was normal except for an intraventricular conduction defect. The patient had neither chest pain nor ectopy during exercise, but he had expiratory wheezes and frequent premature atrial and ventricular contractions early in recovery. The arterial pressure tracing showed a delayed upstroke (200 milliseconds to peak pressure).

TABLE 71-1. *Selected Respiratory Function Data*

MEASUREMENT	PREDICTED	BEFORE BRONCHODILATOR	AFTER BRONCHODILATOR
Age, yr		43	
Sex		Male	
Height, cm		171	
Weight, kg	74	89	
Hemoglobin, g/100 ml		15.4	
VC, L	4.47	3.03	3.14
IC, L	2.98	2.03	2.23
TLC, L	6.32	6.54	
FEV₁, L	3.58	1.65	1.84
FEV₁/VC, %	80	54	
MVV, L/min	154	62	73
D$_{CO}$, ml/mm Hg/min	27.2	19.8	

TABLE 71-2. *Selected Exercise Data*

MEASUREMENT	PREDICTED	MEASURED
Maximum V̇$_{O_2}$, L/min	2.70	1.48
Maximum HR, beats/min	177	140
Maximum O$_2$ pulse, ml/beat	15.3	10.6
ΔV̇$_{O_2}$/ΔWR, ml/min/W	10.3	8.5
AT, L/min	> 1.13	1.0
Blood pressure, mm Hg (rest, max ex)		96/69, 132/69
Maximum V̇$_E$, L/min		59
Exercise breathing reserve, L/min	> 15	14
Pa$_{O_2}$, mm Hg (rest, mod ex)		84, 95
P(A − a)$_{O_2}$ mm Hg (rest, mod ex)		16, 14
P(a − ET)$_{CO_2}$, mm Hg (rest, mod ex)		3, 3
V$_D$/V$_T$ (rest, max ex)		0.33, 0.32
HCO$_3^-$, mEq/L (rest, 2-min recov)		25, 24
Carboxyhemoglobin, %		4.3

Fɪɢ. 71-A.

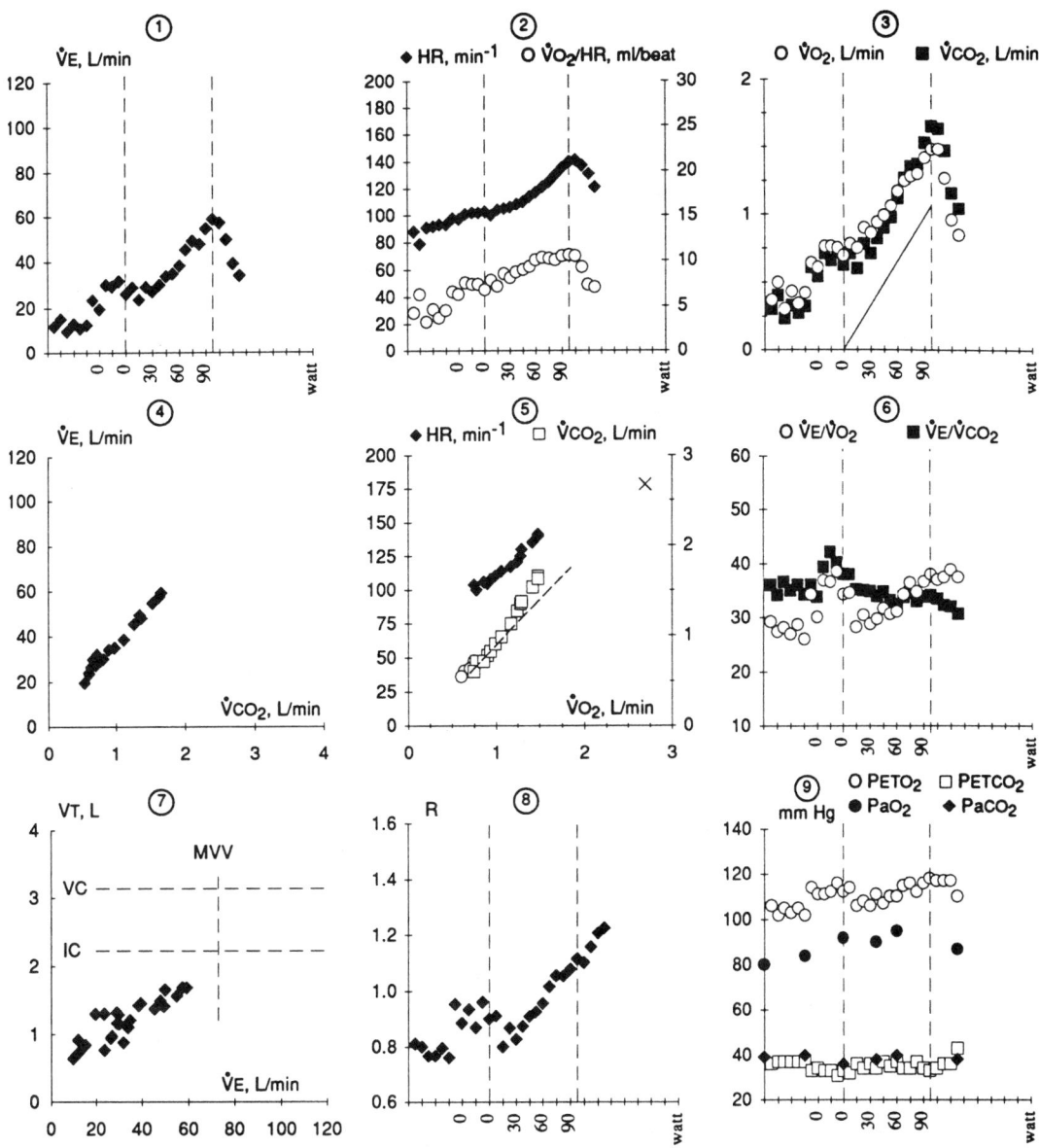

1. Vertical dashed lines in panels 1 to 3 and 6, 8, and 9 indicate the beginning and the end of increasing work period.

2. Unloaded cycling is performed for 3 minutes before the left vertical dashed line.

3. In panel 3, the diagonal line shows the increase of $\dot{V}O_2$ at a slope of 10 ml/min/W.

4. In panel 5, the diagonal dashed line has a slope of 1; the "x" in the upper right is the predicted maximum heart rate and $\dot{V}O_2$ for the subject.

TABLE 71-3.

Time min	Work rate watts	BP mm Hg	HR min⁻¹	f min⁻¹	$\dot{V}E$ L/min BTPS	$\dot{V}CO_2$ L/min STPD	$\dot{V}O_2$ L/min STPD	$\dfrac{\dot{V}O_2}{HR}$ ml/beat	R	pH	HCO3 meq/L	PO2, mm Hg ET	a	(A-a)	PCO2, mm Hg ET	a	(a-ET)	$\dfrac{\dot{V}E}{\dot{V}CO_2}$	$\dfrac{\dot{V}E}{\dot{V}O_2}$	$\dfrac{VD}{VT}$
	Rest	93/63								7.42	25		80			39				
	Rest		88	13	11.9	0.30	0.37	4.2	0.81			106			36			36	29	
	Rest		79	18	15.2	0.40	0.50	6.3	0.80			102			37			34	27	
	Rest		91	15	9.7	0.23	0.30	3.3	0.77			105			37			37	28	
	Rest		92	17	13.0	0.33	0.43	4.7	0.77			103			37			35	27	
	Rest		93	16	11.1	0.27	0.34	3.7	0.79			105			37			36	29	
	Rest	96/69	93	17	12.4	0.32	0.42	4.5	0.76	7.41	25	102	84	16	37	40	3	34	26	0.33
	Unloaded		98	18	23.5	0.61	0.64	6.5	0.95			114			33			36	34	
	Unloaded		97	15	19.6	0.54	0.61	6.3	0.89			111			34			34	30	
	Unloaded		101	26	30.2	0.71	0.76	7.5	0.93			111			33			39	37	
	Unloaded		102	23	29.8	0.66	0.76	7.5	0.87			112			33			42	37	
	Unloaded		102	36	32.0	0.72	0.75	7.4	0.96			116			31			40	39	
	Unloaded	114/75	103	28	26.4	0.63	0.70	6.8	0.90	7.46	25	112	92	19	33	36	3	38	34	0.34
0.5	15		100	25	29.1	0.71	0.78	7.8	0.91			114			32			38	35	
1.0	15		104	31	23.8	0.60	0.75	7.2	0.80			106			36			35	28	
1.5	30		105	22	29.2	0.78	0.90	8.6	0.87			108			34			35	30	
2.0	30		106	28	27.2	0.71	0.86	8.1	0.83			106			36			35	29	
2.5	45	117/78	108	26	30.1	0.82	0.94	8.7	0.87	7.43	25	111	90	18	34	38	4	34	30	0.31
3.0	45		110	31	34.0	0.90	0.99	9.0	0.91			107			37			35	32	
3.5	60		114	29	35.0	0.98	1.06	9.3	0.92			110			35			33	31	
4.0	60	114/69	117	27	38.7	1.12	1.17	10.0	0.96	7.35	22	110	95	14	37	40	3	33	31	0.32
4.5	75		121	33	45.6	1.27	1.25	10.3	1.02			115			34			34	34	
5.0	75		125	35	49.6	1.35	1.28	10.2	1.05			116			34			35	36	
5.5	90		130	32	48.0	1.37	1.30	10.0	1.05			112			37			33	35	
6.0	90	132/69	135	35	54.9	1.53	1.42	10.5	1.08			116			34			34	37	
6.5	105		140	35	59.2	1.65	1.48	10.6	1.11			118			33			34	38	
7.0			141	34	57.6	1.63	1.48	10.5	1.10			117			34			34	37	
	Recovery		137	30	50.0	1.47	1.27	9.3	1.16			117			36			32	37	
	Recovery		131	27	39.5	1.16	0.96	7.3	1.21			117			36			32	39	
	Recovery	114/72	121	29	34.3	1.04	0.85	7.0	1.22	7.42	24	110	87	30	43	38	-5	31	37	0.24

Interpretation

COMMENTS

Resting respiratory function tests reveal moderately severe obstructive lung disease with some response to inhaled albuterol and with a decreased $D_{L_{CO}}$. Wheezing was noted during recovery from exercise. The carboxyhemoglobin level is increased. The patient has known significant valvular heart disease. The systemic blood pressure tracing showed a delayed upstroke (200 milliseconds to peak pressure), pulse pressure was low at rest, and systolic pressure did not increase normally during exercise.

ANALYSIS

In flow chart 1, maximum $\dot{V}O_2$ and the anaerobic threshold are decreased. Proceeding to flow chart 4, the low breathing reserve (branchpoint 4.1) and high exercise VD/VT, (branchpoint 4.2) lead us to the diagnosis of lung disease with impaired peripheral oxygenation. This is an acceptable, but an incomplete, diagnosis because the impaired peripheral oxygenation was not due primarily to the increase in pulmonary vascular resistance, but rather to left-sided failure from valvular heart disease. The low anaerobic threshold, low $\Delta\dot{V}O_2/\Delta WR$, and low, nearly flat O_2 pulse despite β blockade are all evidence of a low maximal cardiac output. Could the low cardiac output be exclusively on the basis of pulmonary vascular disease secondary to mitral valve disease or emphysema? This is possible, but it seems unlikely, considering the symptoms of recurrent lightheadedness and the findings of severe aortic valve disease confirmed by cardiac catheterization and the slow upstroke in the arterial pressure tracing with exercise.

CONCLUSION

Although the patient has obstructive lung disease and accompanying pulmonary vascular disease, the main cause of exercise intolerance is the inability to increase cardiac output appropriately with exertion, primarily related to aortic valvular disease.

CASE 72 *Cardiac disease and mild obstructive airways disease: Cycle and treadmill*

CLINICAL FINDINGS

This 64-year-old shipyard worker was referred for evaluation. He stated that he was not limited in any of his activities; he had no shortness of breath walking on the level and only mild dyspnea after climbing 25 steps. He had smoked a half a pack of cigarettes daily until 1 year prior to this evaluation. Physical examination revealed no abnormality of the cardiovascular or respiratory systems except for a resting blood pressure of 160/84. Questionable pleural thickening was noted on chest x-ray studies. There was a small but consistent improvement in expiratory flow rates and MVV following inhalation of aerosolized isoproterenol.

EXERCISE FINDINGS

The patient performed exercise on a cycle ergometer and, 1 month later, on a treadmill. He first pedalled at 60 rpm, without added load, for 3 minutes. The work rate was then increased 20 W per minute to his symptom-limited maximum. Arterial blood was sampled every second minute, and intra-arterial blood pressure was recorded from a percutaneously placed brachial artery catheter. The resting ECG was normal. He stopped exercising because of leg fatigue. Near the end of cycle exercise, 1 mm horizontal ST depression was noted in leads 2, 3, and AVF. On repeat testing 1 month later on the treadmill, the patient stopped exercising because he "could not get a good deep breath" and felt tired. There were no abnormal ECG findings on that test.

TABLE 72-1. *Selected Respiratory Function Data*

MEASUREMENT	PREDICTED	MEASURED
Age, yr		64
Sex		Male
Height, cm		182
Weight, kg	83	80
Hematocrit, %		47
VC, L	4.49	4.25
IC, L	2.99	3.95
TLC, L	6.94	7.61
FEV_1, L	3.51	2.96
FEV_1/VC, %	78	70
MVV, L/min	140	121
D_{LCO}, ml/mm Hg/min	28.8	28.1

TABLE 72-2. *Selected Exercise Data*

MEASUREMENT	PREDICTED		MEASURED	
	CYCLE	TREADMILL	CYCLE	TREADMILL
Maximum $\dot{V}O_2$, L/min	2.19	2.43	1.56	1.65
Maximum HR, beats/min	156	156	143	157
Maximum O_2 pulse, ml/beat	14.1	15.6	10.9	10.5
$\Delta\dot{V}O_2/\Delta WR$, ml/min/W	10.3		9.7	
AT, L/min	> 0.97	> 1.08	1.0	1.1
Blood pressure, mm Hg (rest, max)			194/98,230/98	
Maximum $\dot{V}E$, L/min			68	77
Exercise breathing reserve, L/min			53	44
Pa_{O_2}, mm Hg (rest, max ex)			98,104	
$P(A-a)_{O_2}$, mm Hg (rest, max ex)			22,18	
$P(a-ET)_{CO_2}$, mm Hg (rest, max ex)			2, −3	
V_D/V_T (rest, heavy ex)			0.30,0.24	
HCO_3^-, mEq/L (rest, 2-min recov)			24,17	

Fig. 72-A. *Cycle ergometry.*

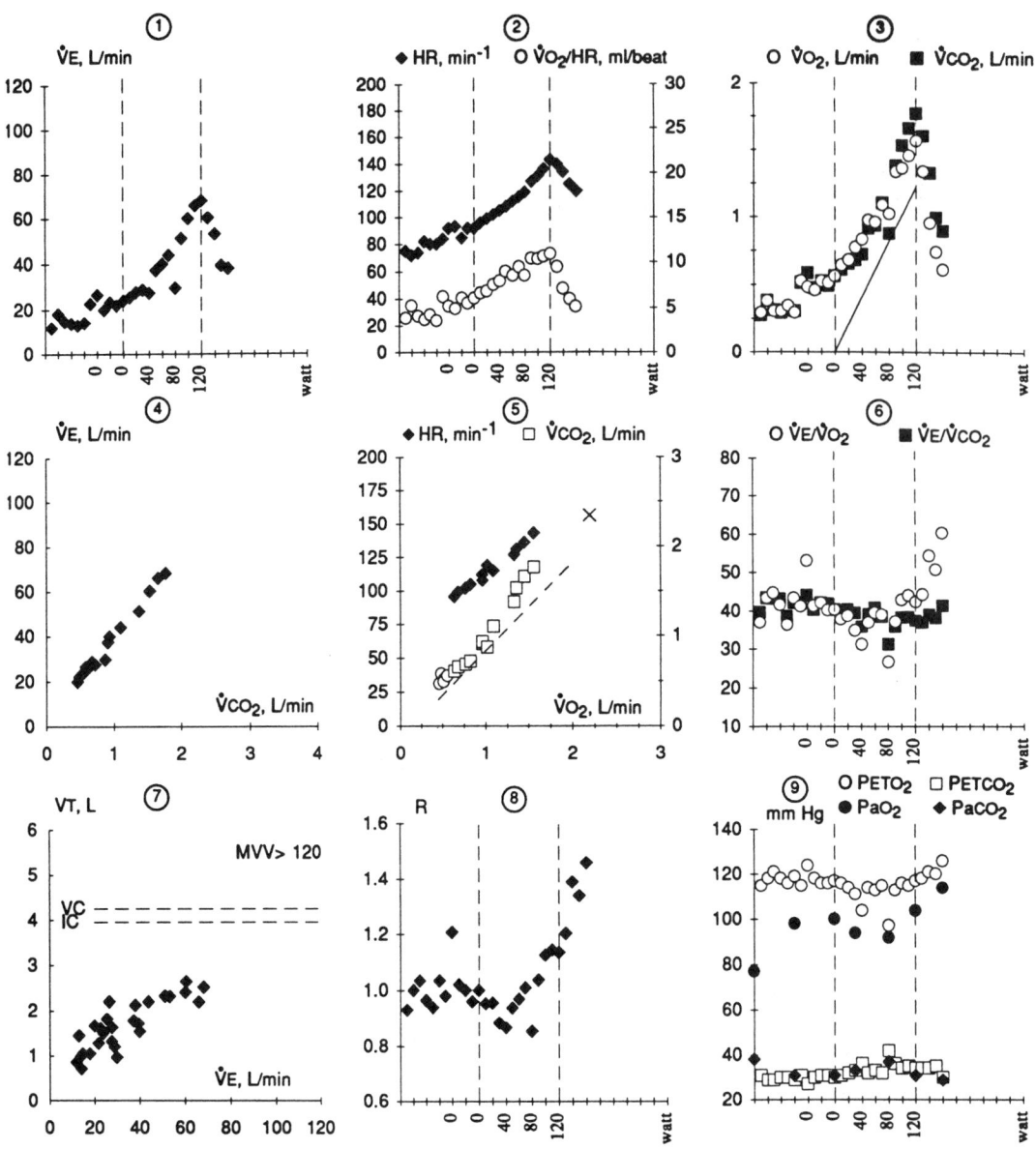

1. Vertical dashed lines in panels 1 to 3 and 6, 8, and 9 indicate the beginning and the end of increasing work period.

2. Unloaded cycling is performed for 3 minutes before the left vertical dashed line.

3. In panel 3, the diagonal line shows the increase of $\dot{V}O_2$ at a slope of 10 ml/min/W.

4. In panel 5, the diagonal dashed line has a slope of 1; the "x" in the upper right is the predicted maximum heart rate and $\dot{V}O_2$ for the subject.

Fig. 72-B. *Treadmill ergometry.*

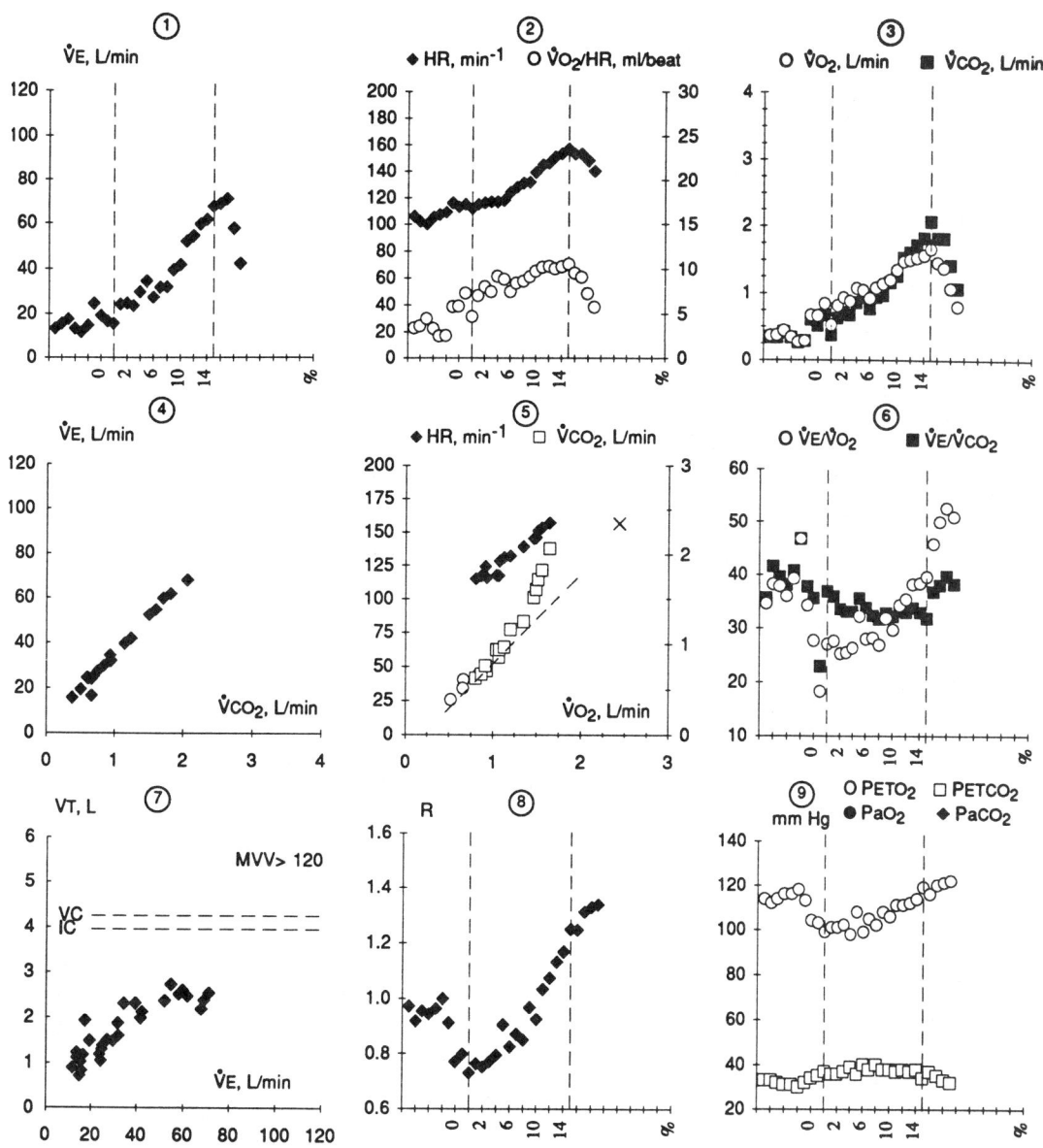

1. Vertical dashed lines in panels 1 to 3 and 6, 8, and 9 indicate the beginning and the end of increasing work period.

2. Zero grade walking is performed for 2 minutes before the left vertical dashed line.

3. In panel 5, the diagonal dashed line has a slope of 1; the "x" in the upper right is the predicted maximum heart rate and $\dot{V}O_2$ for the subject.

TABLE 72-3. *Cycle ergometry.*

Time min	Work rate watts	BP mm Hg	HR min⁻¹	f min⁻¹	$\dot{V}_E$ L/min BTPS	$\dot{V}_{CO_2}$ L/min STPD	$\dot{V}_{O_2}$ L/min STPD	$\frac{\dot{V}_{O_2}}{HR}$ ml/beat	R	pH	HCO₃ meq/L	PO2, mm Hg ET	a	(A-a)	PCO2, mm Hg ET	a	(a-ET)	$\frac{\dot{V}_E}{\dot{V}_{CO_2}}$	$\frac{\dot{V}_E}{\dot{V}_{O_2}}$	VD VT
	Rest	194/98								7.42	24		77			38				
	Rest		75	14	11.9	0.27	0.29	3.9	0.93			115			31			40	37	
	Rest		72	17	17.9	0.38	0.38	5.3	1.00			118			29			43	43	
	Rest		74	14	14.6	0.31	0.30	4.1	1.03			121			29			43	45	
	Rest	176/95	82	14	13.7	0.29	0.30	3.7	0.97			118			30			43	42	
	Rest		80	9	13.1	0.32	0.34	4.3	0.94			116			30			39	36	
	Rest		80	20	14.3	0.30	0.29	3.6	1.03	7.48	23	119	98	22	29	31	2	42	43	0.30
	Unloaded		84	14	22.6	0.51	0.52	6.2	0.98			115			31			42	41	
	Unloaded		92	12	26.5	0.58	0.48	5.2	1.21			124			27			44	53	
	Unloaded		93	12	20.0	0.47	0.46	4.9	1.02			118			30			40	41	
	Unloaded	194/95	85	15	23.2	0.52	0.52	6.1	1.00			116			31			42	42	
	Unloaded		92	17	21.9	0.49	0.51	5.5	0.96			116			31			42	40	
	Unloaded		92	16	24.0	0.56	0.56	6.1	1.00	7.47	22	117	100	19	30	31	1	40	40	0.29
0.5	20		96	14	25.4	0.61	0.64	6.7	0.95			116			31			40	38	
1.0	20	209/92	99	17	27.7	0.65	0.68	6.9	0.96			114			32			40	39	
1.5	40		102	24	28.8	0.68	0.77	7.5	0.88	7.44	22	111	94	20	33	33	0	39	35	0.31
2.0	40		105	21	27.6	0.72	0.83	7.9	0.87			104			36			36	31	
2.5	60		108	21	37.4	0.91	0.97	9.0	0.94			114			32			39	37	
3.0	60	212/92	112	26	40.0	0.93	0.96	8.6	0.97			113			33			41	39	
3.5	80		115	20	44.0	1.10	1.09	9.5	1.01			115			32			38	39	
4.0	80		119	31	29.8	0.87	1.02	8.6	0.85	7.40	23	97	92	16	42	37	-5	31	27	0.23
4.5	100		127	22	51.3	1.38	1.33	10.5	1.04			113			36			36	37	
5.0	100	230/98	131	25	60.3	1.53	1.36	10.4	1.13			116			34			38	43	
5.5	120		136	30	66.1	1.66	1.45	10.7	1.14			115			35			38	44	
6.0	120		143	27	68.2	1.77	1.56	10.9	1.13	7.40	19	117	104	18	34	31	-3	37	42	0.24
	Recovery		140	23	60.7	1.60	1.33	9.5	1.20			118			34			37	44	
	Recovery	221/95	134	23	53.4	1.32	0.95	7.1	1.39			121			34			39	54	
	Recovery		125	23	39.5	0.99	0.74	5.9	1.34			120			35			38	51	
	Recovery		120	18	38.2	0.89	0.61	5.1	1.46	7.38	17	126	114	14	30	29	-1	41	60	0.27

Interpretation

COMMENTS

This case is presented to contrast cycle with treadmill incremental exercise testing. Respiratory function measurements at rest suggest that this patient has mild obstructive lung disease (Table 72-1). Moreover, note that the patient hyperventilated at rest (Pa_{CO_2} and R values in Table 72-3) when first starting to breathe on the mouthpiece.

ANALYSIS

In flow chart 1, the maximum $\dot{V}_{O_2}$ is reduced in both the cycle and treadmill exercise studies while the anaerobic threshold is low normal (Table 72-2). Using flow chart 3, the breathing reserve is high (branchpoint 3.1), whereas the exercise ECGs (branchpoint 3.3) are equivocally abnormal. The patient did not have chest pain and the $\Delta\dot{V}_{O_2}/\Delta WR$ is normal, but the O₂ pulse is abnormally low, indicating a circulatory abnormality— whether pulmonary vascular, peripheral vascular, or cardiac. Although the patient hyperventilates and has obstructive lung disease, he has no evidence of ventilation-perfusion mismatching or pulmonary vascular disease. The significant resting systemic hypertension does not increase unusually during exercise, implying that peripheral vascular disease is not the primary disorder. The ECG findings and steep heart rate-$\dot{V}_{O_2}$ relationship in both forms of ergometry (panel 5 in Fig. 72-A and B) suggest that the primary diagnosis is cardiac disease.

CONCLUSION

Cardiac disease has limited exercise performance. This is confirmed by the absence of a cardiac reserve at the reduced maximum work rate, failure for $\dot{V}_{O_2}$ to rise normally with increasing work rate (treadmill exercise study), and the reduced maximal O₂ pulse.

TABLE 72-4. *Treadmill ergometry.*

Time min	Treadmill grade, %	BP mm Hg	HR min⁻¹	f min⁻¹	$\dot{V}_E$ L/min BTPS	$\dot{V}_{CO_2}$ L/min STPD	$\dot{V}_{O_2}$ L/min STPD	$\dfrac{\dot{V}_{O_2}}{HR}$ ml/beat	R	pH	HCO₃ meq/L	PO2, mm Hg ET	a	(A-a)	PCO2, mm Hg ET	a	(a-ET)	$\dfrac{\dot{V}_E}{\dot{V}_{CO_2}}$	$\dfrac{\dot{V}_E}{\dot{V}_{O_2}}$	VD VT
	Rest		106	12	13.5	0.35	0.36	3.4	0.97			114			33			36	35	
	Rest		102	15	15.4	0.34	0.37	3.6	0.92			112			33			42	38	
	Rest		100	9	17.4	0.42	0.44	4.4	0.95			114			32			40	38	
	Rest		105	11	13.5	0.33	0.35	3.3	0.94			116			31			38	36	
	Rest		107	13	11.7	0.26	0.27	2.5	0.96			116			31			41	39	
	Rest		109	21	14.9	0.28	0.28	2.6	1.00			118			30			47	47	
	0		116	19	24.6	0.61	0.67	5.8	0.91			113			32			38	34	
	0		113	13	19.3	0.51	0.66	5.8	0.77			104			34			36	28	
	0		115	14	16.5	0.67	0.84	7.3	0.80			103			35			23	18	
	0		112	19	15.6	0.38	0.52	4.6	0.73			99			37			37	27	
0.5	2		115	23	24.2	0.62	0.81	7.0	0.77			101			36			36	27	
1.0	2		116	18	24.9	0.70	0.93	8.0	0.75			101			36			33	25	
1.5	4		117	20	23.8	0.67	0.87	7.4	0.77			102			37			33	25	
2.0	4		117	20	29.7	0.85	1.07	9.1	0.79			98			39			33	26	
2.5	6		118	15	34.6	0.94	1.04	8.8	0.90			108			36			35	32	
3.0	6		124	18	27.2	0.76	0.92	7.4	0.83			99			40			34	28	
3.5	8		128	17	31.8	0.94	1.08	8.4	0.87			105			38			32	28	
4.0	8		131	20	32.0	0.96	1.13	8.6	0.85			102			40			32	27	
4.5	10		132	17	39.5	1.16	1.20	9.1	0.97			108			38			33	32	
5.0	10		139	21	41.8	1.25	1.35	9.7	0.93			106			38			32	30	
5.5	12		145	22	52.3	1.52	1.47	10.1	1.03			111			37			33	34	
6.0	12		146	20	54.7	1.61	1.50	10.3	1.07			111			38			33	35	
6.5	14		151	23	59.9	1.72	1.52	10.1	1.13			112			37			34	38	
7.0	14		153	25	61.9	1.82	1.56	10.2	1.17			114			38			33	38	
7.5	16		157	31	67.8	2.06	1.65	10.5	1.25			119			34			32	39	
	Recovery		153	29	69.2	1.82	1.46	9.5	1.25			116			37			37	46	
	Recovery		153	28	71.2	1.81	1.38	9.0	1.31			120			35			38	50	
	Recovery		148	23	58.1	1.42	1.07	7.2	1.33			121			33			40	52	
	Recovery		140	20	42.4	1.07	0.80	5.7	1.34			122			32			38	51	

CASE 73 β-Adrenergic blockade, systemic hypertension, pulmonary vascular disease, and mild chronic bronchitis

CLINICAL FINDINGS

A 55-year-old former shipyard worker had first noted exertional dyspnea and a morning cough with small amounts of sputum approximately 5 years earlier. He retired 3 years previously because of an injury to the left foot. The patient had a 60 pack year smoking history but had stopped 1 year ago. Hypertension, diagnosed 1 year previously, was being treated with hydrochlorothiazide and propranolol. There is no history of angina or congestive heart failure. Examination revealed normal breath sounds, cardiovascular examination, and peripheral pulses. Chest roentgenograms showed minimal pleural plaques without evidence of parenchymal lung disease.

EXERCISE FINDINGS

The patient performed exercise on a cycle ergometer. He pedalled at 60 rpm without added load for 3 minutes. The work rate was then increased 20 W per minute to his symptom-limited maximum. Arterial blood was sampled every second minute, and intra-arterial blood pressure was recorded from a percutaneously placed brachial artery catheter. Resting and exercise ECGs were normal except for relative bradycardia. The patient stopped exercise complaining of general fatigue and shortness of breath.

TABLE 73-1. *Selected Respiratory Function Data*

MEASUREMENT	PREDICTED	MEASURED
Age, yr		55
Sex		Male
Height, cm		173
Weight, kg	76	85
Hematocrit, %		48
VC, L	4.20	4.54
IC, L	2.80	3.66
TLC, L	6.26	6.88
FEV_1, L	3.32	3.16
FEV_1/VC, %	79	70
MVV, L/min	140	121
DL_{CO}, ml/mm Hg/min	28.1	16.6

TABLE 73-2. *Selected Exercise Data*

MEASUREMENT	PREDICTED	MEASURED
Maximum $\dot{V}O_2$, L/min	2.35	1.59
Maximum HR, beats/min	165	113
Maximum O_2 pulse, ml/beat	14.3	14.4
$\Delta\dot{V}O_2/\Delta WR$, ml/min/W	10.3	9.8
AT, L/min	> 1.01	0.95
Blood pressure, mm Hg (rest, max)		182/107,206/113
Maximum $\dot{V}E$, L/min		72
Exercise breathing reserve, L/min	> 15	49
Pa_{O_2}, mm Hg (rest, max ex)		73,71
$P(A-a)_{O_2}$, mm Hg (rest, max ex)		31,46
$P(a-ET)_{CO_2}$, mm Hg (rest, max ex)		3,4
VD/VT (rest, heavy ex)		0.33,0.35
HCO_3^-, mEq/L (rest, 2-min recov)		24,18

Fig. 73-A.

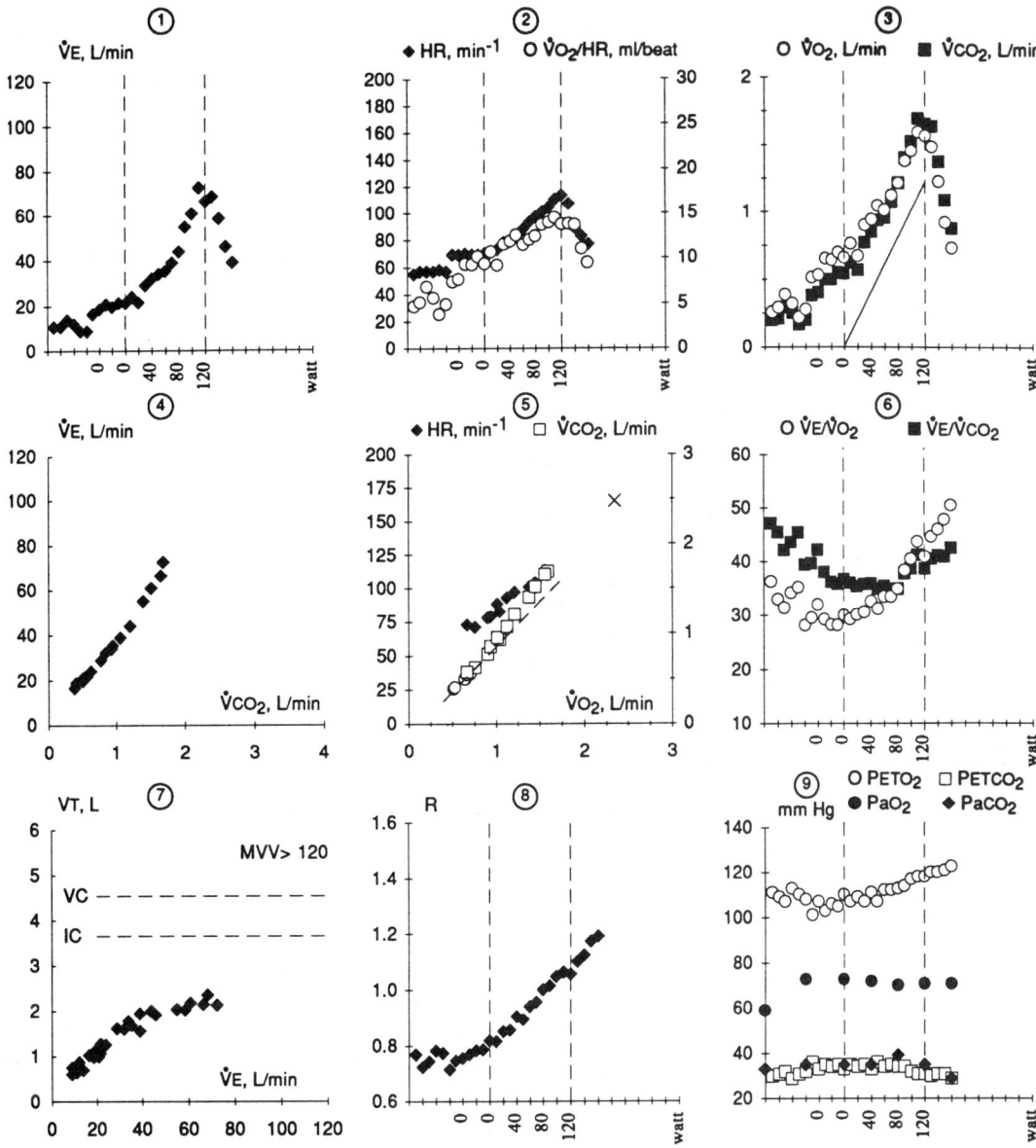

1. Vertical dashed lines in panels 1 to 3 and 6, 8, and 9 indicate the beginning and the end of increasing work period.

2. Unloaded cycling is performed for 3 minutes before the left vertical dashed line.

3. In panel 3, the diagonal line shows the increase of $\dot{V}O_2$ at a slope of 10 ml/min/W.

4. In panel 5, the diagonal dashed line has a slope of 1; the "x" in the upper right is the predicted maximum heart rate and $\dot{V}O_2$ for the subject.

TABLE 73-3.

Time min	Work rate watts	BP mm Hg	HR min⁻¹	f min⁻¹	$\dot{V}E$ L/min BTPS	$\dot{V}CO_2$ L/min STPD	$\dot{V}O_2$ L/min STPD	$\frac{\dot{V}O_2}{HR}$ ml/beat	R	pH	HCO₃ meq/L	PO2, mm Hg ET	a	(A-a)	PCO2, mm Hg ET	a	(a-ET)	$\frac{\dot{V}E}{\dot{V}CO_2}$	$\frac{\dot{V}E}{\dot{V}O_2}$	$\frac{VD}{VT}$
	Rest									7.47	24		59			33				
	Rest		55	15	10.7	0.20	0.26	4.7	0.77			111			30			47	36	
	Rest		57	17	11.0	0.21	0.29	5.1	0.72			109			31			46	33	
	Rest		57	20	13.9	0.29	0.39	6.8	0.74			107			32			42	31	
	Rest	182/107	57	14	12.1	0.25	0.32	5.6	0.78			113			29			44	34	
	Rest		58	15	9.0	0.17	0.22	3.8	0.77			110			31			45	35	
	Rest		57	12	8.9	0.20	0.28	4.9	0.71	7.44	23	108	73	31	32	35	3	39	28	0.33
	Unloaded		69	16	16.4	0.38	0.51	7.4	0.75			101			36			40	29	
	Unloaded	193/107	69	19	18.5	0.40	0.53	7.7	0.75			107			33			42	32	
	Unloaded		70	21	20.8	0.50	0.65	9.3	0.77			103			35			38	29	
	Unloaded		69	17	19.5	0.50	0.64	9.3	0.78			106			34			36	28	
	Unloaded		69	20	21.4	0.55	0.70	10.1	0.79			105			35			36	28	
	Unloaded		70	19	21.4	0.54	0.66	9.4	0.82	7.44	23	110	73	36	33	35	2	37	30	0.30
0.5	20		71	19	23.9	0.62	0.76	10.7	0.82			107			35			36	29	
1.0	20	194/107	73	17	21.6	0.57	0.67	9.2	0.85			109			34			35	30	
1.5	40		78	18	29.0	0.77	0.90	11.5	0.86			107			35			36	31	
2.0	40		79	20	32.2	0.85	0.94	11.9	0.90	7.44	23	111	72	40	33	35	2	36	32	0.30
2.5	60		83	19	33.9	0.93	1.04	12.5	0.89			107			36			35	31	
3.0	60	197/110	88	21	35.4	0.95	1.01	11.5	0.94			112			34			35	33	
3.5	80		93	20	39.0	1.07	1.12	12.0	0.96			112			35			35	33	
4.0	80		97	22	44.0	1.21	1.21	12.5	1.00	7.42	25	113	70	41	34	39	5	35	35	0.35
4.5	100		101	27	55.0	1.40	1.38	13.7	1.01			114			34			38	38	
5.0	100	206/113	104	28	61.0	1.52	1.45	13.9	1.05			117			32			39	40	
5.5	120		110	34	72.4	1.69	1.59	14.5	1.06			118			31			41	44	
6.0	120		113	31	66.4	1.65	1.56	13.8	1.06	7.42	22	118	71	46	31	35	4	39	41	0.35
	Recovery		107	29	68.4	1.63	1.48	13.8	1.10			120			30			40	45	
	Recovery	213/107	89	29	58.6	1.37	1.22	13.7	1.12			120			31			41	46	
	Recovery		83	24	46.0	1.08	0.92	11.1	1.17			121			31			41	48	
	Recovery		77	25	39.0	0.87	0.73	9.5	1.19	7.40	18	123	71	54	29	29	0	42	51	0.28

Interpretation

COMMENTS

The mechanics of breathing are normal, but the diffusing capacity is significantly reduced (Table 73-1). The resting ECG is normal.

ANALYSIS

In flow chart 1, maximum $\dot{V}O_2$ and the anaerobic threshold are reduced (Table 73-2). See flow chart 4. The breathing reserve is high (branchpoint 4.1). The ventilatory equivalent for CO_2 at the anaerobic threshold is high (branchpoint 4.3). This suggests that the patient has an abnormal pulmonary circulation. Confirmation of this is demonstrated by high VD/VT, $P(A-a)_{O_2}$, and $P(a-ET)_{CO_2}$ values (indices of ventilation-perfusion mismatching). Because there is no associated disturbance in respiratory mechanics, we must conclude that these findings are on the basis of primary pulmonary vascular disease. The significant reduction in diffusing capacity (DL_{CO}) is compatible with this conclusion. There is no abrupt decrease in Pa_{O_2} or O_2 saturation at the start of exercise (branchpoint 4.5), indicating that a right to left shunt does not accompany the pulmonary vascular disease. Because the patient is being treated with propranolol, the heart rate response is unusually low for this kind of abnormality. Thus, the low heart rate and the systemic hypertension likely contribute to the low maximum $\dot{V}O_2$ and anaerobic threshold.

CONCLUSION

Exercise limitation is caused by pulmonary vascular disease, systemic hypertension, and impaired heart rate response secondary to β_2 adrenergic blockade.

CASE 74 β-adrenergic blockade, obesity, and asbestosis

CLINICAL FINDINGS

This 61-year-old man was referred for follow-up cardiopulmonary exercise testing because of his 30-year work exposure to asbestos. He had stopped smoking 13 years before but had a 100 pack year history of cigarette smoking. He had noted dyspnea in the past 2 years (associated with an 11 kg weight gain) but denied cough, chest pain, claudication, or ankle edema. He had hypertension; his only medications were atenolol and nifedipine. Examination revealed rare crackles at the right lung base, normal heart sounds, and peripheral pulses. Resting ECG showed a prolonged PR interval, J-point elevations in leads V2 and V3, and nonspecific T wave abnormalities in the lateral chest leads. Chest roentgenograms revealed some diaphragmatic calcification, pleural thickening, and parenchymal scarring.

EXERCISE FINDINGS

The patient performed exercise on a cycle ergometer. He pedalled at 60 rpm without an added load for 3 minutes. The work rate was then increased 15 W per minute to tolerance. Heart rate and rhythm were continuously monitored; 12-lead ECGs were obtained during rest, exercise, and recovery. Blood pressure was measured with a sphygmomanometer and oxygen saturation with an ear oximeter. The patient appeared to give a good effort and stopped exercise because of general fatigue; he denied chest pain or dyspnea during or after the study. The patient had no ectopy or abnormal ECG changes during or after exercise. Ear oximetry studies were normal.

TABLE 74-1. *Selected Respiratory Function Data*

MEASUREMENT	PREDICTED	MEASURED
Age, yr		61
Sex		Male
Height, cm		179
Weight, kg	81	120
Hematocrit, %		42
VC, L	4.41	2.97
IC, L	2.94	2.67
TLC, L	6.75	5.04
FEV$_1$, L	3.46	2.34
FEV$_1$/VC, %	78	78
MVV, L/min	140	92
DL$_{CO}$, ml/mm Hg/min	27.2	26.6

TABLE 74-2. *Selected Exercise Data*

MEASUREMENT	PREDICTED	MEASURED
Maximum V̇O$_2$, L/min	2.50	1.92
Maximum HR, beats/min	159	105
Maximum O$_2$ pulse, ml/beat	15.7	18.8
ΔV̇O$_2$/ΔWR, ml/min/W	10.3	9.6
AT, L/min	> 1.10	1.3
Blood pressure, mm Hg (rest, max ex)		140/90, 160/80
Maximum V̇E, L/min		69
Exercise breathing reserve, L/min	> 15	23

TABLE 74-3.

Time min	Work rate watts	BP mm Hg	HR min^{-1}	f min^{-1}	$\dot{V}E$ L/min BTPS	$\dot{V}CO_2$ L/min STPD	$\dot{V}O_2$ L/min STPD	$\frac{\dot{V}O_2}{HR}$ ml/beat	R	pH	HCO$_3$ meq/L	PO2, mm Hg ET	a	(A-a)	PCO2, mm Hg ET	a	(a-ET)	$\frac{\dot{V}E}{VCO2}$	$\frac{\dot{V}E}{VO2}$	$\frac{VD}{VT}$
	Rest	140/90																		
	Rest		67	13	12.3	0.37	0.42	6.3	0.88			109			36			30	27	
	Rest		67	17	12.7	0.37	0.42	6.3	0.88			110			36			30	27	
	Rest		67	13	12.7	0.37	0.41	6.1	0.90			110			36			31	28	
	Rest	130/80	69	15	13.1	0.37	0.44	6.4	0.84			109			36			32	27	
	Unloaded		76	19	18.5	0.54	0.66	8.7	0.82			104			38			31	26	
	Unloaded		79	22	21.0	0.60	0.72	9.1	0.83			98			42			32	27	
	Unloaded		77	24	19.6	0.58	0.75	9.7	0.77			98			41			30	23	
	Unloaded	130/80	82	20	23.9	0.74	0.90	11.0	0.82			101			40			30	25	
	Unloaded		83	23	29.6	0.93	1.09	13.1	0.85			104			38			30	25	
	Unloaded		80	23	26.9	0.83	0.93	11.6	0.89			106			39			30	27	
0.5	15		83	22	26.7	0.81	0.90	10.8	0.90			93			45			31	28	
1.0	15	145/80	85	23	29.5	0.91	0.99	11.6	0.92			108			38			30	28	
1.5	30		84	23	30.4	0.94	1.05	12.5	0.90			106			38			30	27	
2.0	30		86	24	35.0	1.06	1.15	13.4	0.92			102			40			31	29	
2.5	45		87	24	34.4	1.07	1.18	13.6	0.91			106			38			30	27	
3.0	45	140/80	87	24	36.4	1.14	1.24	14.3	0.92			108			38			30	28	
3.5	60		88	26	36.1	1.15	1.27	14.4	0.91			98			43			29	27	
4.0	60		91	26	40.6	1.28	1.35	14.8	0.95			110			38			30	28	
4.5	75		92	27	45.0	1.41	1.44	15.7	0.98			107			39			30	30	
5.0	75	150/90	96	27	51.6	1.59	1.53	15.9	1.04			111			38			31	32	
5.5	90		100	29	56.1	1.70	1.63	16.3	1.04			112			37			32	33	
6.0	90		100	28	60.0	1.79	1.70	17.0	1.05			112			37			32	34	
6.5	105		105	33	65.5	1.92	1.82	17.3	1.05			113			36			33	34	
7.0	105	160/80	109	37	69.4	2.04	1.92	17.6	1.06			114			36			32	35	
	Recovery		98	32	61.2	1.89	1.78	18.2	1.06			111			39			31	33	
	Recovery		98	27	62.4	1.91	1.56	15.9	1.22			115			39			31	39	
	Recovery		90	25	54.5	1.62	1.23	13.7	1.32			118			37			32	43	
	Recovery		86	20	42.8	1.32	0.94	10.9	1.40			122			35			31	44	

Interpretation

COMMENTS

The reduced lung volumes are compatible with mild restrictive disease due to obesity (reduced ERV) and asbestosis. The nearly normal IC suggests that the restriction is primarily caused by obesity.

ANALYSIS

In flow chart 1, maximum $\dot{V}O_2$ is reduced (branchpoint 1.1), but the anaerobic threshold is normal (branchpoints 1.2 and 1.3), despite the patient's inability to raise his exercise heart rate above 105 beats/min. Going next to flow chart 3, the normal breathing reserve (branchpoint 3.1) and probably normal ECG (branchpoint 3.2) lead one to the diagnosis of poor effort or musculoskeletal disorder. There are no measures of VD/VT or arterial-alveolar pressure differences, but the normal ventilatory equivalents and normal ear oximetry are evidence against any major gas ex-

change abnormality during exercise. The high heart rate reserve might lead one to consider poor effort, but the high recovery R of 1.40 (indicating a significant metabolic acidosis) is evidence against this diagnosis. The low maximum heart rate and accompanying high maximum O_2 pulse are best explained by a high degree of β blockade from atenolol, which gives more time than usual for filling of the ventricles. The high $\dot{V}O_2$ at unloaded pedalling (nearly 1.0 L/min) is typical of obesity.

CONCLUSION

β-adrenergic blockade therapy of hypertension can cause significant reduction in maximum heart rate, maximum $\dot{V}O_2$, and maximum work rate. Usually, as in this patient, the increase in O_2 pulse is an important factor in overcoming the effect of reduction in maximum heart rate and minimizing the effect on maximum $\dot{V}O_2$. Obesity and the limited ability to increase heart rate can lead to the symptom of fatigue, however, as found in this case.

FIG. 74-A.

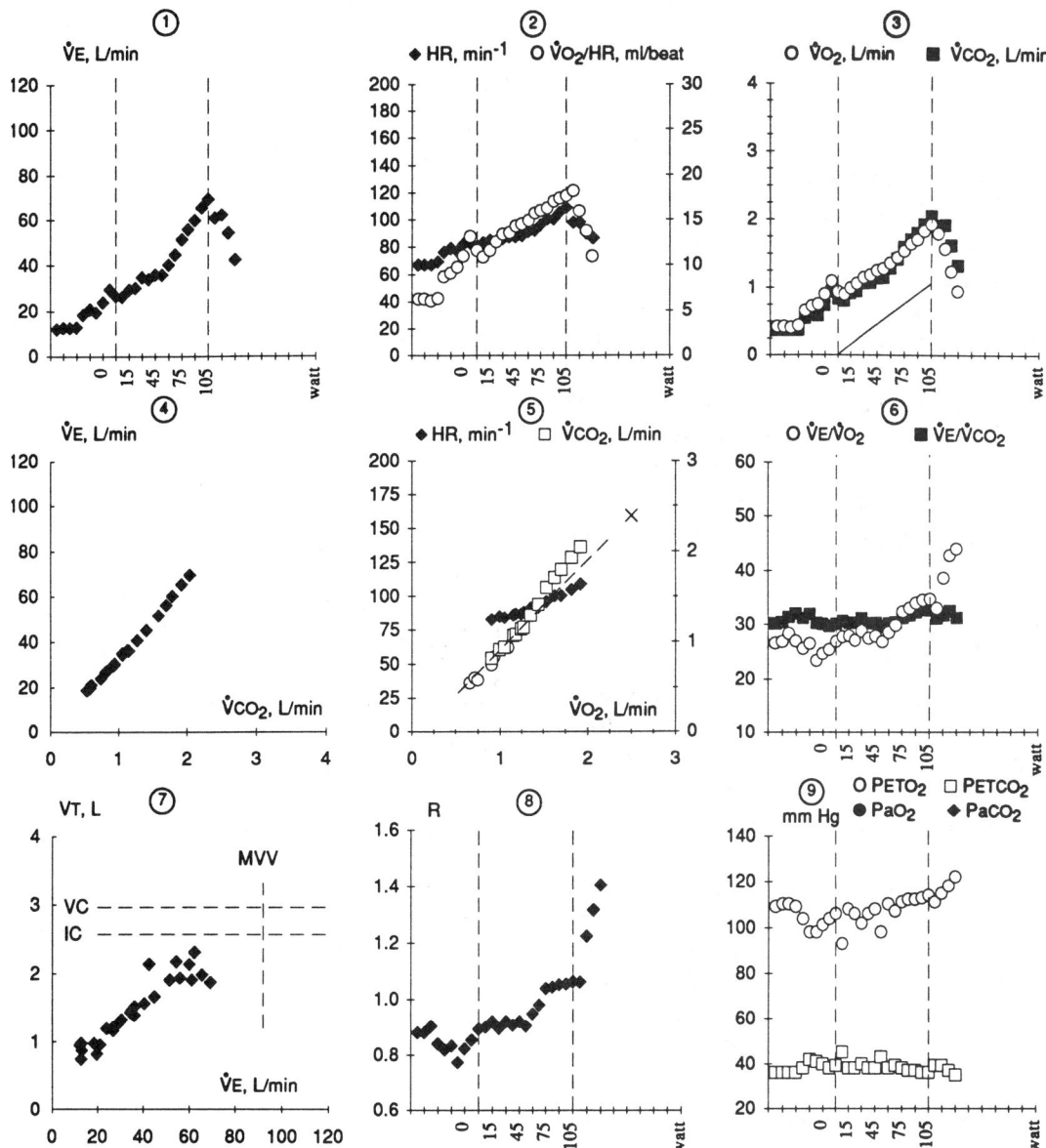

1. Vertical dashed lines in panels 1 to 3 and 6, 8, and 9 indicate the beginning and the end of increasing work period.

2. Unloaded cycling is performed for 3 minutes before the left vertical dashed line.

3. In panel 3, the diagonal line shows the increase of $\dot{V}O_2$ at a slope of 10 ml/min/W.

4. In panel 5, the diagonal dashed line has a slope of 1; the "x" in the upper right is the predicted maximum heart rate and $\dot{V}O_2$ for the subject.

CASE 75 *Pulmonary vascular disease, chronic bronchitis, asbestosis, and myocardial ischemia*

CLINICAL FINDINGS

This 51-year-old shipyard worker had noted increased dyspnea on exertion for 2 years, until he was unable to finish cleaning his one bedroom apartment. For several years he had had a morning cough productive of small amounts of yellow sputum. He had over 40 pack years of cigarette smoking and continued to smoke. He denied chest pain, tightness, or pressure. Chest x-ray studies showed a streaky infiltrate in the lower lung fields with nodular scarring in the upper lung zones. Physical examination of the chest was normal. There was equivocal clubbing of the digits. Peripheral pulses were normal. ECG showed left axis deviation.

EXERCISE FINDINGS

The patient performed exercise on a cycle ergometer. He first pedalled at 60 rpm, without added load, for 3 minutes. The work rate was then increased 15 W per minute to his symptom-limited maximum. Arterial blood was sampled every second minute, and intra-arterial blood pressure was recorded from a percutaneously placed brachial artery catheter. The patient stopped exercising because of severe knee cramps. During incremental exercise he developed premature atrial and ventricular contractions, and 3 to 4 mm ST segment depression in leads V4 and V5. He denied any chest pain or discomfort, dizziness or lightheadedness. The ST segments returned to normal within 1 minute of recovery.

TABLE 75-1. *Selected Respiratory Function Data*

MEASUREMENT	PREDICTED	MEASURED
Age, yr		51
Sex		Male
Height, cm		166
Weight, kg	70	55
Hematocrit, %		49
VC, L	3.88	3.83
IC, L	2.59	2.37
TLC, L	5.71	6.81
FEV_1, L	3.07	2.41
FEV_1/VC, %	79	63
MVV, L/min, direct	136	120
MVV, L/min, indirect	123	96
D_{LCO}, ml/mm Hg/min	26.9	21.5

TABLE 75-2. *Selected Exercise Data*

MEASUREMENT	PREDICTED	MEASURED
Maximum $\dot{V}_{O_2}$, L/min	1.99	1.77
Maximum HR, beats/min	169	150
Maximum O_2 pulse, ml/beat	11.8	11.8
$\Delta\dot{V}_{O_2}/\Delta WR$, ml/min/W	10.3	9.7
AT, L/min	> 0.86	1.2
Blood pressure, mm Hg (rest, max)		132/72,189/99
Maximum $\dot{V}_E$, L/min		79
Exercise breathing reserve, L/min	> 15	17
Pa_{O_2}, mm Hg (rest, max ex)		69,63
$P(A-a)_{O_2}$, mm Hg (rest, max ex)		30,44
$P(a-ET)_{CO_2}$, mm Hg (rest, max ex)		10,6
V_D/V_T (rest, heavy ex)		0.53,0.47
HCO_3^-, mEq/L (rest, 2-min recov)		25,17

Fig. 75-A.

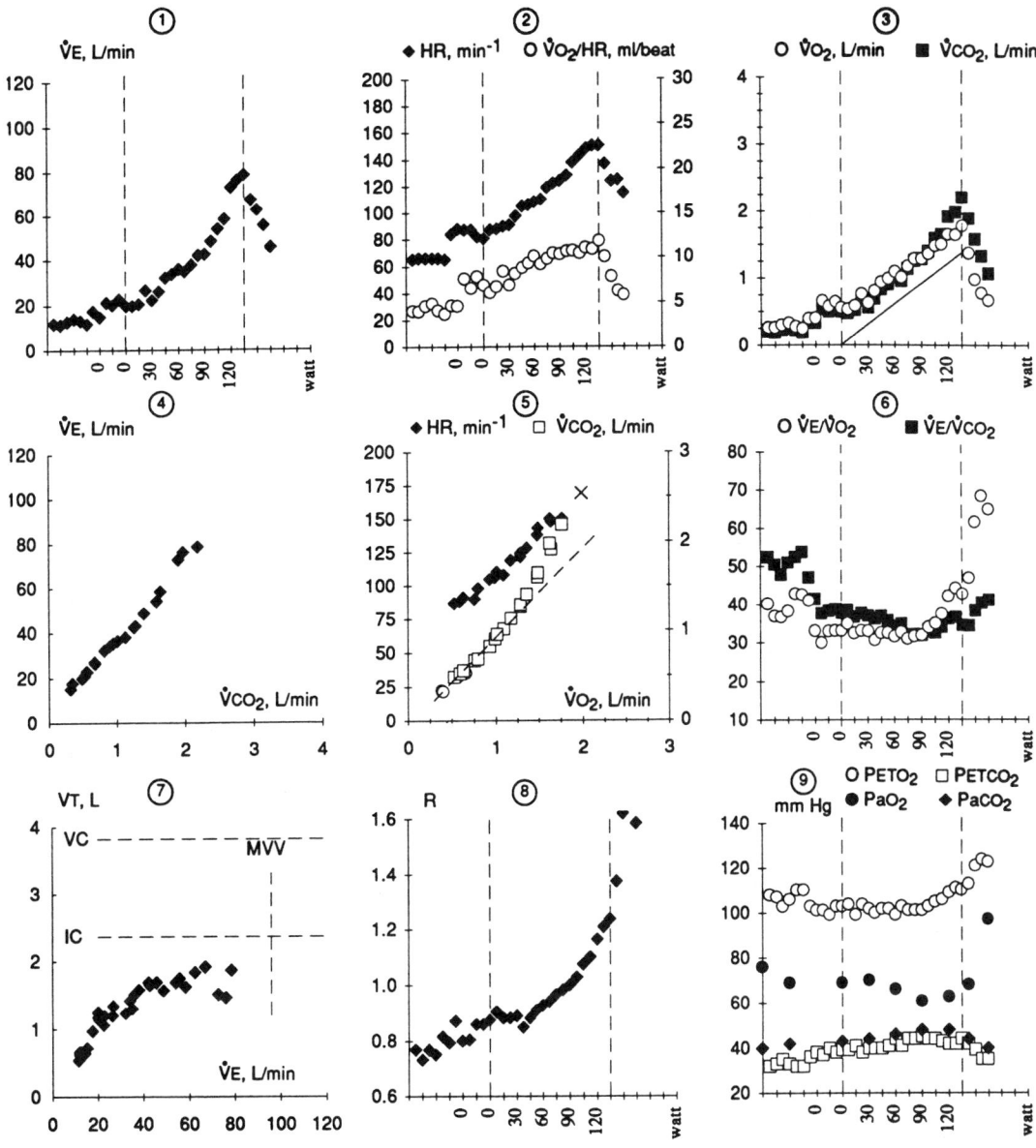

1. Vertical dashed lines in panels 1 to 3 and 6, 8, and 9 indicate the beginning and the end of increasing work period.

2. Unloaded cycling is performed for 3 minutes before the left vertical dashed line.

3. In panel 3, the diagonal line shows the increase of $\dot{V}_{O_2}$ at a slope of 10 ml/min/W.

4. In panel 5, the diagonal dashed line has a slope of 1; the "x" in the upper right is the predicted maximum heart rate and $\dot{V}_{O_2}$ for the subject.

Interpretation

COMMENTS

Resting respiratory function tests are compatible with mild airflow obstruction (Table 75-1). The diffusing capacity is at the lower limits of normal. The resting ECG is essentially normal.

ANALYSIS

In flow chart 1, the maximum $\dot{V}_{O_2}$ and the anaerobic threshold are normal (Table 75-2). See flow chart 2. The ECG at maximum exercise is abnormal suggesting ischemic changes. The arterial blood gases are also significantly abnormal during

TABLE 75-3.

Time min	Work rate watts	BP mm Hg	HR min⁻¹	f min⁻¹	V̇E L/min BTPS	V̇CO₂ L/min STPD	V̇O₂ L/min STPD	V̇O₂/HR ml/beat	R	pH	HCO₃ meq/L	PO2, mm Hg ET	a	(A-a)	PCO2, mm Hg ET	a	(a-ET)	V̇E/V̇CO₂	V̇E/V̇O₂	VD/VT
	Rest	132/72								7.42	25		76			40				
	Rest		65	18	12.0	0.20	0.26	4.0	0.77			108			32			52	40	
	Rest		66	21	11.4	0.19	0.26	3.9	0.73			107			33			51	37	
	Rest		66	19	12.6	0.23	0.30	4.5	0.77			103			35			48	37	
	Rest	159/81	66	22	14.1	0.24	0.32	4.8	0.75	7.39	25	106	69	28	33	42	9	51	38	0.52
	Rest		66	21	13.3	0.22	0.27	4.1	0.81			110			32			52	43	
	Rest		65	19	11.8	0.19	0.24	3.7	0.79			110			32			54	42	
	Unloaded		84	18	17.5	0.34	0.39	4.6	0.87			103			36			47	41	
	Unloaded		88	21	15.0	0.32	0.40	4.5	0.80			101			38			41	33	
	Unloaded		87	18	21.4	0.53	0.66	7.6	0.80			101			37			37	30	
	Unloaded	165/90	87	16	20.1	0.49	0.57	6.6	0.86			99			40			38	33	
	Unloaded		82	19	22.8	0.55	0.64	7.8	0.86			103			38			39	33	
	Unloaded		81	16	19.9	0.49	0.56	6.9	0.88	7.38	25	103	69	33	39	43	4	38	33	0.44
0.5	15		87	17	19.9	0.48	0.53	6.1	0.91			104			39			38	35	
1.0	15	180/93	88	18	20.6	0.52	0.59	6.7	0.88			99			41			37	32	
1.5	30		90	20	26.9	0.67	0.76	8.4	0.88			104			38			38	33	
2.0	30		91	21	22.5	0.56	0.63	6.9	0.89	7.37	25	102	70	32	40	44	4	37	33	0.43
2.5	45		98	22	26.4	0.68	0.80	8.2	0.85			100			40			36	31	
3.0	45	186/93	105	26	32.3	0.82	0.93	8.9	0.88			102			40			37	32	
3.5	60		106	24	34.2	0.90	0.99	9.3	0.91			102			41			36	32	
4.0	60		108	24	36.4	1.01	1.09	10.1	0.93	7.35	25	99	66	35	44	46	2	34	32	0.42
4.5	75		110	27	35.3	0.95	1.01	9.2	0.94			103			41			35	33	
5.0	75	189/93	119	24	38.1	1.13	1.17	9.8	0.97			101			44			32	31	
5.5	90		122	25	42.4	1.26	1.28	10.5	0.98			101			44			32	31	
6.0	90		124	26	43.0	1.28	1.28	10.3	1.00	7.31	24	101	61	41	45	48	3	32	32	0.41
6.5	105		128	31	48.8	1.40	1.36	10.6	1.03			103			44			33	34	
7.0	105	191/99	138	32	54.2	1.59	1.48	10.7	1.07			105			44			32	35	
7.5	120		143	36	58.6	1.64	1.49	10.4	1.10			106			43			34	37	
8.0	120		148	48	72.8	1.91	1.64	11.1	1.16	7.28	22	109	63	44	42	48	6	36	42	0.47
8.5	135		150	52	76.2	1.97	1.63	10.9	1.21			111			42			36	44	
9.0	135	189/99	150	42	78.7	2.19	1.77	11.8	1.24			110			44			34	42	
	Recovery		137	35	67.2	1.88	1.37	10.0	1.37	7.25	19	113	68	47	42	44	2	34	47	0.41
	Recovery	184/84	124	34	62.6	1.57	0.97	7.8	1.62			121			39			38	62	
	Recovery		125	32	55.9	1.32	0.78	6.2	1.69			124			35			40	68	
	Recovery		115	27	45.8	1.06	0.67	5.8	1.58	7.24	17	123	97	25	35	40	5	41	65	0.45

exercise (branchpoint 2.1). The indices of ventilation-perfusion matching (V_D/V_T, $P(a - ET)_{CO_2}$, and $P(A - a)_{O_2}$) (branchpoint 2.3) are clearly abnormal, suggesting that this patient has lung disease and/or pulmonary vascular disease. Because the results of the resting respiratory function tests are not consistent with a diagnosis of restrictive lung disease and suggest that the patient's airflow obstruction is only mild, it is likely that the major abnormalities in ventilation-perfusion mismatching observed in this patient are attributable to pulmonary vascular disease. The ECG abnormalities that this patient developed as he approached his maximum work rate, despite the absence of chest pain, suggest that the patient also develops myocardial ischemia under exercise stress.

CONCLUSION

This study shows normal maximum exercise capacity in a patient with pulmonary vascular disease and myocardial ischemia. There is clear evidence of significant ventilation-perfusion mismatching of the type seen with pulmonary vascular disease; however, his pulmonary mechanics are only mildly abnormal. Presumably, this is an instance of changes in the pulmonary circulation disproportionate to airway or parenchymal disease. Additionally, the exercise induced ST segment depression and arrhythmia, typical of myocardial ischemia, suggest coronary artery disease. The pulmonary vascular disease and exercise hypoxemia possibly contribute to this cardiac abnormality.

CASE 76 *Asthma, obesity, and anemia*

CLINICAL FINDINGS

This 50-year-old meatcutter and former smoker had severe exertional dyspnea and had been hospitalized on several occasions for what had been considered to be congestive failure with wheezing, leg edema, and orthopnea. He was referred for exercise testing to aid in distinguishing between cardiac and respiratory disease. He had been anemic for an unknown period of time but had no dependent edema at the time of testing. Breath sounds were distant.

EXERCISE FINDINGS

The patient performed exercise on a cycle ergometer. He pedalled at 60 rpm without an added load for 3 minutes. The work rate was then increased 15 W per minute to tolerance. Arterial blood was sampled every second minute, and intra-arterial pressure was recorded from a percutaneously placed brachial artery catheter. Heart rate and rhythm were continuously monitored; 12-lead ECGs were obtained during rest, exercise, and recovery. The patient appeared to give an excellent effort and stopped exercise because of severe dyspnea and exhaustion. He denied chest pain during or after the study. No arrhythmias or ischemic changes were noted on ECG.

TABLE 76-1. *Selected Respiratory Function Data*

MEASUREMENT	PREDICTED	MEASURED
Age, yr		50
Sex		Male
Height, cm		174
Weight, kg	77	91
Hemoglobin, g/100 ml		10.3
VC, L	4.40	3.11
IC, L	2.94	2.15
TLC, L	6.44	9.78
FEV_1, L	3.49	1.14
FEV_1/VC, %	79	37
MVV, L/min	147	45
DL_{CO}, ml/mm Hg/min	24.4	28.8

TABLE 76-2. *Selected Exercise Data*

MEASUREMENT	PREDICTED	MEASURED
Maximum $\dot{V}O_2$, L/min	2.55	1.20
Maximum HR, beats/min	170	147
Maximum O_2 pulse, ml/beat	14.3	8.4
$\Delta\dot{V}O_2/\Delta WR$, ml/min/W	10.3	7.6
AT, L/min	> 1.10	0.95
Blood pressure, mm Hg (rest, max)		135/90,180/84
Maximum $\dot{V}E$, L/min		41
Exercise breathing reserve, L/min	> 15	4
Pa_{O_2}, mm Hg (rest, max ex)		84,76
$P(A-a)_{O_2}$, mm Hg (rest, max ex)		19,21
$P(a-ET)_{CO_2}$, mm Hg (rest, max ex)		5,5
VD/VT (rest, max ex)		0.43,0.46
HCO_3^-, mEq/L (rest, max ex)		31,29

TABLE 76-3.

Time min	Work rate watts	BP mm Hg	HR min⁻¹	f min⁻¹	$\dot{V}E$ L/min BTPS	$\dot{V}CO_2$ L/min STPD	$\dot{V}O_2$ L/min STPD	$\frac{\dot{V}O_2}{HR}$ ml/beat	R	pH	HCO₃ meq/L	PO2, mm Hg ET	a	(A-a)	PCO2, mm Hg ET	a	(a-ET)	$\frac{\dot{V}E}{\dot{V}CO_2}$	$\frac{\dot{V}E}{\dot{V}O_2}$	$\frac{VD}{VT}$
	Rest		122	19	16.4	0.41	0.44	3.6	0.93			107			39			36	34	
	Rest		122	21	16.0	0.38	0.42	3.4	0.90			106			39			37	34	
	Rest		122	22	16.4	0.38	0.41	3.4	0.93			108			38			38	35	
	Rest	135/90	123	23	16.8	0.38	0.42	3.4	0.90	7.48	31	107	84	19	38	43	5	39	35	0.43
	Rest		123	25	17.0	0.36	0.40	3.3	0.90			108			38			41	37	
	Rest		123	25	16.4	0.35	0.41	3.3	0.85			106			39			41	35	
	Rest		122	22	16.6	0.39	0.44	3.6	0.89			106			39			38	33	
	Rest	126/84	123	22	15.8	0.37	0.42	3.4	0.88	7.46	31	104	78	22	40	45	5	38	33	0.43
	Unloaded		123	35	18.1	0.32	0.41	3.3	0.78			103			38			47	37	
	Unloaded		123	31	20.1	0.44	0.57	4.6	0.77			99			41			40	31	
	Unloaded		122	28	20.6	0.50	0.64	5.2	0.78			98			42			36	28	
	Unloaded	138/90	122	26	22.2	0.57	0.60	4.9	0.95	7.42	31	99	82	17	41	49	8	35	33	0.45
0.5	15		123	33	22.3	0.49	0.61	5.0	0.80			100			41			40	32	
1.0	15		124	30	24.6	0.63	0.78	6.3	0.81			98			43			35	28	
1.5	30		126	31	25.9	0.68	0.80	6.3	0.85			101			42			34	29	
2.0	30		127	26	25.9	0.79	0.88	6.9	0.90			98			46			30	27	
2.5	45		129	29	30.0	0.92	0.97	7.5	0.95			99			46			30	28	
3.0	45	140/78	132	33	32.9	0.99	1.00	7.6	0.99	7.38	30	103	85	14	46	51	5	30	30	0.41
3.5	60		131	31	33.9	1.11	1.07	8.2	1.04			100			49			28	29	
4.0	60		134	35	36.8	1.14	1.08	8.1	1.06			103			48			30	31	
4.5	75		139	30	36.6	1.24	1.15	8.3	1.08			102			50			27	30	
5.0	75	132/84	142	36	39.6	1.27	1.19	8.4	1.07	7.32	29	100	76	19	51	58	7	29	31	0.45
5.5	90		145	43	40.8	1.25	1.20	8.3	1.04			100			51			30	31	
6.0	90	180/84	147	48	40.4	1.19	1.07	7.3	1.11	7.32	29	95	76	21	53	58	5	31	34	0.46
	Recovery		138	47	32.8	1.02	1.02	7.4	1.00			89			60			28	28	
	Recovery		138	50	30.1	0.81	0.83	6.0	0.98			89			60			32	31	

Interpretation

COMMENTS

Resting respiratory function studies showed severe obstructive lung disease with hyperinflation, no improvement in flow rates following inhaled albuterol, and an above predicted D_{LCO}. (The predicted value for D_{LCO} was adjusted for the patient's anemia; the measured value was not adjusted.) The patient was also overweight, with arterial blood gases and pH suggesting a chronic compensated respiratory acidosis and an acute respiratory alkalosis.

ANALYSIS

In flow chart 1, the maximum $\dot{V}O_2$ and anaerobic threshold were both decreased (Table 76-2). Most striking is the ventilatory limitation accompanied by increasing respiratory acidosis and a low O_2 pulse. We are directed through branchpoints 1.1, 1.2, and 1.3 to flow chart 4. The low breathing reserve (branchpoint 4.1) and the high VD/VT (branchpoint 4.2) lead us to "lung disease with impaired peripheral oxygenation." The patient's data do not fit the conditions listed under this diagnosis perfectly, but he does have a low arterial O_2 content (anemia and slightly decreased arterial O_2 saturation) and many of the factors listed in the pulmonary vascular disease category. If we had used flow chart 5, we might have arrived through branchpoints 5.1, 5.3, and 5.7 to the diagnosis of "obstructive lung disease." This is satisfactory, especially because of the severe respiratory acidosis that developed during exercise, but it accounts poorly for his low $\Delta\dot{V}O_2/\Delta WR$ and flat O_2 pulse, which indicate an O_2 flow problem. These latter abnormalities relate to his anemia.

CONCLUSION

As noted in Chapter 7, the flow charts cannot, and should not, always come to a single diagnosis. This is because the patient may have pathophysiologic features involving more than one organ system. In this patient, the primary problem appears to be severe obstructive lung disease, complicated by anemia and obesity. Associated pulmonary vascular disease cannot be excluded.

Fig. 76-A.

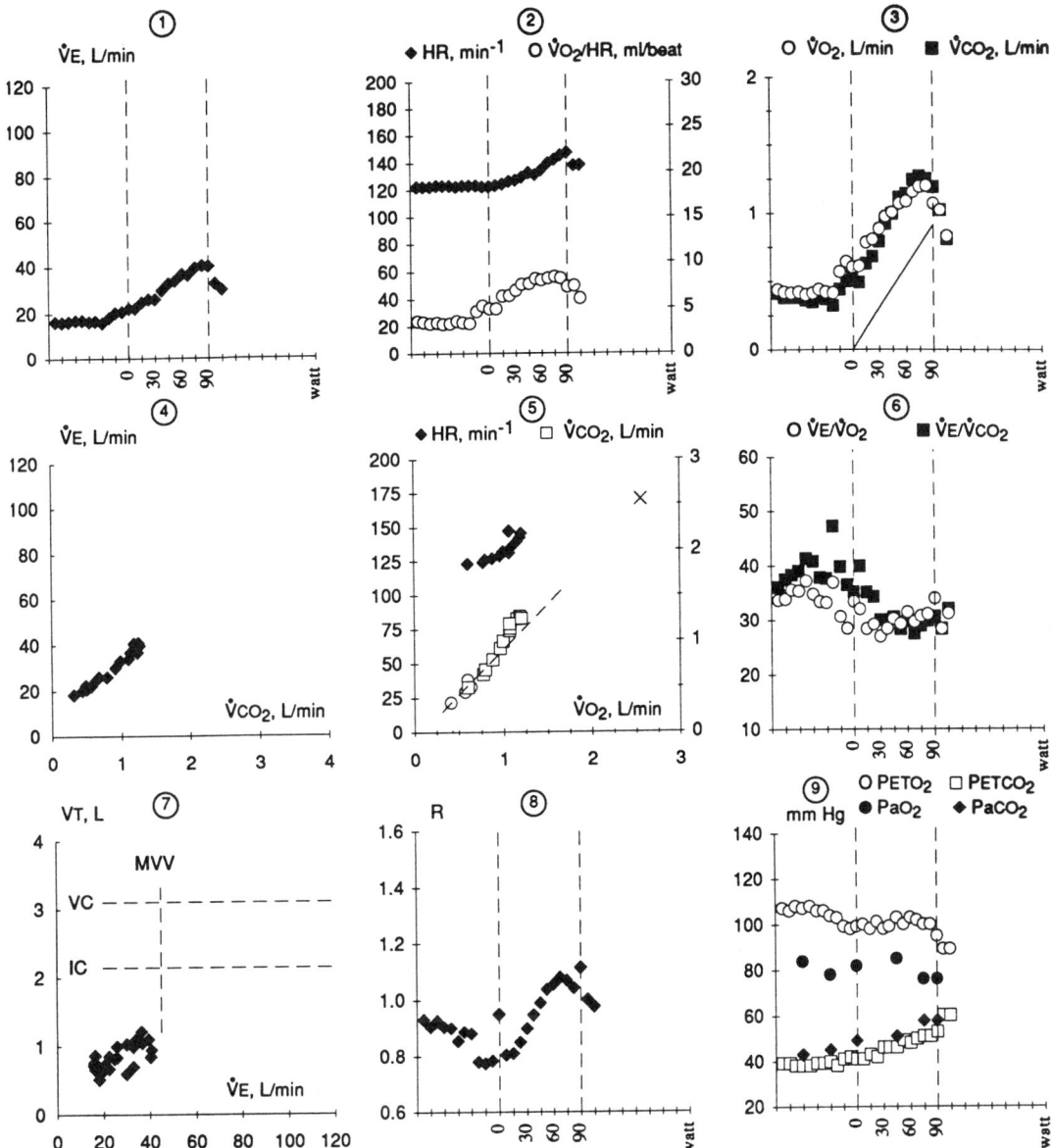

1. Vertical dashed lines in panels 1 to 3 and 6, 8, and 9 indicate the beginning and the end of increasing work period.

2. Unloaded cycling is performed for 2 minutes before the left vertical dashed line.

3. In panel 3, the diagonal line shows the increase of $\dot{V}O_2$ at a slope of 10 ml/min/W.

4. In panel 5, the diagonal dashed line has a slope of 1; the "x" in the upper right is the predicted maximum heart rate and $\dot{V}O_2$ for the subject.

CASE 77 *Obstructive airway and pulmonary vascular disease, with a patent foramen ovale and systemic hypertension*

CLINICAL FINDINGS

This 64-year-old retired shipyard worker was evaluated because of increasing shortness of breath that had begun 7 years previously and had increased to become evident with walking two blocks or climbing a flight of stairs. He had smoked half a pack of cigarettes daily from age 40 to 60. He had been treated with ioniazid and ethambutol for pulmonary tuberculosis for 4 years, 2 decades before. Prostatic carcinoma had been diagnosed 8 months previously while he was having a transurethral prostatectomy. He took triamterene, hydrochlorothiazide, and methyldopa for the treatment of hypertension. Pulse was irregular without other evidence of cardiovascular disease. The chest x-ray studies revealed a single small pleural plaque on the left, evidence of old granulomatous disease in the right apex, and a flat diaphragm. Respiratory function tests done several days prior to exercise showed airway obstruction.

EXERCISE FINDINGS

The patient performed exercise on a cycle ergometer. He pedalled at 60 rpm without added load for 3 minutes. The work rate was then increased 15 W per minute to his symptom-limited maximum. Arterial blood was sampled every second minute, and intra-arterial blood pressure was recorded from a percutaneously placed brachial artery catheter. Resting ECG showed some premature atrial and premature ventricular contractions, poor R wave progression from leads V1 through V3, and

left atrial enlargement. At 90 W there were occasional pairs of premature ventricular contractions and two episodes of ventricular bigeminy. The patient stopped exercising because of shortness of breath. Under questioning, he also conceded that he had felt some substernal tightness at the highest work rate.

TABLE 77-1. *Selected Respiratory Function Data*

MEASUREMENT	PREDICTED	MEASURED
Age, yr		64
Sex		Male
Height, cm		178
Weight, kg	80	82
Hematocrit, %		47
		BEFORE BRONCHODILATOR	AFTER BRONCHODILATOR
VC, L	3.82	4.52	4.75
IC, L	2.55	3.25	
TLC, L	5.93	8.66	
FEV$_1$, L	2.98	2.69	2.78
FEV$_1$/VC, %	78	60	58
MVV, L/min	121	90	112
D$_{LCO}$, ml/mm Hg/min	24.8	14.0	

TABLE 77-2. *Selected Exercise Data*

MEASUREMENT	PREDICTED	MEASURED
Maximum $\dot{V}_{O_2}$, L/min	2.16	1.42
Maximum HR, beats/min	156	159
Maximum O$_2$ pulse, ml/beat	13.9	8.9
$\Delta\dot{V}_{O_2}/\Delta WR$, ml/min/W	10.3	8.1
AT, L/min	> 0.95	1.2
Blood pressure, mm Hg (rest, max)		186/116,263/128
Maximum $\dot{V}_E$, L/min		91
Exercise breathing reserve, L/min	> 15	−1
Pa$_{O_2}$, mm Hg (rest, max ex)		79,57
P(A−a)$_{O_2}$, mm Hg (rest, max ex)		38,65
P(a−ET)$_{CO_2}$, mm Hg (rest, max ex)		4,9
V$_D$/V$_T$ (rest, heavy ex)		0.38,0.47
HCO$_3^-$, mEq/L (rest, 2-min recov)		24,17

Fɪɢ. 77-A.

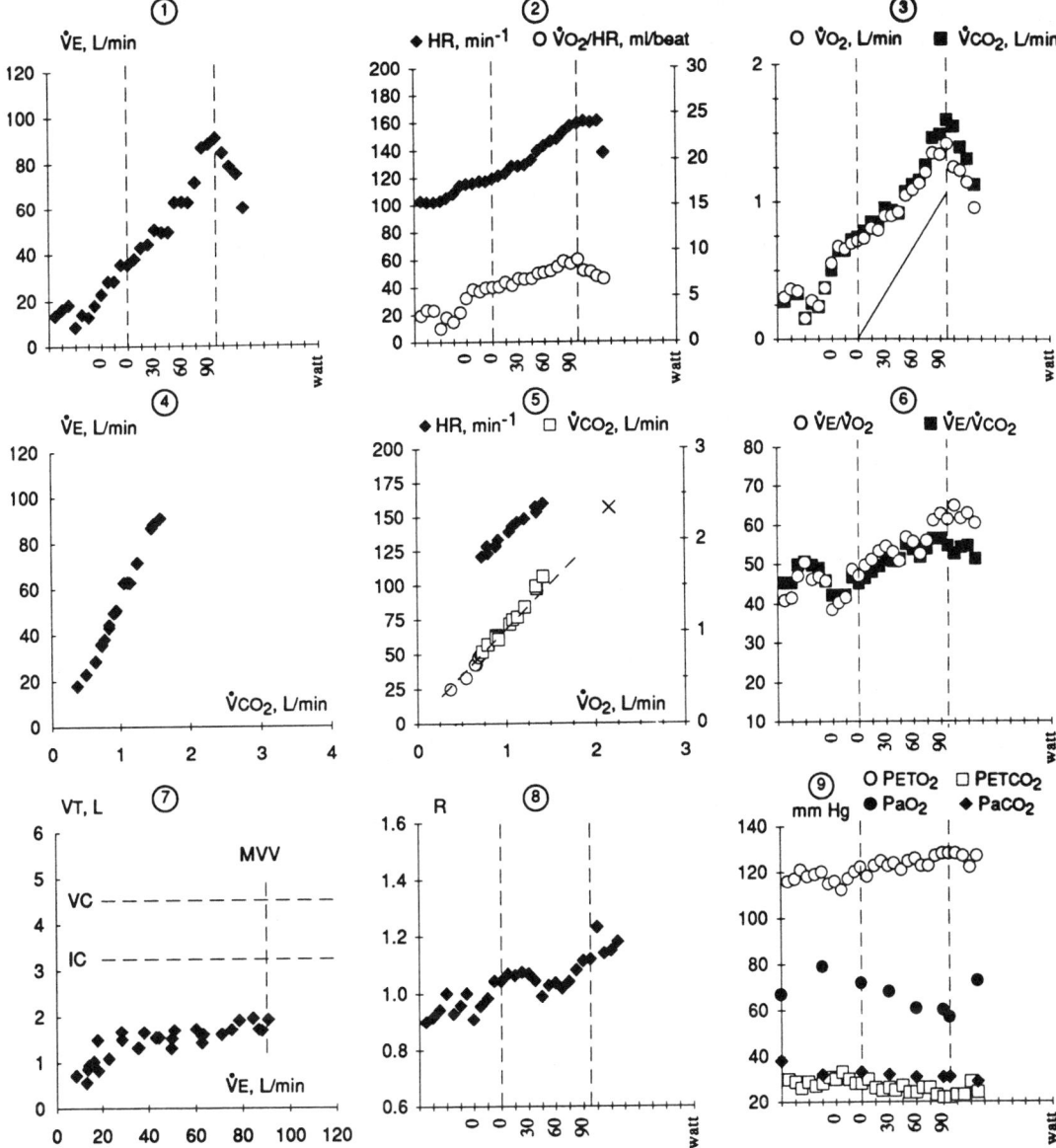

1. Vertical dashed lines in panels 1 to 3 and 6, 8, and 9 indicate the beginning and the end of increasing work period.

2. Unloaded cycling is performed for 3 minutes before the left vertical dashed line.

3. In panel 3, the diagonal line shows the increase of $\dot{V}O_2$ at a slope of 10 ml/min/W.

4. In panel 5, the diagonal dashed line has a slope of 1; the "x" in the upper right is the predicted maximum heart rate and $\dot{V}O_2$ for the subject.

TABLE 77-3.

Time min	Work rate watts	BP mm Hg	HR min⁻¹	f min⁻¹	$\dot{V}_E$ L/min BTPS	$\dot{V}_{CO_2}$ L/min STPD	$\dot{V}_{O_2}$ L/min STPD	$\frac{\dot{V}_{O_2}}{HR}$ ml/beat	R	pH	HCO₃ meq/L	PO2 ET	PO2 a	PO2 (A-a)	PCO2 ET	PCO2 a	PCO2 (a-ET)	$\frac{\dot{V}_E}{\dot{V}_{CO_2}}$	$\frac{\dot{V}_E}{\dot{V}_{O_2}}$	$\frac{V_D}{V_T}$
	Rest	185/116								7.42	24		67			38				
	Rest		103	16	13.6	0.27	0.30	2.9	0.90			116			30			45	41	
	Rest		102	16	16.3	0.33	0.36	3.5	0.92			117			29			45	42	
	Rest		102	22	18.3	0.33	0.35	3.4	0.94			121			26			50	47	
	Rest		103	12	8.6	0.15	0.15	1.5	1.00			118			29			51	51	
	Rest		105	15	14.2	0.26	0.28	2.7	0.93			119			27			50	46	
	Rest	185/116	108	23	13.2	0.23	0.24	2.2	0.96	7.46	22	120	79	38	28	32	4	49	47	0.38
	Unloaded		114	12	17.9	0.37	0.37	3.2	1.00			115			31			46	46	
	Unloaded		115	21	22.9	0.50	0.55	4.8	0.91			116			30			42	38	
	Unloaded		116	17	28.4	0.64	0.67	5.8	0.96			112			33			42	40	
	Unloaded		117	19	28.5	0.64	0.65	5.6	0.98			117			30			42	41	
	Unloaded		117	27	35.8	0.72	0.69	5.9	1.04			120			28			47	49	
	Unloaded	236/126	119	27	35.6	0.74	0.71	6.0	1.04	7.43	22	122	72	46	28	33	5	45	47	0.39
0.5	15		121	23	38.1	0.78	0.73	6.0	1.07			118			30			46	50	
1.0	15		123	28	43.1	0.85	0.80	6.5	1.06			123			26			48	51	
1.5	30		128	29	44.5	0.85	0.79	6.2	1.08			125			25			49	53	
2.0	30	236/128	128	30	50.9	0.95	0.89	7.0	1.07	7.44	21	123	68	52	26	32	6	51	54	0.45
2.5	45		129	33	49.9	0.93	0.89	6.9	1.04			124			25			51	53	
3.0	45		133	38	49.8	0.91	0.92	6.9	0.99			121			27			51	51	
3.5	60		139	44	62.7	1.07	1.04	7.5	1.03			125			24			55	57	
4.0	60		143	39	63.2	1.12	1.08	7.6	1.04	7.44	21	126	61	59	24	31	7	53	55	0.45
4.5	75		146	40	62.7	1.15	1.13	7.7	1.02			123			26			52	52	
5.0	75		148	44	71.3	1.26	1.21	8.2	1.04			123			26			54	56	
5.5	90		153	50	86.6	1.46	1.35	8.8	1.08			127			23			56	61	
6.0	90		157	52	88.2	1.49	1.34	8.5	1.11	7.42	20	128	60	61	22	31	9	56	63	0.48
6.5	105	263/128	159	47	90.8	1.59	1.42	8.9	1.12	7.41	19	128	57	65	22	31	9	55	61	0.47
	Recovery		161	43	84.4	1.54	1.25	7.8	1.23			128			23			52	65	
	Recovery		160	41	78.6	1.39	1.22	7.6	1.14			127			23			54	62	
	Recovery		161	44	75.2	1.31	1.14	7.1	1.15			122			29			55	63	
	Recovery	233/139	138	35	60.3	1.12	0.95	6.9	1.18	7.39	17	127	73	51	24	29	5	51	60	0.40

Interpretation

COMMENTS

This case is presented to illustrate the considerable amount of gas exchange abnormality that can occur during exercise, even with only mild abnormalities in spirometry.

The results of the resting respiratory function studies indicate that this patient has mild airflow obstruction, hyperinflation, and a moderately severe abnormality in diffusing capacity (Table 77-1). The resting ECG is abnormal, as evidenced by premature atrial and ventricular contractions and poor R wave progression from V1 to V3. The intra-arterial blood pressure is elevated. In such instances, one might have considered deferring the exercise test until blood pressure was under better control. The cuff-measured blood pressure is on the average 10 mm Hg lower than the directly recorded blood pressure, as described in Chapter

6. Because of the blood pressure elevation, the patient was exercised especially cautiously. The objective was to determine if this patient was primarily limited by his heart or lung disorder.

ANALYSIS

In flow chart 1, the maximum $\dot{V}_{O_2}$ is reduced while the anaerobic threshold is normal (Table 77-2), which directs us through branchpoints 1.1, 1.2, and 1.3 to flow chart 3. The breathing reserve is low (branchpoint 3.1). The patient has evidence of lung disease with ventilation-perfusion mismatching (high V_D/V_T, $P(a-ET)_{CO_2}$, and $P(A-a)_{O_2}$), but the heart rate reserve is low, not high. Further, at branchpoint 3.2, although his ventilatory frequency at maximal exercise is less than 50, consistent with his obstructive (low FEV_1/VC) lung disease, he does not develop a respiratory acidosis during exercise. However, it is not necessary to confirm every physiologic abnormality accompanying a disorder. Therefore, we use flow chart 5 through branchpoints 5.1, 5.3, and 5.7 to the diagnostic box entitled "obstructive lung disease." Here, the systematic increase in $P(A-a)_{O_2}$, the absence of respiratory acidosis, the negative heart rate reserve, and the prominent findings of ventilation-perfusion mismatching should cause us to consult the diagnostic box entitled "pulmonary vascular disease." Here, one can find that the confirmatory data are all present, i.e., decreasing Pa_{O_2} with increasing work rate, a steep heart rate response, a normal heart rate reserve, a low $\Delta\dot{V}_{O_2}/\Delta WR$, a significant *metabolic* acidosis rather than a respiratory acidosis at maximum exercise, and a low $D_{L_{CO}}$, which is disproportionately reduced compared to the degree of airflow obstruction.

Finally, it appears that this patient's abnormality in gas exchange is largely accounted for by the opening of a foramen ovale during exercise. (See the last item in the pulmonary vascular disease diagnostic box.) R is greater than 1 throughout exercise (panel 8, Fig. 77-A). $P_{ET_{CO_2}}$ decreases with increasing work rate (panel 9, Fig. 77-A) in contrast to that observed for patients with obstructive lung disease, and the calculated V_D/V_T and $P(a-ET)_{CO_2}$ not only remain abnormal but become more abnormal as work rate is increased (Table 77-3) because venous blood bypasses the lungs and mixes with arterialized blood. Decreasing $P_{ET_{CO_2}}$ and increasing $P(a-ET)_{CO_2}$ and V_D/V_T with work rate, and a sustained high R are all characteristic of a right to left shunt during exercise. 100% oxygen breathing during the exercise test might have confirmed the development of the right to left shunt. The cardiac ectopy that became more significant as exercise progressed was probably due to myocardial ischemia consequent to systemic hypertension (documented) and pulmonary hypertension (undocumented).

The patient has a low breathing reserve, not because his ventilatory capacity is significantly reduced but rather because his ventilatory requirement is high consequent to the increasing V_D/V_T and the maintenance of a low alveolar P_{CO_2}.

CONCLUSION

This patient has pulmonary vascular disease, possibly secondary to obstructive lung disease, with a probable opening of a foramen ovale during exercise. Cardiac ectopy could be caused by myocardial ischemia consequent to systemic and/or pulmonary hypertension.

CASE 78 *Talc pneumoconiosis and obstructive airway disease with pulmonary vascular disease*

CLINICAL FINDINGS

This 63-year-old man had complained of progressive dyspnea for 10 years, but denied cough, sputum, wheezing, chest pain, or ankle edema. He had hypertension of 5 years' duration and was being treated with clonidine and dyazide. For several months he had noted epigastric burning pain, occasionally relieved by meals. He had been exposed to talc for over 40 years in his work and was an ex-smoker with a 40 pack year history of cigarette smoking. He had no heart murmurs. The chest roentogenogram showed pulmonary fibrosis. Resting ECG showed left anterior hemi-block and T-wave abnormalities in the anteroseptal region suggestive of ischemia. The patient had a cardiopulmonary exercise test to evaluate the pathophysiology of his exertional dyspnea.

EXERCISE FINDINGS

The patient performed exercise on a cycle ergometer. He pedalled at 60 rpm without an added load for 3 minutes. The work rate was then increased 20 W per minute to tolerance. Arterial blood was sampled every second minute, and intra-arterial pressure was recorded from a percutaneously placed brachial artery catheter. The patient stopped exercise because of shortness of breath. He had no chest pain and no further ECG abnormalities.

TABLE 78-1. *Selected Respiratory Function Data*

MEASUREMENT	PREDICTED	MEASURED
Age, yr		63
Sex		Male
Height, cm		163
Weight, kg	68	67
Hematocrit, %		53
VC, L	3.28	3.56
IC, L	2.19	2.28
TLC, L	5.17	6.00
FEV_1, L	2.55	2.20
FEV_1/VC, %	78	62
MVV, L/min	115	96
DL_{CO}, ml/mm Hg/min	23.9	10.7

TABLE 78-2. *Selected Exercise Data*

MEASUREMENT	PREDICTED	MEASURED
Maximum $\dot{V}_{O_2}$, L/min	1.84	1.02
Maximum HR, beats/min	157	161
Maximum O_2 pulse, ml/beat	11.7	6.7
$\Delta\dot{V}_{O_2}/\Delta$WR, ml/min/W	10.3	5.2
AT, L/min	> 0.81	0.8
Blood pressure, mm Hg (rest, max)		162/84,249/145
Maximum $\dot{V}_E$, L/min		66
Exercise breathing reserve, L/min	> 15	30
Pa_{O_2}, mm Hg (rest, max ex)		79,57
$P(A-a)_{O_2}$ mm Hg (rest, max ex)		33,64
$P(a-ET)_{CO_2}$, mm Hg (rest, max ex)		4,6
V_D/V_T (rest, max ex)		0.42,0.44
HCO_3^-, mEq/L (rest, 2-min recov)		22,17

Fɪɢ. 78-A.

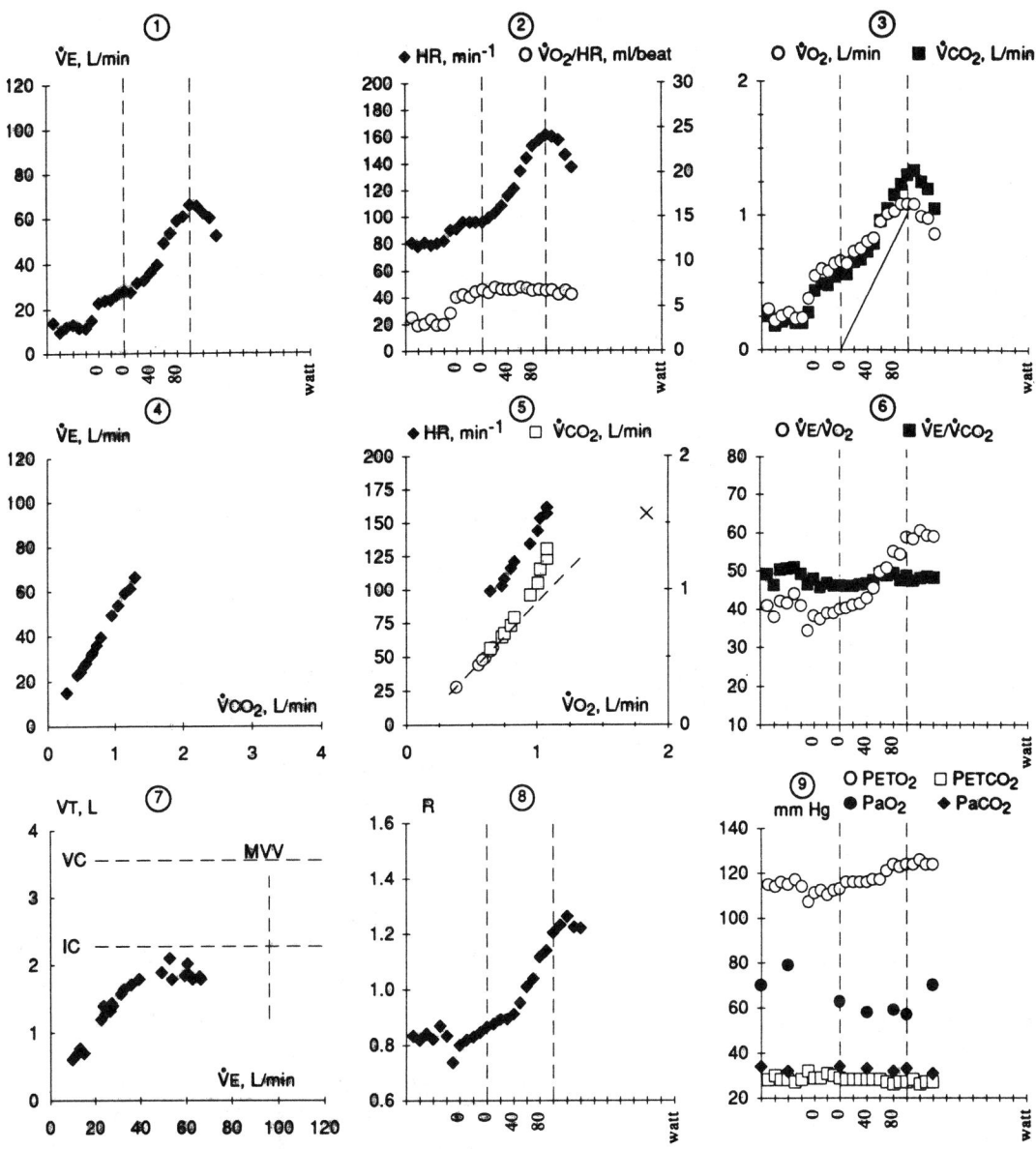

1. Vertical dashed lines in panels 1 to 3 and 6, 8, and 9 indicate the beginning and the end of increasing work period.

2. Unloaded cycling is performed for 3 minutes before the left vertical dashed line.

3. In panel 3, the diagonal line shows the increase of $\dot{V}_{O_2}$ at a slope of 10 ml/min/W.

4. In panel 5, the diagonal dashed line has a slope of 1; the "x" in the upper right is the predicted maximum heart rate and $\dot{V}_{O_2}$ for the subject.

TABLE 78-3.

Time min	Work rate watts	BP mm Hg	HR min⁻¹	f min⁻¹	$\dot{V}_E$ L/min BTPS	$\dot{V}_{CO_2}$ L/min STPD	$\dot{V}_{O_2}$ L/min STPD	$\dfrac{\dot{V}_{O_2}}{HR}$ ml/beat	R	pH	HCO₃ meq/L	PO2, mm Hg ET	a	(A-a)	PCO2, mm Hg ET	a	(a-ET)	$\dfrac{\dot{V}_E}{\dot{V}_{CO_2}}$	$\dfrac{\dot{V}_E}{\dot{V}_{O_2}}$	$\dfrac{V_D}{V_T}$
	Rest	162/84								7.43	22	70			34					
	Rest		81	19	13.9	0.25	0.30	3.7	0.83			115			28			49	41	
	Rest		78	16	9.7	0.18	0.22	2.8	0.82			114			30			46	38	
	Rest		81	17	12.0	0.21	0.25	3.1	0.84			116			28			50	42	
	Rest		79	17	13.1	0.23	0.28	3.5	0.82	7.46	22	115	79	33	28	32	4	51	42	0.42
	Rest		80	17	11.6	0.20	0.23	2.9	0.87			117			27			51	44	
	Rest	192/96	82	17	11.3	0.20	0.24	2.9	0.83			114			28			49	41	
	Unloaded	240/117	90	21	14.8	0.28	0.38	4.2	0.74			107			32			46	34	
	Unloaded		91	19	22.7	0.44	0.55	6.0	0.80			111			29			48	38	
	Unloaded		96	17	23.8	0.49	0.60	6.3	0.82			112			29			46	37	
	Unloaded		96	19	24.1	0.48	0.58	6.0	0.83			110			31			47	39	
	Unloaded		96	20	26.6	0.54	0.64	6.7	0.84			112			30			46	39	
	Unloaded	237/111	96	20	28.0	0.57	0.66	6.9	0.86	7.44	23	113	63	49	29	34	5	46	40	0.42
0.5	20		99	19	27.4	0.56	0.64	6.5	0.88			116			28			46	40	
1.0	20		103	20	31.6	0.65	0.73	7.1	0.89			116			28			46	41	
1.5	40		108	20	32.7	0.67	0.75	6.9	0.89			116			28			46	41	
2.0	40	240/114	116	21	35.9	0.73	0.80	6.9	0.91	7.45	23	116	58	56	28	33	5	47	43	0.42
2.5	60		121	22	39.4	0.79	0.83	6.9	0.95			117			28			48	45	
3.0	60		134	26	49.3	0.96	0.95	7.1	1.01			117			28			49	50	
3.5	80		144	30	53.7	1.05	1.01	7.0	1.04			121			27			49	51	
4.0	80	246/123	153	32	59.2	1.15	1.03	6.7	1.12	7.44	21	124	59	62	26	32	6	49	55	0.43
4.5	100		157	33	61.2	1.23	1.08	6.9	1.14			123			27			47	54	
5.0	100	249/145	161	37	66.4	1.30	1.08	6.7	1.20	7.40	20	124	57	64	27	33	6	49	59	0.44
	Recovery		160	36	65.8	1.33	1.08	6.8	1.23			124			28			47	58	
	Recovery		157	35	62.8	1.25	0.99	6.3	1.26			126			26			48	60	
	Recovery		146	30	60.5	1.20	0.98	6.7	1.22			124			27			48	59	
	Recovery	234/108	137	25	52.6	1.05	0.86	6.3	1.22	7.35	17	124	70	53	27	31	4	48	59	0.40

Interpretation

COMMENTS

Resting studies showed a mild obstructive ventilatory defect with a severely reduced $D_{L_{CO}}$. The patient had systemic hypertension at rest with a mildly abnormal ECG.

ANALYSIS

In flow chart 1, maximum $\dot{V}_{O_2}$ is decreased. The anaerobic threshold is borderline abnormal. If one goes next to flow chart 3, the high breathing reserve and mildly abnormal ECG lead to the diagnosis of myocardial ischemia, but this is unsatisfactory because it does not take into account the severe gas exchange disturbances elicited. Flow charts 4 or 5 are preferable. Referring to flow chart 5, at branchpoint 5.1 we note abnormal V_D/V_T, $P(a-_{ET})_{CO_2}$, and $P(A-a)_{O_2}$. The breathing reserve is normal (branchpoint 5.3), and the $P(A-a)_{O_2}$ progressively decreases (branchpoint 5.6), leading to the category of pulmonary vascular disease, with many confirmatory findings. The patient does have mild obstructive lung disease, but this is physiologically less important than the pulmonary vascular disease, as evidenced by the high V_D/V_T, increased $P(A-a)_{O_2}$, positive $P(A-a)_{O_2}$, high ventilatory equivalents, and low and unchanging O_2 pulse. The systemic hypertension could also be contributing to a high afterload and low cardiac output state.

CONCLUSION

This patient has pulmonary vascular disease that is more severe than can be explained by uncomplicated obstructive lung disease, as well as coexistent systemic hypertension. A subsequent lung biopsy demonstrated talc pneumoconiosis.

CASE 79 *Systemic sclerosis and primary lung cancer: Preoperative evaluation*

CLINICAL FINDINGS

This 59-year-old woman with progressive systemic sclerosis was found to have a potentially operable squamous cell carcinoma of the lung by fiberoptic bronchoscopy. She had a 26 pack year history of cigarette smoking, complained of dyspnea after walking one block, and denied having a productive cough or hemoptysis. She had no history or overt signs or symptoms of heart disease. Her only medications were thyroid supplements and estrogens. A cardiopulmonary exercise test was done to evaluate cardiac and lung function reserves in response to stress.

EXERCISE FINDINGS

The patient performed exercise on a cycle ergometer. She pedalled at 60 rpm without an added load for 3 minutes. The work rate was then increased 5 W per minute to her symptom-limited maximum. Arterial blood was sampled every second minute, and intra-arterial blood pressure was recorded from a percutaneously passed brachial artery catheter. Resting and exercise ECGs were normal. The patient stopped exercise complaining of tired thighs.

TABLE 79-1. *Selected Respiratory Function Data*

MEASUREMENT	PREDICTED	MEASURED
Age, yr		59
Sex		Female
Height, cm		165
Weight, kg	62	75
Hematocrit, %		43
VC, L	2.73	2.26
IC, L	1.82	1.36
TLC, L	4.57	3.34
FEV_1, L	2.18	1.58
FEV_1/VC, %	80	70
MVV, L/min	82	73
DL_{CO}, ml/mm Hg/min	18.0	8.4

TABLE 79-2. *Selected Exercise Data*

MEASUREMENT	PREDICTED	MEASURED
Maximum $\dot{V}O_2$, L/min	1.43	0.86
Maximum HR, beats/min	161	135
Maximum O_2 pulse, ml/beat	8.9	6.4
$\Delta \dot{V}O_2/\Delta WR$, ml/min/W	10.3	9.1
AT, L/min	> 0.7	0.7
Blood pressure, mm Hg (rest, max ex)		135/69,180/81
Maximum $\dot{V}E$, L/min		38
Exercise breathing reserve, L/min	> 15	35
PaO_2, mm Hg (rest, max ex)		66,55
$P(A-a)O_2$ mm Hg (rest, max ex)		24,51
$P(a-ET)CO_2$, mm Hg (rest, max ex)		7,13
VD/VT (rest, max ex)		0.40,0.47
HCO_3^-, mEq/L (rest, recov)		25,23

TABLE 79-3.

Time min	Work rate watts	BP mm Hg	HR min⁻¹	f min⁻¹	$\dot{V}E$ L/min BTPS	$\dot{V}CO_2$ L/min STPD	$\dot{V}O_2$ L/min STPD	$\dfrac{\dot{V}O_2}{HR}$ ml/beat	R	pH	HCO₃ meq/L	PO2, mm Hg ET	a	(A-a)	PCO2, mm Hg ET	a	(a-ET)	$\dfrac{\dot{V}E}{\dot{V}CO_2}$	$\dfrac{\dot{V}E}{\dot{V}O_2}$	$\dfrac{VD}{VT}$
	Rest	132/69								7.40	24		69			40				
	Rest		68	26	9.8	0.16	0.24	3.5	0.67			103			34			47	32	
	Rest		73	25	7.6	0.13	0.21	2.9	0.62			94			39			42	26	
	Rest		71	22	8.4	0.15	0.24	3.4	0.63			99			36			44	27	
	Rest	135/69	71	21	9.0	0.18	0.27	3.8	0.67	7.38	25	98	66	24	36	43	7	40	27	0.40
	Rest		72	19	7.8	0.15	0.23	3.2	0.65			98			36			41	27	
	Rest		74	20	7.8	0.15	0.24	3.2	0.63			95			37			41	25	
	Unloaded		88	27	14.7	0.32	0.46	5.2	0.70			99			36			39	27	
	Unloaded		93	34	19.8	0.39	0.50	5.4	0.78			109			33			43	34	
	Unloaded		98	29	19.3	0.43	0.56	5.7	0.77			107			34			39	30	
	Unloaded		102	33	22.8	0.50	0.61	6.0	0.82			108			34			40	33	
	Unloaded		106	33	21.2	0.48	0.59	5.6	0.81			108			35			38	31	
	Unloaded	171/81	109	31	23.2	0.55	0.63	5.8	0.87	7.37	24	110	53	49	34	43	9	37	33	0.41
0.5	5		111	29	22.4	0.55	0.65	5.9	0.85			107			36			36	31	
1.0	5		112	28	23.2	0.58	0.66	5.9	0.88			109			35			36	32	
1.5	10		113	27	22.8	0.58	0.65	5.8	0.89			108			36			35	32	
2.0	10	174/78	115	33	27.2	0.63	0.67	5.8	0.94	7.35	23	110	54	52	36	42	6	39	36	0.42
2.5	15		121	34	28.3	0.67	0.71	5.9	0.94			112			35			38	36	
3.0	15		123	33	28.1	0.66	0.71	5.8	0.93			109			37			38	36	
3.5	20		124	40	35.5	0.80	0.79	6.4	1.01			116			32			40	41	
4.0	20		126	32	30.5	0.76	0.80	6.3	0.95			112			35			37	35	
4.5	25		131	42	38.3	0.88	0.86	6.6	1.02			116			33			39	40	
5.0	25	180/81	131	39	37.0	0.86	0.82	6.3	1.05	7.35	25	116	55	51	33	46	13	39	41	0.47
5.5	30		135	38	36.9	0.87	0.84	6.2	1.04			116			33			39	40	
	Recovery		126	39	37.2	0.86	0.83	6.6	1.04			116			33			39	41	
	Recovery		122	36	30.5	0.70	0.70	5.7	1.00			112			35			39	39	
	Recovery		119	36	30.5	0.71	0.70	5.9	1.01			113			35			39	39	
	Recovery	162/69	114	40	30.9	0.68	0.64	5.6	1.06	7.32	23	116	63	44	34	45	11	40	43	0.47
	Recovery		111	43	28.1	0.58	0.55	5.0	1.05			116			34			42	44	
	Recovery		110										118			30					

Interpretation

COMMENTS

The resting respiratory function studies show mild restriction and mild obstruction, severe loss of available pulmonary capillary bed, and mild hypoxemia. She had no known cardiac disease.

ANALYSIS

In flow chart 1, the patient had a low maximum $\dot{V}O_2$ and borderline anaerobic threshold (Table 79-2). If we use flow chart 3, we proceed through branchpoint 3.1 (normal breathing reserve) and through branchpoint 3.3 (normal ECG) to poor effort or musculo-skeletal disorder. This impression does not fit our patient well because she has unequivocal evidence of gas exchange abnormalities. If her anaerobic threshold were indeterminate (flow chart 5) or low (flow chart 4), we would be directed to impaired pulmonary circulation as her primary problem. Because her breathing reserve is normal (branchpoint 4.1), we are directed to the right branch. Because the $\dot{V}E/\dot{V}CO_2$ is high (branchpoint 4.3), we are given the diagnosis of "abnormal pulmonary circulation." The patient has all the physiologic abnormalities that define this disorder. The patient does have a low arterial O_2 saturation (of approximately 85%) during exercise. She also meets all the qualifications for pulmonary vascular disease without a clear right to left shunt (branchpoint 4.5).

CONCLUSION

This patient, with both restrictive and obstructive lung disease, does not have ventilatory limitation during exercise, but she demonstrates significant gas exchange abnormalities characteristic of pulmonary vascular disease. This may be part of her systemic sclerosis and associated interstitial lung disease. Her $\dot{V}O_2$max of 11.5 ml/min/kg places her in an extremely high risk category for pulmonary resection.

Fɪɢ. 79-A.

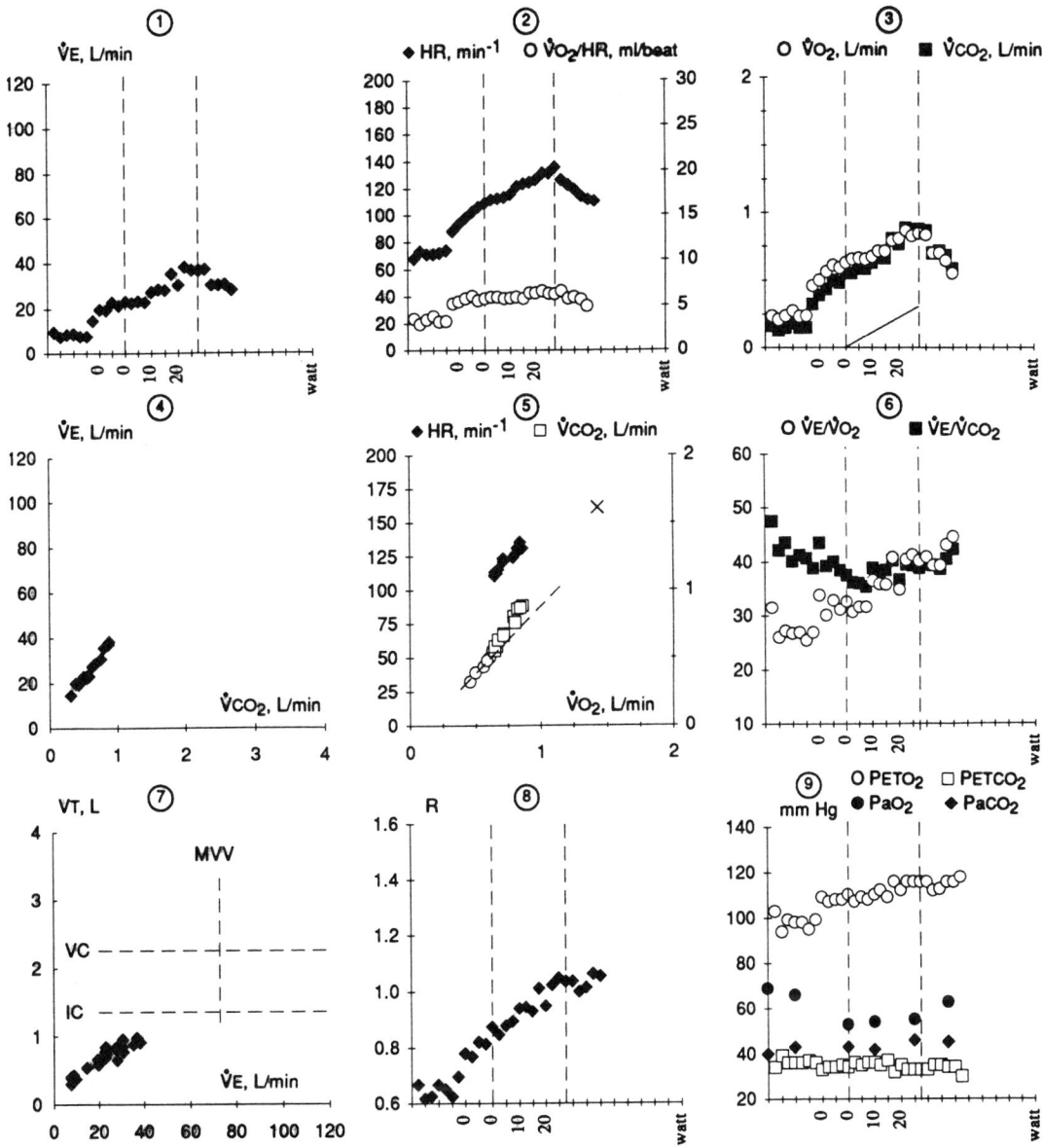

1. Vertical dashed lines in panels 1 to 3 and 6, 8, and 9 indicate the beginning and the end of increasing work period.

2. Unloaded cycling is performed for 3 minutes before the left vertical dashed line.

3. In panel 3, the diagonal line shows the increase of $\dot{V}O_2$ at a slope of 10 ml/min/W.

4. In panel 5, the diagonal dashed line has a slope of 1; the "x" in the upper right is the predicted maximum heart rate and $\dot{V}O_2$ for the subject.

Symbols and Abbreviations

Dash ($^-$) above any symbol indicates a *mean* value
Dot (˙) above any symbol indicates a *time derivative*

GASES

PRIMARY SYMBOLS		EXAMPLES	
V	gas volume	V_A	volume of alveolar gas
$\dot{V}$	gas volume/unit time	$\dot{V}_{O_2}$	O_2 uptake/minute
P	gas pressure	$P_{A_{O_2}}$	alveolar O_2 pressure
$\bar{P}$	mean gas pressure	$\bar{P}_{C_{O_2}}$	mean capillary O_2 pressure
F	fractional concentration of a particular gas	$F_{I_{O_2}}$	fractional concentration of O_2 in inspired gas
f	respiratory frequency		
D	diffusing capacity	D_{CO}	diffusing capacity for CO
R	respiratory exchange ratio		
RQ	respiratory quotient		
Q	gas quantity		
$\dot{Q}$	gas quantity/unit time (gas flow)	$\dot{Q}_{O_2}$	O_2 consumed/minute
STPD	standard temperature and pressure (0°C, 760 mm Hg), dry		
BTPS	body temperature and pressure, saturated with water vapor		

SECONDARY SYMBOLS (small capitals)		EXAMPLES	
I	inspired gas	$F_{I_{O_2}}$	fractional concentration of O_2 in inspired gas
E	expired gas	V_E	volume of expired gas
A	alveolar gas	$\dot{V}_A$	alveolar ventilation/minute
ET	end tidal	$P_{ET_{CO_2}}$	end-tidal CO_2 tension
T	tidal gas	V_T	tidal volume
D	dead space gas	V_D	physiological dead space volume
B	barometric	P_B	barometric pressure

BLOOD

PRIMARY SYMBOLS		EXAMPLES	
$\dot{Q}$	volume flow of blood/ unit time	$\dot{Q}c$	blood flow through pulmonary capillaries/ minute
C	concentration of gas in blood phase	Ca_{O_2}	content of O_2 in arterial blood
S	% saturation of Hb with O_2	$S\bar{v}_{O_2}$	saturation of Hb with O_2 in mixed venous blood

SECONDARY SYMBOLS		EXAMPLES	
a	arterial blood	Pa_{CO_2}	partial pressure of CO_2 in arterial blood
v	venous blood	$P\bar{v}_{O_2}$	partial pressure of O_2 in mixed venous blood
c	capillary blood	Pc_{O_2}	partial pressure of O_2 in pulmonary capillary blood

VARIABLES AND PARAMETERS

$\dot{V}_{O_2}$	oxygen uptake
$\dot{V}_{O_2}max$	maximal aerobic power
$\dot{V}_{CO_2}$	carbon dioxide output
$\dot{Q}_{O_2}$	O_2 consumption
$\dot{Q}_{CO_2}$	CO_2 production
AT	anaerobic threshold
LT	lactate threshold
LAT	lactic acidosis threshold
R	gas exchange ratio
RQ	respiratory quotient
$\dot{V}_E/\dot{V}_{O_2}$	ventilatory equivalent for O_2
$\dot{V}_E/\dot{V}_{CO_2}$	ventilatory equivalent for CO_2
V_D/V_T	physiological dead space/tidal volume ratio
V_D	physiological dead space
BR	breathing reserve
HR	heart rate
HRR	heart rate reserve
WR	work rate
$\Delta\dot{V}_{O_2}/\Delta WR$	change in $\dot{V}_{O_2}$/change in WR

LUNG VOLUMES AND FLOWS

V_T	tidal volume = volume of air inhaled or exhaled with each breath
VC	vital capacity = maximal volume that can be expired after maximal inspiration
IC	inspiratory capacity = maximal volume that can be inspired from the resting end-expiratory level
ERV	expiratory reserve volume = maximal volume that can be expired from the resting end-expiratory level
FRC	functional residual capacity = volume of gas in lungs at end-expiration
RV	residual volume = volume of gas in lungs after maximal expiration
TLC	total lung capacity = volume of gas in lungs after maximal inspiration
FEV_x	forced expired volume in x seconds, e.g., FEV_1 (one second)
MVV	maximal voluntary ventilation

Glossary

Aerobic: Having molecular oxygen present; describes metabolic process utilizing oxygen.

Alveolar to arterial P_{O_2} difference ($P(A-a)_{O_2}$): The difference between the ideal alveolar P_{O_2} and the mean arterial P_{O_2}. This difference is considered to be an index of the lungs' inefficiency with respect to oxygen exchange.

Alveolar ventilation ($\dot{V}_A$): Conceptionally, this is the volume of inspired gas that reaches the alveoli per minute, or the volume of gas that is evolved from the alveoli per minute. In practice, it is computed as the theoretic alveolar ventilation necessary to produce the arterial level of CO_2 tension at the current CO_2 output level.

Anaerobic: Lacking or inadequate molecular oxygen; describes any metabolic process that does not use molecular oxygen.

Anaerobic threshold *(AT)*: The exercise $\dot{V}_{O_2}$ above which anaerobic high-energy PO_4 production supplements aerobic high-energy PO_4 production, with consequential lowering redox state, increase in lactate/pyruvate (L/P) ratio, and net increase in lactate production at the site of anaerobiosis. Exercise above the *AT* is reflected in the muscle effluent and central blood by an increase in lactate concentration and L/P ratio, and a metabolic acidosis. Gas exchange is also affected by characteristic slowing of $\dot{V}_{O_2}$ kinetics and an increase in CO_2 output over that produced from aerobic metabolism, resulting from HCO_3^- buffering of lactic acid.

Analog to digital converter: A device for transforming continuously changing information into discrete units over some small time frame, within which the value is considered to be relatively constant. This transforms continuous signals to a form that can be analyzed by a digital computer.

Arterial to end-tidal P_{CO_2} difference ($P(a-ET)_{CO_2}$): The difference between the mean arterial P_{CO_2} and the end-tidal P_{CO_2}. This is positive when the arterial P_{CO_2} is higher than the end-tidal P_{CO_2}.

Arterial-mixed venous O_2 content difference

$(C(a - \bar{v})_{O_2})$: The difference in the O_2 content of the arterial and venous blood, usually expressed in milliliters of O_2 per deciliter or liter of blood.

ATPS: Gas volume conditioned to the ambient (e.g., room) temperature and pressure, and saturated with water vapor at ambient temperature.

Breath-by-breath: The expression of a particular physiologic value averaged over one entire respiratory cycle. These are usually expressed as the value that physiologic variable would have if maintained over an entire minute (e.g., ventilation expressed as L/min). Breath-by-breath is also used to describe a method for measurement of respiratory gas exchange in which respired gas volume and simultaneously measured expired gas concentration are integrated and reported.

Breathing reserve (BR): The difference between the maximum voluntary ventilation and the maximum exercise ventilation. Hence, this represents the body's residual potential for further increasing ventilation at maximum exercise.

BTPS: Gas volume conditioned to body temperature and the ambient atmospheric pressure and fully saturated with water vapor at the subject's body temperature.

Carbon dioxide output ($\dot{V}_{CO_2}$): The amount of CO_2 exhaled from the body into the atmosphere per unit time, expressed in milliliters or liters per minute, STPD. This differs from CO_2 production rate under conditions in which additional CO_2 may be evolved from the body's stores or CO_2 is added to the body's stores. In the steady-state, CO_2 output equals CO_2 production rate. In rare circumstances, appreciable quantities of CO_2 can be eliminated from the body as bicarbonate via the gastrointestinal tract or by hemodialysis.

Carbon dioxide production ($\dot{Q}_{CO_2}$): The amount of carbon dioxide produced by the body's metabolic processes and in some circumstances released by buffering reactions within the body, expressed in milliliters or liters per minute, STPD.

Cardiac output ($\dot{Q}$): The flow of blood from the heart in a particular period of time, usually expressed as liters per minute. It is the product of the average stroke volume per beat and the heart rate, i.e., number of beats per minute.

Constant work rate test: An exercise test in which a constant power output is required of the subject.

Dead space or physiologic dead space (V_D): This is the theoretic volume of gas taken into the lung that is not involved in gas exchange, assuming that the gas tensions in the alveolar volume equilibrate with those of the pulmonary capillary blood as it leaves the lung. Thus, the physiologic dead space is made up of the anatomic dead space (the volume of the upper airways, trachea, and bronchi) and the alveolar dead space (the volume of alveoli that are ventilated but unperfused and a certain portion of those that are underperfused).

Dead space/tidal volume ratio (V_D/V_T): The proportion of the tidal volume that is made up of the physiologic dead space. This is an index of the relative inefficiency for pulmonary gas exchange to eliminate CO_2.

Diffusing capacity: This is a measure of the rate of uptake of a particular gas across the alveolar-capillary bed for a specified driving pressure for that gas. It is measured, therefore, as the volume of gas per unit time per pressure difference (e.g., ml/min/mm Hg). It is also referred to as the pulmonary gas transfer index (a term that more properly reflects the measurement). It is most practical to use carbon monoxide as the test gas for measurement of diffusing capacity of the lungs, in which case it is referred to as $D_{L_{CO}}$.

Diffusion defect: A defect in the lungs' ability for gas diffusion. This is typically caused either by an abnormally increased diffusion path length or by conditions in which the transit time of the red cell through the pulmonary capillary bed is so fast that insufficient time is available for complete diffusion equilibrium.

Disability: A legal term that considers the effect of a functional impairment on the patient's ability to perform a specific work task and other factors such as age, sex, education, social environment, job availability, and the energy requirements of the occupation.

End-tidal P_{CO_2}($P_{ET_{CO_2}}$): The P_{CO_2} of the respired gas determined at the end of an exhalation. This is commonly the highest P_{CO_2} measured during the alveolar phase of the exhalation.

End-tidal P_{O_2} ($P_{ET_{O_2}}$): The P_{O_2} determined in the respired gas at the end of an exhalation. This is typically the lowest P_{O_2} determined during the alveolar portion of the exhalation.

Exponential: A process in which the instantaneous rate of change of a variable is proportional to the "distance" from a steady-state or required level; hence, the rate of change of the function under consideration is rapid when it is far from its steady-state value and slows progressively as the function approaches its steady-state. If the process is known to be, or may be reasonably estimated to be, exponential, the time to reach 63% of the final value, i.e., to approach within 37% of the final value, is termed the time constant (τ) of the response. If the process is exponential, this time constant is related to the half time (the time to reach 50% of the final value) by the equation $t\frac{1}{2} = 0.693 \times \tau$.

Fick method for cardiac output: A means of estimating cardiac output from the uptake of O_2 by the lungs and the arterial − mixed venous O_2 content difference. $\dot{Q} = \dot{V}_{O2}/C(a - \bar{v})_{O_2}$. When the same principle is used to measure cardiac output with CO_2 as the test gas, the CO_2 output is divided by the $C(\bar{v} - a)_{CO_2}$.

Frequency response: This reflects the fidelity with which a device can track rapidly changing physiologic information. The frequency response of the device is usually determined by applying some rapidly changing signals of a particular amplitude, spanning a range of frequencies, and then establishing the range over which the device accurately tracks the signal.

Gas exchange ratio (R): The ratio of the carbon dioxide output to the oxygen uptake per unit time. This ratio reflects not only tissue metabolic exchange of the gases, but also the influence of transient change in gas storage of O_2, and especially of CO_2; e.g., the gas exchange ratio exceeds the respiratory quotient during hyperventilation as additional CO_2 is evolved from the body's stores, whereas the gas exchange ratio is less than the respiratory quotient during transient hypoventilation when CO_2 is retained in the body's stores.

Half time (t½): Unlike the time constant, which requires evidence of exponentiality for its determination, the half time of a response is a simple description of the time to reach half of the change to the final value, regardless of the function. It is, therefore, generally representative of the speed of approaching the steady-state.

Heart rate reserve (HRR): The difference between the predicted highest heart rate attainable during maximum exercise and the actual highest heart rate, usually during exercise testing involving large muscle masses, such as during cycle or treadmill ergometry.

Ideal alveolar P_{O2}: A term that describes the alveolar P_{O2} that would be obtained if the lung were an ideal gas exchanger, i.e., with ventilation uniformly matched to perfusion.

Impairment: A medical term reflecting an abnormality of physiologic function that persists after treatment. For exercise, it could represent any defect in the ventilatory-circulatory-metabolic coupling of external to internal respiration.

Incremental exercise test: An exercise test designed to provide gradational stress to the subject. The work rate is usually increased over uniform periods of time, for example, every 4 minutes, every minute, every 15 seconds, or even continuously (e.g., ramp pattern increment).

Lactate: The anion of lactic acid.

Lactate threshold *(LT)*: The exercise $\dot{V}_{O2}$ above which a net increase in lactate production results in a sustained increase in central blood lactate concentration.

Lactic acid: A three-carbon carboxylic acid ($CH_3CHOHCOOH$) that is one of the potential end-products of glucose oxidation. Another major product is pyruvic acid ($CH_3COCOOH$), which can undergo conversion to acetyl coenzyme A and can thereby be further oxidized. The relative amounts of lactic acid and pyruvic acid are determined by the cytosolic redox state; a low redox state, reflected by a high ratio of $NADH/NAD^+$, favors the generation of lactic acid, which in turn maintains the supply of NAD^+ necessary for glycolysis to continue. The presence of lactic acid is a marker of anaerobic metabolism.

Lactic acidosis threshold *(LAT)*: The exercise $\dot{V}_{O2}$ above which arterial standard HCO_3^- decreases because of a net increase in lactate production. This can be detected by an increase in CO_2 output (from dissociation of H_2CO_3 as HCO_3^- buffers lactic acid) above that which would be predicted from aerobic metabolism alone during a progressively increasing work rate exercise test.

Laminar flow: A condition in which the flow of a fluid (gas or liquid) through a conduit is characterized by the uniform direction of flow of any plane sheet of the fluid, each of which flows parallel to any other in the direction of flow. Under conditions of laminar flow, the pressure difference between two fixed points upstream and downstream is directly proportional to flow and inversely proportional to resistance of the conduit.

Mass spectrometer: A device that separates and measures molecules of gas of a particular type, in a mixed gas stream, on the basis of their mass. Two types are commonly used. The fixed collector uses a magnetic means of separating the gases; these are then counted at different specific sensors. Alternatively, a quadrapole mass spectrometer utilizes shifts in an electromagnetic field to separate the gases such that only one gas arrives at the counter at a particular time.

Maximum exercise heart rate: The highest obtainable heart rate during a maximum effort test.

Maximum exercise ventilation: The highest minute ventilation achieved during a maximum work rate test. This is usually determined by tests that tax large muscle masses, such as cycle or treadmill ergometry.

Maximum voluntary ventilation (MVV): The upper limit of the body's ability to ventilate the lungs. This is conventionally measured from maximal volitional effort for short periods of time, e.g., 12 seconds, and expressed in units of liters per minute, BTPS.

Mets: Oxygen uptake required for a given task divided by resting oxygen uptake.

Minute ventilation ($\dot{V}_I$ or $\dot{V}_E$): The volume of air taken into or exhaled from the body in one minute. This is conventionally expressed at body temperature, saturated with water at atmospheric pressure (BTPS).

Mixed venous blood: A sample of blood representative of the flow-weighted venous blood returning from all the organs of the body. Usually, blood obtained from the pulmonary artery is considered to be mixed venous blood.

Mixed venous O_2 or CO_2: The average partial pressure, or gas content, of the blood returning from all the tissues of the body and, having been fully mixed in the right heart, is normally represented by the concentration or partial pressure of that substance in the pulmonary arterial blood.

Mixing chamber: A device that mixes the dead space and alveolar gas to produce a gas that is representative of the mixed expired gas. This is typically achieved by exhaling into a baffled chamber that mixes several breaths. The mixed expired concentration of a gas can be measured downstream from the chamber. Considerable care, however, must be taken when using such a device

to measure metabolic rate to align the delayed mixed expired value with the appropriate volume measurement.

O_2 content (C_{O_2}): The volume of O_2 (STPD) in a given volume (L, dl, ml) of blood. This includes the major component that is bound to hemoglobin and that amount physically dissolved in the blood.

O_2 debt: The additional oxygen utilized in excess of the baseline needs of the body following a bout of exercise.

O_2 deficit: The oxygen equivalent of the total energy utilized to perform the work that did not derive from reactions utilizing atmospheric oxygen taken into the body after the start of the exercise. Consequently, for moderate intensity exercise, this O_2 deficit represents the energy equivalent of the depletion of the high-energy phosphate stores and oxygen stored in the body at the start of the work. For heavy or severe exercise, the oxygen deficit includes, in addition, the energy equivalent of the anaerobic processes.

O_2 delivery: The amount of oxygen delivered to a tissue per unit time. It is, therefore, the product of the oxygen content of arterial blood and the blood flow to that tissue.

O_2 difference: The difference between the O_2 uptake predicted for a work rate during an incremental exercise test and the highest O_2 uptake attained.

O_2 flow: The amount of oxygen actually flowing per unit time, either from the heart or into a region of interest, such as a muscle or a muscle fiber. This, therefore, is a product of the oxygen content of the arterial blood and the total or regional blood flow.

O_2 pulse: The oxygen uptake divided by the heart rate. Hence, it is the amount of oxygen extracted by the tissues of the body from the O_2 carried in each stroke volume.

Oximeter: A device that uses transmission techniques to estimate the saturation of hemoglobin with oxygen. Direct oximetry is done on blood samples. For indirect oximetry, a site for measurement, such as the earlobe or finger, is selected because blood comes close to the skin, traverses the capillary bed with little loss of oxygen, and hence, the mean capillary value will reflect arterial values. See pulse oximeter.

Oxygen consumption ($\dot{Q}O_2$): The amount of oxygen utilized by the body's metabolic processes in a given time, expressed in milliliters or liters per minute, STPD.

Oxygen uptake ($\dot{V}O_2$): The amount of oxygen extracted from the inspired gas in a given period of time, expressed in milliliters or liters per minute, STPD. This can differ from oxygen consumption under conditions in which oxygen is flowing into or being utilized from the body's stores. In the steady-state, oxygen uptake equals oxygen consumption.

Phase I: The period of time following the onset of exercise that is required for the products of exercise metabolism to reach the lungs. During Phase I, the mixed venous blood entering the pulmonary capillary bed has not changed its composition. Phase I is a result of the transit delay from the site of increased metabolism. Normally, this period is 15 to 20 seconds.

Phase II: The period of time following the onset of exercise when the mixed venous blood gas concentrations continue to change because of changes in the effluent from the exercising muscles. It, therefore, reflects the "kinetic phase" of the gas exchange that begins at the end of Phase I and continues until a steady-state is obtained.

Phase III: The steady-state phase of gas exchange during exercise. For moderate exercise, it reflects the period in which the mixed venous gas concentrations have become constant. For heavy exercise, $\dot{V}O_2$ is observed to increase slowly during this phase, likely related to lactate metabolism.

Physiologic dead space: See dead space.

Pneumotachograph: A device used to measure gas flow. It is typically composed of a screen across which the pressure drop stemming from the flow of gas may be measured. This determines the instantaneous gas flow. Flow may be integrated over time to yield the volume of air respired.

Power: See work rate.

Pulse oximeter: A noninvasive device for estimating arterial blood oxygen saturation using a combination of spectrophotometry and pulse plethysmography. The pulse oximeter probe is designed to be placed on the earlobe or finger tip.

Pulse pressure: The difference between the systolic and the diastolic blood pressure.

Pump calibrator: A device that simulates the airflow and gas concentration waveforms encountered during respiration. Because the "metabolic rate" of such a device can be precisely calculated, it is useful for calibration of an exercise gas exchange measurement system.

R: See gas exchange ratio.

RQ (respiratory quotient): The ratio of the rate of carbon dioxide production to oxygen consumption. This ratio reflects the metabolic exchange of the gases in the body's tissues and is dictated by substrate utilization.

Ramp exercise test: see incremental exercise test. An exercise testing protocol in which the work rate is continuously increased at a constant rate, e.g., 10 W/min.

Response time: A means of characterizing the rate at which a device or system responds to a given signal. For example, in response to a sudden application of a constant level of input, how long does the output take to become constant? This can be characterized by the time constant, half time, or the time to reach 90% of the final value.

STPD: Gas volume at standard conditions of temperature and pressure, free of water vapor. The standard conditions are 0°C, 760 mm Hg, and dry gas.

Set-point: This is a term used in control system theory that reflects the particular value of a regulated variable that the output of the system regulates. For example, a CO_2 set point is considered to be the operating level of arterial P_{CO_2}, which is maintained at its relatively constant (i.e., set-point) value by changes in ventilation at a given level of CO_2 output.

Steady-state: This is a characteristic of a physiologic system in which its functional demands are being met such that its output per unit time becomes constant. The time to achieve a steady-state commonly differs for different physiologic systems. For example, following the onset of constant load exercise, oxygen uptake rises to reach its steady-state appreciably faster than CO_2 output or ventilation. A constant value attained by the system is not sufficient, however, to determine that the system is in a steady-state. If the system reaches the limit of its output, and, as a result, its output becomes constant, as in the case of oxygen uptake reaching its maximum value, a steady-state does not prevail. The system in this instance is in a limited state, not a steady-state.

Stroke volume: The volume of blood ejected from either ventricle of the heart in a single beat.

Sustainable work rate: This is a relative term that reflects the extent to which a particular work rate may be sustained for sufficient time for the successful completion of a particular occupational, recreational, or laboratory-induced work rate. Therefore, at a sustainable work rate, the subject does not fatigue within the time constraints of the requirements of the test.

Thermodilution blood flow measurement: A technique in which a measured bolus of physiologic fluid of known temperature, usually at 0°C, is injected into a vascular stream, such as in the right atrium, and the temperature of the blood is measured at a mixed downstream point, such as in the pulmonary artery. The addition of the cold bolus of fluid decreases the blood temperature at the downstream point; the amount of cooling is a function of the blood flow. Thermodilution cardiac output measurements are usually performed using a thermistor-tipped pulmonary artery catheter (Swan-Ganz type).

Tidal volume to inspiratory capacity ratio (V_T/IC): The ratio of the volume of air actually breathed during a breath to the air potentially available for that breath, the latter measured from the end-expiratory lung volume to the maximum inspiratory volume. Hence, it reflects the proportion of the potential inspiratory volume excursion that is actually utilized for a particular breath.

Transcutaneous gas tension: The technique for estimating the partial pressure of the gas in the capillary blood perfusing a region of skin with high flow and low metabolic rate. When the intent of this measurement is to estimate arterial blood gases, it must be interpreted with caution.

Transducer: A device that transforms energy from one form to another. Consequently, a pressure transducer is a device that changes fluid pressure into an electrical signal that can be analyzed and used for display or recording.

Turbulent flow: A condition in which the fluid (gas or liquid) flow has characteristic eddies, whorls, and diverse directional currents, such that additional energy needs to be applied to create a given fluid flow. Under conditions of turbulent flow, the relationship between flow and pressure is nonlinear.

V-slope method: A technique that allows detection of the onset of lactic acidosis during an incremental exercise test when one notes an accelerated rate of CO_2 output generated from bicarbonate buffering of lactic acid.

$\Delta \dot{V}O_2(6 - 3)$: The difference in oxygen uptake between the sixth and the third minute of a constant load exercise test. Normal subjects typically attain a steady-state for constant load exercise within 3 minutes during moderate exercise; hence, the $\Delta \dot{V}O_2(6 - 3)$ is zero. A positive value for this index reflects a degree of continuing non-steady-state for the work and usually signals fatiguing exercise.

$\dot{V}O_2$max: The highest oxygen uptake obtainable for a given form of ergometry despite further work rate increases and effort by the subject. This is characterized by a plateau of oxygen uptake despite further increases in work rate.

$\Delta \dot{V}O_2/\Delta$ work rate: The increase in oxygen uptake in response to a simultaneous increase in work rate. Under appropriate conditions (e.g., steady-state aerobic work), this may be used to estimate the efficiency for muscular work.

Wasted ventilation ($\dot{V}D$): The difference between the computed alveolar ventilation and the measured minute ventilation. Also known as the physiologic dead space ventilation, this term is meant to reflect the volume of the respired air that did not participate in alveolar capillary gas exchange, and it is equal to $V_D \times f$.

Work: A physical quantification of the force operating on a mass that causes it to change its location. Under conditions where force is applied and no movement results (e.g., during an isometric contraction), no work is performed, despite increased metabolic energy expenditure. The unit of work is the joule $= \text{kg m}^2/\text{sec}^2$.

Work rate or power: This reflects the rate at which work is performed, i.e., work per unit time. Work rate is usually measured in watts (kg m^2/sec^3 or joule/sec) or alternatively in kilopond meters per minute (kp·m/min); 1 W is equivalent to 6.12 kp·m/min.

Devices and Systems for Collecting and Analyzing Physiologic Data

Systems

THE PROPER interpretation of exercise test data depends on accurate data collection and correct calculations. A variety of systems, measuring devices, recorders, calculation devices, and other equipment have been used for these purposes. Computer techniques have been incorporated to facilitate data storage and calculation. A number of commercial systems are available that make considerable use of computerization. However, useful information can be obtained from even very simple systems.

SYSTEM WITH "MINIMAL" EQUIPMENT

Exercise testing can be performed with little or no equipment. A measured course, stairway, or hallway provides a reproducible and functional exercise stress. Data collected can include review of symptoms, physical examination, and heart rate and blood pressure at the conclusion of exercise. Arterial blood gases may be obtained, albeit with some inconvenience, while the subject is exercising. Sampling of arterial blood once exercise has ceased does not reflect the exercise condition however, because of the rapid change in Po_2 at the conclusion of exercise.

SYSTEM WITHOUT ANALYSIS OF EXPIRED GASES

A treadmill or cycle ergometer permits a more controlled and reproducible exercise stress. Because the subject is relatively stationary, blood pressure and heart rate may be obtained repeatedly, and a continuously monitored electrocardiogram (ECG) incorporating 1, 3, or 12 leads may be used. Oxygen administration may be conveniently given during exercise for some forms of testing. Some authors have asserted that the work rate on a cycle or treadmill can be translated into an estimate of oxygen uptake, but this procedure is subject to potentially important errors.

Manually Operated System for Expired Gas Analysis

Expired gas can be collected during exercise by using a suitable breathing valve and an attached meteorologic-type balloon, gas-impermeable plastic bag, or Douglas-type bag. Gas is collected for 1 to 2 minutes at intervals during exercise. Although it is most often used during constant work rate exercise testing, this method can be used to collect repeated samples of expired gas over relatively short intervals. Thus, it may be used during some non-steady conditions. If desired, a series of bags can be connected to stopcocks for sequential sampling. After collection, bags can be emptied into a spirometer or through a dry gas meter to determine volume. Mixed expired CO_2 and O_2 can be determined using appropriate individual analyzers or a respiratory mass spectrometer.

Collection bags or balloons should be light in weight and hung vertically to avoid added resistance to the expired breathing circuit. Care must be taken to ensure that bags or balloons are leak-free. A small amount of approximately mixed expired gas should be put into the bags and the bags emptied as much as possible before expired gas collection. This will reduce errors caused by room air trapped in the bags inadvertently before collection. In addition, changes in expired gas composition may occur from diffusion of gas through the bags if analysis is greatly delayed.

A semi-automated system using bags to collect expired gas was described by Wilmore and Costill.[1] This system used a rotating valve to deliver gas to one of three collection bags. The other two bags were simultaneously either having their contents analyzed or, after analysis, being evacuated. Ventilation could be determined by a gas meter or pneumotachograph in series with the collection bags. Thus, sequential samples could be automatically obtained and analyzed.

System Using a Mixing Chamber

In this type of system, expired minute ventilation is determined using a pneumotachograph or other type of in-line flow or volume measurement device. Expired gas is then passed into a mixing chamber from which gas is sampled and analyzed for O_2 and CO_2 concentrations. With proper mixing of expired gas from each breath, differences in O_2 and CO_2 concentration from the beginning to the end of each breath are smoothed, and the resultant O_2 and CO_2 concentrations are equal to the volume-weighted average concentrations or "mixed expired" O_2 and CO_2 concentrations. These are equivalent to the O_2 and CO_2 concentrations that would have been obtained from a bag collection of expired gas.

In an ideal mixing chamber, with instantaneous and complete mixing of gas added, the introduction of a constant flow of a given gas eventually results in the gas in the mixing chamber having a composition identical to that of this gas. The time course by which the concentration of the gas approaches that of the input gas is approximately exponential, and for this ideal mixing chamber, the mixing characteristics can be described by a time constant = $V_{mc}/\dot{V}$, where V_{mc} is the volume of the mixing chamber and $\dot{V}$ is the constant flow of gas into and out of the chamber. The time constant is related to the time the mixing chamber takes to reach the new gas concentration after a step-change in the input gas is introduced. The change reaches about 95% of its final value after three time constant intervals have elapsed.

A large gas flow (or minute ventilation) or a mixing chamber of small size has a short time constant. Under these conditions, this chamber would respond rapidly to a change in gas concentration; that is, a step-change in input would be quickly reflected in a change in concentration sampled from the chamber; however, the small volume of such a mixing chamber means that a subject with a large tidal volume relative to mixing chamber volume will produce marked fluctuations in instantaneous O_2 and CO_2 concentrations in the chamber. In other words, the intra-breath changes in gas concentration would not be adequately dampened in such a mixing chamber. On the other hand, too large a mixing chamber volume compared to tidal volume results in an impractically long time to reach any new equilibrium, making the mixing chamber poorly responsive to changes in gas concentration of the expired gas. Thus, a compromise among stability of concentration, mixing, and equilibration time is usually chosen. Most authors suggest a mixing chamber volume of 5 to 6 L for testing adults during exercise.[2,3] At rest, the time constant for a chamber of this size would be about 1 minute (a 95% concentration change would be reached in about 3 minutes). The time constant decreases as ventilation increases during exercise, making this suitable for most exercise protocols.

These factors suggest that fixed volume mixing chambers may be satisfactory during exercise in which $\dot{V}E$, F_{ECO_2} and F_{EO_2} are changing slowly, but may not be satisfactory when rapid changes are expected. In the latter situation, an alteration in actual mixed expired gas concentration is not reflected in the mixing chamber until after a new equilibrium is reached. Thus, if ventilation is continuously measured, some time or volume adjustment must be made to match the correct mixed expired gas concentrations with the correct ventilation when calculating $\dot{V}O_2$ and $\dot{V}CO_2$. Because it is possible to predict the response of a given mixing chamber with changes in minute ventilation, a mixing chamber that changes in size as a function of minute ventilation may be one way of addressing changes in response during exercise. Some exercise testing systems incorporate this feature, but the accuracy of this method is not clear.

Variables measured using such a system may include expired ventilation, mixed-expired CO_2 and O_2, $\dot{V}O_2$ and $\dot{V}CO_2$, heart rate, and respiratory rate. All these may be recorded on a calibrated multichannel physiologic recorder. An automated system using a mixing chamber can also be designed to record these data and to calculate variables periodically during exercise.

BREATH-BY-BREATH SYSTEMS

Gas exchange variables change rapidly at the onset of exercise, during exercise in which work rate changes more frequently than every 3 to 4 minutes, and at the beginning of recovery from exercise. The ability to measure these rapidly changing values makes it possible to utilize several useful work rate protocols such as 1-minute incremental increases in work rate. Because mixed expired bag collection and mixing chamber systems may not be suitable with these protocols, breath-by-breath systems for measuring gas exchange are often used.

A breath-by-breath system measures airflow or volume continuously and simultaneously determines instantaneous expired CO_2 and O_2 concentration. The CO_2 output and O_2 uptake during each breath are calculated and the cumulated totals of all breaths over a measured time period are $\dot{V}CO_2$ and $\dot{V}O_2$. To make accurate measurements, ventilation and gas concentrations must be determined as near to continuously as possible. The number of different measurements and the large number and frequent sampling of data make a breath-by-breath system impractical without the aid of computer-controlled sampling and calculation.

We have used breath-by-breath systems for both research applications and for evaluation of patients.[4–6] These systems make it possible to determine gas exchange rapidly and accurately under many conditions. By interpolating breath-by-breath expired volume, O_2 uptake, and CO_2 output second-by-second, it is possible to reduce the variability in breath-by-breath measurements. The second-by-second values can then be time-averaged using replicate studies,[4–6] thereby reducing the noise in measurement and enhancing the physiologic responses to transient changes in work rate.

Measurement of Volume, Flow Rate, or Ventilation

Several methods of measuring respired gas volume and flow rates during exercise can be used. Each has advantages and disadvantages that make them suitable for different types of systems. Whereas expired ventilation or flow is usually measured, many of the physiologic variables desired can be calculated from inspired volume or flow with the appropriate adjustments. Devices for measuring volume or flows may be used directly as part of the breathing circuit, or they may be used to measure volumes from a collecting container. If the device is used directly, then flow resistance, linearity, and frequency response may be important considerations.[7] If flow is measured rather than volume, e.g., with a pneumotachograph, then flow rate must be electrically or mathematically integrated over time to determine volume per unit time. Volume can be measured directly using a gas meter, spirometer, or volume transducer. Although, theoretically, flow can be determined from the volume signal by differentiation, this is usually not done because differentiation is inherently noisy compared to integration.

DRY GAS METER

A dry gas meter, such as a Parkinson-Cowan type, can be used to measure the volume collected in Douglas bags or rubber meteorologic balloons. Thus, it is suitable for a manually operated system with intermittent collection of expired gas. Alternatively, the dry gas meter can be used directly in either the inspired or expired side of a breathing valve circuit. The dry gas meter is reasonably accurate, especially if used with constant flow, but it may be subject to mechanical leaks and maladjustment. Moisture in the expired gas has also been recognized as a potential cause of error.[7]

SPIROMETER

A large spirometer, such as a Tissot-type water-sealed spirometer of 120-, 350-, or 600-L capacity, is an extremely useful device in the exercise laboratory. It can be used to measure volumes collected in bags or balloons, used for calibration of other volume and flow devices, or used directly in a manually operated system. The advantages of a large spirometer include accuracy, simplicity, and ease of quality control. Disadvantages are its size and bulk, the difficulty connecting recording devices, and, if used as a direct measurement device, poor frequency response and potential resistance to breathing.

PNEUMOTACHOGRAPH

Pneumotachographs are devices used to measure instantaneous gas flow. The most commonly used devices consist of either a number of parallel tubes (Fleisch) or a series of fine wire mesh screens. Each device, therefore, offers a small resistance to airflow that is usually undetectable by the subject. The change in pressure measured across this known resistance is measured and related to the gas flow rate.

Gas flow is directly proportional to pressure drop when flow is laminar, and the relationship is given by Poiseuille's law. With laminar flow, the only energy loss from the moving gas occurs because of frictional resistance from the walls of the structure containing the gas and a small amount of frictional loss caused by differences in forward velocity for adjacent gas molecules. The proportionality coefficient between flow and pressure is conductance, the inverse of resistance, which is constant for constant dimensions of the resistive element for a given gas viscosity. When flow becomes nonlaminar or turbulent, energy of the gas (pressure) is lost in acceleration of the gas molecules, and the relationship between flow and pressure becomes nonlinear and unpredictable. In general, conditions approximating laminar flow in smooth walled tubes will be met if the gas velocity is low compared to the cross-sectional area of the tube. In addition, laminar flow is disrupted by changes in the size or direction of conducting tubing. The resultant turbulent flow can be restored to laminar if the gas is allowed to flow through a relatively long, straight, smooth-walled tube of appropriate size. In a pneumotachograph, laminar flow is necessary to maintain a known relationship between pressure and flow, so flow can be determined from pressure measurements.

In a Fleisch pneumotachograph, laminar flow is encouraged by small flow channels and low velocities of gas. This is accomplished by making the resistance element a bundle of parallel channels. A small, flexible, plastic tube is connected at each end of the resistance element, and these two tubes are connected to a differential pressure transducer. During gas flow through the pneumotachograph, the differential pressure is proportional to the flow. The electrical signal from the transducer can be further processed or displayed directly. The pressure transducer must be relatively sensitive because the approximate pressure difference at the usually recommended maximal flow rate is only 1.2 to 1.3 cm H_2O.

The pneumotachograph, by definition, introduces additional resistance into the breathing circuit. Because the Fleisch pneumotachograph is made in several different sizes, with larger sizes intended for measuring higher flow rates, the resistance is minimal and appears to be undetectable by the subject (on the order of 0.2 to 0.6 cm H_2O/L/sec).

Linearity

The size of the pneumotachograph, the upstream gas flow geometry, the range of flow to be measured, and the method of measurement determine its linearity. For a given pneumotachograph, pressure drop can be shown to be a satisfactory linear function of gas flow rate until flow rate exceeds some particular value. The flow at which pressure becomes nonlinear depends on the size of the pneumotachograph. For exercise testing in adults, flows encountered generally indicate that a No. 3 Fleisch pneumotachograph is appropriate. This device has a reasonably linear response for flows up to 5 to 10 L per second and adequate sensitivity in the low flow range.

A known constant flow of air can be generated by an airpump (such as a vacuum cleaner), appropriate valves, and a calibrated flow meter. From this a curve of pressure drop across the pneumotachograph versus flow can be derived.[8] Yeh et al.[9] used a weighted-averaging technique and calibrated syringe to determine the pneumotachograph pressure-flow characteristics, a method that avoids the use of a flow generator. This method should prove satisfactory for a computer-aided data acquisition system. Generally, pneumotachograph manufacturers provide data on expected pressure-flow characteristics of their products, but these should be rechecked after installation and after attachment of devices needed for actual measurements.

Finucane et al.[7] studied the influence of upstream geometry using Fleisch pneumotachographs. They found that the pressure-flow relationship was linear over the widest gas flow range when the immediate upstream geometry was a pipe of the same internal diameter as the pneumotachograph. They suggested that for a No. 3 Fleisch, 11 cm length of straight pipe, and for a No. 4 Fleisch, 12 cm of straight pipe were optimal. A rough guide would be to use a straight smooth pipe with a length of 5 to 6 times the diameter of the flow meter immediately in front of the pneumotachograph in the entering air stream.

Compensation for documented nonlinearities in the pressure-flow relationship can be made by altering the output of the differential pressure transducer either electrically or, in computer-based systems, mathematically. The linear flow range has been increased by as much as 50 to 100% with, generally, less than 2% inaccuracy at recommended maximal flow. In commercial systems, empiric calibration curves may be used to optimize pneumotachograph performance.

Frequency Response

Rapidly changing flow rates may not be measured with perfect fidelity if the pneumotachograph is unable to respond instantaneously. Because the pneumotachograph has no moving parts, any delay is due solely to the inertia of gas movement. This inertia is the result of an additional pressure difference needed to accelerate the gas within the pneumotachograph and would appear as a greater pressure difference at a given flow rate. Finucane et al.[7] found that, for Fleisch pneumotachographs, flow values did lag behind pressure changes for sinusoidal flow at frequencies up to 10 Hz; however, the lag was small and in all probability is insignificant compared to the frequency response of other parts of the breathing circuit used for exercise studies. It is necessary also to consider the frequency characteristics of the differential pressure transducer and any linearizing circuit, the response of the chart recorder if used, and the sampling frequency of digital sampling if a computerbased system is used. In addition, a minimum number of interconnecting fittings should be used.[10]

Temperature

Pneumotachographs used for measuring flow of ambient air are usually kept at ambient temperature. Because expired gas is usually warmer and contains more water vapor than ambient air, contact of this gas with an ambient-temperature pneumotachograph would result in condensation and obstruction of the pneumotachograph resistance elements. These pneumotachographs, therefore, are often used with an electric heater to warm the pneumotachograph to a temperature slightly above expired gas temperature. Too high a temperature results in significant cooling during calibration and use, with resultant inconsistent errors.

The problem is more complicated, however, because a heated pneumotachograph not only warms the expired gas (if the gas is cooler than the pneumotachograph), but also warms it by a variable amount depending on the flow of gas. Warming the gas increases its volume and thereby alters the pressure-flow relationship. Whereas theoretic methods can be used to estimate the degree of warming, two practical methods may eliminate the problem. Both methods make the expired gas temperature as it enters the pneumotachograph and the pneumotachograph temperature equal. Either the expired gas can be kept warm prior to entering a heated pneumotachograph, or the expired gas can be allowed to cool to ambient temperature before reaching an ambient temperature pneumotachograph. In the first method, the temperature of the pneumotachograph should be only slightly warmer (0.5° C) than the temperature of the gas passing through it. If the expired gas is cooled, then the method must guarantee that even a large flow of expired gas can be quickly cooled to ambient temperature. This can generally be assumed if several feet of wide-bore tubing are interposed between the breathing valve and the pneumotachograph. The ease of pneumotachograph calibration is also a consideration; the ambient-temperature pneumotachograph is simpler to use.

Gas Density and Viscosity

Oxygen is significantly more viscous than nitrogen. Because viscosity is a direct factor in Poiseuille's law relating pressure difference and flow rate for a given straight tube, it follows that air and 100% oxygen would have different pressure-flow relationships. Calibration and calculation methods need to consider this effect or unexpected errors will arise. For 100% oxygen breathing, flows are measured approximately 11% higher for a pneumotachograph calibrated with a known flow rate of air (21% O_2). In systems that use a pneumotachograph, appropriate adjustment at the time of calibration or during calculation of ventilation and gas exchange is necessary. These should be performed automatically in commercial systems that offer protocols for exercise testing with oxygen breathing. Although only gas viscosity is a direct factor in Poiseuille's law, gas density is a determinant of whether laminar or turbulent flow will exist at a given gas velocity in a given straight tube. A low-density, high-viscosity gas, such as a mixture consisting of a high proportion of helium, maintains laminar flow at higher velocities, and therefore, pressure difference and flow rate remain linear at higher flow rates.

NONLAMINAR FLOWMETER

A relatively new device for measurement of flow uses the principle of the Pitot tube, a device for measuring flow velocity in fluids. The Pitot tube measures the difference in pressure at an opening placed directly facing the fluid stream compared to the pressure at an opening perpendicular to the fluid stream (static pressure). From Bernoulli's law, the velocity of fluid movement is proportional to the square root of the pressure difference. From the cross-sectional area of the device, the flow can be calculated. The Pitot tube has the advantage of being non-resistive. It is also dependent on turbulent flow rather than on laminar flow conditions.

A flowmeter suitable for exercise gas exchange measurements based on the Pitot tube principle uses a differential pressure transducer to determine the pressure difference between the static and mid-stream ports. A suitable algorithm calculates the flow from the pressure signal and could also correct for any nonlinearities over the flow measurement range. Advantages of such a device compared to a conventional pneumotachograph

include low resistance and lack of a requirement for laminar flow. Problems with heating or cooling of expired gas should also be minimized with such a device.

OTHER FLOW AND VOLUME MEASURING DEVICES

The turbine volume transducer places a lightweight impeller in the gas stream and measures the volume of gas flow directly by measuring the speed of the impeller. It has been used for measuring bidirectional gas flows, i.e., both inspiratory and expiratory gas. Because of gas temperature changes, however, a correction must be used to obtain expired volume using the principle of nitrogen balance between inspired and expired gas. Moreover, the speed of the impeller may be sensitive to water or saliva deposition. In a comparison between a turbine flowmeter system and a pneumotachograph system (which was independently calibrated), the turbine system had as much as a 20% error for resting $\dot{V}O_2$ and $\dot{V}CO_2$ even though the accuracy of minute ventilation determination was similar for both devices.[11] During exercise, the accuracy of $\dot{V}O_2$ and $\dot{V}CO_2$ improved. The investigators attributed the error in gas exchange measurements to a lag between gas flow and impeller rotation (impeller inertia), both at the start and end of gas flow.

The mass of gas rather than the volume or flow is measured using a hot-wire anemometer.[12,13] This device determines the change in amount of electrical current, compared to baseline, needed to maintain a constant temperature of a wire placed in the air stream. The wire material is selected so the wire resistance is strongly influenced by the wire temperature. The rate of mass movement of gas and its thermal capacity relate to the current change and, by using an appropriate model, the flow of gas can be calculated. This method is inherently nonlinear, but this can be adjusted using suitable digital computer algorithms.

CALIBRATION

Validation of any flow or volume device is essential for confidence in the ability of the device to measure accurately and reproducibly under testing conditions. A water-sealed spirometer is recommended as a primary standard for volume measurements, and spirometer volume change over a timed period can be used as a flow standard. Secondary standards include calibrated large-volume syringes of 1 to 4 L and various gas flowmeters. These secondary standards should be calibrated against a spirometer before use. If flow or volume signals are further processed by analog or digital means, the results will be subject to the response characteristics and calculation methods of these instruments as well.[10] The accuracy of flow and volume can also be determined using a calibrated pump calibrator (see later).

Pneumotachographs have special calibration considerations related to the problems of temperature, water vapor, viscosity, and geometry. The simplest method is to calibrate the pneumotachograph under conditions identical to those of the testing process. Thus, a known volume or flow of gas of essentially identical temperature, relative humidity, and gas composition to the anticipated measured gas should be delivered to the pneumotachograph through identical upstream geometry. The flow range at which a linear pressure drop is expected should be determined rather than assumed from manufacturers' specifications.

Breathing Valves

Breathing valves separate inspired from expired gas flows so expired gas can be collected and analyzed. The ideal valve prevents contamination of either gas flow by the other. The ideal valve also has low resistance to both inspiration and expiration, has low rebreathed volume (low valve dead space), and operates silently. Other advantages would include low size and weight, lack of generation of turbulence in the air stream, ease of cleaning and sterilization, and low cost.

As expected, no valve design is ideal. For testing healthy, fit, exercising adults, however, a low resistance valve is preferred because of the high levels of ventilation that must be accommodated. These valves usually consist of two or three sets of one-way "J valves" each for inspiration and expiration. The small "J valves" allow rapid opening and closing. Examples include triple J valves, double J valves, and Otis-McKerrow type valves. All these have dead space volumes of 100 to 320 ml that should be considered if calculation of V_D/V_T is intended. A high-capacity Rudolph valve may also be suitable for high flow applications. At lower flow rates, Koegel and Hans-Rudolph valves with smaller dead space volumes and slightly higher flow resistances may be used.

Characteristics of valves should be determined in the laboratory prior to use. Dead space can be determined for the valve plus attached mouthpiece by measuring the amount of water it can contain. Valve resistance can be determined during constant airflow using a pressure transducer, vacuum cleaner, and flowmeter and is expressed as cm H_2O/L/sec. This value may be different between inspiration and expiration. Commonly, dry gas or room air is used for calibration. This can cause underestimation of valve resistance during exercise testing, because the valve flaps can require additional pressure to open when wet and gas flow is pulsatile. Some valves, even if they have low resistance to constant airflow, may appear to subjects to "stick" closed temporarily, perhaps altering their pattern of breathing. Finally, valves may develop back-leaks, especially when subjected to high flows and pressures during heavy exercise. These leaks should be suspected for any valve, but especially after prolonged use, infrequent cleaning, excessive secretions, or damage to component parts. Errors in ventilation or gas exchange measurements may be important clues to a leaking breathing valve. If a leak is suspected, simultaneous recording of inspiratory and expiratory flow during exercise may reveal the presence and location of the leak.

Gas Analyzers

Details of Scholander and Haldane analysis of expired gases can be found in standard references.[14] These methods are accurate but time consuming and tedious, making them impractical for large numbers of repeated measurements. Nevertheless, they are useful for initial calibration of other gas analyzers and primary analysis of stored gases used for calibration.

Carbon dioxide analyzers measure absorption by CO_2 at appropriate wavelengths of infrared light. Infrared light is passed through a cell containing the gas to be measured, and the amount of light transmitted is compared to a reference value. Absorption is proportional to the fractional CO_2 concentration. The measurement cell must be kept clean and free of water condensation.

Oxygen analyzers operate using several different principles. Two types have been used. The Pauling-type or paramagnetic analyzer measures the change in a given magnetic field introduced by changes in oxygen quantity in a chamber located within the magnetic field. Because other respiratory gases have little paramagnetic susceptibility, these will not affect the magnetic field. More commonly used, the electrochemical O_2 analyzer depends on chemical reactions between O_2 and a substrate that generates a small electrical current. This current is proportional to the rate of O_2 molecules reacting with the substrate and thus to the concentration of O_2. Because a current is produced, these analyzers are sometimes called fuel cell O_2 analyzers.

Both these types of devices measure partial pressure of the gas and therefore are affected by water vapor, pressure in the sampling systems, and changes in barometric pressure and altitude. Thus, for a given fractional concentration of O_2, changes in any of these conditions at the sensor location will erroneously result in different measured O_2 fractions. Because the sample flow rate delivering gas to the analyzer is generally held constant, a change in sampling site pressure may result from changes in resistance of the delivery tubing. Constant sample flow and constant pressure at the measurement site can be maintained by using a high-pressure suction pump and a large resistance in the connection between the analyzer and the pump. The large resistance and high pressure tend to make flow and pressure independent of changes in sample tube resistance. Nevertheless, care must be taken to ensure that sample tube resistance is identical during calibration and measurement, and water condensation, saliva, or foreign bodies are not trapped in the delivery tubing.

CO_2 analyzers are sensitive to pressure but less sensitive to flow or resistance changes, but both CO_2 and O_2 analyzers report the fraction of CO_2 or O_2 of the total gas, including any water vapor present. This is important during calibration because ambient air usually contains some water vapor, resulting in a measured O_2 concentration below that of dry air, i.e., less than the 20.93% of dry air. Carbon dioxide analyzers are affected in the same way. Expired gas, if water is not removed prior to analysis, will become saturated with water vapor at the lowest temperature that it reaches before being analyzed. Because temperature determines the partial pressure of water in a saturated gas, this temperature must be accurately known or estimated if expired CO_2 and O_2 are to be accurately determined using these analyzers. An alternative is to pass the gas over anhydrous calcium sulfate. This substance removes water vapor and allows determination of CO_2 and O_2 concentrations as if the gas were dry. This method

introduces a substantial delay between the time the gas is exhaled and the time the sample reaches the analyzer. This may be a disadvantage in breath-by-breath gas exchange measurement systems. Recently, tubing has been introduced that selectively transports water vapor out of the sample as it is transported to the analyzer. In effect, the water vapor partial pressure of the gas delivered to the analyzer is equal to that of ambient air and is not influenced by temperature of the gas at the point of sampling. Additional consideration of the significance of water vapor in calculating $\dot{V}_{O_2}$ can be found in Appendix D.

In a mass spectrometer of the fixed collector type, sampled gases are ionized to positively charged ions by an electron beam. Then, in a near vacuum, the ions are accelerated by an electric field and are then subjected to a magnetic field. The direction the ions take in the magnetic field is dependent on their mass/charge ratios. The different ions representing different gases then are detected by appropriately located detectors that produce a voltage output proportional to the number of ions that strike the collector per unit time. The individual detector voltages can be electronically divided by the total voltage. This quotient is the fractional concentration of each gas. Note that, because the total voltage is dependent on the sum of the individual detector voltages, any gas for which there is no detector does not contribute to the total. For respiratory mass spectrometry, detectors for O_2, CO_2, and N_2 are typically used; ordinarily there are no detectors for water vapor, argon, or other inert gases present in trace amounts in air. Thus, the O_2 or CO_2 concentrations given by a mass spectrometer are concentrations relative to a dry gas containing no water vapor or inert gas, regardless of whether the originally sampled gas contained water or inert gas.

Gas analyzers, including mass spectrometers, should be checked for linearity within the range of needed values. This can be done by analyzing gases of known concentration of O_2 and CO_2. If an analyzer is nonlinear, a calibration curve can be constructed by observing the analyzer output at several gas concentrations.[15]

Calibration of gas analyzers should be performed using gases of known concentration. The analyzers should be warmed up for sufficient time to ensure against electrical drift, an identical sampling arrangement to that used during testing should be used, and the sample cells should be cleaned if necessary. A device for drying gas prior to analysis may or may not be used during calibration procedures. Most often, a two-point calibration can be used if the analyzer is sufficiently linear. It is convenient to use dry room air as one calibration point, assuming an O_2 of 20.93% and CO_2 of 0.04% (essentially zero). A calibration gas of approximately 15% O_2, 5% CO_2, and balance N_2 (but whose actual values are accurately known) is appropriate for the second point because these concentrations are in the middle of the anticipated range of expired gas concentrations. The concentrations of the calibration gas mixture may be analyzed independently by Haldane or Scholander techniques or by a carefully calibrated mass spectrometer. Alternatively, gas having O_2 and CO_2 concentrations of acceptable precision can be obtained from a reliable gas supplier, but these high precision gases are expensive. A useful procedure is to keep for long-term use a tank of gas for which O_2 and CO_2 are accurately known (high precision), then to use this gas periodically to calibrate a mass spectrometer. Subsequently, the mass spectrometer can be used to measure concentrations of less expensive gases used for day-to-day calibration.

The gas transport delay time and the response time of each analyzer to the introduction of a new gas are important aspects of breath-by-breath exercise systems. This is further addressed in Appendix D. For manual analysis of mixed expired gases, delay and response times are not critical.

Validation and Maintenance of Exercise Gas Exchange Systems

In the past, systems of analyzers and computers for determination of gas exchange during exercise were often assembled by individual laboratories. Validation often comprised the majority of the time required for development of these systems. Now, most often, commercially manufactured exercise systems are used by clinicians and investigators. Though it is tempting to consider these automated devices fool-proof, these systems should undergo validation and should have periodic monitoring for accuracy and reproducibility of results.

Validation can be performed by simultaneous collection of mixed expired gas (see earlier) while the exercise system is collecting data on normal subjects.[4–5,16] For mixing chamber and breath-by-breath systems, extremes of tidal volume and flow are particularly challenging. It is easiest to collect expired gas during the steady-state of constant work exercise; but such validation may not provide evidence of accurate measurement during rapidly changing exercise protocols or when the major focus is on the short-term time course of gas exchange (gas exchange kinetics).

The reproducibility of a system can be monitored by having a small group of subjects, e.g., laboratory personnel, available for periodic exercise testing using an identical protocol. Clinically significant differences in results should indicate the need for review of the instrument calibration procedures, review of calibration factors, checking of analyzer performance, and other troubleshooting.

A useful device is a calibrator that simulates gas exchange at a known and reproducible rate. One simulator uses a sinusoidal pump of known volume and measurable frequency to provide an accurate "expired minute ventilation."[17] Gas exchange (O_2 uptake and CO_2 output) is simulated by the introduction of a gas mixture containing 21% CO_2 in nitrogen to the room air pumped into the exercise system. $\dot{V}O_2$ and $\dot{V}CO_2$ measured by the system should be equal to 0.21 × the flow rate of 21% CO_2 into the pump calibrator and the respiratory gas exchange ratio should equal 1; however, adjustment of the exercise system algorithms may be necessary to accommodate the nearly dry, room temperature expirate in a system set up to measure body temperature, saturated expirate. The pump calibrator has been demonstrated to provide an accurate simulation of gas exchange that can be used for validation. In addition, the device is useful for routine periodic checks of reproducibility. If an error (or change) in measured minute ventilation, $\dot{V}O_2$, or $\dot{V}CO_2$ is found, analysis of the differences in the measurements may also suggest the nature of the problem.

Validation and reproducibility data, along with any additional data, should be kept for future reference. Many commercially manufactured systems have an option to print a listing of the current status of gas analyzers, environmental conditions, calibration gas concentrations, temperature, and other important system variables. This information can be helpful in identifying a problem and in resolving problems with the help of the manufacturer.

Arterial Blood Gases and Arterial Catheters

Arterial blood gases may be obtained by arterial puncture or drawn through indwelling arterial catheters. Arterial punctures may be difficult to perform if the subject is moving, usually cannot be obtained repeatedly, and, if uncomfortable, may affect the subject's response to exercise and the results of the blood gases. Arterial punctures may be particularly difficult at or near a subject's exhaustion. In some laboratories, arterial punctures are performed just after the completion of exercise. This practice is to be discouraged because these results may be significantly different from those obtained immediately prior to cessation of work,[18-20] especially for Pa_{O_2} and $P(A-a)_{O_2}$. Nevertheless, arterial punctures are useful if the exercise protocol permits and if only a few blood samples are needed.

Indwelling arterial catheters make the repeated sampling of arterial blood for blood gases simpler, faster, and painless, and they permit continuous monitoring of blood pressure during exercise as well. The most common insertion sites are the brachial and radial arteries. The radial artery site has the theoretic advantage that the ulnar artery can supply blood to the hand if the radial artery is blocked, whereas the brachial artery is the sole blood supply of the lower arm. With meticulous care, however, we have never had a serious complication of brachial artery catheterization in several thousand insertions over a 20-year period. The disadvantage of the radial artery site is that it may interfere with gripping of the cycle ergometer handlebars; in addition, referring direct blood pressure measurements to the left atrial level may be more difficult. A description of the insertion of a brachial artery catheter is included in Appendix E.

Arterial punctures and catheterization are rarely complicated by pain or other discomfort, bleeding, arterial spasm, distal arterial thromboembolism, thrombosis, and infection. Most frequently, subjects complain of mild discomfort and hematoma formation following puncture. Sufficient pressure for an adequate amount of time after puncture or removal of the catheter and an elastic pressure dressing can help to avoid this problem. Arterial catheters should be used with special care or avoided in patients with known peripheral vascular disease.

Noninvasive Measurement of Blood Gases

PULSE OXIMETRY

Pulse oximetry estimates arterial blood oxygen saturation. In the past, in vivo oximetry using transmission spectrophotometry through the antihelix of the ear required multiple wavelengths of light, a heater to increase and maintain blood flow, and a heavy, complex device attached to the subject's ear. Since the late 1970s, the principle of pulse oximetry has been widely used.[21] With this technique, an estimate of arterial oxygen saturation is derived from a combination of spectrophotometry and pulse plethysmography. Current devices use two wavelengths of light produced by light-emitting diodes, one in the red and one in the infrared spectrum, and a detector that measures light intensity passing through the ear lobe or fingertip. Pulsatile (maximum compared to minimum) absorption of light at these two wavelengths can be theoretically shown to provide enough information to determine the ratio of oxyhemoglobin to total hemoglobin, assuming that all the pulsatile change is due to arterial blood. In practice, manufacturers of pulse oximeters use empiric calibration curves to determine the coefficients used in calculation.

Pulse oximetry is theoretically independent of skin pigmentation and the thickness of the ear lobe or finger; however, some studies have shown that dark skin pigmentation may affect results.[22,23] Pulse oximeters cannot distinguish carboxyhemoglobin (and methemoglobin) from oxyhemoglobin; it may be convenient to think of the percentage of oxygen saturation reported from a pulse oximeter as being equal to (100 − % deoxyhemoglobin). In general, pulse oximetry becomes more inaccurate when oxygen saturation is less than 75%.[21]

During exercise, pulse oximetry has additional potential problems. Movement artifact and stray incidental light interfere with pulse oximetry accuracy, and these may be particularly bothersome during vigorous exercise. Although some studies have found acceptable accuracy of pulse oximeters during exercise,[22-25] Hansen and Casaburi[26] have shown that overestimation and underestimation of arterial blood oxygen saturation may occur at maximum exercise using one particular pulse oximeter. Reasons for this include dependence of the pulse oximeter on sufficient blood flow to the vascular bed measured, a change in the shape of the arterial pulse waveform, a change in empirically determined calibration factors, movement artifact, or other problems. Another study using two different pulse oximeters, however, concluded that pulse oximetry was accurate in normal subjects breathing hypoxic gas during exercise.[25] Escourrou and co-workers[27] found significantly different pulse oximetry estimates of oxygen saturation compared to measured values with three different pulse oximeters.[27] These authors concluded, however, that changes in pulse oximeter O_2 saturation from rest to exercise were useful for clinical decision making.

The major disadvantage of pulse oximetry is that saturation rather than arterial Po_2 is measured. Thus, although the correlation between measured arterial O_2 saturation and pulse oximetry O_2 saturation is often good, significant decreases in arterial Po_2 in the range of $Po_2 > 60$ mm Hg result in only small decreases in O_2 saturation. For patients whose Pa_{O_2} decreases to below 60 mm Hg during exercise, pulse oximetry proves useful. For other patients whose resting and exercise Pa_{O_2} is greater than 60 mm Hg but who are suspected of significant decreases in Pa_{O_2} during exercise, one approach is to use pulse oximetry during a preliminary test. If arterial oxygen saturation decreases by more than 3 to 5%, then an arterial catheter is placed for direct measurement of Pa_{O_2} and $P(A-a)_{O_2}$ during a repeat exercise study. Nevertheless, clinically important decreases in Pa_{O_2} may occur that could be undetectable by pulse oximetry alone.

TRANSCUTANEOUS Po_2 MEASUREMENTS

Transcutaneous Po_2 (Ptc_{O_2}) is measured using a Clark electrode attached to the skin. A current proportional to the number of oxygen molecules diffusing out of the skin beneath the electrode is produced. This current is determined and reported as partial pressure in mm Hg. The Ptc_{O_2} reflects not only arterial Po_2, but also the blood flow to the skin under the electrode, the hemoglobin concentration and oxyhemoglobin dissociation curve, and the distance from the epidermal capillaries. To improve blood flow, the electrodes in use heat the skin under the sensor to 43 to 45° C. This necessitates correction of the Ptc_{O_2} for the rightward shift of the oxyhemoglobin dissociation curve. This is often done automatically by the instrument. Reports by Schonfeld et al.[28] and by McDowell and Theide[29] on normal subjects and patients suggest that transcutaneous Po_2 may be a reasonable estimate of arterial Po_2; however, it has been generally concluded that the response time of transcutaneous Po_2 devices is unacceptably slow for useful measurements during exercise.[21]

Pulmonary Artery Catheters

A pulmonary artery catheter can add valuable information during exercise testing in some kinds of patients. Possible measurements include pulmonary artery pressure, pulmonary artery wedge pressure, mixed venous blood gases, and cardiac output by thermal indicator dilution. The Swan-Ganz catheter is balloon-tipped and flow-directed, and a physician can pass it through a large vein in the arm through the right atrium, right ventricle, and into the pulmonary artery with or without fluoroscopic guidance. Because arrhythmias and heart block potentially occur during placement, this should be done only with ECG monitoring and appropriate resuscitation equipment and medications standing by. For pressure measurements, a calibrated transducer and recorder are needed for continuous recordings. Note that during exercise, especially in patients with lung disease, large swings in intrathoracic pressure with respiration may be transmitted to the pulmonary artery and wedge pressures. Intravascular pressures restricted to measurement at end-exhalation are usually most relevant. Samples of blood can be drawn from the catheter tip for mixed venous blood gases needed for the calculation of cardiac output using the Fick equation (see Appendix D) or calculation of venous admixture.

The thermodilution method introduces a bolus of physiologic fluid (usually isotonic saline or 5% dextrose in water) of known volume (10 ml), temperature (usually 0° C), and specific heat and specific gravity into a blood vessel transporting the total cardiac output. The temperature change downstream reflects the volume of dilution of the bolus and cardiac output can be calculated. The injection site is usually in the right atrium, and temperature sensor is at the tip of the pulmonary artery catheter. The integral of temperature over time is inversely proportional to cardiac output. Although this calculation can be done manually, a dedicated computer unit is most often used.

Stetz et al.[30] reviewed several studies and concluded that thermodilution cardiac outputs in catheterization laboratories and intensive care units were of comparable accuracy to Fick or dye-dilution methods. These authors suggested, however, that a 20 to 26% difference in cardiac output should be found before concluding that two single determinations were different. Advantages of thermodilution include safety, lack of recirculation, speed, and repeatability.

The disadvantages of a pulmonary artery catheter include increased risks, costs, and preparation time. Uncommon complications can include arrhythmias, heart block, bleeding, perforation of the right ventricle or pulmonary artery, and infections. Under specific circumstances, however, the benefits gained from information obtained from these catheters may outweigh the risks.

Ergometers

TREADMILLS

Treadmills allow subjects to perform familiar walking and running exercise at measured speeds and grades of incline. A variety of protocols for increasing work performed have been reported, and both low and high work rates may be obtained.

Treadmills have some advantages over cycle ergometers. A subject performing on a treadmill generally has a maximum $\dot{V}O_2$ approximately 5 to 10% higher than on a cycle ergometer. Some subjects and patients are simply not able to cycle because of problems of coordination.

On the other hand, treadmills require more space than a cycle ergometer, demand extra caution during testing, and may introduce movement artifacts in measurement of ventilation and pulmonary gas exchange. Subjects must not hold on tightly to any part of the treadmill, such as a hand railing, because this may decrease the oxygen uptake required for a given speed and grade. Because work rate can only be approximated from body weight, speed, and grade, oxygen uptake measurements are highly desirable during exercise. Work efficiency during treadmill walking cannot be precisely determined because of the difficulty in estimating work rate. Because of the advantages of an exercise test in which there is a constant increase in work rate (power output) with time, a treadmill protocol that produces a linear increase in work rate is desirable. Constant speed with a fixed increase in grade per time interval (e.g., 1% per minute) comes closest to providing a linear increase in work rate, but this treadmill protocol is unlikely to be perfect for all subjects.

Treadmill speed and grade should be routinely checked for accuracy and reproducibility. Grade may be determined by using a plumb line and tape measure. Speed can be accurately determined by using a stopwatch to time the movement of a mark made on the treadmill belt.

CYCLE ERGOMETERS

Cycle ergometers enable one to make a precise estimation of the work rate. Leg cycling may be performed sitting or supine. Advantages of the cycle ergometer over the treadmill include the ability to vary the work rate in step, incremental, or ramp fashion; the ability to determine work efficiency; smaller size; potentially greater safety because the subject is supported at all times; and less effect of movement artifact on measurements. Some subjects and patients, however, may not be able to pedal the cycle because of lack of coordination and experience. The seat may become uncomfortable during a prolonged exercise study.

When the patient is in the upright position, seat height is important and should be carefully adjusted. When the patient is seated, the foot at the lowest point of the pedalling cycle should be such that the knee is almost but not completely straight. It is useful to record the seat height in the subject's records so future studies may be done identically. Subjects should be asked to wear tennis shoes suitable for the types of pedals on the cycle. Toe clips may or may not be used, as desired.

Two types of cycle ergometers are in general use. Mechanically braked devices use an adjustable brake to provide resistance to pedalling. The adjustment is made by increasing or decreasing contact of a friction belt on a moving flywheel attached to the pedals. The work rate achieved is proportional to the cycling frequency or speed of the flywheel. As such, a particular work rate is only achieved if the subject cycles within a narrow range of pedalling rate. Electrically braked cycle ergometers use a variable electromagnetic field to produce a resistance to pedalling that is made to vary appropriately with flywheel speed, varying the resistance to cycling to maintain work rate at the set level. A work rate set on this type of cycle ergometer is thereby present at a wide range of cycling speeds. The work rate on the electrically braked devices may be set by a remote controller, or it may be adjusted automatically by a digital computer controller.

When subjects must pedal at a particular rate, metronomes and/or tachometers can be used to assist subjects' performance.

Calibration of the cycle is highly desirable both when used initially and periodically thereafter. Manufacturers' specifications and calibration procedures should be followed. Commercially available or specially built devices that generate known amounts of power can act as standards for calibration and verification.[31] Other methods have been devised to provide for cycle calibration and validation.[32–34] In addition, because oxygen uptake in an individual maintains a constant relationship to work rate, a group of readily available subjects (e.g., laboratory staff) may be used for rough checks on cycle work rate accuracy.

When a subject pedals on the cycle with "no resistance added," work is obviously performed. In addition to the work rate necessary to move the legs, the work rate performed to keep the cycle flywheel in motion is usually about 15 W for electromagnetically braked ergometers, and it may be as much as 20 to 30 W for mechanically braked cycle ergometers (and may vary considerably with pedalling rate). This work rate may exceed the maximal capacity of some severely limited patients. Manufacturer specifications may provide information on the work rate of "unloaded cycling," but users should make this determination for themselves.

Work and Power

During exercise, the muscles require delivery of oxygen appropriate for the work performed. The rate of oxygen utilization is related to the physical energy required to perform exercise. In basic physical units, force ($kg \cdot m/sec^2$ or newton) = mass (kg) $\times$ acceleration (m/sec^2). When this force is applied over a distance, work is performed. Thus, work ($kg \cdot m^2/sec^2$ or newton $\cdot$ m or joule) = force ($kg \cdot m/sec^2$ or newton) $\times$ distance (m); however, we are most often interested in the rate of work or power = work ($kg \cdot m^2/sec^2$ or newton $\cdot$ m or joule)/sec. The unit of power is the watt. A watt (W) is equal to 1 joule/sec = 1 newton $\cdot$ m/sec = 1 $kg \cdot m^2/sec^3$.

For a cycle ergometer, a rotating flywheel is restrained by a friction belt or electromagnet. The work rate is the distance traveled by a point on the circumference of the wheel $\times$ the rotational frequency of the flywheel $\times$ the restraining force. This force can be expressed as newtons or, commonly, as kiloponds, where 1 kilopond (kp) = 1 kg $\times$ 9.81 m/sec^2. Work rate or power can be expressed as joules/sec = W = 6.12 kp m/min. To convert from kp m/min to W, divide by 6.12. Thus, a work rate of 612 kp m/min equals 100 W.

Computer Systems

Tremendous amounts of information are obtained during exercise testing with gas exchange mea-

surements, depending on the types and numbers of variables measured. Because of this large amount of information, computers are extremely useful in the exercise laboratory.

For manually operated systems, the volume and complexity of data are manageable using a hand-held or desktop calculator. Programmable calculators and personal computers can make calculations less tedious and less subject to error.[35] These may be programmed using readily available programming languages.

Automated exercise gas exchange systems use computer-controlled data collection, rapid data sampling frequency, multiple calculations, and complex display of data. Nonlinear analyzers, including gas analyzers and flowmeters, can be adjusted using appropriate computer algorithms or tables of empiric corrections. Computers can be programmed to control the ergometer so pre-programmed protocols can be used with treadmills and cycles. Data can be calculated on line and displayed in tabular and graphic form during the exercise test. Usually, computerized systems provide quality control information before and during the exercise test, so inconsistent results suggesting an equipment or computer problem can be identified as early as possible. Finally, computer systems allow for great flexibility in data display, both on screen and in printed copies.

Typically, data sampling from a flow meter and transducer, gas analyzers, pulse oximeter, heart rate monitor, or other device undergoes analog-to-digital conversion. The analog-to-digital converter requires adequate sampling rate; for most gas exchange data, a sampling rate in the range of 50 to 100 Hz is adequate.

References

1. Wilmore, J.H., and Costill, D.L.: Semiautomated systems approach to the assessment of oxygen uptake during exercise. J. Appl. Physiol., 36:618–620, 1974.
2. Poole, G.W., and Maskell, R.C.: Validation of continuous determination of respired gases during steady-state exercise. J. Appl. Physiol., 38:736–738, 1975.
3. Spiro, S.G., Juniper, E., Bowman, P., and Edwards, R.H.T.: An increasing work rate test for assessing the physiological strain of submaximal exercise. Clin. Sci. Mol. Med., 46:191–206, 1974.
4. Beaver, W.L., Wasserman, K., and Whipp, B.J.: On-line computer analysis and breath-by-breath graphical display of exercise function tests. J. Appl. Physiol., 34: 128–132, 1973.
5. Sue, D.Y., Hansen, J.E., Blais, M., and Wasserman, K.: Measurement and analysis of gas exchange during exer-

cise using a programmable calculator. J. Appl. Physiol., 49:456–461, 1980.

6. Sietsema, K.E., Cooper, D.M., Rosove, M.A., Perloff, J.K., Child, J.S., Canobbio, M.M., Whipp, B.J., and Wasserman, K.: Dynamics of oxygen uptake during exercise in adults with cyanotic congenital heart disease. Circulation, 73:1137–1144, 1986.

7. Finucane, K.E., Egan, B.A., and Dawson, S.V.: Linearity and frequency response of pneumotachographs. J. Appl. Physiol., 32:121–126, 1972.

8. Wilmore, J.H., Davis, J.A., and Norton, A.C.: An automated system for assessing metabolic and respiratory function during exercise. J. Appl. Physiol., 40:619–624, 1976.

9. Yeh, M.P., Gardner, R.M., Adams, T.D., and Yanowitz, F.C.: Computerized determination of pneumotachometer characteristics using a calibrated syringe. J. Appl. Physiol., 53:280–285, 1982.

10. Jackson, A.C., and Vinegar, A.: A technique for measuring frequency response of pressure, volume, and flow transducers. J. Appl. Physiol., 47:462–467, 1979.

11. Yeh, M.P., Adams, T.D., Gardner, R.M., and Yanowitz, F.G.: Turbine flowmeter vs. Fleisch pneumotachometer: a comparative study for exercise testing. J. Appl. Physiol., 63:1289–1295, 1987.

12. Yoshiya, I., Nakajima, T., Nagai, I., and Jitsukawa, S.: A bidirectional respiratory flowmeter using the hot-wire principle. J. Appl. Physiol., 38:360–365, 1975.

13. Yoshiya, I., Shimada, Y., and Tanaka, K.: Evaluation of a hot-wire respiratory flowmeter for clinical applicability. J. Appl. Physiol., 47:1131–1135, 1979.

14. Consolazio, C.F., Johnson, R.E., and Pecora, L.J.: Physiological Measurements of Metabolic Function in Man. New York, McGraw-Hill, 1963.

15. Gabel, R.A.: Calibration of nonlinear gas analyzers using exponential washout and polynomial curve fitting. J. Appl. Physiol., 34:400–401, 1973.

16. Versteeg, P.G., and Kippersluis, G.J.: Automated systems for measurement of oxygen uptake during exercise testing. Int. J. Sports Med., 10:107–112, 1989.

17. Huszczuk, A., Whipp, B.J., and Wasserman, K.: A respiratory gas exchange simulator for routine calibration in metabolic studies. Eur. Respir. J., 3:465–468, 1990.

18. Ries, A.L., Fedullo, P.F., and Clausen, J.L.: Rapid changes in arterial blood gas levels after exercise in pulmonary patients. Chest, 83:454–456, 1983.

19. Frye, M., DiBenedetto, R., Lain, D., and Morgan, K.: Single arterial puncture vs. arterial cannula for arterial gas analysis after exercise. Chest, 93:294–299, 1988.

20. O'Neill, A.V., and Johnson, D.C.: Transition from exercise to rest. Ventilatory and arterial blood gas responses. Chest, 99:1145–1150, 1991.

21. Clark, J.S., Votteri, B., Arriagno, R.L., Cheung, P., Eichhorn, J.H., Fallat, R.J., Lee, S.E., Newth, C.J.L., and Sue, D.Y.: Noninvasive assessment of blood gases. Am. Rev. Respir. Dis., 145:220–232, 1992.

22. Zeballos, R.J., and Weisman, I.M.: Reliability of ear oximetry during exercise and hypoxia in black subjects. Chest, 96:162S, 1989.

23. Smyth, R.J., D'Urzo, A.D., Slutsky, A.S., Galdo, B.M., and Rebuck, A.S.: Ear oximetry during combined hypoxia and exercise. J. Appl. Physiol., 60:716–719, 1986.

24. Ries, A.L., Farrow, J.T., and Clausen, J.L.: Accuracy of two ear oximeters at rest and during exercise in pulmonary patients. Am. Rev. Respir. Dis., 132:685–689, 1985.

25. Powers, S.K., Dodd, S., Freeman, J., Ayers, G.D., Samson, H., and McKnight, T.: Accuracy of pulse oximetry to estimate HbO_2 fraction of total Hb during exercise. J. Appl. Physiol., 67:300–304, 1989.

26. Hansen, J.E., and Casaburi, R.: Validity of ear oximetry in clinical exercise testing. Chest, 91:333–337, 1987.

27. Escourrou, P.J.L., Delaperche, M.R., and Visseaux, A.: Reliability of pulse oximetry during exercise in pulmonary patients. Chest, 97:635–638, 1990.

28. Schonfeld, T., Sargent, C.W., Bautista, D., Walters, M.A., O'Neal, M.H., Platzker, A.C.G., and Keens, T.C.: Transcutaneous oxygen monitoring during exercise stress testing. Am. Rev. Respir. Dis., 121:457–462, 1980.

29. McDowell, J.W., and Thiede, W.H.: Usefulness of the transcutaneous P_{O_2} monitor during exercise testing in adults. Chest, 78:853–855, 1980.

30. Stetz, C.W., Miller, R.G., Kelly, G.E., and Raffin, R.A.: Reliability of the thermodilution method in the determination of cardiac output in clinical practice. Am. Rev. Respir. Dis., 126:1001–1004, 1982.

31. Clark, J.H., and Greenleaf, J.E.: Electronic bicycle ergometer: a simple calibration procedure. J. Appl. Physiol., 30:440–442, 1971.

32. Van Praagh, E., Bedu, M., Roddier, P., and Coudert, J.: A simple calibration method for mechanically braked cycle ergometers. Int. J. Sports Med., 13:27–30, 1992.

33. Russell, J.C., and Dale, J.D.: Dynamic torquemeter calibration of bicycle ergometers. J. Appl. Physiol., 61:1217–1220, 1986.

34. Giezendanner, D., Di Prampero, P.E., and Cerretelli, P.: A programmable electrically braked ergometer. J. Appl. Physiol., 55:578–582, 1983.

35. Powles, A.C.P., and Jones, N.L.: A pocket calculator program for noninvasive assessment of cardiorespiratory function. Comput. Biol. Med., 12:163–173, 1982.

Calculations, Formulae, and Examples

THIS APPENDIX presents the most essential formulae for calculating gas exchange and other related variables during exercise. An example accompanies the formula for each variable, using typical data acquired during exercise testing. Whereas the calculation of these variables uses well-defined and tested formulae, several areas deserve particularly close attention. Thus, at the end of this appendix, we address the specific problems of water vapor in the calculation of $\dot{V}O_2$, the problem of making corrections for the dead space of the breathing valve, and aspects of breath-by-breath gas exchange analysis.

Formulae and Example of Gas Exchange Calculation

The formula for calculating each variable must take into account the conditions under which measurements are made and certain conventions that are followed. For the example calculation, we assume that expired gas is collected for 2 minutes into, a meteorologic balloon or a Douglas bag. Volume is measured in a large spirometer; fractional concentrations of O_2 and CO_2 are measured to within 0.04% using gas analyzers or a mass spectrometer. For the gas analyzers, the gas is passed through a column of anhydrous calcium sulfate to remove water vapor prior to analysis. An arterial blood sample is obtained during the collection of expired gas.

The measurements used for the example calculation are given in Table D-1.

MINUTE VENTILATION ($\dot{V}E$)

The volume of gas exhaled is divided by the time of exhalation in minutes to determine minute ventilation ($\dot{V}E$). By convention, $\dot{V}E$ is reported at body temperature saturated with water vapor at ambient pressure (BTPS), as in formula 1. It may be necessary during calculation to obtain $\dot{V}E$ (STPD) using formula 2, or from the appropriate tables (see Appendix F).

TABLE D-1. *Measurements Used for Example of Calculation of Gas Exchange*

measured volume: 54.2 L (ATPS)
collection time: 2 min
number of breaths: 41 in 2 min
heart rate (HR) = 120/min
body temperature = 37° C
F_{IO_2} = 0.2093 (20.93%)
F_{ICO_2} = 0.0004 (0.04%)
F_{EO_2} = 0.162 (16.2%)
F_{ECO_2} = 0.041 (4.1%)
(Fractions of dry gas volume)

Hemoglobin-15 g/100 mL
valve dead space = 64 ml
ambient temperature (T) = 22° C
barometric pressure (PB) = 760 mm Hg
partial pressure of water, saturated at 22° C (P_{H_2O}) = 19 mm Hg

Pa_{O_2} = 91 mm Hg
Pa_{CO_2} = 36 mm Hg
pH = 7.44
Sa_{O_2} = 95%

P_{ETCO_2} = 38 mm Hg
$P\bar{v}_{O_2}$ = 27 mm Hg
$S\bar{v}_{O_2}$ = 50%

A. Most commonly, ventilation is measured at ambient temperature and gas is fully saturated with water vapor at that temperature (ATPS). Formula 1 is used to adjust volume from ATPS to BTPS. The temperature and water vapor correction factors can also be found in Appendix F.

$$\dot{V}_E \text{ (L/min, BTPS)} = \dot{V}_E \text{ (L/min, ATPS)}$$
$$\times \frac{(273 + 37)}{273 + T} \quad (1)$$
$$\times \frac{P_B - P_{H_2O} \text{ (at T)}}{P_B - 47}$$

where T is ambient temperature (° C), body temperature is 37° C, P_{H_2O} at 37° C is 47 mm Hg, and P_B is barometric pressure.

B. Once $\dot{V}_E$ (BTPS) is found, $\dot{V}_E$ (STPD) can be obtained using formula 2. This converts $\dot{V}_E$ (BTPS) to STPD (273° K, barometric pressure = 760 mm Hg, and no water vapor present) for $\dot{V}_{CO_2}$ and $\dot{V}_{O_2}$ calculations.

$$\dot{V}_E \text{ (L/min, STPD)} = \dot{V}_E \text{ (L/min, BTPS)}$$
$$\times \frac{273}{(273 + 37)}$$
$$\times \frac{(P_B - 47)}{760}$$

which becomes,

$$\dot{V}_E \text{ (L/min, STPD)} = \dot{V}_E \text{ (L/min, BTPS)} \times 0.826,$$
$$\text{if } P_B = 760 \text{ mm Hg.} \quad (2)$$

Example:

$$\dot{V}_E \text{ (L/min, ATPS)} = \frac{\text{Total Volume (ATPS)}}{\text{Total Collection Time}}$$
$$= \frac{54.2}{2 \text{ min}} = 27.1$$

then, from formula 1

$\dot{V}_E$ (L/min, BTPS)

$$= 27.1 \times \frac{310}{(273 + 22)} \times \frac{(760 - 19)}{(760 - 47)} = 29.6$$

and, from formula 2,

$$\dot{V}_E \text{ (L/min, STPD)} = 29.6 \times 0.826 = 24.3$$

RESPIRATORY FREQUENCY (f)

$$f \text{ (min}^{-1}) = \frac{\text{number of complete breaths}}{\text{total time for complete breaths}} \quad (3)$$

Example:

$$f \text{ (min}^{-1}) = \frac{41 \text{ breaths}}{2 \text{ min}} = 20.5$$

TIDAL VOLUME (VT)

$$V_T \text{ (L, BTPS)} = \frac{\dot{V}_E \text{ (L/min, BTPS)}}{f} \quad (4)$$

Example:

$$V_T \text{ (L, BTPS)} = \frac{29.6}{20.5} = 1.44$$

CO_2 OUTPUT ($\dot{V}_{CO_2}$)

The CO_2 output and O_2 uptake are reported under STPD conditions. If $\dot{V}_E$ and $\dot{V}_I$ are measured at or converted to STPD conditions, F_{ECO_2} is the fraction of dry gas volume, and F_{ICO_2} is zero or negligible:

$$\dot{V}_{CO_2} \text{ (L/min, STPD)} = \dot{V}_E \text{ (L/min, STPD)} \quad (5)$$
$$\times F_{ECO_2}$$

or, for $P_B = 760$ mm Hg,

$$\dot{V}_{CO_2} \text{ (L/min, STPD)} = \dot{V}_E \text{ (L/min, BTPS)} \quad (6)$$
$$\times\ 0.826 \times F_{ECO_2}$$

Example: Substituting $\dot{V}_E$ and F_{ECO_2} (Table D-1) into formula 5,

$$\dot{V}_{CO_2} \text{ (L/min, STPD)} = 24.3 \times 0.041 = 0.997$$

O_2 Uptake ($\dot{V}_{O_2}$)

For the derivation of the formula for $\dot{V}_{O_2}$ and consideration of water vapor, see Appendix D, Special Considerations. Formula 7 should be used only after calculating the dry expired gas fraction (if an electrochemical O_2 analyzer is used) or with a mass spectrometer.

If $\dot{V}_E$ is measured at or converted to STPD, F_{IO_2} is 0.2093 (dry room air), F_{ECO_2} and F_{EO_2} are fractions of CO_2 and O_2 in dry gas, and $F_{ICO_2} = 0$, then:

$$\dot{V}_{O_2} \text{ (L/min, STPD)} = \dot{V}_E \text{ (L/min, STPD)} \quad (7)$$
$$\times\ (\Delta F_{O_2})\text{true,dry}$$

where (ΔF_{O_2}) true, dry $= 0.265 - 1.265 \times F_{EO_2} - 0.265 \times F_{ECO_2}$ for a person breathing room air. The (ΔF_{O_2}) true,dry can also be obtained from the nomogram in Appendix F.

Example: Substituting from Table D-1 into formula 7:

$$(\Delta F_{O_2})\text{true,dry} = 0.265 - 0.205 - 0.0108$$
$$= 0.049$$
$$\dot{V}_{O_2} \text{ (L/min, STPD)} = 24.3 \times 0.049 = 1.19$$

Gas Exchange Ratio (R)

$$R = \frac{\dot{V}_{CO_2} \text{ (L/min, STPD)}}{\dot{V}_{O_2} \text{ (L/min, STPD)}} \quad (8)$$

Example:

$$R = \frac{0.997}{1.19} = 0.84$$

Ventilatory Equivalent for CO_2 and O_2 ($\dot{V}_E/\dot{V}_{CO_2}$, $\dot{V}_E/\dot{V}_{O_2}$)

The ventilatory equivalents for CO_2 and O_2 are measurements of ventilatory requirement for a given metabolic rate. Thus, by convention they are expressed as $\dot{V}_E$ (L/min, BTPS) divided by $\dot{V}_{CO_2}$ or $\dot{V}_{O_2}$ (L/min, STPD). Because the portion of the ventilation wasted in clearing the breathing valve deadspace is irrelevant in determining the ventilatory requirement, the valve deadspace (V_{Dm}) per breath is subtracted from the total $\dot{V}_E$:

$$\dot{V}_E/\dot{V}_{CO_2} = \frac{\dot{V}_E \text{ (L/min, BTPS)} - [f\ min^{-1} \times V_{Dm} \text{ (L)}]}{\dot{V}_{CO_2} \text{ (L/min, STPD)}} \quad (9)$$

$$\dot{V}_E/\dot{V}_{O_2} = \frac{\dot{V}_E \text{ (L/min, BTPS)} - [f\ min^{-1} \times V_{Dm} \text{ (L)}]}{\dot{V}_{O_2} \text{ (L/min, STPD)}} \quad (10)$$

Example:

$$\dot{V}_E/\dot{V}_{CO_2} = \frac{29.6 - [20.5 \times 0.064]}{0.997} = 28.4$$

$$\dot{V}_E/\dot{V}_{O_2} = \frac{29.6 - [20.5 \times 0.064]}{1.19} = 23.8$$

Oxygen Pulse ($\dot{V}_{O_2}$/HR)

$$\dot{V}_{O_2}\text{/HR (ml, STPD/beat)}$$
$$= \frac{\dot{V}_{O_2} \text{ (L/min, STPD)} \times 1000 \text{ ml/L}}{\text{HR (beats/min)}} \quad (11)$$

Example:

$$\dot{V}_{O_2}\text{/HR (ml, STPD/beat)} = \frac{1.19 \times 1000}{120} = 9.9$$

Alveolar P_{O_2} ($P_{A_{O_2}}$)

$$P_{A_{O_2}} \text{ (mm Hg)} = F_{I_{O_2}} \times (P_B - 47) \quad (12)$$
$$- \frac{P_{A_{CO_2}}}{R} (1 - F_{I_{O_2}} (1 - R))$$

where P_B is barometric pressure in mm Hg, $P_{A_{CO_2}}$ is ideal alveolar P_{CO_2} in mm Hg, R is the gas exchange ratio, and $F_{I_{O_2}}$ is the fraction of inspired O_2, dry. Usually, the assumption that $P_{A_{CO_2}} = Pa_{CO_2}$ is used and the term $F_{I_{O_2}} \times (1 - R)$ may be dropped because it is so small that it has an insignificant effect on the calculated $P_{A_{O_2}}$, especially during air breathing. This simplifies the formula to:

$$P_{AO_2} \text{ (mm Hg)} = F_{IO_2} \times (P_B - 47) - \frac{Pa_{CO_2}}{R} \tag{13}$$

Whereas R is often assumed to be 0.8 at rest, this assumption may be incorrect; it should certainly be measured during exercise.

Example: Substituting into formula 13,

$$P_{AO_2} \text{ (mm Hg)} = (0.2093 \times 713) - \frac{36}{0.84} = 106$$

ALVEOLAR-ARTERIAL P_{O_2} DIFFERENCE ($P[A-a]_{O_2}$)

$$P(A-a)_{O_2} \text{ (mm Hg)} = P_{AO_2} - Pa_{O_2} \tag{14}$$

where P_{AO_2} is determined as above and Pa_{O_2} is arterial P_{O_2}.

Example:

$$P(A-a)_{O_2} \text{ (mm Hg)} = 106 - 91 = 15$$

ARTERIAL END-TIDAL P_{CO_2} DIFFERENCE ($P[a-ET]_{CO_2}$)

$$P(a-ET)_{CO_2} = Pa_{CO_2} - P_{ETCO_2} \tag{15}$$

where Pa_{CO_2} is arterial P_{CO_2} and P_{ETCO_2} is end-tidal P_{CO_2}.

Example:

$$P(a-ET)_{CO_2} = 36 - 38 = -2 \text{ mm Hg}$$

PHYSIOLOGIC DEAD SPACE (V_D)

$$V_D \text{ (L)} = V_T \text{ (L)} \times \frac{(Pa_{CO_2} - P\bar{E}_{CO_2})}{Pa_{CO_2}} - V_{DM} \text{ (L)} \tag{16}$$

where V_T is tidal volume, Pa_{CO_2} is arterial P_{CO_2}, $P\bar{E}_{CO_2}$ is mixed expired P_{CO_2}, and V_{DM} is breathing valve dead space. Mixed expired P_{CO_2} can be calculated from:

$$P\bar{E}_{CO_2} = \frac{\dot{V}_{CO_2} \text{ (L/min, STPD)}}{\dot{V}_E \text{ (L/min, STPD)}} \times (P_B - 47 \text{ mm Hg})$$

Example:

$$P\bar{E}_{CO_2} = \frac{0.997 \times 713}{24.3} = 29$$

$$V_D \text{ (L)} = 1.44 \times \frac{36 - 29}{36} - 0.064 = 0.22$$

PHYSIOLOGIC DEAD SPACE/TIDAL VOLUME RATIO (V_D/V_T)

$$\frac{V_D}{V_T} = \frac{(Pa_{CO_2} - P\bar{E}_{CO_2})}{Pa_{CO_2}} - \frac{V_{DM} \text{ (L)}}{V_T \text{ (L)}} \tag{17}$$

Example:

$$\frac{V_D}{V_T} = \frac{36 - 29}{36} - \frac{0.064}{1.44} = 0.15$$

There has been an unfortunate trend of calculating V_D/V_T "noninvasively" by substituting P_{ETCO_2} for Pa_{CO_2} in the foregoing formulas. This practice is to be condemned, because the relationship between Pa_{CO_2} and P_{ETCO_2} is unpredictable during exercise and is influenced strongly by the presence of lung disease.[1] Furthermore, small errors in Pa_{CO_2} may result in clinically important differences in the calculated V_D/V_T.

CARDIAC OUTPUT

The cardiac output ($\dot{Q}$) can be determined by thermal indicator dilution (see Appendix C) or by the Fick method using $\dot{V}_{O_2}$ and arterial-mixed venous O_2 content difference:

$$\dot{Q} \text{ (L/min)} = \frac{\dot{V}_{O_2} \text{ (ml/min, STPD)}}{(Ca_{O_2} - C\bar{v}_{O_2}) \text{ ml } O_2/\text{L blood}} \tag{18}$$

where Ca_{O_2} is O_2 content in arterial and $C\bar{v}_{O_2}$ is O_2 content in mixed venous blood. These can be calculated from:

$$C_{O_2} \text{ (ml } O_2/100 \text{ ml)} = (S_{O_2} \times 0.01$$
$$\times 1.34 \text{ ml } O_2/\text{g Hb} \times [\text{Hb}]) \tag{19}$$
$$+ (0.003 \text{ ml } O_2/\text{mm Hg}/100 \text{ ml} \times P_{O_2})$$

where [Hb] is hemoglobin concentration in g/100 ml blood and S_{O_2} is the oxyhemoglobin saturation. Note that this calculation gives O_2 content in ml $O_2/100$ of blood and needs to be converted to ml O_2/L blood by multiplying by 10.

Example:

$$Ca_{O_2} (ml\, O_2/100\, ml) = (95\% \times 0.01 \times 1.34 \times 15)$$
$$+ (0.003 \times 91) = 19.4$$
$$C\overline{v}_{O_2} (ml\, O_2/100\, ml) = (50\% \times 0.01 \times 1.34 \times 15)$$
$$+ (0.003 \times 27) = 10.1$$
$$(Ca_{O_2} - C\overline{v}_{O_2}) = 19.4 - 10.1$$
$$= 9.3\, ml\, O_2/100\, ml$$
$$= 93\, ml\, O_2/L$$

$$\dot{Q}\, (L/min) = \frac{1190\, (ml/min,\, STPD)}{93\, ml\, O_2/L\; blood} = 12.8$$

The foregoing method of cardiac output measurement requires a sample of mixed venous blood. A noninvasive determination of cardiac output can be made, however, using an analogous formula for CO_2 and an estimate of mixed venous CO_2 content (indirect Fick). The mixed venous P_{CO_2} can be approximated by several techniques, for example, single-exhalation[2] and rebreathing.[3] With the rebreathing method, a mixture of CO_2 and high inspired O_2 is rebreathed, and the P_{CO_2} of the rebreathed gas rapidly approaches that of mixed venous blood. The mixed venous content of CO_2 ($C\overline{v}_{CO_2}$) can then be estimated using hemoglobin concentration and the CO_2 dissociation curve adjusted for estimated oxygen saturation.[4] The arterial P_{CO_2} is used to determine arterial CO_2 content (Ca_{CO_2}) and, using $\dot{V}_{CO_2}$, cardiac output is:

$$\dot{Q}\, (L/min) = \frac{\dot{V}_{CO_2}\, (ml/min,\, STPD)}{(C\overline{v}_{CO_2} - Ca_{CO_2})\; ml\, CO_2/L\; blood}$$
(20)

The arterial P_{CO_2} must be used in this calculation rather than the end-tidal P_{CO_2}. This is because the CO_2 content versus P_{CO_2} curve (CO_2 dissociation curve) is steep, and a small error in P_{CO_2} results in a large error in CO_2 content. In addition, the $P_{ET_{CO_2}}$ is higher than Pa_{CO_2} in normal subjects but usually lower than Pa_{CO_2} in patients with a substantial alveolar dead space during exercise. The accuracy of the cardiac output also depends on an extremely accurate blood gas analysis for both arterial and mixed venous P_{CO_2} values. In addition, the oxygen content of the blood greatly affects the relationship between P_{CO_2} and CO_2 content (Haldane effect), and the mixed venous oxygen is not known using these estimates. Additionally, above the AT, the CO_2 dissociation curve is displaced downward. This results in a reduced mixed venous CO_2 content for a given $P\overline{v}_{CO_2}$. Because of these reasons, cardiac output measure-

ments by this indirect, noninvasive method should be considered approximate and used with caution.

Calculations at Maximum Exercise

BREATHING RESERVE (BR)

BR (L/min)
$$= MVV\, (L/min) - \dot{V}_E\, (L/min)\, at\, maximum\, exercise$$
(21)

BR (%)
$$= \frac{MVV\, (L/min) - \dot{V}_E\, (L/min)\, at\, maximum\, exercise}{MVV\, (L/min)}$$
$$\times 100$$
(22)

where MVV is maximum voluntary ventilation at rest.

Example: If MVV is 82 L/min and $\dot{V}_E$ at maximum exercise is 65 L/min, then:

$$BR\, (L/min) = 82 - 65 = 17\, L/min$$
$$BR\, (\%) = \frac{82 - 65}{82} \times 100 = 21\%$$

HEART RATE RESERVE (HRR)

$$HRR\, (beats/min) = Predicted\, maximum\, HR$$ (23)
$$- HR\, at\, maximum\, exercise$$

$$HRR\, (\%) = Predicted\, maximum\, HR$$
$$\frac{- HR\, at\, maximum\, exercise}{Predicted\, maximum\, HR}$$ (24)
$$\times 100$$

where predicted maximum HR (adults) = 220 − age (years). Example: For a 60-year-old man, predicted maximum HR = 220 − 60 = 160 beats/min. If HR at maximum exercise is 145 beats/min, then:

$$HRR\, (beats/min) = 160 - 145 = 15$$
$$HRR\, (\%) = \frac{160 - 145}{160} \times 100 = 9\%$$

Special Considerations of Calculation of Gas Exchange Variables

WATER VAPOR AND OXYGEN UPTAKE ($\dot{V}_{O_2}$)

Oxygen uptake ($\dot{V}_{O_2}$) is often determined by collection and analysis of expired gas. The usual calculation method determines $\dot{V}_{O_2}$ using expired ventilation, expired CO_2 fraction, and expired O_2 fraction and is based on the assumption that the volumes of nitrogen (and other inert gases) inspired and expired do not differ over the collection period. During rest and exercise, this method has been found to be satisfactory.[5,6] Nevertheless, errors may be introduced if careful attention to methods and calculations is not taken. This is especially true of how water vapor is handled because this variable can greatly affect the end result.

If the Scholander or Haldane method of gas analysis or a mass spectrometer is used, or water vapor is removed by drying the gas prior to measurement, then measured gas concentration is relative to total gas excluding the volume of water vapor. Thus, the dilution of the concentration of each gas caused by water vapor can be ignored and calculations are relatively simple:

$$\dot{V}_{O_2} \text{ (L/min, STPD)} = (F_{I_{O_2}} \times \dot{V}_I \text{ [L/min, STPD])}$$

$$- (F_{E_{O_2}} \times \dot{V}_E \text{ [L/min, STPD]})$$

where $F_{I_{O_2}}$ and $F_{E_{O_2}}$ are the O_2 fractions of dry gas volumes. If over the period of collection, the volumes of inspired and expired nitrogen (and other inert gases) are equal during breathing, then:

$$\dot{V}_I \times F_{I_{N_2}} = \dot{V}_E \times F_{E_{N_2}}, \text{ and}$$
$$\dot{V}_I = (F_{E_{N_2}}/F_{I_{N_2}}) \times \dot{V}_E$$

where $F_{I_{N_2}}$ and $F_{E_{N_2}}$ are the fractional concentrations of nitrogen and other inert gases.

Because $(F_{I_{N_2}} + F_{I_{O_2}} + F_{I_{CO_2}}) = 1$ and $(F_{E_{N_2}} + F_{E_{O_2}} + F_{E_{CO_2}}) = 1$, then:

$$\dot{V}_I = \frac{(1 - F_{E_{O_2}} - F_{E_{CO_2}})}{(1 - F_{I_{O_2}} - F_{I_{CO_2}})} \times \dot{V}_E$$

and

$$\dot{V}_{O_2} \text{ (L/min, STPD)}$$

$$= \left[\frac{F_{I_{O_2}} \times (1 - F_{E_{O_2}} - F_{E_{CO_2}})}{(1 - F_{I_{O_2}} - F_{I_{CO_2}})} - F_{E_{O_2}} \right]$$

$$\times \dot{V}_E \text{ (L/min, STPD)}$$

The quantity in brackets is called the true O_2 difference, (ΔF_{O_2}) true.

If we assume that $F_{I_{CO_2}} = 0$, or is negligible, then:

$$(\Delta F_{O_2})\text{true} = \frac{(F_{I_{O_2}} - F_{E_{O_2}} - F_{I_{O_2}} \times F_{E_{CO_2}})}{(1 - F_{I_{O_2}})}$$

and

$$\dot{V}_{O_2} \text{ (L/min, STPD)} = \dot{V}_E \text{ (L/min, STPD)}$$
$$\times (\Delta F_{O_2})\text{true}$$

For room air inspired gas, $F_{I_{O_2}}$ (dry) $= 0.2093$, and:

$$\dot{V}_{O_2} \text{ (L/min, STPD)} = \dot{V}_E \text{ (L/min, STPD)}$$

$$\times (0.265 - 1.265 \times F_{E_{O_2}} - 0.265 \times F_{E_{CO_2}}) \quad (25)$$

If water vapor is not removed from the gas and the method of gas analysis measures gas fraction of the total gas volume including water vapor, as is the case for most O_2 analyzers, then the water vapor will reduce each dry gas fraction by the factor:

$$\frac{(P_B - P_{H_2O})}{P_B} \text{ or } (1 - F_{H_2O})$$

In this case, the determination of $\dot{V}_{O_2}$ is affected by water vapor as follows. First, $\dot{V}_{O_2}$ can be expressed using $\dot{V}_I$ and $\dot{V}_E$ measured under the conditions of measurement, i.e., at temperature T and containing some water vapor:

$$\dot{V}_{O_2} \text{ (L/min, STPD)} = \frac{273}{273 + T} \times \frac{P_B}{760}$$

$$\times (\dot{V}_I \times F_{I_{O_2}} - \dot{V}_E \times F_{E_{O_2}})$$

$$(26)$$

where $\dot{V}_I$ and $\dot{V}_E$ are L/min at temperature T, and $F_{I_{O_2}}$ and $F_{E_{O_2}}$ are fractions of $\dot{V}_I$ and $\dot{V}_E$ respectively, including the volume of water vapor.

Because $\dot{V}_I = (F_{E_{N_2}}/F_{I_{N_2}}) \times \dot{V}_E$, and

$$(F_{E_{N_2}} + F_{E_{O_2}} + F_{E_{CO_2}} + F_{E_{H_2O}}) = 1 \text{ and}$$
$$(F_{I_{N_2}} + F_{I_{O_2}} + F_{I_{CO_2}} + F_{I_{H_2O}}) = 1,$$

then substituting into equation 26 gives:

$$\dot{V}_{O_2} \text{ (L/min, STPD)} = \dot{V}_E \text{ (L/min at T)}$$

$$\times k(T, P_{H_2O}) \times (\Delta F_{O_2}) \text{ true} \quad (27)$$

where

$$k(T, P_{H_2O}) = \frac{273}{273 + T} \times \frac{P_B}{760}$$

and

$$(\Delta F_{O_2})\ true = \frac{F_{I_{O_2}} \times (1 - F_{E_{CO_2}} - F_{E_{H_2O}}) - F_{E_{O_2}} \times (1 - F_{I_{H_2O}})}{(1 - F_{I_{O_2}} - F_{I_{H_2O}})}$$

The calculation of $\dot{V}_{O_2}$ is simpler if the expired gas is dried prior to analysis for O_2 and CO_2. Beaver[8] provides a nomogram for calculation of oxygen uptake in the presence of water vapor, however, that can be used to determine $\dot{V}_{O_2}$ and R from a sample of mixed expired gas assumed to be fully saturated with water vapor at a known temperature (see Appendix F). The subject is assumed to be breathing room air and the O_2 and CO_2 analyzers display the fractions of total expired gas including water vapor. Substantial errors would result if water vapor were not taken into account. Again, the correction is not needed when gas fractions are measured as fractions of dry gas.

Breath-by-breath measurement systems must deal with the effect of water vapor on calculation of $\dot{V}_{O_2}$. Rapidly responding gas analyzers or a respiratory mass spectrometer are used. A mass spectrometer may be adjusted to "ignore" water vapor if the sum of ion voltages is made up of only those measuring N_2, O_2, CO_2, and argon, with water vapor ignored in both inspired and expired gases. If this method is used, then the volume to be multiplied by true O_2 fraction should be adjusted to the dry volume.

Rapidly responding O_2 analyzers and infrared CO_2 analyzers used without drying the analyzed gas read fractions of total gas volume and therefore read lower concentrations than if the same gas were measured after being dried. As shown in equation 27, the values can be used in a breath-by-breath system if $F_{E_{H_2O}}$ and $F_{I_{H_2O}}$ are known.[8] The assumption that expired gas is fully saturated at some known temperature is the starting point for several approaches to dealing with this in breath-by-breath systems.

First, the expired gas sample can be kept warm to prevent condensation. If gas is fully saturated at a known temperature, $F_{E_{H_2O}}$ can be estimated. A heated sampling tube is necessary and the temperature must be accurately known. For example,

assuming a value of 37° C when actual expired gas temperature is 32° C can result in a 7 to 8% error in $\dot{V}_{O_2}$. During exercise, expired gas rapidly cools in the mouthpiece and breathing valve to as low as 32° C. Because gas for analysis is most often sampled at this location in breath-by-breath systems, then, even if the gas is rewarmed, there will have been some unknown loss of water vapor to condensation.

A second approach is to allow the sampled gas to cool to a known temperature. This avoids the problem of indeterminate loss of water vapor from cooling followed by rewarming. Auchincloss et al.[9] described a water bath that cooled expired gas to 15° C prior to rewarming and analysis. If a small-diameter sampling tube and low flow rate can be used, then gas may be allowed to cool to ambient temperature. This latter method is convenient and simple, but care should be taken that water droplets do not alter resistance and flow characteristics of the sampler and do not affect the linearity and response of the analyzer.

Deno and Kamon described a dryer for use in on-line breath-by-breath systems.[10] Removing water vapor by passing gas through a tube containing calcium sulfate is generally unsuitable for breath-by-breath methods because it introduces unacceptable delay times, may distort the gas concentration profile, and cannot meet the challenge of large gas sample flows. Deno and Kamon used a copper condenser tube and separator immersed in an ice bath at 1° C. Even at flow rates of saturated 38° air up to 1 L/min, P_{H_2O} was maintained at 5 mm Hg. Response times were compatible with those reported for breath-by-breath systems albeit at moderately high sample flow rates (1 L/min).

Another approach uses special conducting tubing that allows water vapor to pass into and out of the gas being conveyed to the gas analyzer until equilibrium is reached with the atmosphere. Thus, water vapor partial pressure in the gas analyzers is assumed to be equal to the ambient P_{H_2O} rather than saturated at some temperature. This method avoids the need to know the precise temperature and temperature changes of the respired gas and does not adversely affect the response time.

Oxygen Uptake ($\dot{V}_{O_2}$) and Oxygen Breathing

The use of the foregoing equations during breathing of oxygen-enriched inspired gas mixtures has potential problems. The relationship of V_I to V_E is subject to large differences for small measurement errors when F_{IO_2} and F_{EO_2} are high and F_{IN_2} and F_{EN_2} are low. In addition, the assumption that $\dot{V}_I \times F_{IN_2} = \dot{V}_E \times F_{EN_2}$ is not valid for a transient wash-out period during which hyperoxic gas is inspired and more nitrogen is removed during expiration than is added during inspiration. In addition, while the subject is breathing 100% oxygen, the equations given previously cannot be used because there is no inspired or expired nitrogen after the wash-out period.

Although calculation of $\dot{V}_{O_2}$ during enriched oxygen breathing is theoretically possible, the accuracy of $\dot{V}_{O_2}$ using conventional equations and measurements is almost certainly less than when the subject is breathing room air. $\dot{V}_{O_2}$ calculated with $F_{IO_2} > 0.21$ should be interpreted with caution.

An alternative approach to testing subjects during oxygen breathing is to ignore or not make measurements of $\dot{V}_{O_2}$. Most often, a reason for exercise testing is to determine the need for supplemental oxygen in a particular patient. This question can usually be answered by comparison of maximum work rate, heart rate, respiratory frequency, minute ventilation, $\dot{V}_E/\dot{V}_{CO_2}$, and exercise endurance between a maximum exercise test on room air with a similar test during oxygen breathing. An objective improvement in exercise capacity and decreased $\dot{V}_E$ and $\dot{V}_E/\dot{V}_{CO_2}$ are encouraging signs of a beneficial effect of supplemental O_2.

Valve Dead Space and Physiologic Dead Space/Tidal Volume Ratio

The physiologic dead space consists of the anatomic dead space and the alveolar dead space. During measurement, the volume of the breathing valve and mouthpiece apparatus is considered to be in series with the anatomic dead space. This apparatus dead space is usually subtracted from the V_D calculated by the Engoff modification of the Bohr equation:

$$V_D = V_T \, (L) \times \frac{Pa_{CO_2} - P\bar{E}_{CO_2}}{Pa_{CO_2}} - V_{Dm} \, (L)$$

where V_D is subject dead space, V_T is tidal volume, and V_{Dm} is the volume of the apparatus (or valve dead space).

Bradley and Younes,[11] Suwa and Bendixen,[12] and Singleton et al.[13] reported that the effective dead space of the valve (the correction term

$[V_{Dm}]$) may be different from the measured mechanical dead space. The reader is referred to their thorough analyses of the proper correction value under various conditions.

In practice, most reports of V_D during exercise have corrected for apparatus dead space by subtracting the entire mechanical dead space. Any potential error can be minimized if the valve dead space is small and the subject's tidal volume is relatively large compared to V_{Dm}. Valves with large dead spaces may be necessary, however, because they usually offer smaller breathing resistances at high inspiratory and expiratory flows. These high flows would be encountered when studying healthy normal subjects with large tidal volumes during exercise. On the other hand, patients with small tidal volumes will usually not generate high flows during exercise and the small dead space valves are recommended.

Calculations for Breath-by-Breath Analysis

Breath-by-breath methods use the same formulae as for mixed expired gas collections. Conceptually, the expired volume is divided into small sequential samples. The volume of each is determined and, when multiplied by the gas concentrations appropriate for that sample adjusted for the time difference between the flow and gas concentration signals, gives the volume of CO_2 eliminated or O_2 taken up for that sample. The results are summed mathematically and then reported either per breath or per unit time. Thus, the term "breath-by-breath" applies to the method of expired gas analysis and data reduction and does not necessarily mean that each breath is individually reported.

If V_E is the sum of all volume exhaled between time 0 and time T then:

$$V_E = \sum_{t=0}^{T} Vexp(t + \Delta t)$$

where $Vexp(t + \Delta t)$ is the volume expired between time t and $t + \Delta t$, Δt is a time interval, and T is the total time of expiration for single or multiple breaths.

This is satisfactory if volume is directly measured over small time intervals. If expired flow rather than volume is measured, then:

$$V_E = \int_0^T \dot{V}exp(t)dt$$

where $\dot{V}exp(t)$ is the expired flow over the infinitesimally small time interval dt at time t. The volume exhaled over that time is the product $\dot{V}exp(t) \times dt$. In practice, a small constant Δt is substituted for dt and the mean flow during the time interval $(t + \Delta t)$ is used as $\dot{V}exp(t)$:

$$V_E = \sum_{t=0}^{T} \dot{V}exp(t + \Delta t) \times \Delta t$$

where $\dot{V}exp(t + \Delta t)$ is the mean flow rate during the time interval $t + \Delta t$. The minute ventilation ($\dot{V}_E$) is the volume per unit time.

In a breath-by-breath system, the V_{CO_2} is calculated by multiplying the nearly instantaneous F_{ECO_2} for each small time interval by the simultaneous expired volume during that interval. These products are then integrated:

$$V_{CO_2} = \int_{t=0}^{T} \dot{V}exp(t)dt \times F_{ECO_2}(t)$$

where $\dot{V}exp(t)dt$ is the instantaneous expired volume and $F_{ECO_2}(t)$ is the instantaneous expired CO_2 concentration at time t, adjusted for the delay between when the gas is sampled and when the analyzer reads the appropriate concentration. In practice, the small time interval Δt is substituted for dt:

$$V_{CO_2} = \sum_{t=0}^{T} \dot{V}exp(t + \Delta t) \times \Delta t \times F_{ECO_2}(t)$$

where $\dot{V}exp(t + \Delta t)$ is the mean flow for the time period t to $t + \Delta t$, $F_{ECO_2}(t)$ is the mean expired CO_2 during this time period, and Δt is a small time interval. For the volume of O_2 taken up, the true O_2 difference $[(\Delta F_{O_2})true]$ is substituted for F_{ECO_2} in this equation. The $\dot{V}_{CO_2}$ and $\dot{V}_{O_2}$ are equal to the volume of CO_2 or O_2 divided by the time during exhalation, whether expressed per breath or per minute or other time unit.

An analog integrator or analog-to-digital converter and digital computer can perform the necessary multiplication and summation. The respired gas is not, strictly speaking, measured and analyzed continuously, but instead is rapidly sampled, e.g., every 20 milliseconds. The resultant expired flow versus time curve is, therefore, made up of sequential points sampled at intervals Δt or at a frequency $f = 1/\Delta t$. The rate of sampling is important because rapid and large changes in expired flow (or gas concentration) may occur during exercise and could be missed if the data are sampled at too slow a rate. Bernard,[14] using generalized simulated curves of expired flow and expired CO_2, found that a sample rate of 30 Hz was adequate during exercise, and that rates of 40, 50, and 100 Hz achieved little improvement in fidelity. Beaver et al.,[15] in their analysis, suggested that a sampling frequency equal to twice the highest frequency occurring in the signal to be measured should be used. They suggested that for human exercise testing a frequency of 50 Hz is satisfactory to record flow and mass spectrometer signals.

A minor consideration is the method of summation or numeric integration. Bernard[14] suggested that the trapezoidal rule was adequate for integration of respiratory signals. This assumes, as previously, that the mean expired flow and gas concentrations during the time period between t and $t + \Delta t$ is equal to the average of the values measured at the beginning and end of the time period.

A serious potential problem deals with time alignment of the appropriate expired flow (or volume) and expired gas concentration because of the appreciable time required for gas transport and measurement by most gas analyzers. For breath-by-breath analysis, it is essential that the appropriate instantaneous flow rate be multiplied by the proper time-matched expired gas concentration. Whereas flow rates can be determined accurately and nearly instantaneously with good fidelity, gas analyzer measurements cannot with current technology be made without some delay and distortion inherent to the transport of gas to the analyzer and the intrinsic characteristics of the analyzer. The accuracy of a breath-by-breath system is dependent on the ability of the system to match flow rate and appropriate gas concentration prior to integration. Thus, each flow sampled must be stored until the appropriate expired gas concentration value has been determined. This matching process is usually performed as part of the computer program for on-line exercise systems.

Bernard[14] used simulated curves of expired CO_2 and expired flow to estimate potential error caused by the time delay between measurements of these two variables. Using perfectly time-matched hypothetic curves as standard, less than a 5% difference in calculated $\dot{V}_{CO_2}$ was found if the time misalignment was less than 25 milliseconds. Of importance is that the theoretic sampling rate was 100 Hz, the signals were given random noise, and the product of flow and CO_2 was integrated using the trapezoid rule.

Two factors contribute to the time alignment problem. Most systems use a capillary tube with a pump to draw a continuous expired gas sample into the analyzer. The gas transport time is dependent on the dimensions of the tube and the pump flow rate; transport time is typically on the order of 100 to 200 milliseconds. Second, the gas analyzer output itself has an intrinsic response time that further adds to the delay. For infrared CO_2 analyzers, electrochemical O_2 analyzers, and respiratory mass spectrometers the time constants for response are in the range of 50 to 100 milliseconds. The net result is that an instantaneous change in gas concentration at the sampling end of the tubing is accurately measured but only after introducing corrections to account for these delays. The mixing and diffusion of gas within the sampling tubing may further distort the result. These must also be accounted for in these corrections.

In most solutions to this problem, an instantaneous or step change in gas concentration is introduced at the sampling inlet and the time course of the gas analyzer output is observed. Attempts are then made to determine optimal methods of compensating for the gas transport delay and gas analyzer response characteristics.

Although the gas analyzer response time component is certainly important, matching of flow and gas concentration signals for gas transport delay, i.e., the time simply to reach the analyzer, alone considerably improves results. Using this method, Bates et al.[16] found a 10-fold reduction in error from the uncorrected value and suggested that this simple adjustment might be sufficient.

To account for the gas analyzer response time, an additional correction function is usually used. This function is derived from analysis of the total response of the gas analyzer system. Beaver et al.[15] indicated that the most significant wave shape distortion is removed by a total delay correction equal to transport delay plus one time constant and analyzed the magnitude of potential errors. Investigators have used various functions to describe the response characteristics of their gas analyzers or mass spectrometers.[16–19] We[20] found that an equal area method for analyzer delay time adds a one time constant delay if the analyzer response curve is exponential and an empirically determined longer delay time if the curve is sigmoid. Factors that affect selection of an optimal method included the level of noise in the measured signal, the sampling rate, and the type of calculation desired.

The importance of matching flow rate and ap-

propriate gas concentration cannot be overly stressed for a breath-by-breath system. Although not all investigators agree on the optimal way of dealing with gas analyzer response time, a satisfactory balance among degree of accuracy, speed, and reproducibility can be reached.

References

1. Lewis, D., Sietsema, K.E., Casaburi, R., and Sue, D.Y.: Inaccuracy of noninvasive estimates of V_D/V_T in clinical exercise testing. Am. Rev. Respir. Dis., 147:A185, 1993.
2. Kim, T.S., Rahn, H., and Farhi, L.E.: Estimation of the true venous and arterial P_{CO_2} by gas analysis of a single-breath. J. Appl. Physiol., 21:1338–1344, 1966.
3. Jones, N.L., Campbell, E.J.M., McHardy, G.J.R., Higgs, B.E., and Clode, M.: The estimation of carbon dioxide pressure of mixed venous blood during exercise. Clin. Sci., 32:311–327, 1967.
4. McHardy, G.J.R.: The relationship between the differences in pressure and content of carbon dioxide in arterial and venous blood. Clin. Sci., 32:299–309, 1967.
5. Wagner, J.A., Horvath, S.M., Dahms, T.E., and Reed, S.: Validation of open-circuit for the determination of oxygen consumption. J. Appl. Physiol., 34:859–863, 1973.
6. Wilmore, J.H., and Costill, D.L.: Adequacy of the Haldane transformation in the computation of exercise $\dot{V}_{O_2}$ in man. J. Appl. Physiol., 35:85–89, 1973.
7. Beaver, W.L., Wasserman, K., and Whipp, B.J.: On-line computer analysis and breath-by-breath graphical display of exercise function tests. J. Appl. Physiol., 34:128–132, 1973.
8. Beaver, W.L.: Water vapor corrections in oxygen consumption calculations. J. Appl. Physiol., 35:928–931, 1973.
9. Auchincloss, J.H., Gilbert, R., and Baule, G.H.: Control of water vapor during rapid analysis of respiratory gases in expired air. J. Appl. Physiol., 28:245–247, 1970.
10. Deno, N.S., and Kamon, E.: A dryer for rapid response on-line expired gas measurements. J. Appl. Physiol., 46:1196–1199, 1979.
11. Bradley, P.W., and Younes, M.: Relation between respiratory valve dead space and tidal volume. J. Appl. Physiol., 49:528–532, 1980.
12. Suwa, K., and Bendixen, H.H.: Change in Pa_{CO_2} with mechanical dead space during artificial ventilation. J. Appl. Physiol., 24:556–563, 1968.
13. Singleton, G.J., Olsen, C.R., and Smith, R.L.: Correction for mechanical dead space in the calculation of physiological dead space. J. Clin. Invest., 51:2768–2772, 1972.
14. Bernard, T.E.: Aspects of on-line digital integration of pulmonary gas transfer. J. Appl. Physiol., 43:375–378, 1977.
15. Beaver, W.L., Lamarra, N., and Wasserman, K.: Breath-by-breath measurement of true alveolar gas exchange. J. Appl. Physiol., 51:1662–1675, 1981.
16. Bates, J.H.T., Priak, G.K., Tanner, T.E., and McKinnon, A.E.: Correcting for the dynamic response of a respiratory mass spectrometer. J. Appl. Physiol., 55:1015–1022, 1983.

17. Noguchi, H., Ogushi, Y., Yoshiya, I., Itakura, N., and Yambayashi, H.: Breath-by-breath $\dot{V}_{CO_2}$ and $\dot{V}_{O_2}$ require compensation for transport delay and dynamic response. J. Appl. Physiol., 52:79–84, 1982.
18. Mitchell, R.R.: Incorporating the gas analyzer response time in gas exchange computations. J. Appl. Physiol., 47: 1118–1122, 1979.

19. Arieli, R., and Van Liew, H.D.: Corrections for the response time and delay of mass spectrometers. J. Appl. Physiol., 51:1417–1422, 1981.
20. Sue, D.Y., Hansen, J.E., Blais, M., and Wasserman, K.: Measurement and analysis of gas exchange during exercise using a programmable calculator. J. Appl. Physiol., 49:456–461, 1980.

Preparation for the Exercise Test

Requesting the Test

W E USE a request form for exercise studies. On this form the referring physician gives us the:

1. Patient's name, address, and telephone number.
2. Patient's weight, height, sex, and age.
3. Tentative diagnosis and the reason for the study.
4. Type of test and special requirements.

Most often, the exercise test should be discussed with the referring physician, so the type of test and the reason for doing it are clear before the day of the test. In addition, the discussion helps one to decide whether the cycle or treadmill is the preferable form of ergometry, whether an arterial catheter or pulse oximeter is desired, and whether 12-lead electrocardiograms (ECGs) are needed during exercise. This is also a time at which the patient's medications, previous studies, special needs or limitations, and other details can be discussed.

Preparing the Patient

We give the patient an appointment slip on which we remind the patient of the date and time of the procedure. We have also found it useful to include:

1. A brief explanation of the procedure.
2. A reminder to wear loose-fitting, comfortable clothes and shoes suitable for exercise.
3. A suggestion to avoid eating a heavy meal before the exercise test.

Preparation of the Physician

The physician in attendance during the test obtains a brief history of the patient's medical problems and the specific symptoms limiting exercise. The history should include a list of medications, an idea of physical activity status, and some estimate of the safety of exercising the patient. A brief physical examination should include blood pressure and pulse, cardiopulmonary examination, peripheral pulses, and upper and lower extremity muscles and joints. Before the exercise test begins, the physician should obtain and evaluate pertinent resting studies such as the chest roentgenogram, ECG, arterial blood gases, and pulmonary function. Then, the physician is in position to inform the patient of the risks and benefits of the exercise study and to obtain consent.

Preparation of the Laboratory

The laboratory should be air-conditioned and regulated at a comfortable temperature and humidity. The patient's view should be pleasant and not cluttered with tubing, wires, or a bulletin board with distracting papers hanging from it. If blood is to be sampled, the syringes should be prepared and placed in a convenient location to avoid confusion or extra motion during the time of the study. The number of people in the laboratory should be limited to those needed for making the measurements and for safety. Finally, extra sounds should be kept to a minimum. Soft background music helps to dampen noise but does not interfere with communication between the examiner and the technician. In summary, a pleasant, professional environment is needed to obtain the maximum confidence and therefore performance by the patient.

ECG LEAD PLACEMENT

The ECG leads should be placed on appropriate, stable areas of the body. We use adhesive silver-silver chloride gel ECG patches such as those used in intensive care units. The skin is shaved if necessary and is wiped with rubbing alcohol before the patches are applied.

The site of the three leads for monitoring heart rate and rhythm is shown in Figure 5-1; however, we do not hesitate to move the site of the leads as necessary to obtain an optimal tracing.

We use the 12-lead ECG in addition for patients in whom we suspect myocardial ischemia. The positions of the leads are shown in Figure 5-1. The arm leads are placed close to the monitoring lead patches above the scapulae; the leg leads are placed on the low back above the iliac crests. These locations minimize movement artifact. The

chest (V-leads) are positioned in standard locations on the anterolateral chest wall. Again, adhesive ECG patches are used. A technician obtains an ECG while the patient is at rest, approximately every other minute during exercise, and more often if an arrhythmia is noted or the patient complains of chest pain.

Brachial Artery Catheter Placement

EQUIPMENT

1. Appropriate catheter.
2. Cournand-type needle with sharp, hollow stylus.
3. A 2-ml syringe with a 26-gauge needle for local anesthesia.
4. Sterile saline suitable for intravascular injection.
5. Heparinized saline, 50 ml, for catheter flushing.

SELECTION OF CATHETER

We use a polyethylene catheter that is 25 cm long and has a diameter of 1.37 mm. The tip is tapered to fit a guidewire (50 cm × 0.63 mm) that fits through a 19-gauge thin-walled Cournand needle. The catheter is long enough so the end used for collection can be brought around to the back of the arm and sampling can be done without the subject's altering the position of his or her arm or being aware of when blood is sampled.

ARTERY SELECTION AND ARM POSITIONING

The brachial or radial artery is generally used. Complications such as thrombosis are exceedingly rare when appropriate precautions are taken. We find the brachial artery to be preferable, however, because it is larger and the catheter has less effect on compromising its lumen. Moreover, the patient's arm need not be secured to a board, and sliding of the catheter in and out of the artery when the patient moves is not a problem. The radial pulse should be palpated to ensure continued patency.

Positioning the arm is extremely important:

1. Extend the arm; place a rolled towel or cushion under the elbow for maximum extension.
2. Pronate the hand.
3. Palpate the brachial artery on the medial side of the antecubital fossa.

ANESTHESIA

If the patient is not allergic to the local anesthetic agent, anesthetize the skin and area around the artery. It is more humane, and the likelihood of arterial spasm is reduced. We use 1 to 2% lidocaine without epinephrine. After positioning the arm, inject local anesthetic (1) intradermally above the artery, (2) subcutaneously just above the artery, and (3) subcutaneously on either side of the artery. The total amount should be about 1 to 2 ml.

ARTERIAL PUNCTURE AND CATHETER INSERTION

1. Use a 19-gauge Cournand needle.
2. Locate the artery between the fingers in the area of anesthesia.
3. Insert the sharp, hollow stylus in the needle.
4. Holding the needle by its shield, while keeping the stylus in the needle with one's thumb (be sure not to cover the hole in the stylus), penetrate the skin over the artery. Position the tip of the needle above the artery. Then abruptly insert the stylus and the needle tip into the artery.
5. When the tip of the stylus enters the artery, blood may flow out of the stylus.
6. Advance the needle another 2 to 3 mm to be sure that the tip of needle is in the artery (the stylus protrudes a little beyond the tip of the needle).
7. Remove the stylus. Blood should shoot out of the needle with arterial pressure. If it does not, withdraw the needle slightly (it might have gone into the posterior wall of artery). Once a clear stream of arterial blood is evident, it is safe to advance the needle further into the lumen of the artery using the continuous stream of blood to document the needle's position. The needle advance may be facilitated by depressing the hub slightly to reduce the possibility of impaling the posterior wall of the artery with the needle tip. DO NOT ADVANCE THE NEEDLE WITHOUT THE STYLUS IN PLACE IF THERE IS NO FLOW OF BLOOD. It may damage the artery. If there is no blood flow, slowly withdraw the needle without the stylus because the needle tip may have passed through the inner wall of the artery. If there is still no blood flow, withdraw the tip of the needle to the skin.
8. If unsuccessful, clear the needle and stylus of any blood or clot, then try again.

9. With the needle tip in the lumen of the artery, documented by freely flowing blood, thread the guidewire for the catheter through the needle and slide it about 3 inches into the lumen of the artery. If the guidewire does not slip EASILY past the needle tip, the needle lumen is not centered in the lumen of the artery, and the needle must be repositioned.
10. Remove the needle, leaving the guidewire in place. Compress for hemostasis over the site at which the needle was inserted because the guidewire is narrow relative to the withdrawn needle.
11. Slide the smoothly tapered end of the catheter over the wire. When the catheter reaches the skin, slide it through the skin and arterial wall using a gently rotating motion.
12. When the catheter position is well established several inches into the artery, remove the guidewire. Blood should flow out the end of the catheter.
13. Attach a Luer-lock stopcock to the end of catheter and flush with heparinized saline.
14. Cover the site of insertion with sterile gauze and fix with tape. Tape the catheter to the skin. Now the catheter is ready for use.

FOR DIFFICULT PUNCTURES

Limit yourself to 15 minutes of effort. If you are not successful by then, stop trying and ask someone with more experience to help, or just rely on noninvasive measurements. The latter will provide a considerable amount of information.

Blood Pressure

It is most accurate to measure blood pressure directly from an indwelling arterial catheter. The reason is that the background noise of the cycling or treadmill (especially) can make it difficult to hear the Korotkoff sounds. The patient's swinging arm during walking also makes the measurement of blood pressure by the cuff method difficult. Direct arterial blood pressure recording is convenient when an arterial catheter is in place. A pressure transducer should be located at the level of the left atrium (approximately the fourth intercostal space with the patient upright), and the transducer should be carefully calibrated. Cuff-measured systolic and diastolic blood pressures average about 10 mm Hg less than directly recorded brachial artery pressures during cycle ergometry (see Table 6-3).

APPENDIX F
Tables and Nomogram

TABLE F-1. *Partial Pressure of Water of Saturated Gas at Centigrade Temperature T.*

T	PH₂O	T	PH₂O	T	PH₂O
10	9.20	20	17.53	30	31.83
11	9.84	21	18.65	31	33.70
12	10.51	22	19.82	32	35.67
13	11.23	23	21.07	33	37.73
14	11.98	24	22.38	34	39.90
15	12.78	25	23.76	35	42.18
16	13.63	26	25.21	36	44.57
17	14.53	27	26.74	37	47.08
18	15.47	28	28.35	38	49.70
19	16.47	29	30.04	39	52.45
20	17.53	30	31.83	40	55.34

TABLE F-2. *Factors for Conversion from ATPS to BTPS (37° C)*

	T° C	16	17	18	19	20	21	22	23	24	25	26	27	28	29	30
	600	1.138	1.132	1.126	1.120	1.115	1.109	1.103	1.097	1.090	1.084	1.078	1.071	1.065	1.058	1.051
	610	1.136	1.131	1.125	1.119	1.114	1.108	1.102	1.096	1.090	1.083	1.077	1.071	1.064	1.058	1.051
	620	1.135	1.130	1.124	1.118	1.113	1.107	1.101	1.095	1.089	1.083	1.076	1.070	1.064	1.057	1.050
	630	1.134	1.129	1.123	1.117	1.112	1.106	1.100	1.094	1.088	1.082	1.076	1.069	1.063	1.056	1.050
	640	1.133	1.128	1.122	1.116	1.111	1.105	1.099	1.093	1.087	1.081	1.075	1.069	1.062	1.056	1.049
	650	1.132	1.127	1.121	1.116	1.110	1.104	1.098	1.092	1.087	1.081	1.074	1.068	1.062	1.056	1.049
	660	1.131	1.126	1.120	1.115	1.109	1.103	1.098	1.092	1.086	1.080	1.074	1.068	1.061	1.055	1.049
	670	1.130	1.125	1.119	1.114	1.108	1.103	1.097	1.091	1.085	1.079	1.073	1.067	1.061	1.055	1.048
	680	1.129	1.124	1.118	1.113	1.107	1.102	1.096	1.090	1.085	1.079	1.073	1.067	1.060	1.054	1.048
PB	690	1.128	1.123	1.118	1.112	1.107	1.101	1.095	1.090	1.084	1.078	1.072	1.066	1.060	1.054	1.047
	700	1.128	1.122	1.117	1.111	1.106	1.100	1.095	1.089	1.083	1.077	1.072	1.066	1.059	1.053	1.047
	710	1.127	1.121	1.116	1.111	1.105	1.100	1.094	1.088	1.083	1.077	1.071	1.065	1.059	1.053	1.047
	720	1.126	1.121	1.115	1.110	1.104	1.099	1.093	1.088	1.082	1.076	1.070	1.065	1.059	1.052	1.046
	730	1.125	1.120	1.115	1.109	1.104	1.098	1.093	1.087	1.082	1.076	1.070	1.064	1.058	1.052	1.046
	740	1.124	1.119	1.114	1.109	1.103	1.098	1.092	1.087	1.081	1.075	1.070	1.064	1.058	1.052	1.046
	750	1.124	1.118	1.113	1.108	1.102	1.097	1.092	1.086	1.080	1.075	1.069	1.063	1.057	1.051	1.045
	760	1.123	1.118	1.113	1.107	1.102	1.096	1.091	1.086	1.080	1.074	1.069	1.063	1.057	1.051	1.045
	770	1.122	1.117	1.112	1.107	1.101	1.096	1.090	1.085	1.079	1.074	1.068	1.062	1.057	1.051	1.045
	780	1.122	1.116	1.111	1.106	1.101	1.095	1.090	1.084	1.079	1.073	1.068	1.062	1.056	1.050	1.044

T° C is ambient temperature in degrees centigrade; PB is barometric pressure.

TABLE F-3. *Factors for Conversion from ATPS to STPD*

T° C	16	17	18	19	20	21	22	23	24	25	26	27	28	29	30
600	0.729	0.725	0.722	0.718	0.714	0.710	0.706	0.703	0.699	0.695	0.691	0.686	0.682	0.678	0.674
610	0.741	0.738	0.734	0.730	0.726	0.723	0.719	0.715	0.711	0.707	0.703	0.698	0.694	0.690	0.685
620	0.754	0.750	0.746	0.742	0.739	0.735	0.731	0.727	0.723	0.719	0.715	0.710	0.706	0.702	0.697
630	0.766	0.762	0.759	0.755	0.751	0.747	0.743	0.739	0.735	0.731	0.727	0.722	0.718	0.714	0.709
640	0.779	0.775	0.771	0.767	0.763	0.759	0.755	0.751	0.747	0.743	0.739	0.734	0.730	0.726	0.721
650	0.791	0.787	0.783	0.779	0.775	0.771	0.767	0.763	0.759	0.755	0.751	0.746	0.742	0.737	0.733
660	0.803	0.800	0.796	0.792	0.788	0.784	0.780	0.775	0.771	0.767	0.763	0.758	0.754	0.749	0.745
670	0.816	0.812	0.808	0.804	0.800	0.796	0.792	0.788	0.783	0.779	0.775	0.770	0.766	0.761	0.757
680	0.828	0.824	0.820	0.816	0.812	0.808	0.804	0.800	0.795	0.791	0.787	0.782	0.778	0.773	0.768
PB 690	0.841	0.837	0.833	0.829	0.824	0.820	0.816	0.812	0.807	0.803	0.799	0.794	0.790	0.785	0.780
700	0.853	0.849	0.845	0.841	0.837	0.832	0.828	0.824	0.820	0.815	0.811	0.806	0.802	0.797	0.792
710	0.866	0.861	0.857	0.853	0.849	0.845	0.840	0.836	0.832	0.827	0.823	0.818	0.813	0.809	0.804
720	0.878	0.874	0.870	0.865	0.861	0.857	0.853	0.848	0.844	0.839	0.835	0.830	0.825	0.821	0.816
730	0.890	0.886	0.882	0.878	0.873	0.869	0.865	0.860	0.856	0.851	0.847	0.842	0.837	0.833	0.828
740	0.903	0.899	0.894	0.890	0.886	0.881	0.877	0.872	0.868	0.863	0.859	0.854	0.849	0.844	0.840
750	0.915	0.911	0.907	0.902	0.898	0.894	0.889	0.885	0.880	0.875	0.871	0.866	0.861	0.856	0.851
760	0.928	0.923	0.919	0.915	0.910	0.906	0.901	0.897	0.892	0.887	0.883	0.878	0.873	0.868	0.863
770	0.940	0.936	0.931	0.927	0.923	0.918	0.913	0.909	0.904	0.900	0.895	0.890	0.885	0.880	0.875
780	0.953	0.948	0.944	0.939	0.935	0.930	0.926	0.921	0.916	0.912	0.907	0.902	0.897	0.892	0.887

T° C is ambient temperature in degrees centigrade; PB is barometric pressure.

TABLE F-4. *Estimated $\dot{V}_{O_2}$ for Various Activities*

ACTIVITY	ESTIMATED $\dot{V}_{O_2}$ (ml/kg/min)	ACTIVITY	ESTIMATED $\dot{V}_{O_2}$ (ml/kg/min)
Basic postures		Hitching trailers, operating jacks or heavy levers	12.25
Sitting only (desk work, writing, calculating)	4.25	Masonry, painting, paperhanging	14.0
Standing only (bartending)	8.75		
Walking 3.0 mph	10.5	*Walking: moderate work*	
3.5 mph	14.0	Carrying trays, dishes	14.70
		Gas station mechanical work (changing tires, etc.)	15.75
Sitting: light or moderate work			
Driving a car	4.25	*Heavy arm work*	
Driving a truck	5.30	Lifting and carrying	
Hand tools, light assembly	5.30	(a) 20–44 lbs	15.75
Working heavy levers	7.0	(b) 45–64 lbs	21.0
Riding mower	8.75	(c) 65–84 lbs	26.25
Crane operator	8.75	(d) 85–100 lbs	29.75
Driving heavy truck (including frequent on and off with some arm work)	10.5	*Heavy tools*	
		Jackhammers, pneumatic drills	21.0
Standing: moderate work		Shovel, pick	28.0
Light assembly at slow pace	8.75		
Gas station operator	9.45	*Carpentry*	
Scrubbing, waxing, polishing (floors, walls)	9.45	Light interior repair (tile laying)	14.0
Heavy assembly (farm machinery, plumbing)	10.5	Building and finishing interior	15.75
Light welding	10.5	Putting in sidewalk	17.5
Stocking shelves (light objects)	10.5	Exterior remodeling (hammering, sawing)	21.0
Janitorial work	10.5		
Assembly line with light or medium parts at moderate pace	12.25	*Miscellaneous*	
		Pushing objects of 75 lb or more (desks, file cabinets)	28.0
Assembly line with brief lifting every 5 minutes (45 lbs or less)	12.25	Laying railroad track	24.5
		Cutting trees—chopping wood	
Same as above (parts > 45 lbs)	14.0	Hand saw	19.25
		Automatic	10.5

(From Tennessee Heart Association: Physician's Handbook for Evaluation of Cardiovascular and Physical Fitness. Nashville, Tennessee Heart Association, 1972; reprinted with permission.)

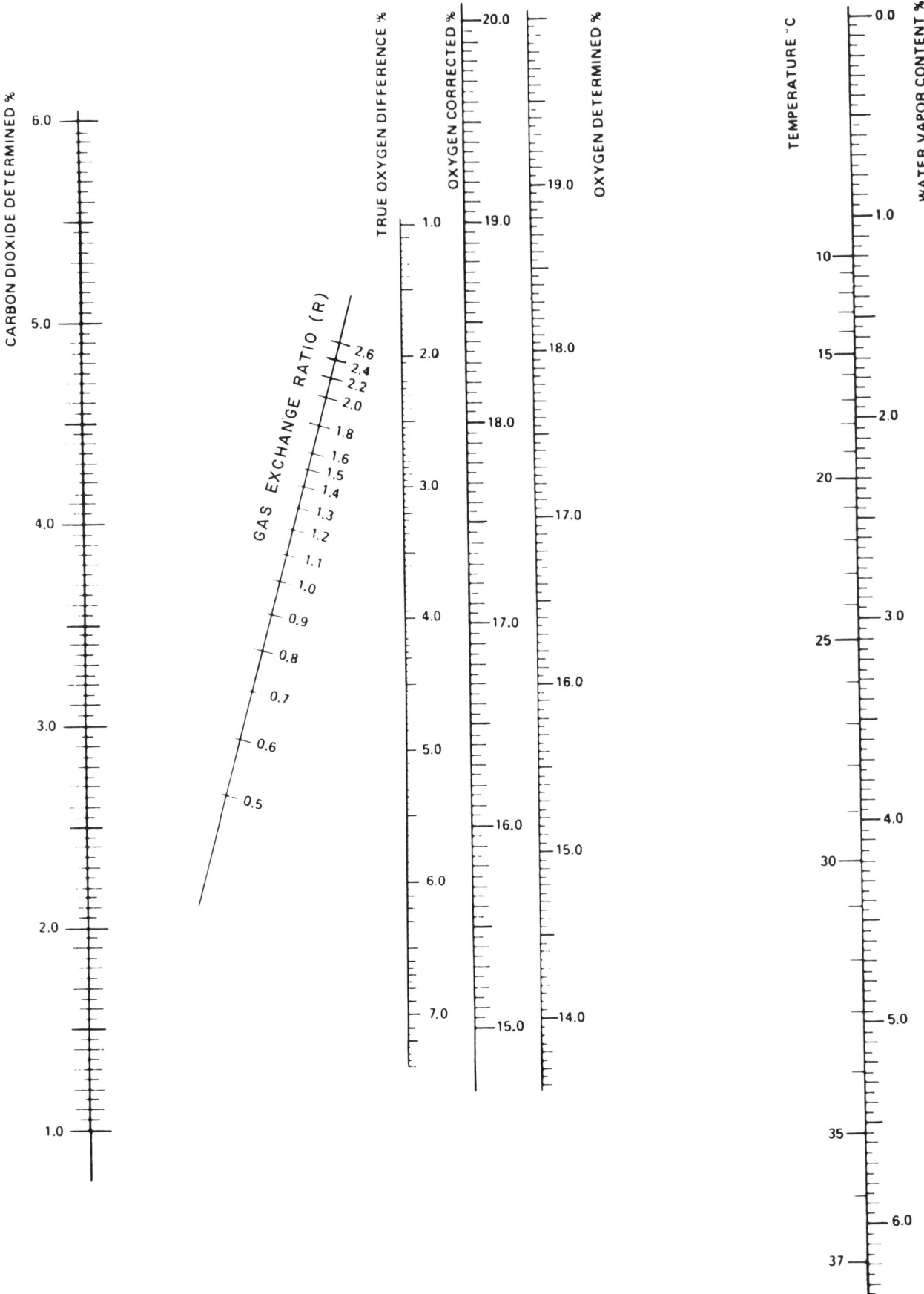

Fig. F-1. Nomogram for computing true O_2 difference ($[\Delta F_{O_2}]$ true) and gas exchange ratio (R) from a sample of expired gas, using values of expired CO_2 ($F_{E_{CO_2}}$) and expired O_2($F_{E_{O_2}}$) present in a wet sample whose water vapor content is known, or, if the sample is saturated with water, whose temperature is known. (Modified from Beaver, W.L.: Water vapor corrections in oxygen consumption calculations. J. Appl. Physiol., 35:928–931, 1973.)

Index

Page numbers in *italics* refer to illustrations; numbers followed by t indicate tables.